BIBLIOGRAPHY OF AUSTRALIAN MEDICINE
1790–1900

BIBLIOGRAPHY OF AUSTRALIAN MEDICINE 1790–1900

EDWARD FORD

SYDNEY UNIVERSITY PRESS

Exclusive Distributor
ISBS, Inc.
P.O. Box 555
Forest Grove, OR 97116

SYDNEY UNIVERSITY PRESS
Press Building, University of Sydney

UNITED KINGDOM, EUROPE, MIDDLE EAST, AFRICA, CARIBBEAN
Prentice/Hall International, International Book Distributors Ltd
Hemel Hempstead, England
NORTH AND SOUTH AMERICA
International Scholarly Book Services, Inc., Forest Grove, Oregon

National Library of Australia Cataloguing-in-Publication data

Ford, *Sir* Edward, 1902–.
Bibliography of Australian medicine 1790–1900.

Index.
ISBN 0 424 00022 9.

1. Medicine—Australia—Bibliography. I. Title.

016.610994

First published 1976

This book is funded by money from
THE ELEANOR SOPHIA WOOD BEQUEST

Printed in Australia by Macarthur Press (Books) Pty Limited, Parramatta

CONTENTS

LIST OF PLATES

(between pages 144 and 145)

ACKNOWLEDGEMENTS

It is a pleasure to acknowledge my indebtedness to the libraries and private collections that have made this work possible, and to express my sincerest thanks for the assistance so generously furnished.

This compilation was based primarily on the unparalleled Australian collection of the Mitchell Library and the associated Dixson and Reference Collections of the Library of New South Wales, together with the National Library of Australia and the State Library of Victoria. Special acknowledgement is gratefully made to the Principal Librarians and staffs for invaluable help and facilities.

I am deeply grateful also to the Principal Librarians of the State Libraries of South Australia, Tasmania, Western Australia, and the Oxley Memorial Library of the State Library of Queensland, to the librarians of the various university and medical libraries, and to many collectors of medical Australiana, for generous and unfailing assistance.

To my dear friends the late Sir John Ferguson of Sydney and Professor K. F. Russell of the University of Melbourne, whose bibliographical advice and encouragement made this work possible, my gratitude cannot be adequately expressed.

To the late Dr. G. A. M. Heydon of the University of Sydney, of happy memory, I am deeply grateful for many kindnesses, including the generous provision of secretarial help.

For assistance in many ways, I am indebted particularly to: Mr Harrison Bryan, University of Sydney; Mr. A. H. Chisholm, Sydney; the late Mr. E. M. Christie, Melbourne; Mr. J. E. Claffey, Sydney; Mr. R. L. Cope, Parliamentary Library of New South Wales; Dr. C. Craig, Launceston; Sir William Crowther, Hobart; Dr. C. J. Cummins, Sydney; Mr. G. Dennes, Sydney; Miss Jessie Dobson, Royal College of Surgeons of England; Dr. F. M. C. Forster, Melbourne; Dr. C. Fortune, Perth; Mrs Pauline Fanning, National Library; Professor B. Gandevia, University of New South Wales; Mrs Alison Holster, Royal Australasian College of Physicians; Mr. E. F. Kunz, National Library; Mr. W. R. Le Fanu, Royal College of Surgeons of England; Miss Judith Lloyd, Medical Library, University of Adelaide; Mrs M. Macgregor, Queensland Institute of Medical Research, Brisbane; Dr. L. J. T. Murphy, Melbourne; Dr. D. M. O'Sullivan, Ballarat; Mr. L. M. Payne, Royal College of Physicians of London; Dr. F. N. L. Poynter and Mr. R. Price, Wellcome Institute of History of Medicine, London; Miss Patricia Reynolds, Latrobe Library, Melbourne; Miss A. M. H. Rolleston, Australian Medical Association, Sydney; Miss J. Short, State Library of South Australia; Mr. G. T. Stilwell, State Library of Tasmania; Miss Ann Tovell, Medical Society of Victoria Museum, Melbourne; Mrs Joan Martin, Royal Children's Hospital, Melbourne; Dr. Ronald Winton, Sydney. Acknowledgement is also made to the Australian Academy of the Humanities for a grant towards production costs.

Finally, I must thank Mrs Bill Cantwell for her skilled and arduous secretarial assistance, and Mr. Malcolm Titt and Mr. David New of Sydney University Press for their editorial guidance and advice.

E. F.

LIBRARY SYMBOLS

AMAN	Australian Medical Association (New South Wales Branch), Sydney
AMAQ	Australian Medical Association (Queensland Branch), Brisbane
AMAV	Australian Medical Association (Victorian Branch), Melbourne
BG	Associate Professor B. Gandevia, Sydney
CC	Dr. Clifford Craig, Launceston
DL	Dixson Library (Library of New South Wales), Sydney
DOS	Dr. D. M. O'Sullivan, Ballarat
EF	Author's collection
FC	Ferguson Collection (National Library of Australia)
FF	Dr. F. M. C. Forster, Melbourne
HDN	Health Department of New South Wales, Sydney
HDV	Health Department of Victoria, Melbourne
KFR	Professor K. F. Russell, Melbourne
LNSW	Library of New South Wales, Sydney
ML	Mitchell Library (Library of New South Wales), Sydney
MLWA	Medical Library of Western Australia, Perth
NL	National Library of Australia, Canberra
OL	Oxley Memorial Library (State Library of Queensland), Brisbane
RACP	Royal Australasian College of Physicians, Sydney
RACS	Royal Australasian College of Surgeons, Melbourne
SLS	State Library of South Australia, Adelaide
SLT	State Library of Tasmania, Hobart
SLV	State Library of Victoria, Melbourne
SLW	State Library of Western Australia, Perth
SPH	School of Public Health and Tropical Medicine, University of Sydney
UA	University of Adelaide (Barr Smith Library)
UM	University of Melbourne, Melbourne
UQ	University of Queensland, Brisbane
US	University of Sydney, Sydney
WLC	Sir William Crowther, Hobart

ABBREVIATIONS

abbrev.	abbreviated
Aberd.	Aberdeen
Adel.	Adelaide
advt	advertisement
AIF	Australian Imperial Force
AMA	Australian Medical Association
Amer.	American
an. rep.	annual report
anaesth.	anaesthetist
anat.	anatomy
ann.	annals
anon.	anonymous
anthrop.	anthropological
assn	association
asst	assistant
Aust.	Australia Australian
Aust. Enc.	*Australian Encyclopaedia*, 1–10, Syd., 1958
Austsia	Australasia
Austsn	Australasian
b.	born
bact.	bacteriologist bacteriology
bd	board
benev.	benevolent
bibliog.	bibliography
biog.	biography
biol.	biological biology
BMA	British Medical Association
BMC	*British Museum General Catalogue of Printed Books*
BPCMUS	*Bulletin of the Post-Graduate Committee in Medicine of the University of Sydney*
Bris.	Brisbane
Brit.	British
Brux.	Brussels
bull.	bulletin
Camb.	Cambridge
cat.	catalogue
chancr	chancellor
chem.	chemistry
clin.	clinical
CMO	chief medical officer
col.	colonial column
coll.	collection college
com.	committee
cong.	congress
cons.	consulting
d.	died
dent.	dental dentistry
dep.	deputy
dept	department
dict.	dictionary
dis.	disease diseases
dispens.	dispensary
dist	district
dir	director
Dub.	Dublin
ed.	edited edition editor
Edin.	Edinburgh
Eng.	England English
engr.	engraved
epidem.	epidemiological
Ferguson	Ferguson, J. A., *Bibliography of Australia*, 1–7, Syd., 1941–69, facs. reprint, Canberra, 1975–6
fig.	figure
flg	folding
frontis.	frontispiece
gaz.	gazette
gen.	general
geog.	geographical
Glas.	Glasgow
GMO	government medical officer
govt	government
gynaec.	gynaecologist gynaecology
Heaton	Heaton, J. H., *Australian Dictionary of Dates and Men of the Time*, Lond., 1879
hist.	historical
HO	health officer
hon.	honorary
hosp.	hospital
HRA	*Historical Records of Australia*
HRNSW	*Historical Records of New South Wales*
hyg.	hygiene

illustn	illustration
infirm.	infirmary
inspr	inspector
inst.	institute
instn	institution
intdn	introduction
intercol.	intercolonial
J.	journal
lab.	laboratory
l.b.	last page blank
lect.	lecturer
leg.	legislative
litho.	lithograph
Lond.	London
mat. med.	materia medica
med.	medical
Melb.	Melbourne
Mennell	Mennell, P., *The Dictionary of Australasian Biography*, Lond., 1892
microbiol.	microbiology
Miller	Miller, E. M., *Australian Literature ... to 1935*, 1–2, Melb., 1940; facs. reprint, Syd., 1975
MO	medical officer
MOH	medical officer of health
ms. mss	manuscript manuscripts
ND	no date on title
NG	New Guinea
NI	no imprint on title
no	number
ns	new series
NS	item not seen
NSW	New South Wales
NT	Northern Territory
N.Y.	New York
NZ	New Zealand
obit.	obituary
obst.	obstetrician obstetrics
ophth.	ophthalmologist ophthalmology
p. pp.	page pages
P., proc.	proceedings
parlt	parliament parliamentary
path.	pathological pathology
pharm.	pharmacy pharmaceutical
phys.	physician
physiol.	physiology physiological
pl.	plate plates
post-grad.	post-graduate

pr	printer
prelim.	preliminary
pres.	president presidential
prof.	professor
pt	part
pub.	public
p.w.	paper wrappers
Qd	Queensland
quart.	quarterly
QUI	Queen's University, Ireland
r.	recto
RAHS	Royal Australian Historical Society
r.b.	recto blank
RCP	Royal College of Physicians
RCS	Royal College of Surgeons
rec.	records
ref.	reference
reg.	registrar
regs.	regulations
repr.	reprint
rptd	repeated
roy.	royal
SA	South Australia
sci.	science
sec.	secretary
Sel. Com.	select committee
ser.	series
Serle	Serle, P., *Dictionary of Australian Biography*, 1–2, Melb., 1940
SGC	*Index Catalogue of the Library of the Surgeon General's Office, United States Army*
soc.	society
SSAL	*Scientific Serials in Australian Libraries* (1971)
St And.	St Andrew's
stn	station
supp.	supplement
surg.	surgeon surgery surgical
Syd.	Sydney
Tas.	Tasmania
TCD	Trinity College Dublin
trans.	transactions
transl.	translated translation
Univ.	University
US	United States of America
v.	verso
V&P	*Votes and Proceedings*

v.b.	verso blank
VDL	Van Diemen's Land
vet.	veterinary
Vic	Victoria
vol.	volume
WA	Western Australia

INTRODUCTION

THE AIM OF THIS WORK is to describe the printed material relating to Australian medicine which appeared from 1790, when Surgeon-General John White's first Australian medical contribution was published, up to and including the year 1900. This span of one hundred and eleven years covers a period of national formation, from the early years of the struggling penal colony on Sydney Cove, through the ensuing hundred years of settlement, exploration and development. It concludes as the present century, with the foundation of the Australian Commonwealth in 1901, introduces a new era of nationhood.

Practitioners of medicine played an essential part in every phase of this development. They were of many origins—some were surgeons of convict or immigrant ships, a few were convicts, some officials, some migrants who sought gold or adventure or a place in a new land, others, including some who were highly qualified and already distinguished, were sufferers from tuberculosis who sought health. In the early penal days government officers provided a general medical service, established the first hospitals, and gave paid part-time service to free settlers as these appeared. In 1815 the first private practice was established in Sydney by Dr. William Bland, and independent doctors, growing in numbers with expanding population and settlement, increased greatly during the gold rushes and the bursting immigration of the mid-century. They laid the foundations for stable practice in the bustling centres and accompanied and shared the hardships and the often heartbreaking disappointments of every advance. They combined medicine with gold-seeking in mining camps, and practised single-handed in isolated settlements where long visits on horseback or buggy through often trackless country were essential, and drought, flood and bush-fire added to the difficulties of settlers. The pioneers were, as a class, courageous and enterprising, and despite their often combative independence, their quarrels and feuds and their share of human failings, were united in the service of their profession.

The early doctors brought British medical practice to a country which differed widely from their homeland in its inhospitable vastness, climate, conditions of living and occupation, and pattern of disease, and adapted it, of necessity, to the needs of their changed environment. Practice in the widely separated settlements throughout the colonies demanded well-trained general practitioners of broad competence and self-reliance; the poorly trained and incompetent inevitably failed. This consideration was paramount in shaping the teaching of the first Australian medical school, established in the University of Melbourne in 1862, only 27 years after the Port Phillip district received its first settler. Here the medical course was extended a year beyond that required for similar qualification in British schools, to give added training in medicine, surgery and obstetrics to all graduates. The medical schools of Sydney and Adelaide, founded before the end of the century, adopted similar courses. The Australian medical profession, at the end of the period covered by this work, was firmly based on this locally fashioned form of general practice. Their brass plates noted them all as 'physician and surgeon', and as an author has correctly stated, 'they might equally reasonably have added obstetrician, gynaecologist and anaesthetist'. General practice supplied the honorary staffs of hospitals, clinical teachers in medical schools, part-time appointees to the developing health services, and the emerging specialism budded from its ranks. The hall-marks of the profession were all-round proficiency, self-reliance and independence.

The term 'Medicine', as applied in this bibliography, is used in a comprehensive sense to embrace all aspects of health and healing. It refers, firstly, to the content and practice of orthodox medicine in all its branches, and to its practitioners, institutions, associations and societies, and includes dentistry, nursing and pharmacy. It contains also official medicine, as displayed in items as those relating to the early colonial medical service, the surgeons and surgeon-superintendents of the convict transport service, and the fore-runners of the present day governmental health and welfare organizations. Various aspects of life and livelihood which affected the public health and welfare also find a place. Domestic medicine is included, with its profuse output of direction and advice on home treatment in illness and emergency, infant care and home nursing, which held an especially valued place in the years of widely scattered population, sparse settlement and hardship. The vagaries and often roguery of quack medicine, which flourished almost without restraint to the end of last century, are also represented, together with various cults and fads, both professional and popular, which had their day.

The present compilation follows the general plan of the concluding three volumes (1851–1900) of Sir John Ferguson's *Bibliography of Australia*, in which an alphabetical arrangement of items is adopted. The work was commenced following Sir John's reluctant but necessary decision to generally omit medical material from his volumes of these crowded years. It is the direct result of this revered Master's kindly persuasion, tuition and help.

The works described include books, pamphlets, periodicals, broadsides and leaflets. Items printed in Australia relate to medicine in general, and those published anywhere outside Australia refer particularly to some aspect of Australian medicine. Occasionally history or travel books containing indicated passages of special pertinence or interest, and accounts of medical visitors, are included.

Since the medical practitioners of the time enter the purview of the work, occasional non-medical items are added as displaying aspects of the extra-professional interests or activities of these. For reason of personal history, also, the early works of medical authors who published prior to settling in Australia are usually shown with their local productions, and in general the main publications of listed authors, appearing after 1900, are noted.

All dates in titles, printed in Roman numerals, are here for convenience shown in Arabic figures. Measurements are in millimetres.

Many institutions have changed their names, often repeatedly, in the course of the period covered. These are consequently recorded under the title shown in their latest entry, and prior or subsequent names appear in cross references or notes.

Material of the following categories has been excluded from the content of the present volume:

(a) Statutes relating to medicine.

(b) Medical statistics. These are covered by the *Bibliography of Vital Statistics in Australia and New Zealand*, by H. O. Lancaster, *Aust. J. Statistics*, 1964, 6 : 33–99.

(c) Veterinary medicine in general, though including numerous items directly pertinent to human medicine

(d) Articles from periodicals, unless subsequent issue as independent publications is clearly indicated.

(e) Items relating to New Zealand and New Guinea, without Australian reference.

Occasional exceptions to the above occur, however, for special reasons.

Selection has been exercised in two areas, the first in regard to items from the Parliamentary Papers of the various states, due to the voluminous extent of these important records. In the second, which refers to water supplies and sanitation, certain reports, usually of large-scale schemes of engineering rather than medical interest, have been omitted.

Brief biographical notes on authors, with references preferably from medical sources, are added. Works consulted for this include J. H. Heaton, *Australian Dictionary of Dates and Men of the Time*, 1879; P. Mennell, *The Dictionary of Australian Biography*, 1892; P. Serle, *Dictionary of Australian Biography*, 1949; *Australian Encyclopaedia*, 10 vols, 1958; *Australian Dictionary of Biography*, 4 vols, 1966–72; and the medical directories of the period. These are rarely cited in the notes.

An endeavour has been made to show the holdings of listed items by the various libraries and private collections indicated above. This protracted task was impelled by long experienced frustration encountered in the search for titles noted, without location, in various publications. Though references have been checked with catalogues, omissions are inevitable.

Titles appear which have not been found in any collection, their only trace being a reference in some printed work. These 'ghost' publications—named representatives of printings that have disappeared—are listed with available details. Such losses were inevitable for reasons that have caused only single or few copies of early medical pamphlets to survive, and certain medical periodicals and almanacs to exist in rare and broken sets. For many were of ephemeral interest, conditions inimical to the care of books prevailed, libraries as repositories of local works were totally lacking or in their infancy, and small issues and hard usage common.

A number of works of promised publication, lacking all evidence of the actual achievement of this, are also noted. Attention has usually been drawn to these by advertisement as 'shortly to be published' or 'to be published by subscription.' These are of interest as the pursuits of local medical authors.

Plagiarism was rife in publications of the period, especially in the treatises of unqualified practitioners, though certain professional authors were also involved. Attention was drawn to this in 1873 by C. E. Reeves MD, *Heart Diseases in Australia*, in an angry statement that 'men who can scarcely put twelve words together daily advertise themselves as authors of works, paraphrased from some American edition of a German or French author. In Europe, these quasi authors would quickly be exposed, but here these robberies pass unchallenged'. Literary 'piracy'—republication of a work without the authority of its author—also existed here, as elsewhere, during this period. It may consequently be expected that many pirated editions appear among the reprinted overseas publications listed, particularly those of American authors.

Numerous bibliographical and reference works, and catalogues of libraries, institutions and booksellers, have been consulted. Special reference must be made to J. A. Ferguson, *Bibliography of Australia*; E. Morris Miller, *Australian Literature . . . to 1935*, Melb., 1940; B. Gandevia, *An Annotated Bibliography of the History of Medicine in Australia*, Syd., 1956; and the library catalogues of the British Museum, and the Surgeon-General's Office, United States Army.

To the memory of

FREDERIC WOOD JONES

JOHN ALEXANDER FERGUSON

A

Abbott, Francis
See Hall, Edward Swarbreck and Abbott, F.

Adam, George Rothwell Wilson
Ideals in the pursuit of medicine: an address delivered at the Annual Meeting of the Medical Students' Society ... [Arms] Melbourne: October, 1900. Ernest S. Fysh ... At the Press of Alma Mater.
171 × 98. Pp. [ii] (v.b., 34 (l.b.). Title varied in red. P. w. (title rptd, abbrev., and with cut).
For G. R. W. Adam (1853–1924) MB, ChM Edin., MD Melb., Hon. Obst. Women's Hosp., see obit., *Med. J. Aust.*, 1925, 1 : 149.
Copies: FF. 1

Adelaide and Parkside Lunatic Asylums
South Australia. Annual Report of the Resident Medical Officer of the Lunatic Asylums. 1871. Adelaide: ... W. C. Cox, Govt Printer ... 1872.
207 × 138. Pp. 16. P. w. (title rptd).
For Adel. and Parkside Asylums. Signed A. S. Paterson, MD.
Copies: SLS. 2

[No. 136. South Australia. Report of Commission appointed to report upon the Adelaide and Parkside Lunatic Asylums; together with minutes of proceedings, evidence, and appendices. ... Adelaide: ... E. Spiller, Govt Printer ... 1884.
330 × 204. Pp. xvi, 238 (l.b.).
On management, and treatment of patients.
Copies: LNSW, SLS, SLV. 3

Adelaide Chamber of Manufactures
South Australian industries and manufactures. Papers read before the Chamber of Manufactures, and reprinted by authority of the Government. Adelaide: W. C. Cox, Govt Printer ... 1875.
206 × 138. Pp. [vi], 294. P. w. (title rptd). Includes 'Winegrowing in South Australia', by A. C. Kelly MD, pp. 1–3, and W. L. Cleland MB, ChM, pp. 4–14.
Copies: ML, SLS, SLV. 4

Adelaide Children's Hospital
The proposed Children's Hospital. Reprinted from the "South Australian Register". Adelaide: Printed by William Kyffin Thomas ... 1876.
157 × 100. Pp. 20 (l.b.). P. w. (title rptd).
Copies: SLS. 5

The constitution and by-laws of the Adelaide Children's Hospital and Training School for Nurses. Adelaide: William Kyffin Thomas, Printer ... 1876.
190 × 128. Pp. 18 (2, 4 blank). Includes list of officers.
Copies: SLS. 6

Proceedings at the ceremony of laying the foundation stone of the Adelaide Children's Hospital ... June 20, 1878. ... Adelaide: Printed by W. K. Thomas ... 1878.
163 × 100. Pp. 20.
For history, see *Nursing in SA. First hundred years*, Adel., 1938; 2 ed. 1939.
Copies: SLS. 7

The Adelaide Children's Hospital by "Vid". Reprinted from the "S. A. Register" ... Adelaide: R. K. Thomas, Printer ...
160 × 102. Pp. [ii] (v.b.), 18. ND. [1880.] P. w. (variation of title, with verses; notice on v. of back wrapper).
Copies: SLS. 8

Rules for the guidance of the officers, nurses, & servants of the Adelaide Children's Hospital and Training School for Nurses, Incorporated. Adopted 5th February, 1891. Adelaide: Printed by Vardon and Pritchard ... 1891.
210 × 135. Pp. 16 (last 2 blank). P. w. (title rptd).

Copies: SLS. 9

Adelaide City Baths

The City Baths, Adelaide. Swimming baths, tepid baths, Turkish baths. The Turkish baths: under the distinguished patronage of His Excellency the Governor ... The Board of Management of the Adelaide Hospital, and the leading medical men of the Colony. T. Bastard, Lessee. ... Adel.: Printed by Waddy, Botting & Co. ...

168 × 104. Pp. 8. P. w. (cover title).

Includes therapeutic uses of Turkish baths.

Copies: SLV. 10

Adelaide Homoeopathic Dispensary

The First Annual Report of the Adelaide Homoeopathic Dispensary for the year ending May 22, 1868. Established 1867. Adelaide: Andrews, Thomas, & Clark ... 1868.

212 × 130. Pp. 14.

Copies: SLS (1868–9), SLV (1868–9). 11

Adelaide Hospital

The Adelaide Hospital. Subscriptions have been opened towards a fund for the erection of a permanent hospital, to be built on the site reserved for that purpose by the late Colonel Light ... [Text continues.]

Fcap folio. Pp. [4] (last 3 blank). Colophon—Robert Thomas and Co., Printers, Adel. ND. [1839.]

For history, see J. Estcourt Hughes, *A history of the Royal Adel. Hosp.*, Adel., 1967; also *Nursing in SA. First hundred years*. Adel., 1938; 2 ed. 1939. Re-named Royal Adel. Hosp. in 1939.

Copies: SA Archives. 12

———

Some account of the Adelaide Hospital, with the rules and regulations, dietary and statistics. Adelaide, G. Dehane, Printer ...

180 × 108. Pp. 22 (l.b.). ND. [1841.]

Copies: SLS. 13

———

Rules and regulations for the management of the Adelaide Hospital, with formulary of prescriptions, and table of diseases for medical returns. Adelaide: ... W. C. Cox, Govt Printer. 1850.

181 × 105. Pp. 22 (l.b.). Stiff p. w., cloth back-strip, paper label.

Later editions—1860 (SLS); 1868 (ML, NL); 1876 (SLS); 1899 (ML).

Copies: ML, SLS, SLV. 14

———

[No. 31. South Australia. Report on Adelaide Hospital by Commission appointed to inquire into and report on the management, etc., of the Lunatic Asylum and Hospital. ... Adelaide: ... W. C. Cox, Govt Printer ... 1864.

324 × 203. Pp. x, 42. Blue paper.

Copies: LNSW, SLS, SLV. 15

———

[No. 101. South Australia. Minutes of evidence and appendices taken by the Board of Management of the Adelaide Hospital respecting charges made by Dr. Leith Napier against Professor Watson; together with resolutions of the Board. Ordered by the House of Assembly to be printed ... Adelaide: ... C. E. Bristow, Govt Printer ... 1896.

326 × 210. Pp. 48.

For Watson's defence, see No. 2455.

Copies: LNSW, ML, SLS, SLV. 16

———

[No. 116. South Australia. Professor Watson's charges against Dr. Napier. Laid on table of Legislative Council, November 26th, 1896, and ordered to be printed December 8th, 1896. ... [Text begins.]

325 × 206. Pp. 4. NI.

Copies: LNSW, SLS, SLV. 17

———

[No. 116 A. South Australia. Report of Dr. Napier on Professor Watson's charges. Laid on the table of the Legislative Council, November 26th, 1896, and ordered to be printed ... [Text begins.]

325 × 206. Single leaf, v.b. NI.

Rep. to Bd of Management, Adel. Hosp.

Copies: LNSW, SLS, SLV. 18

———

The Adelaide Hospital dispute. The case for the Government. By the Hon. F. W. Holder, Treasurer of South Australia. Reprinted from the "Review of Reviews" for November [1896].

178 × 125. Pp. 16. 2 portraits. Colophon: ... T. Shaw Fitchett ... Melb. P. w. (cover title).

Copies: SLS, RACP. 19

———

The Adelaide Hospital ... A short account of

the circumstances which led to the resignation of the honorary staff. Published under the authority of the South Australian Branch of the British Medical Association. Adelaide: W. K. Thomas & Co. . . . 1896.

215 × 140. Pp. 30. P. w. (title rptd).

Account of dispute between SA Govt and Adel. Hosp. Bd, leading to resignation of the hon. staff, with events of two years.

Copies: SLS. 20

[No. 101A. South Australia. Report of the Select Committee of the Legislative Council on the Adelaide Hospital; together with minutes of proceedings, evidence, and appendices . . . Adelaide: . . . C. E. Bristow, Govt Printer . . . 1897.

329 × 202. Pp. xvi (l.b.), 196. 4 pl. (with 9 anatomical diagrams).

On management, care and treatment of patients.

Copies: LNSW, ML, SLS, SLV. 21

South [Royal Arms] Australia. Rules for the officers, nurses, and attendants of the Adelaide Hospital. Adopted, July 21st, 1899. Adelaide: C. E. Bristow, Govt Printer . . . 1899.

212 × 138. Pp. 24 (l.b.). P. w. (title rptd).

Copies: ML. 22

South [Royal Arms] Australia. Rules for the nurses and attendants of the Adelaide Hospital. . . . Adelaide: C. E. Bristow, Govt Printer . . . 1899.

214 × 137. Pp. 12 (l.b.).

Copies: SLS. 23

The Adelaide Hospital. The Adelaide Hospital dispute is at last, and happily, ended. It began . . . over a trifle; but it rose to a furious height, spread over the whole colony, and has lasted for years. It furnished the text for grave Parliamentary debate, overflowed all the journals, threatened to wreck a Cabinet, did actually put the entire medical profession in quarrel with the one great hospital of the colony, and temporarily destroyed the medical school . . . [Text continues.]

252 × 209. Single leaf, v.b. [1900.]

Proof sheet, with 'Review of Reviews 15 March 1900' in pencil; and ms. note in hand of Prof. F. Wood Jones FRS.

Copies: EF. 24

Adelaide Lunatic Asylum

[No. 30. South Australia. Report on Lunatic Asylum by Commission appointed to inquire and report upon the management, etc., of the Lunatic Asylum and Hospital. . . . Adelaide: . . . W. C. Cox, Govt Printer . . . 1864.

324 × 203. Pp. x, 38. Blue paper.

Copies: LNSW, SLS, SLT, SLV. 25

See also Adelaide and Parkside Lunatic Asylum.

Adelaide Medical Students' Society

No. 1. Vol. 1. The Medical Students' Society Review. May, 1889. Contents. . . . Adelaide: T. S. Carey & Co., Printers . . .

218 × 138. Pp. 24. P. w. (cover title, advts on v. of both wrappers).

Title later became *The Review*. The formation of the Society is briefly referred to in *Med. J. Aust.*, 1924, 2 : 462.

Copies: UA (Vol. 1–, 1889–). 26

Aesculapius Peripateticus

Cancer—a result of vaccination. . . . with introduction and notes by Ernst Meyer, B.A., Ph.D. Melbourne: . . . J. C. Stephens. 1898.

204 × 132. Pp. 8.

Noted as chapter from unpublished book on small-pox and vaccination by a medical scientist. Claims that 'where the so-called human lymph is employed, syphilis, leprosy and tuberculosis follow in its train; and wherever calf lymph is used, tuberculosis and cancer spread like a conflagration.'

Copies: NL. 27

Ahearne, Joseph

Presidential address . . . at the First Annual Meeting of the North Queensland Medical Society. 1890 Townsville: . . . Hastings & Jones . . .

213 × 137. Pp. 20 (l.b.). P. w. (amended title).

Health and living conditions in Queensland tropics.

Copies: ML. 28

Albury Hospital

See Andrews, Arthur.

Alfred Hospital, Melbourne

Prince Alfred Hospital. [Note follows from John Blair, Hon. Sec., Executive Committee ... 29th April, 1868.] Proposed General Committee. [Names follow.]

Folio. Pp. 7. No title page.

Copies: SLV. 29

The Prince Alfred Hospital. Correspondence between the Government and the Committee of the Prince Alfred Hospital on the subject of the grant asked for that institution. Melbourne: Stillwell and Knight ... 1868.

206 × 132. Pp. 8. P. w. (title rptd, letter inside back wrapper).

Govt demands that projected role of Hosp. should be changed from general to convalescent and incurable, which is opposed.

Copies: SLV. 30

Progress Report of the Executive Committee of the Prince Alfred Hospital ... Melbourne: Mason, Firth & McCutcheon ... 1870.

8vo. Pp. 12 (l.b.).

Copies: SLV. 31

The proposed constitution & rules of the Alfred Hospital. Melbourne: Mason, Firth, & M'Cutcheon ... 1870.

204 × 132. Pp. 8. Printer's error in date (MDCCLXX). P. w.

Copies: SLV. 32

The constitution & rules of the Alfred Hospital. As adopted at a meeting of contributors held in October 14, 1870. Melbourne: Mason, Firth & M'Cutcheon ... 1870.

8vo. Pp. 8. P. w.

Copies: NL. 33

Alfred Hospital, St. Kilda Road. Report of the Admission Committee.

204 × 132. Pp. 8. ND. (?1871.) Colophon—Fergusson and Moore ... Melb.

Copies: SLV. 34

The First Annual Report of the Managers of the Alfred Hospital, and a list of subscriptions and donations for 1871. Melbourne: Fergusson and Moore ... 1872.

234 × 178. Pp. 16. P. w. (title rptd).

Copies: Alfred Hosp. (1871–), EF (1887, 1896), ML (1889–1891), SLV (1871–). 35

Alfred Hospital. Rules, &c., for nurses under training. 1880. Melbourne: Bones & Watt, Printers ...

8vo. Pp. 8.

Copies: SLV. 36

Alfred Hospital Pharmacopoeia

Issued 1871. Noted in *Aust. med. J.*, 1871, 16: 128. NS.

37

Allen, Sir Harry Brookes

The University of Melbourne. 14th March, 1891. The Dean of the Faculty of Medicine ... I have the honour to report ... concerning the re-organisation of the Departments of Anatomy and Pathology [Text continues.]

204 × 110. Pp. 6 (l.b.). Melb., Edgerton & Moore, 1891.

Recommends separate chairs of anatomy and pathology and establishment of an institute of preventive medicine.

Copies: BG. 38

1891. Victoria. First general report on recognition of Melbourne University degrees; Mr. Mansergh's scheme for drainage of Melbourne; necessity for re-survey of Melbourne; the Metropolitan Board of Works; sewerage works and disposal of sewage ... Presented to both Houses ... Robt S. Brain, Govt Printer, Melbourne.

306 × 204. Pp. 18.

First of three reports made to Vic. Govt after author's official visit to Europe.

Copies: AMAV, EF, KFR, ML, NL, SLV, UM. 39

1891. Victoria. Second general report on Metropolitan water supply; pollution of rivers; unhealthy areas and dwellings; results obtained by sanitary works; the great avoidable mortalities; isolation of infectious disease; disinfection; milk supply; preparation and conservation of calf lymph; abattoirs and noxious trades; health officers and inspectors; hygienic museum; institute of preventive medicine . . . Presented to both Houses . . . Robt S. Brain, Govt Printer, Melbourne.

306 × 204. Pp. 26.

Copies: AMAV, EF, KFR, ML, NL, SLV, UM. 40

1891. Victoria. Final general report on hospital construction and management . . . Presented to both Houses . . . Robt S. Brain, Govt Printer, Melbourne.

306 × 204. Pp. 32. 17 plans.

Includes, in addition to overseas hospitals, sections on Prince Alfred Hosp. Syd., and Melb. Hosp.

Copies: AMAV, BG, KFR, ML, NL, SLV, UM. 41

1891. Victoria. Professor Koch's remedy for tuberculosis. . . . Report . . . Presented to both Houses of Parliament . . . Robt S. Brain, Govt Printer, Melbourne.

326 × 204. Pp. 20 (l.b.).

Author was sent by Vic. Govt to Germany to report on the newly announced tuberculin cure. He advises that tuberculin has indisputable diagnostic value; it is probably a valuable therapeutic agent, though 'months and probably years must pass before . . . we can estimate (its) true value . . .'

Copies: AMAV, KFR, ML, NL, SLV, UM. 42

Intercolonial Medical Congress of Australasia, Third Session, Sydney. 1892. Section of Anatomy, Physiology, Pathology and Pharmacology. President's address . . . Melbourne: Stillwell and Co. . . . 1892.

204 × 135. Pp. 24. Repr. *Aust. med. J.*, 15 Nov. 1892.

Copies: SLV, UM. 42a

Tabular list of medical periodicals in Melbourne libraries. Prepared by Professor Allen, M.D. . . . with the assistance of the librarians. [Text begins.]

NS. Reprinted in *Aust. med. J.*, 1893, ns 15 : 97–112. Lists holdings of SLV, Med. Soc. Vic., Univ. Melb. Noted in T. S. Hall's *Catalogue*, 1899, as the only catalogue of this nature published in Melbourne.

43

University of Melbourne. Elementary pathological histology. Methods and description of sections. Melbourne: Rae Bros. . . . 1895.

236 × 153. Pp. [ii] (v.b.), 102. Alternate leaves blank after p. 10; included in numbering. P. w. (cover title).

Class notes for students.

For Sir Harry Brookes Allen (1854–1926) MD Melb., Prof. Anat. and Path. (later Path.) and Dean Med. Univ. Melb., see obit., *Med. J. Aust.*, 1926, 1 : 414; King, E. S. J. (1951), 'The story of the Melb. School of Pathology', *Med. J. Aust.*, 2: 101.

Later publications: 'A history of the Med. School', in *Univ. Melb. Med. School Jubilee*, Melb., 1914; *Pathology. Notes of lectures and demonstrations*, Melb., 1919; 2 ed., 1921.

Copies: ML, SLV, UM. 44

Alleyne, Haynes Gibbes

1852. New South Wales. Health Officer. . . . Letter from the Health Officer, to the Colonial Secretary. Sydney, 11th December, 1852.

322 × 190. Pp. 4 (l.b.). Pale blue paper. Signed: H. G. Alleyne MD. *NSW*, *Leg. Council*, *V&P*, 1852.

Quarantine Officer, after censure, outlines the difficulties of his post and applies for boat and crew for his use.

H. G. Alleyne (d. 1882) MD Edin. was HO Port Jackson for 30 years, Med. Adviser to NSW Govt, Hon. Phys. Syd. Infirm., and a local pioneer of chloroform anaesthesia. See obit., *Austsn med. Gaz.*, 1882, 1: 165; McCallum F. (1926), 'An early Aust. Quarantine Officer', *Health*, 4 : 1; Dunlop, N. J. (1927), *Med. J. Aust.*, 1 : 141 (for anaesthesia).

Copies: LNSW, NL. 45

'Alma Mater' Medical Supplement

Brownless Memorial Supplement. Being a special medical supplement to "Alma Mater" Vol. 3, No. 6. Septr. 1898.

242 × 178. Pp. 36. P. w. (cover title, decorated and with portrait).

Memorial issue for Sir A. C. Brownless MD, Chancellor Melb. Univ. Contains illustrated history of Melb. Med. School.

Copies: ML, SLT, SLV, UM, US, UT. 46

Anatomical Museum, Melbourne

See Kreitmayer and Wiseheart's Anatomical Museum.

Anderson, William John

The causes, symptoms, and treatment of eccentric nervous affections. London: J. Churchill . . . 1850.

8vo. Pp. xiii, 199. Cloth. NS.

Copies: British Museum. 47

The symptoms & treatment of the diseases of pregnancy. By William John Anderson, F.R.C.S. District Accoucheur to St. Mary's Hospital [Emblem] London: John Churchill . . . 1852.

196 × 125. Pp. x, 120 (last—colophon only). Cloth.

Noted in No 50, as republished by Sherriff and Downing, Syd. NS.

Copies: US. 48

"Continued fever in children", reprinted from the *Association Medical Journal* of August 25, 1854. With which is: "On the use of nitro-sulphuric acid in cholera and diarrhoea" . . . London: T. Richards. 1854.

8vo. Pp. 35. NS.

For note of reissue by Sherriff and Downing, Syd., see No 50.

Copies: Wellcome Inst. Med. Hist., Lond. 49

Hysterical and nervous affections of women. Read before the Harveian Society. By William John Anderson, Sydney. . . . New edition. Sydney: Sherriff & Downing, 256, George Street. 1864.

186 × 120. Pp. [ii] (book notice, r.b.), 40, 4 (book notices). Limp cloth, paper label.

1 ed., Lond., Churchill, 1853. Pp. 40 (l.b.). NS.

Notes reissue by Sherriff and Downing of following works by W. J. Anderson FRCS of 124 Phillip St, Sydney, with extracts of press reviews of earlier eds: *Hysterical, hypochondriacal, epileptic, and other nervous affections*, post 8vo., cloth; *The symptoms and treatment of the diseases of pregnancy*, post 8vo., cloth; *Continued fever in children.* N.S.

W. J. Anderson (1821–71) FRCS, Accoucheur to St Mary's Hosp. and to St George's and St James's Dispens., and Sec. and Vice-Pres. Harveian Soc., came to Aust., probably for health reasons, between 1856 and 1859. He was in Balmain up to 1862, and thence practised at various Syd. addresses. He died on a voyage home from Syd. in 1871. See *Plarr's Lives of Fellows of RCS*, 1930, 1 : 25.

Copies: ML. 50

Andrews, Alexander (editor)

A sketch of the colony of Western Australia, containing a brief narrative of its resources and prospects, and designed for the guidance of persons contemplating emigration. Edited by Alexander Andrews, Esq. . . . Reprinted from the Swan River News and Western Australian Chronicle . . . London: Edward Colyer . . .

4to. Pp. 16. ND. [1849].

Includes climate and medical refs, noting W. P. Dineley, Surgeon, Fremantle Gaol. 'Measles, smallpox, typhoid or puerperal fevers, or any of those dread diseases to which the mother country is subject are here unknown. . . . peculiarly adapted to those . . . who suffer from affections of the chest'.

Copies: ML, SLW. 50a

Andrews, Arthur

The early years and struggles of the Albury Hospital and Benevolent Asylum. . . . [Text begins.]

204 × 147. Pp. 6. Galley proofs laid down. ND. NI. History, 1858–70.

Copies: ML. 51

Anthrax and Inoculation

Anthrax and inoculation. Reprinted from "The Australasian Pastoralists' Review." Melbourne: M'Carron, Bird & Co . . . 1899.

186 × 120. Pp. 12. P. w. (cover title).

Article (anon.) states that Pasteur anthrax vaccine deteriorates more rapidly than a locally developed product. Letters appended from F. Zimmermann of Pasteur Vaccine Lab., and J. A. Gunn of M'Garvie Smith and Gunn, manufacturers of local product.

Copies: ML, NL. 52

The Same. Another ed., 1899, pp. 16 (l.b.). Adds further Zimmermann letter.

Copies: ML. 53

Anthropological Museum (Jordan & Beck), Melb.

See Jordan and Beck, Drs.

Ararat Hospital, Vic.

The Second Annual Report of the ... Ararat Hospital: with the rules and regulations ... and a statistical table of cases treated, etc. Ararat: Printed by Nuthall and Banfield, Advertiser Office ... 1861.

204 × 127. Pp. 24.

Copies: SLV (1860–71). 54

Archer, W. A.

See No. 2424.

Archer, William Henry

Abstracts of English and colonial patent specifications relating to the preservation of food, etc. Compiled from original documents ... in the Patent Office ... Melbroune ... Melbourne: ... John Ferres, Govt Printer; also by H. T. Dwight ... 1870.

209 × 135. Pp. xvi, 66. 4 flg sheets of drawings.

Includes J. Bancroft's method for desiccation of meats and vegetables (No 155).

Copies: CC, ML, UM. 55

———

Supplement to abstracts of English and Colonial patent specifications relating to the preservations of food, etc. Compiled from original documents ... in the Patent Office ... Melbourne ... Melbourne: ... John Ferres, Govt Printer; also ... by H. T. Dwight ... 1870.

209 × 135. Pp. [ii] (v.b.), [67]–74, 1 flg sheet of drawings. Errata slip.

For Wm Henry Archer (1825–1909) FIA, Reg. Gen. of Vic., see McCallum, F. (1928) 'An Aust. pioneer in vital statistics', *Health*, 6, (2) : 33.

Copies: CC. 56

Armstrong, William George

Metropolitan Combined Sanitary Districts. Annual report of the Medical Officer of Health ... for the year ending 31st December, 1898. [Text begins.]

331 × 214. Pp. 12. Colophon—Syd.: William Applegate Gullick, Govt Pr—1899. Signed: W. G. Armstrong, MB, DPH.

Copies: EF. 57

———

[No. 81. South Australia. The alleged cases of bubonic plague. Ordered by the House of Assembly to be printed, August 3rd, 1900 ... Alleged cases of bubonic plague at the Adelaide Hospital. Report by Dr. W. G. Armstrong, of Sydney. [Text begins.]

325 × 206. Pp. 2. NI.

Consultant's examination of three suspect cases.

W. G. Armstrong (1860–1942) MB, ChM Syd., DPH Camb., was MOH Syd. from 1898 and later Dir Gen. Pub. Health NSW and Pres. Bd of Health (1920–4). He was associated with Ashburton Thompson in his able plague control and worked notably for reduction of infant mortality. See obit., *Med. J. Aust.*, 1942, 1 : 272.

Copies: LNSW, SLS, SLV. 58

Arthur, Richard

Hypnotic suggestion. ... Reprinted from the "Australasian Medical Gazettee" for December, 1891. L. Bruck ... Sydney. 1891.

186 × 122. Pp. 14. P. w. (cover title).

Author studied hypnotism in Europe, presented Edin. MD thesis on 'Hypnotism and its therapeutic uses', used method in his practice, and wrote and lectured on it. See his 'In defence of hypnotism', *Austsn med. Gaz.*, 1893, 12 : 238.

Copies: ML. 59

———

The innocence of children ... Sydney: S. D. Townsend & Co. ... 1894.

135 × 107. Pp. 8.

On sex education for children.

Copies: FC, ML. 60

———

The needed change in the age of consent. An appeal for the better protection of our girls. ... Sydney: The Christian World Press ... 1896.

153 × 90. Pp. 12.

An appeal for raising the 'age of consent' from 14 to 18 years.

For Richard Arthur (1865–1932) MD, MLA, Hon. Otolarygologist Syd. Hosp. and Minister for Health NSW, see obit., *Med. J. Aust.*, 1932, 2 : 95.

Copies: FC, ML. 61

Ashworth, Louis Naish

See Turner, A. J. and Ashworth, L. N.

Astles, Harvey Eustace

Fermented liquors: shall I use them, or not? ... Adelaide: Scrymgour & Sons, Printers ... Published by George Robertson & Co. ... 1886.

161 × 102. Pp. [viii] (l.b.), 32, [2] (colophon, v.b.). Errata slip. Stiff p. w. (abbrev. title).

On good and bad effects of alcohol, which is regarded as a valuable drug, and use in hospitals supported.

H. E. Astles MD, FRCPE, GMO NT, later settled in Adel. (Pres. BMA); about 1896 was in Perth (Hon. Phys. Perth Hosp., Pres. BMA); and about 1900 in Melb. (Phys. Melb. Hosp.).

Copies: ML, SLS. 62

Asylum for Blind, Sydney

Asylum for Blind. It is proposed to establish an asylum in which to receive and educate the blind . . . [Text continues.]

204 × 130. Single leaf, v.b. ND. NI.

Signed: H. G. Douglass, George F. Wise, Hon. Secs.

Copies: LNSW. 63

Atherton, Ebenezer

See Notes on homoeopathy.

Atkins, G. Purcell

See South Aust.—Parliament, No 1986.

Atkinson, J. Fife

What shall we do with our dead? Discussed as a sanitary question. Melbourne: W. H. Williams, Printer . . . 1878.

206 × 130. Pp. 12 (l.b.).

Discusses insanitary state of current burial practices, and recommends cremation. Author was the Sec., Vic. Funeral Reform Assn.

Copies: ML. 64

Austin, George

How to be beautiful. A book for women. by Dr. Geo. Austin, M.R.C.S.E. Adelaide: Modern Printing Company . . . 1891.

185 × 125. Pp. 64 (l.b.).

Includes hygiene, diet, exercise, bathing, clothing and topical measures.

Copies: SLS. 65

Austin Hospital for Incurables, Melbourne

The Second Annual Report of the Austin Hospital for Incurables, Melbourne. Founded 1881. ... From June, 1883, to June 1884. Melbourne: J. J. Miller, Printer . . . 1884.

206 × 132. Pp. 20 (l.b.).

Hosp. opened 14 Aug. 1882; later named Austin Hospital.

Copies: Austin Hosp. (1882–), SLV (1883–1900 incomplete). 66

Australasian Homoeopathic Medical Gazette

The Australasian Homoeopathic Medical Gazette [Motto] A record of the Progress of Homoeopathy in the Australian Colonies—Published Quarterly. ... No. 1, Vol. 1]. Dunedin, July 15, 1895. [Price, 2/6 Per Annum, Post Free.

282 × 220. Pp. 12.

Vol. 1, nos 1–4, July 1895–April 1896 only seen.

Copies: ML. 67

Australasian Journal of Pharmacy

The Australasian Journal of Pharmacy. The organ of pharmacy in the Australasian Colonies, devoted to the advancement of pharmaceutical knowledge. Volume 1.—January—December, 1886. Melbourne: A. H. Massina & Co., Printers and Publishers . . .

350 × 235. Vols 1–34, 1886–1919; ns, 1920–.

Official journal of the associated pharmaceutical organisations of Australasia. In 1934 incorporated *The Chemist and Druggist and Pharmacist of Australasia*.

Copies: See *SSAL*. 68

Australasian Medical Association (proposed)

See Ballarat Med. Assn; also Ballarat and Goulburn Valley Med. Assns.

Australasian Medical Directory and Hand-Book

The Australasian Medical Directory and Hand-Book. Edited and compiled by Ludwig Bruck. First year of publication. Sydney : Published at the "Australasian Medical Gazette" Office. London: Bailliere, Tindall, & Cox . . . 1883.

214 × 132. Pp. [10] (advts), viii, 194, [8] (advts). Cloth.

Copies: EF, KFR, ML, NL, SLV, UA. 69

The Same. 2 ed., 1886. Adds appendix of unregistered medical practitioners and list of American medical colleges 'not recognized.' Pp. [8] (advts), vi, 270, [4] (advts). Cloth.

Copies: BG, EF, KFR, ML, NL, SLV, UA, US. 70

The Same. 3 ed., 1892. Pp. [24] (advts), [vi], 238 (last advt), [8] (advts).

Copies: BG, EF, KFR, ML, NL, SLV, UA. 71

The Same. 4 ed., 1896. Pp. [4] (advts), [vi], 196, [2] (advts).
Copies: EF, KFR, ML, NL, OL, SLV, UA. 72

The Same. 5 ed. 1900. Pp. [x] (advts, prelim.), 224, [4] (advts).
Copies: BG, EF, KFR, ML, NL, OL, SLV, UA. 73

Australasian Medical Gazette

The Australasian Medical Gazette: being the official organ of the Combined Australasian Branches of the British Medical Association. Vol. 1. Edited by Frederick Milford, M. D. From October, 1881, to September, 1882. Sydney: L. Bruck, Medical Publisher . . . 1882.
255 × 210. Pp. 170.
Vols. 1–35; 1881/2–1914. Monthly; weekly in 1911.
Founded in 1881 by Ludwig Bruck, as official organ of BMA branches; purchased in 1894 by BMA (NSW); combined with *Australian Medical Journal* in 1914 to form the *Medical Journal of Australia*. See Cumpston, J.H.L. (1939), 'The history of med. journalism in Aust.', *Med. J. Aust.*, 2 : 1.
Copies: See *SSAL*. 74

Australasian Quarantine Conference of Melbourne

1896. Victoria. Proceedings of the Australasian Quarantine Conference of Melbourne, 1896. Presented to both Houses . . . Robt S. Brain, Govt Printer, Melbourne.
336 × 209. Pp. 24.
Recommends uniform law and practice, compulsory notification of infectious diseases, isolation accommodation at ports, med. examination of overseas ships.
Copies: LNSW, ML, NL, SLV. 75

The Same. Queensland. 1896. Presented to both Houses. Pp. 16 (l.b.). Govt Pr, Brisbane.
Copies: LNSW, NL, OL, SLV. 76

Australasian Sanitary Conference of Sydney

1884. Legislative Assembly. New South Wales. The Australasian Sanitary Conference of Sydney, N.S.W., 1884. Report, minutes of proceedings, and appendix. . . . Sydney: Thomas Richards, Govt Printer. 1884.
331 × 208. Pp. 70. 5 plans. P. w. (title rptd).
An especially important conference of Govts of all states, to consider quarantine and health measures—an early step towards federation.
Recommends uniform quarantine procedures, compulsory vaccination, infectious disease notification, and federal quarantine stations in N. and W. Australia. Reported at length in *Austsn med. Gaz.*, 1884, 4 : 18.
Copies: BG, EF, HDN, HDV, KFR, ML, NL, SLV, US, UM. 77

Australasian Trained Nurses' Association

Report of the Council of the Australasian Trained Nurses' Association, presented at the annual meeting . . . [Text begins.]
212 × 135. Pp. 4. (1900.)
Formed 1899 as NSW Trained Nurses' Assn.
Copies: ML. 78

Australasian Trained Nurses' Association. June, 1900. We beg to inform you that at a meeting of the Council . . . [Text continues.]
212 × 135. Pp. [4] (last 3 blank).
On benevolent fund for members.
Copies: ML. 79

Australasian Trained Nurses' Association. Founded 1899. Register of members, 1900. Sydney: R. T. Kelly . . . 1900.
212 × 135. Pp. 42, [iv] (l.b.). P. w. (abbrev. title).
Copies: ML. 80

Australia As It Is

Australia as it is. New South Wales. Climates and diseases [Text begins.]
171 × 105. Pp. ii, 3–48. No title p. Bristol, 1840.
Advice to migrants. Climate and diseases, pp. 3–16.
Copies: LNSW. 81

Australia Felix

Australia Felix: happy homes for happy people. 1. Under the ground; a story of the bottle. . . . R. Mackay, Melbourne.
178 × 122. Pp. 32. ND. (c. 1874.)

The murderous activities of Burke and Hare, Edinburgh 'resurrectionists', with a moral on the evils of alcohol.

Copies: SLV. 82

Australian and Tasmanian Intercolonial Plague Conference

Australian and Tasmanian Intercolonial Plague Conference. Melbourne . . . 1900.

331 × 204. Pp. 30. Colophon—Robt S. Brain, Govt Pr, Melb.

Recommends adoption of Venice Plague Convention.

Copies: NL. 83

———

Melbourne Plague Convention, 11th April, 1900. This Conference recommends that the Venice Plague Convention be adopted by the Governments of Australia and Tasmania, subject to the following alterations and additions:- [Text continues.]

331 × 204. Pp. 2. Colophon—Robt S. Brain, Govt Pr, Melb.

Copies: NL. 84

Australian Biological Station

Australian Biological Station. Biology Department, University of Sydney, 12th December, 1890. [Text follows.]

263 × 212. Pp. 4. Title head p. 1. [Sydney, 1890.]

Letter signed W. A. Haswell, Univ. Syd., appeals for funds for re-establishment of Syd. Biological Stn, Watsons Bay, the site of which had been resumed for military purposes in 1886. See Syd. Biol. Station.

Copies: ML, US. 85

Australian Botanic Practitioner

The Australian Botanic Practitioner and Journal of the Australasian Society of Medical Botanists. Vol. 1.—No. 1. March, 1889. Sixpence. [Text begins.]

273 × 204. Pp. 8. NI.

Published each second month. Editor—John Broadbent.

Copies: SLV (v. 1–3; 1889/90–1891/2). 86

Australian Children

Australian children. How to keep them well, and how to treat them when ill. Price 6d.

NS. Advertised in *Dr. Hall's pocket health guide*, published for Health Protection League of Vic. by W. T. Pyke, Hawthorn Vic. [?1892.] 87

Australian Chivalry

Australian chivalry; or fire-side knight errantry. [Poem begins.]

288 × 206. Single leaf. Double cols. ND. [c. 1832.]. Colophon: A. Hill, Printer . . . Syd.

A satirical poem describing an attack made with a poker by a knight (Sir John Jamison MD) upon his dinner guest S——e (Savage), at his home at Regentsville. The actors are identified by Ferguson, 2 : 1507, which suggests Rev. John Dunmore Lang as author. One verse (of 12) follows:

> I shall not follow Homer's plan,
> By telling how the row began,
> Or how, in argument, folks ran–
> On pork, salt beef and cabbage;
> What odds, how first commenced the fight,
> Or who was wrong or who was right?
> Enough to know, one was a knight,
> And t'other was a S—e!

Sir John Jamison (1776–1844), Surg. RN, son of Princ. Surg. Thos Jamison, knighted by King of Sweden for services in a cholera epidemic, settled in Sydney in 1814 and engaged in pastoral pursuits. See *Aust. Enc.*; Campbell, J. F. (1932), 'Early settlement on Lower Nepean River, NSW', *JPRAHS*, 18 : 264.

Copies: ML. 88

Australian College of Dentistry

The Australian College of Dentistry, 191 Lonsdale Street, Melbourne. Syllabus. 1899–1900. Printers: J. T. Harty & Co. . . . Melbourne.

217 × 138. Pp. 16. ND. P. w. (cover title).

Copies: SLV. 89

Australian College of Dentistry and Melbourne Dental Hospital

The Australian College of Dentistry and Melbourne Dental Hospital First Annual Report. (Presented . . . 14th July, 1898.) . . . Melbourne: J. T. Harty & Co. . . . 1898.

206 × 130. Pp. 8 (last colophon only). P. w. (cover title).

College opened 1 July 1897, affiliated Melb. Dental Hosp. founded 1895. For notes—with Odontological Soc. and Dental Bd—see *A brief resume of dental education in Vic. A souvenir . . . of new Melb. Dental Hosp. and the Aust. College of*

Dentistry, Melb., 1907 (SLV).
Copies: SLV (1–5; 1897–1903). 90

See also Dental and Oral Hosp. of Vic.; Iliffe, John.

Australian Health Society

Australian Health Society. First Annual Report read at the General Meeting of the Society, held at the Town Hall, Melbourne, on 19th September, 1876. ... Melbourne: Sands and McDougall, Printers ... 1876.

212 × 140. Pp. 16 (last 3 blank). P. w. (title rptd).

Society, founded 1875, engaged in popular health education and campaigns for improved health legislation. Educational programme was conducted by public lectures, classes, pamphlets and wall-sheets.

Copies: AMAV (5–8 reps.), CC (4,8), EF (1–10), ML (1–10), NL (1–8), SLS (1–10), SLV (1–8). 91

No. 1. October 1873. (Tenth thousand.) Australian Health Society. Hints for the prevention of scarlet fever. (Adapted from a paper by the Health Committee of Glasgow). [Text begins.]

183 × 122. Pp. 4.

Also issued as:

No. 1, revised, ND., with title: *Instruction on what to do in cases of scarlet fever*. Pp. 4.........

2 ed., with title: *Prevention of scarlet fever and measles*. NS.

3 ed., 1880. Pp. 8 (1. b.). Melb.: Mason, Firth & M'Cutcheon.

Re-issued 1883. Pp. 4. Melb.: M'Carron, Bird.

Copies: EF, ML, NL, SLS, SLV, US. 92

No. 2.] [December, 1875. Australian Health Society. Melbourne. Pure air and ventilation. Melbourne: H. Cordell, Printer ...

180 × 122. Pp. 8.

2 ed., 1878. Melb.: H. Cordell. Reprinted 1879.

3 ed., ND. Sandhurst: Burrows & Co.

Another ed., 1888. Melb.: Walker, May & Co.

Copies: EF, LNSW, ML, NL, SLS, SLV. 93

No. 3.] [February 1876. Australian Health Society, Melbourne. Rules for the prevention of typhoid fever ... (Eighth thousand. Feb., 1880.) Melbourne: H. Cordell ...

206 × 138. Pp. 8.

1 ed., 1876. Reissued 1880, 1883, 1887.

Issued 1889 in combination with treatise on diphtheria; reprinted 1890.

Copies: EF, ML, NL, SLS, SLV. 94

No. 5. February 1878. Australian Health Society, Melbourne. Rules for the general management of infants, as prepared by the Obstetrical Society of London. (From the "Australian Medical Journal" of May, 1877.) Melbourne: H. Cordell ...

186 × 122. Pp. 8 (l.b.).

Another issue, Feb. 1878. 2 ed., ND, pp. 4, Sandhurst: Burrows. Revised ed., 1888.

Copies: CC, EF, LNSW, ML, NL, SLS, SLV. 95

No. 10] [August, 1880. Australian Health Society. Melbourne. ... A bad smell. [Woodcut of two workmen, holding noses, as they pass a filthy drain.] [Text begins.]

214 × 138. Pp. 4. Colophon—Walker, May & Co. ... Melb.

Another issue (7th thousand), 1883.

'What is the use of a smell? Its use is to warn people of their ill-kept houses and filthy drains, of rotting heaps and stinking cesspools; for in those places grow the poisons that give rise to dysentery, and scarlet fever, and measles, and diphtheria, and typhoid fever.' EF copy has pencil note: 'Author, Alexr. Sutherland, M.A.'

Copies: EF, ML, NL, SLS, SLV. 96

No. 12.] [March 1881. Australian Health Society, Melbourne. The infectious and contagious diseases of children. (This paper has been courteously supplied to the Society by the Central Board of Health for distribution.) Melbourne: Stillwell & Co. ... 1881.

200 × 130. Pp. 8 (l.b.). P. w. (cover title).

Early symptoms, for parents and teachers.

Also as Cent. Bd of Health pamphlet.

Copies: EF, CC, LNSW, ML, NL, SLV. 97

No. 18.] [July 1883. Australian Health Society, Melbourne. ... Soap and water. [Woodcut figure] [Text begins.]

214 × 138. Pp. 4. Colophon—Walker, May and Co. . . . Melb.

A moral tale on the benefits of bathing.

Copies: EF, ML, SLS, SLV. 98

No. 20.] [April, 1884. Australian Health Society, Melbourne. . . . The meetings for wives and daughters. Melbourne: Walker, May & Co. . . . 1884.

222 × 140. Pp. 8.

Health meetings for women at Collingwood.

Copies: EF, ML, NL, SLS, SLV. 99

Society's pamphlets of anonymous authorship are listed above.

For others, see under authors: 4. Girdlestone, T. M.; 6. Gibbons, Sydney; 6. (misnumbered) [Stawell, R. R.]; 7. Hunter, Chas. D.; 8. Jamieson, J.; 9. Rudall, J. T. and Jamieson, J.; 11. Moon, Alice Caroline; 13. Ryan, J. P.; 14. Smith, James; 15. Sutherland, A.; 16. Bartrop, Mrs. and Moon, A.C.; 17. Bromby, J.E.; 19. Blackett, C. R.; 21. Springthorpe, J. W.; 22. Cutts, W. H.; 23. Hughes, W. Kent; 24. Bage, Charles; Gresswell, D. A. (un-numbered). 100

Sanitary tracts issued by the Australian Health Society, Melbourne. First Series Nos. 1 to 13, with "Sanitary Alphabet" and Sixth Annual Report. Published by the Society . . . Melbourne. . . . 1882.

204 × 127. Pp. [ii] (title, v.b.), [ii] (contents, v.b.), pamphlets and report. At foot of 'Contents': 'Bound for presentation to Public Libraries, Mechanics' Institutes, &c. of Victoria.' Cloth.

ML has a further collection of tracts, bound in morocco for presentation to Sanitary Inst of Gt Britain.

Copies: CC, EF, ML, NL, SLV. 101

The sanitary alphabet. Australian Health Society. [Text begins.]

210 × 135. Single coloured leaf, v.b. Melb., August, 1877 (at foot).

Reissued 1881. Health rules in rhyme.

Copies: EF, ML, NL, SLV. 102

Australian Health Society Melbourne Health lectures for the people First Series George Robertson & Company Melbourne, Sydney, Adelaide, and Brisbane 1886

183 × 122. Pp. xiv, [ii], 128 (l.b.). Stiff p. w. (variation of title, advts all other sides).

Contents:

1. What is disease? by W. Simpson Flett.
2. Food and drink as carriers of disease, by James Jamieson.
3. Cheerfulness as a factor in health, by James Smith.
4. The mortality and management of infancy, by T.R.H. Willis.
5. The results of unhealthy education, by J. W. Springthorpe.
6. The food we eat and how to cook it, by C. R. Blackett.

Copies: EF, LNSW, ML, NL, SLS, SLV. 103

Australian Health Society Melbourne Health lectures for the people Second Series George Robertson & Company Melbourne and Sydney 1889

186 × 125. Pp. [14] (advts), viii, 128, [2] (advts). Stiff p. w. (variation of title, with contents; advts all other sides).

Contents:

1. Healthy homes, by J. W. Springthorpe.
2. Worry as a factor of disease, by James Smith.
3. Brain-growth and education, by F. A. Nyulasy.
4. Microbes—a result of fifty years' investigations, by A. N. Pearson.
5. Health and education, by Alexander Sutherland.
6. The causes of blindness, by J. W. Barrett.

Copies: DOS, EF, LNSW, NL, SLS, SLT, SLV. 104

Wall posters:

1. Hints on your health. Melb.: H. Cordell, 1877. Reissued 1880, 1888. (EF, ML).
2. Accidents and emergencies: what to do till the doctor comes. Melb.: Sands & McDougall, 1884. Reissued 1888. Calico copies placed in all Vic. schools and railway stations. (EF, ML).
3. Prevention of infectious diseases (J. W. Springthorpe), 1888. NS.
4. How to prevent the spread of consumption, 1894. NS.

5. The treatment of snake-bite, ND. NS. 105

The Australian Health Society, Melbourne.—Established 1875. President: D. Astley Gresswell . . . A twenty-five years record of the work and progress . . . with list of subscribers, library catalogue, Society's publications, &c. . . . Office and Library: . . . Melbourne.

208 × 138. Pp. 32. [1900] P.w. (shortened title, 2 cuts).

Copies: NL, SLV. 106

Australian Homoeopathic Progress

See *Homoeopathic Progress in Australia*.

Australian Journal of Dentistry

The Australian Journal of Dentistry. A Monthly Review of Dental Science. The only journal published solely in the interest of the Dental Profession in the Australasian Colonies. Volume 1. August, 1897, to July, 1898. Publishing Offices: Australian College of Dentistry and Melbourne Dental Hospital . . . Melbourne: J. T. Harty & Co., Printers . . .

205 × 130. Pp. 294.

Published: Vols 1–59, 1897/8–1955. Superseded in 1956 by *Aust. dental J.*

Copies: See *SSAL*. 107

Australian Medical and Surgical Infirmary

Australian Medical & Surgical Infirmary B. O. Holterman, Esq. M. P., President. Elton Boyd, Ph.D., M. D., Gy.L. . . . Physician-in-Chief. Consulting Rooms: 52 Castlereagh Street, Sydney. [Text begins.]

163 × 98. Pp. [2]. ND. [c. 1884]

'Infirmary' was founded in 1883, with its 'laboratory and manufacturing section' at 674 George St (listed elsewhere as B. O. Holtermann & Co., Import Agents), and existed in 1887. *NSW Leg. Council, Rep. Sel. Com. on . . . Practice of Med. and Surg.*, Syd., 1887, shows that N. P. Allison, clerk without med. training, acted for Boyd during absence in US. (He is noted in an advt as 'Res. Cons. Physician.') He said the Infirmary had no in-patients; treatment was given in boarding houses.

Bernard Otto Holtermann (1838–85), shown as Holterman in above, gold miner, pioneer of photography, and merchant, dealt, *inter alia*, in patent medicines and surgical appliances.

Copies: Geo. Mackaness coll. 108

See also Boyd, Elton.

Australian Medical Association

The laws, a sketch of the origin and formation, and a list of the original fellows, of the Australian Medical Association. 1859. Sydney: . . . Joseph Cook and Co. . . . 1859.

201 × 135. Pp. x (l.b.), 11–18 (l.b.). P. w. (title rptd).

Founded 1859, disbanded 1869. For history see *NSW med. Gaz.*, 1874, 4 : 175; McIntosh, A. M. (1951), *Med. J. Aust.*, 1 : 533.

Copies: ML. 109

Code of ethics recommended by the Council of the Australian Medical Association. Sydney: Printed by Joseph Cook and Co. . . . 1859.

204 × 138. Pp. [ii] (v.b.), 16 (l.b.).

Copies: LNSW, NL. 110

The Medical Directory, for New South Wales, and Queensland. 1860. Published under the auspices of the Australian Medical Association. Sydney: . . . Joseph Cook and Co. . . . 1860.

209 × 138. Pp. 28 (last 2 blank). P. w. (title rptd).

Includes names and location of 230 practitioners; historical sketch and 1st an. rep. of Aust. Med. Assn; note of Aust. Med. Library (1000 vols).

The second Aust. med. directory. For first (1842), see Baker, W.

Copies: DL, LNSW, ML, SLV. 111

The Same, 1861. Pp. 26. Includes 2nd an. rep.

Copies: SLV. 112

Australian Medical Gazette

The Australian Medical Gazette. A journal of medical science, literature, and news. For 1869. Melbourne: Clarson, Massina, & Co., Printers . . . 1870.

242 × 183. Vol. 1 : pp. [iv], 280, 8. Issued twice monthly.

3 vols, nos 1–47; 30 Jan. 1869–30 Dec. 1871. In 1870 size increased and issued monthly.

Official organ of the Med. Assn of Vic. See Gandevia, B. (1952), 'A review of Victoria's early med. journals', *Med. J. Aust.*, 2 : 184; Cumpston, J.H.L. (1914), *Med. J. Aust.*, 1 : 14 (reprinted *ibid*, 1939, 2 : 1).

Copies: See *SSAL*. 113

Australian Medical Journal (1846-1847)

Australian Medical Journal. Edited by George Brooks, Esq., Senior Colonial Surgeon, New South Wales. Vol. 1., Sydney ... August 1, 1846. No. 1. Terms of subscription ... [Text follows.]

272 × 212. Pp. 12. Printed and published by William Baker, at Hibernian Printing Office ... Syd.

The first Australian med. journal. Monthly. Vol. 1, no 1., 1 Aug. 1846—vol. 2, no 3, 1 Oct. 1847 (15 issues). See Crowther, W.E.L.H. (1947), *Med. J. Aust.*, 2: 561; Ford, E. (1972), *Med. History*, 16 : 205.

Copies: LNSW (v. 1, 1–9), ML (v. 1, 1–9, 11–12; v. 2, 1–3). 114

Australian Medical Journal (1856-1896)

The Australian Medical Journal Edited under the superintendence of the Medical Society of Victoria. Vol. 1.—1856. Melbourne: T. M. Buzzard ... Geelong: Brown.—Sydney: Waugh & Cox.—Adelaide: E. S. Wigg.—Hobert Town: Huxtable & Deakin.—Launceston: A. Duthie.

209 × 132. Pp. 308, iv (index).

Quarterly; monthly after 1864. Vols 1–23, 1856–78; vols 1–17 (New Series), 1879–95.

Established by the Med. Soc. of Vic. In 1896 amalgamated with *Intercolonial Quarterly Journal of Medicine and Surgery* to form *Intercolonial Medical Journal of Australasia*. In 1910 title of the latter reverted to *Australian Medical Journal*, and this, in 1914, was united with *Australasian Medical Gazette* to form *The Medical Journal of Australia*.

Copies: See *SSAL*. 115

Australian Medical Subscription Library

Rules and regulations of the Australian Medical Subscription Library. Established in 1846. ... Sydney: A. Mason ... 1850.

157 × 93. Pp. 8 (l.b.). Blue tinted paper. P.w. (title rptd).

Library existed 1846 to 1869. See McIntosh, A. M. (1951), *Med. J. Aust.*, 1 : 533; Gandevia, B. and Tovell, Ann. (1964), 'The first Aust. medical libraries', *Med. J. Aust.*, 2 : 314.

Copies: ML. 116

Catalogue of the Australian Medical Subscription Library, established in 1846. With rules and regulations. Sydney: A Mason ... 1855.

217 × 135. Pp. 18, [4] (l.b.). P. w. (title rptd).

Lists about 200 books and numerous journals.

NL copy inscribed: 'To Dr. Muskett from Dr. Bland, 24 Jan. 64.'

Copies: FC, LNSW, ML, NL, SLV. 117

Australian Mutual Provident Society

For the private use of the Society's medical referees. Australian Mutual Provident Society. Instructions to medical referees. To be returned to the Society on the termination of the engagement [along left margin].

178 × 110. Pp. 100 (l.b.), iv (l.b.). (1886.) Limp cloth.

Society also published: *Report on the mortality experience of the A.M.P. Society. 1849–1878*, Syd., 1882; the same, 1849–88, pt 1, Syd., 1891; the same, pt 2, Syd., 1892.

Copies: ML. 118

Australian Practitioner

The Australian Practitioner. A Quarterly Journal of Medical, Surgical, and Sanitary Science, for the Australian Colonies. [Motto] Vol. 1.—1877–78. Edited by Samuel T. Knaggs, M. D., Ch.M. ... George Robertson, Sydney, Melbourne, Adelaide, and Brisbane.

212 × 132. Pp. xii, 270. 3 pl., 1 flg chart.

Vol. 1 (nos 1–4), Oct. 1877–Oct. 1878. Quarterly.

Dr S. T. Knaggs, of Newcastle NSW, ed. and proprietor. See Cumpston, J.H.L. (1939), *Med. J. Aust.*, 2 : 1.

Copies: See *SSAL*. 119

Australian Wife's Advice Book ...

See Healthy Mothers and Sturdy Children.

Avondale Health Retreat, Cooranbong, NSW

See Caro, Edgar R.

B

Bage, Charles

No. 24. Australian Health Society . . . Consumption. A lecture . . . With a note on the tuberculin text. . . . Melbourne: J. C. Stephens . . . 1899.

217 × 143. Pp. 16. P. w. (title rptd).

For Charles Bage (1859–1930) MD Melb., Hon. Phys. Melb. Hosp., see obit., *Med. J. Aust.*, 1931, 1 : 181.

Copies: SLV. 120

Bailey, Frederick Manson

Plants reputed poisonous to stock. . . . [Text begins.]

244 × 158. Pp. 2. 1 pl. Colophon— . . . Edmund Gregory, Gov. Pr . . . Brisbane. From *Qd Agric. J.*, Nov. 1898.

On the Noogoora burr (*Xanthium strumarium*). Experiments by Dr Joseph Bancroft are mentioned.

Also published: *The weeds and suspected poisonous plants* of *Queensland*, 1906.

Copies: EF, ML. 120a

Bailey, Frederick Manson, and Gordon, Patrick Robertson

Plants reputed poisonous and injurious to stock. . . . [litho. of plant] . . . Bris.: James C. Beal, Govt Pr . . . 1887.

214 × 135. Pp. [ii] (v.b.), iv, 112 (mainly v.b.). 44 litho. pl. Cloth or paper boards.

For review see 2283a.

Copies: EF, FC, ML, NL, OL, SLS, SLV, SLW, UA, UM, UQ, US. 121

Bailliere, Ferdinand F.

F. F. Bailliere's catalogue of the British, American, foreign new & standard works . . . [List of subjects, mainly med. and scientific.] F. F. Bailliere . . . Melbourne. . . .

204 × 130. Pp. 36. ND.

Copies: ML. 122

A catalogue of English and foreign medical, chemical, & natural history works, at London prices nett. . . . Melbourne: F. Bailliere . . . London: H. Bailliere. New York: Bailliere Brothers. Paris: J. B. Bailliere. Madrid: Bailley Bailliere. 1862.

214 × 135. Pp. 4 (incomplete).

F. F. Bailliere established his Melb. medical book-selling and publishing house in 1860. He was killed in a railway accident at Jolimont Vic. in 1881 (*Bulletin*, 3 Sept. 1881).

Copies: LNSW. 123

Gratis. No. 111. A catalogue of British and foreign medical & other scientific books, at London prices nett . . . Melbourne: F. F. Bailliere . . . London, Paris, New York, and Madrid. . . . 1863.

209 × 140. Pp. 16.

Copies: EF. 124

See also Beaney, James George, No. 224.

Baker, J. R.

The people's meat supply. The case for public abattoirs. By J. R. Baker, Chairman of the Special Health Committee of the City Council. From *The Register*. [Adelaide.]

272 × 218. Pp. 8 (last 2 blank). 3 columns. ND. [?1899.]

An appeal for reform of the meat trade; unhygienic conditions; diseases transmitted by infected meat.

Copies: SLS. 125

Baker, W.

The New South Wales Medical Act; together with a list of the legally qualified medical practitioners of the Colony: which is respectfully dedicated to the President of the New South Wales Medical Board, by W. Baker, Clerk to the New South Wales Medical Board. Sydney, October 1st, 1842. Published at Baker's Hibernian Office . . .

173 × 110. Pp. [2] (woodcut frontis. with 'List of legally qualified medical practitioners of the Colony of New South Wales . . .' and arms

of RCS Edin., v.b.), 3–18, [2] (advts, v.b.). P. w. (frontis. rptd, advts on verso of front wrapper).

List of 234 persons registered in NSW (including Port Phillip and Moreton Bay) is the first Aust. medical directory.

AMAV copy, bound in morocco, was gift of Dr Thomas Black to the Med. Soc. Vic. in 1885.

Copies: AMAV. 126

Balfour, J. O.

A sketch of New South Wales. By J. O. Balfour ... for six years a settler in the Bathurst district. Printed by J. and F. C. Mathieson, Telegraph Street, E.C.

201 × 122. Pp. vi (l.b.), 120. ND. (Aug. 1845 in preface.) Cloth.

Includes non-professional notes on current diseases, pp. 5–7.

Copies: ML. 127

The Same. Lond., Smith, Elder and Co., 1845.

Copies: DL, FC, LNSW, ML, NL, SLS, UA, UQ. 128

Ballantyne, James

Homes and homesteads in the land of plenty: a handbook of Victoria as a field for emigration. By the Rev. James Ballantyne. Melbourne: Mason, Firth, and M'Cutcheon, General Printers ... 1871.

183 × 115. Pp. xvi, 184 (171–184 advts). Frontis. (flg), 26 pl. Cloth.

Includes chapters on: climate; health and longevity; influence of Vic. climate on consumptive patients; poverty in Victoria.

Copies: DL, FC, ML, NL, SLV, UM, UQ. 129

The Same. 2 ed. Melb., 1871. Pp. 224. Frontis. (flg), 26 pl.

Copies: EF, NL, SLT. 130

The Same. 2 ed. Lond.: Cassel, Petter, and Galpin; Melb: Mason, Firth, and M'Cutcheon. 1872.

Copies: LNSW, ML, SLV. 131

The Same. Supplemented ed. 2 ed., 1871 with added pp. 24, dated 1874 at end.

Copies: DL, FC, NL. 132

Ballarat and Goulburn Valley Medical Associations, Vic.

Ballarat Medical Association (established 1887) and Goulburn Valley Medical Association (established 1893). [Letter begins.]

260 × 209. Pp. [4] (l.b.). ND.

Circular letter on proposed 'Australasian Medical Association', embracing societies of all colonies, with note of meeting.

Copies: DOS. 133

Ballarat District Hospital, Vic.

The First Annual Report ... of Ballarat Hospital; with the rules and regulations ... and statistical table of cases treated during the year 1857. Ballarat: Printed at the "Times" Office ... 1858.

204 × 127. Pp. 12.

Named as Ballarat District Hosp. in 2nd rep.; now Ballarat and District Base Hosp.

See Mackay, E. A. (1936), 'Med. practice during the goldfields era', *Med. J. Aust.*, 2 : 421 (for foundation and early Ballarat practice).

Copies: Ballt Base Hosp. (1857–), KFR (1868–79), SLV (1857–71, 1885). 134

Bye-laws for the internal management of the Ballarat District Hospital. Revised and adopted February, 1871. Ballarat: Charles J. Evans, Printer ... 1871.

220 × 140. Pp. 8. P. w. (title rptd, decorative frame).

Copies: SLV. 135

Ballarat District Medical Society, Vic.

Rules of the Ballarat District Medical Society. Ballarat: Charles Boyd, Printer ... 1886.

220 × 140. Pp. 8 (l.b.). Amended in ink.

Laid down in minute book of Soc. (7 July 1887–25 Jan. 1900) in possession of D. O'Sullivan, Ballarat. Also includes circular letters to members. Soc. is at times referred to as Ballarat Med. Assn.

Foundation of an earlier Medico-Chirurgical Soc. was announced in *Ballarat Times*, 28 Oct. 1854.

Copies: DOS. 136

The Second Annual Report of the Ballarat District Medical Society, submitted at the meeting held at Craig's Hotel ... 31st July, 1896.

275 × 204. Single leaf, v.b. NI.

Copies: DOS (2–4, 1896–8). 137

Ballarat Medical Association, Vic.

Ballarat Medical Association ... Ballarat, 21st October, 1893. Dear Sir, A movement has been started ... in this District and in the Goulburn Valley and North Eastern District, to hold a Conference ... [on] the desirability of forming an "Australasian Medical Association". ... [Letter continues.]

265 × 204. Single leaf, v.b. NI.

Meeting to be held at Pt Phillip Club Hotel, Melb., on 8 Nov. 1893. Signed: Robert Scott, Hon. Soc. See No 133.

Copies: DOS. 138

Ballarat Psychological Association, Vic.

Report of the Ballarat Psychological Association; referring to a series of seances held with Mr. Jesse Shepard, the celebrated musical and physical medium. By R. Lorimer, Hon. Secretary ...

212 × 135. Pp. 20. Title from head p. 1. ND. [1879.] Colophon—James Curtis, Printer ... Ballarat.

Copies: ML. 139

Balls-Headley, Walter

See Headley, Walter Balls—

Bancroft, Joseph

The Queensland Philosophical Society. (From the *Queensland Guardian*, November 24, 1866.) Poisonous animals. [Text begins.]

217 × 138. Pp. 2. Double cols. Colophon— ... 'Guardian Office', Brisbane.

On the common tick and its effects on animals.

Copies: FC. 140

Queensland Philosophical Society. (From the *Queensland Daily Guardian*, February 21, 1867.) Poisonous animals, No. 2. Snakes. [Text begins.]

198 × 132. Pp. 2. Single leaf. Colophon— ... 'Guardian Office', Bris.

Snake-bites: mechanism and treatment.

Copies: Aust. Museum, Syd. 141

The Queensland Philosophical Society. (From the *Queensland Daily Guardian*, June 29, 1867.) [Text begins.]

217 × 138. Pp. 2. Double cols. Colophon— ... 'Guardian Office', Brisbane.

On 'sheep scab', describing parasite and eradication.

Copies: FC. 142

Queensland Philosophical Society. The pituri poison. A paper read ... 28th March, 1872:- [Text begins.]

217 × 138. Pp. 4 (last 2 blank). Double cols. Colophon— ... Courier Office ... Bris.

Initial report of Bancroft's pharmacological investigation of pituri, an aboriginal plant stimulant from Cooper's Creek. Animal experiments are described. Reprinted in *Aust. med. J.*, Nov. 1876, and author's 'Pituri and Duboisia.'

Copies: EF, FC. 143

Queensland. Pituri and Duboisia. Paper read before the Queensland Philosophical Society ... Brisbane: ... James C. Beal, Govt Printer ... 1877.

204 × 132. Pp. 14. 3 photographs, 1 litho. pl.

Identifies pituri, the leaves chewed as a stimulant by certain aboriginal tribes, with the genus *Duboisia*, and indicates pharmacological action, with experimental and botanical notes.

Copies: ML, NL, OL, SLS, UA, US. 144

1877. Queensland. Report on sickness amongst employees, Dalby and Roma Line. Presented to both Houses ... To the ... Colonial Secretary. [Text begins.]

320 × 209. Pp. 2. Colophon—James C. Beal, Govt Pr, Bris. Signed: Joseph Bancroft, M.D., at foot.

On inspection (30 May–4 June) of workers engaged in railway construction between Dalby and Roma, and their families, general malarial infection was found. Recommends distribution of quinine, establishment of 30 bed hospital at Dalby, and conveyance of workers to healthy camp sites for sleeping. Appends text of suggested leaflet on treatment.

Copies: LNSW, ML, NL, OL, SLV. 145

Further remarks on the Pituri group of plants ... Brisbane, 10th October, 1878. Read before the Queensland Philosophical Society. [Text begins.]

214 × 132. Pp. 4 (l.b.). Title at head of p.l. 1 litho. pl., 1 photograph. Colophon— . . . James C. Beal, Govt Pr. . . .

Copies: NL. 146

Pituri and tobacco. (Read before the Queensland Philosophical Society . . . September 4th, 1879.) [Text begins.]

218 × 133. Pp. 16. 2 litho. pl. Colophon— . . . James C. Beal, Govt Pr . . . Bris.

Futher information on properties, native use, and botanical characters of pituri. The mydriatic effects of the alkaloid had established its ophthalmological use in Europe. It is regarded as identical with nicotine, and properties and use compared with those of tobacco.

See also forward note, No. 1421.

Copies: ML, NL, UA. 147

Diseases of animals and plants that interfere with colonial progress. . . . [Text begins.]

209 × 135. Pp. 14. ND. From *Divinity Hall Record*, Dec. 1879, Brisbane.

Copies: UA, UM. 148

Lecture on the miscroscope in our gardens. . . . [Text begins.]

209 × 135. Pp. 8. ND. (1879.). NI. From *Divinity Hall Record*, Dec. 1879, Brisbane.

Copies: UM. 149

The newly introduced poisonous burr, Xanthium Strumarium. (Read before the Queensland Philosophical Society, 22nd January, 1880 . . . [Text begins.]

8vo. Pp. 4 (l.b.). 1 pl. Colophon— . . . James C. Beal, Govt. Pr . . . Bris.

Copies: Parlt Library of Qd. 150

Papers on pituri and Duboisia.

210 × 140. Pp. 32 (l.b.). 3 litho. pl. ND. (c. 1881.) Colophon—Warwick & Sapsford . . . Bris. P. w. (cover title).

Contains three Bancroft papers (Nos 144, 146–7), and Liversidge, A. (No 1169).

Copies: UA. 151

On the mode of birth of the kangaroo, communicated by the Hon. L. Hope, with remarks on the Echidna and Platypus. By J. Bancroft, M. D. President of the Queensland Philosophical Society. (Read 22nd June, 1882.) [Text begins.]

204 × 127. Pp. 4. Colophon—James C. Beal, Govt Pr . . . Bris.

Copies: ML. 151a

Experiments with Indian wheats in Queensland. By J. Bancroft, M. D., President.

215 × 125. Pp. 8 (l.b.). Read 12 Dec., 1884. Repr. *Proc. Roy. Soc. Qd*, vol 1, pt 4.

Copies: SLS. 151b

Queensland Philosophical Society. Coccus Insects. The following paper was read . . . August 1869:— [Text begins.]

217 × 138. Pp. 4 (l.b.). Double cols. Colophon— . . . Courier Office . . . Bris.

Copies: FC. 151c

Colonial and Indian Exhibition, 1886. Contribution to pharmacy from Queensland . . . London: William Clowes and Sons, Limited. . . . 1886.

214 × 137. Pp. ii (title, v.b.), 16 (l.b.). 1 map. P. w. (cover title).

Includes notes on native species investigated by author, including *Alstonia constricta* (bitter bark) as tonic, *Neodaphne obtusifolia* as astringent for dysentery and diarrhoea, *Duboisia myoporoides* as mydriatic, and *D. hopwoodii* (pituri).

Copies: ML, SLV, SLW. 152

The Same. Pp. 16 (l.b.). Colophon—Warwick & Sapsford . . . Bris. 1886.

Copies: NL, SLS, SLV, SLW, UA. 153

On filaria . . . [Text begins.]

242 × 153. Pp. 8 (last 2 blank). Colophon—Melb.: Stillwell and Co., P. w. Repr. *Trans Intercol Med. Cong. Austsia*, 1889 : 49.

Describes author's discovery of the parent *Filaria bancrofti* at Brisbane in Dec. 1876, with clinical and pathological features of infestation in Brisbane.

Specimens were sent to Cobbold in London, with notes that appeared in *Lancet*, 1877, 2 : 70;

Cobbold's description was published in *Lancet*, 1877, 2 : 495; Bancroft's account in *Trans Path. Soc. Lond.*, 1878, 29 : 407.

Copies: EF, US. 154

Australian pemmican concentrated beef, prepared by Dr. J. Bancroft, Brisbane . . . July, 1891 . . . Brisbane : Warwick & Sapsford . . . 1891.

214 × 138. Pp. 14. 1 pl., 2 figs. P. w. (title rptd, with cut).

Advertises Bancroft's venture in meat preserving, by a process invented by him, at works established at Deception Bay Qd. For method, see No 55.

For Joseph Bancroft (1836–1894) MD St And., MRCS, of Brisbane, see obit., *Austsn med. Gaz.*, 1894, 13 : 250; also Cleland, J. B. (1950), *Med. J. Aust.*, 1 : 549; Ford, E. (1961), 'The life and influence of J. B.', *Med. J. Aust.*, 1 : 153 (with bibliog.).

Copies: ML, NL. 155

Bancroft, Thomas Lane

Preliminary notes on some new poisonous plants discovered on the Johnstone River, North Queensland. . . . (Read before the Royal Society of N.S.W., 2 June, 1886.) [Text begins.]

212 × 134. Pp. 4 (l.b.). P. w. (title rptd).

For T. L. Bancroft (1860–1933) MB, ChM Edin., FLS, who made important contributions on Aust. flora and fauna, see obit., *Med. J. Aust.*, 1934, 1 : 512; also Ford, E. (1961), *Med. J. Aust.*, 1 : 160.

Copies: EF. 156

Notes on the Birdsville Horse Disease: by Thos. J. Bancroft. Adelaide: Scrymgour & Sons, Printers. 1892.

182 × 122. Pp. 10, [ii] (colophon, v.b.). Stiff p. w. (title rptd).

Investigation of lethal horse disease in SA.

UQ copy has name amended in ink to Thos. L. Bancroft.

Copies: UQ. 157

[Banks, Samuel Hawker]

Vice and its victims in Sydney. The cause and cure. By a pupil of the late Prof. John Woolley, D.C.L., Principal of Sydney University. . . . Sydney: Published, for the proprietor, at Edwin H. Becke's . . . 1873.

214 × 136. Pp. iv, [iv] (ii blank), 78 (l.b.), [2] (advts).

Drunkenness, poverty, prostitution and crime, and their abatement. Ascribed by *Austsn Bibliog.*, Syd., 1893, to Samuel Hawker Banks.

Copies: FC, LNSW, ML. 158

Banting, William

Corpulence. A letter addressed to the public . . . Melbourne: W. B. Stephens . . . 1864.

183 × 120. Pp. 24. P. w. (title rptd). Reprint of 3 Eng. ed.

Four English eds appeared in 1864.

A dietetic regime reducing carbohydrate, by author, a layman, for the control of obesity. His system is discussed by Thomas, D. J. (1868, No 2171); and Southwood, A. R. (1960), 'Correct weight: the return to Bantingism', *Med. J. Aust.*, 2 : 525.

Method is reprinted (1864) by L. L. Smith (No 1935), who notes its wide adoption and use under the cant term 'Doing the Banting.' 'Banting' has since gained accepted usage, with the meaning 'treatment of obesity by abstinence from sugar, starch and fat' (*Concise Oxford Dict.*), and has the derivative verb 'to bant.'

Copies: FC, ML, NL, SLS, SLV. 159

Banyer, R. B.

Animal magnetism, or mesmerism: being a reply to the lecture delivered by the Rev. W. T. Carter. By R. B. Banyer. Kapunda: Scandrett & Elliott, Printers . . . 1884.

8vo. Pp. 14, [4] (advts, yellow paper). P. w. (title rptd).

Copies: SLS. 160

Barkas, William James

On the Genus Ctenodus, a fish found in the true coal measures of Great Britain. . . . (Read before the Royal Society of N.S.W., 6 September, 1876.) [Text begins.]

204 × 132. Pp. 26 (l.b.). 5 litho. pl. Colophon—Syd.: Charles Potter, Acting Govt Pr—1877.

A bound collection of author's articles in ML includes items on tooth growth, microscopic structure of fossil teeth, and teeth and bones of fossil fish.

W. J. Barkas LRCP, MRCS (1868) practised at Bombala and Paddington NSW.

Copies: ML. 161

Barker, Edward

A case of extroversion of the bladder in a female

treated by operation. ... From Volume LIII of the "Medical-Chirurgical Transactions ..." London: Printed by J. E. Adlard ... 1870.

204 × 132. Pp. [ii] (v.b.), 14. 1 litho. pl.

For Edward Barker (1818–85) MD, FRCS, Hon. Surg. Melb. Hosp., first Lecturer in Surg. Melb. Univ., see obits, *Austsn med. Gaz.*, 4 : 256 and *Aust. med. J.*, 1885, ns 7 : 319; for his first essay on med. history published in Australia, *Aust. med. J.*, 1864, 9 : 152 and 180.

Copies: SLV. 162

Barker, Walter Herbert

Our lunatic asylum. ... Melbourne: Stillwell and Co. ... 1888.

173 × 122. Pp. 16 (l.b.).

Opinions on asylum accommodation.

For W. H. Barker (1856–1924) MRCS, LRCP, Med. Supt of Ararat and later Ballarat Hosp. for Insane, see obit., *Med. J. Aust.*, 1924, 2 : 538. He published: *Mental diseases, a manual for students*, Lond., 1902.

Copies: EF. 163

Barnard, C. E., and Mault, A.

(No. 21.) 1896. ... Parliament of Tasmania. Diphtheria in Hobart and neighbourhood: report by C. E. Barnard, M. D., and A. Mault, with appendices. Presented to both Houses ...

344 × 217. Pp. 10. 1 map. Colophon—William Grahame, Govt Pr. ...

On suspected milk-borne epidemic of 36 cases with 7 deaths.

C. E. Barnard MD Aberd., MRCS, of Hobart, was Port HO, Supt Vaccination, Memb. Cent. Bd Health. See also No 2502.

Copies: BG, ML, NL, SLT, SLV. 164

Barnett, Henry Calvert

Suggestions respecting sanitary improvement in Western Australia ... Perth: R. Pether, Govt Printer, 1876.

204 × 134. Pp. 20. P. w. (title rptd).

H. C. Barnett (1831–97) MRCS, LRCP, lived in China for some years and edited a newspaper at Foochow in 1858. He arrived in WA in 1868 and became GMO at York. From 1872 until his death, he was Col Surg. and Med. Supt of Lunatic Asylum at Fremantle.

Copies: ML, NL. 165

Barraden, R. H.

Lesson No. 1. Hypnotism easily learned. Prof. R. H. Barraden's complete course of 20 illustrated lessions in hypnotism. [Text begins.]

280 × 204. 20 loose leaves, v.b. Figs. ND. (?1900). NI.

Copies: ML. 166

A key to the mysteries of hypnotism. The marvel of the century Prof. R. H. Barraden ... Sydney ... The World's greatest hypnotist. ... 4th edition.

204 × 140. Pp. 32, 7 coloured leaves inserted, un-numbered. ND. (?1900.) P. w. (title rptd with fig. and decorations).

Advt for course of instruction.

Copies: ML. 167

Barrett, Sir James William

Typhoid fever in Victoria ... Section 1 George Robertson Melbourne ... 1883

212 × 140. Pp. 44. 11 graphs (2 flg). P. w. (title rptd.).

A mainly statistical study. Includes: continued fevers, relationship of diarrhoeal affections, seasonal prevalence, climatic influence, mortality, causation. Further parts projected, NS. Rev., *Aust. med. J.*, 1883, ns 5 : 457.

Copies: NL, SLV, UM. 168

Victoria and Tasmania as resorts for consumptives and persons afflicted with lung disease. ... London: ... Harrison and Sons ... 1884.

178 × 107. Pp. 8 (last colophon only). 1 flg map. P. w. (cover title).

Copies: NL. 169

Abstracts from papers on hydatid diseases, Victoria and Tasmania as health resorts, the cause of the first heart sound, Leirnur's system of sewage, antiseptic treatment, and neuro-fibromata. ... London: Wyman & Sons ... 1884.

209 × 138. Pp. 40. 1 flg map.

Copies: NL, UM. 170

The future of the Melbourne University. A lecture ... at the annual meeting of the Medical Students' Society ... [Text begins.]

209 × 127. Pp. 16 (l.b.). ND. Colophon—Austral Co., Printers ... Melb.

Copies: UM. 171

List of original communications. [Text begins.]

201 × 130. 8 leaves, printed on recto of 1–7, versos and last blank. ND. (c. 1898.) NI. P. w.
19 publications listed, with English testimonials.
Copies: EF. 172

———

The physical basis of conduct [Text begins.]
209 × 138. Pp. 8 (l.b.). From *Hermes*, 1898. Address to the Syd. Univ. Med. Soc.
For Sir James Barrett (1862–1945) MD, MS, FRCS, FRACS, a leading figure in the medical, educational and public life of Melbourne, see his *Eighty eventful years*, Melb., 1945; *Med. J. Aust.*, 1945; 2 : 58; *Brit. med. J.*, 1945, 1 : 572.
Later publications include: *Lectures on physiology of the special senses*, 2 vols, Melb., 1910; another ed., 1930; *The Aust. Army Medical Corps in Egypt* (with P. E. Deane), Lond., 1918; *The twin ideals, an educated Commonwealth*, 2 vols, Lond., 1918; *A vision of the possible, what the R.A.M.C. might become*, Lond., 1919; *The war work of the Y.M.C.A. in Egypt*, Lond., 1919.
Copies: UM. 173

———

See also Australian Health Society, No 104 (6).

——— **and Lang, W.**

The use of homatropine as a substitute for atropine in estimating lesions of refraction of the eye. By W. Lang . . . and James W. Barrett . . . London: . . . Harrison and Sons . . . 1885.
183 × 112. Pp. 12. P. w. (title rptd).
Copies: NL, UM. 174

———

The refractive character of the eyes of mammalia, and the action of myotics on the accommodation. By W. Lang, F.R.C.S., Ophthalmic Surgeon to the Middlesex Hospital; and James W. Barret, M. B. . . . London: . . . Harrison and Sons . . . 1886.
212 × 140. Pp. 86 (l.b.). 2 flg charts. P. w. (cover title). Reprint from *Roy. Lond. Ophth. Hosp. Rep.*
Copies: UM. 175

———

On convergent strabismus. By W. Lang . . . Ophthalmic Surgeon to the Middlesex Hospital; and James W. Barrett . . . University of Melbourne. [Text begins.]
204 × 135. Pp. 28. ND. Colophon—Harrison & Sons, St Martin's Lane . . .
Copies: UM. 176

Bartlett, Thomas

New Holland: its colonization, productions & resources, with observations on the relations subsisting with Great Britain. By Thomas Bartlett Assistant-Surgeon 51st Light Infantry. . . . London: Longman, Brown, Green, and Longmans . . . 1843.
201 × 125. Pp. x, 312. Cloth.
Discusses disease and effect of climate in Australia (pp. 190–200).
Copies: DL, FC, LNSW, ML, NL, SLS, SLV, SLW, UA, UM, US. 177

Barton, E. A.

The colonist's medical handbook with directions for treatment of fractures, dislocation and the principal medical and surgical diseases. . . . Second Edition. Cassell & Company, Limited: London, Paris & Melbourne. 1891. . . .
165 × 110. Pp. xii (l.b.), 13–160 (last two blank), [16] (book advts). 23 figs. Cloth.
'Written . . . for the use of Colonists and Squatters who are entirely out of reach of medical assistance. There are only three drugs mentioned . . .—opium, quinine and Epsom Salts—and the appliances for the treatment of emergencies are only those likely to be found in any Squatter's hut.' Preface from Kensington, London.
Copies: ML. 178

Barton, Frederick J.

Queensland Philosophical Society. Asphyxia. A paper read . . . July, 1859 . . . [Text begins.]
214 × 135. Pp. 4. Double cols. Colophon—G. Wright, 'Guardian Office', Brisbane.
Includes section on drowning and resuscitation.
Copies: FC. 179

———

Lecture on climate. (From the Moreton Bay Courier, August 30, 1860.) [Text begins.]
217 × 138. Pp. 8. Double cols. Qd Phil. Soc. lecture.
'The diseases occurring in Queensland from atmospheric causes . . . are, ague, continued fever, chronic rheumatism, and influenza; the first two being caused by the exhalation of vegetable miasm, the next by undue exposure to wet and night air, the last by some unknown

state of the atmosphere, producing at first ordinary colds which soon become infectious and epidemic.'

F. J. Barton (d. 1864) settled in Brisbane prior to 1845 and in 1851 became Surg. Supt Brisbane Hosp., retaining this post to his death. See E. S. Jackson (1923), 'Historical notes ... of Bris. Hosp.', *Med. J. Aust.*, 1 : 281.

Copies: FC. 180

Barton, J.

Forms and features as indicative of character, being an introduction to the study of physiognomy ... Melbourne: ... Upham, Pater & Knapton ... 1885.

183 × 127. Pp. 50 (l.b.). P. w. (title rptd).

Copies: EF. 181

Bartrop, Mrs, and Moon, Alice Caroline

No. 16. June, 1882. Australian Health Society ... "Kitchen physic". ... Melbourne: M'Carron, Bird & Company ... 1882.

214 × 138. Pp. 8.

Invalid diet.

Copies: EF, ML, SLS, SLV. 182

Bassett, William Frederick

Energy; or, thoughts on inductive reasoning in its bearing on natural religion. Bathurst: Glyndwr Whalan, Printer ... 1886.

220 × 138. Pp. 18 (l.b.). P. w. (title rptd).

For W. F. Bassett (1824–1910) MRCS, Asst Col Surg. Parramatta and Hon. MO Bathurst Hosp., see obit., *Austsn med. Gaz.*, 1910, 29 : 228.

Copies: ML. 183

Bathurst District Hospital, NSW

The report of the Bathurst District Hospital, for the fifteen months ending 31st December, 1844. Sydney: Printed by Kemp and Fairfax ... 1845.

217 × 138. Pp. 16. P. w. (title rptd; erratum on verso of front wrapper).

Copies: DL (1844), LNSW (1868). 184

Baume & Kreitmayer's Grand Anatomical Museum

Catalogue of Messrs. Baume & Kreitmayer's Grand Anatomical Museum. ... Lectures for gentlemen by a medical gentleman, and for ladies by Mrs. Kreitmayer. Only adults admitted. Melbourne: ... Shaw, Harnett & Co ... 1861.

206 × 130. Pp. iv, 20. Cover title.

A similar catalogue, in which proprietors are shown as Kreitmayer and Wiseheart, also appeared in Melb., 1861 (No 1112).

Copies: SLV. 185

Bay View Private Hospital for Mental Diseases, Sydney

Bay View House and surroundings. [5 litho. views.] John Sands.

252 × 186. [4]. [c. 1888.]

The first private asylum in NSW, situated at Cook's River (Tempe), was opened in 1865 by G. A. Tucker PhD, proprietor till 1886.

For instn, see Dawson, W. S. (1965), *Annals of psychiatry in NSW. 1850–1900*, Syd., typescript (ML, RACP); also *Austsn med. Gaz.*, 1886, 5 : 158; Oliver, T. J. (1871), *NSW med. Gaz.*, 2 : 6.

Copies: HDN. 186

———

1894–5. New South Wales. Report of the Royal Commission appointed to inquire into the conduct and management of the licensed house for insane at Cook's River, near Sydney, known as "Bayview House", and ... the treatment of certain patients ... Appointed 18th October, 1894. [Royal Arms] ... Sydney: Charles Potter, Govt Printer ... 1895.

331 × 209. Pp. 106 (l.b.), 378. 1 coloured flg map, 3 plans. P. w. (title rptd).

Copies: LNSW, ML, NL, SLV. 187

———

See also Tucker, George Alfred.

[Bayer, Frederick Charles]

In memorium Frederick Charles Bayer, M. D. The following pages have been printed by his relatives with the hope that they may be valued and esteemed by those who knew his worth.

163 × 102. Pp. 28. Adel.: Sands & McDougall Limited, Printers ... ND. (1867.) Black p. w. (title in gold).

Dr. Bayer settled in Adel. in 1847, and died 'after twenty years incessant toil', aged 52.

Copies: NL. 188

Bayes, T.

On the diseases of women. By Dr. Bayes, M. D., &c., &c., late Surgeon to the West London Dispensary. Cloth. Price 10s 6d.

NS. Advertised in *Syd. Morning Herald*, 24 and 29 Sep. 1847, by author, late of London, who announces arrival and commencement of practice in Sydney.

Also noted as 'sold by all booksellers, and at author's residence, 124 Prince-street, Sydney': *On chronic and local diseases of the mucous passages, including directions for the treatment of hemorrhoids, fistulae, strictures &c.*, 8vo.; *On the anatomy of the prostate, bladder, and urethra, obstructions and diseases which they are subject to*, 8vo. Further titles are listed in a frequently repeated advt (*Syd. Morning Herald*, 6 Oct. 1847, p. 1): *On consumption; On diseases of the rectum and urinary organs*, 8vo., price 5s., *On venereal diseases*, 8vo., cloth. Footnote to this advt (14 Oct. 1847) states that Dr Bayes will visit Singapore and Calcutta.

189

Bayldon, John

Obituary. Dr. John Bayldon. (From the "Australian Medical Journal", April, 1872.) [Text begins.]

212 × 135. Pp. 4 (l.b.). Colophon—Stillwell and Knight . . . Melb. Author: J. E. Neild.

Copies: UM. 190

Beaney, James George

Original contributions to the practice of conservative surgery; being a selection from the surgical cases occurring in the practice of James G. Beaney, M.R.C.S.E. . . . Melbourne: George Robertson, 85 & 87 Collins Street East; and . . . London. 1859.

218 × 140. Pp. xx (iv, viii blank), 168. Cloth.

The first surgery book published in Australia. Chapters: disease of hip joint: chronic hydrarthrosis; obstruction of bowels, with tympanites; obstructive dysmenorrhoea; neuralgia of epididymis; varicocele; abscess of bone; traumatic stricture of urethra; exsections of maxillary bones; anaesthesia.

Notice in *The generative system* (1872) states that 2 ed. was preparing for publication, and includes list of contents which varies from that of 1 ed. NS.

See Russell, K. F. (1938), 'The first book on surgery to be published in Vic.', *Aust. NZJ. Surg.*, 8 : 17.

Copies: EF, KFR, NL, SLV, RACS. 191

Contributions to practical surgery, pathological, therapeutic, and operative. . . . Melbourne: Wilson and Mackinnon . . . 1861.

202 × 133. Pp. viii (l.b.), 48 (l.b.). Frontis., 1 pl. Limp cloth.

Though states to be the first of a series on practical surgery, Part 1 only appeared. Contains: (i) A new method of performing excision of the knee-joint, (ii) Stricture of urethra.

Copies: EF, ML, NL, SLV, RACS. 192

Dr. Beaney's vindication: with reflections on the inquest held upon the body of Mary Lewis. [Quotation] Melbourne: W. L. Ambler . . . 1866.

202 × 130. Pp. 44 (l.b.). Leaf following title bears: A Vindication by James George Beaney.

In 1866 Beaney was charged with the murder of a young woman by procuring abortion. In a first trial the jury disagreed; in a second the verdict was 'Not Guilty.' This work attacks Crown medical witnesses.

Leading article from *Lancet*, 29 Sep. 1866 is quoted: '. . . the trial . . . has been less honourable to the medical than the legal profession. In fact, so conflicting was the medical evidence, so carelessly had the post mortem . . . been performed—nay, so obvious was the animus of certain members of the medical profession . . . that nothing short of the highest legal ability could have saved an innocent man from the gallows . . .'

For inquest and trials, see Reeves, C. E., *Queen v Beaney*; for autopsy evidence: Thomas, David John, No 2175.

Copies: LNSW. 193

The Same. Pp. [4] (2, 4 blank), 5–32. Melb., W. B. Stephens, 1866.

Copies: AMAV, SLV. 194

The Same. 2 ed. Pp. 52. Melb., R. N. Henningham, 1870.

Copies: ML, NL, OL, SLV. 195

Syphilis. Its nature & diffusion popularly considered. . . . With fifteen coloured plates. Melbourne George Robertson . . . 1869.

218 × 138. Pp. [xvi] (ii, iv blank), 304. 15 coloured litho. pl. Cloth.

Referred to as a plagiarism by Reeves, C. E. (1873), *Heart diseases in Australia*, p. xv: 'There has been for some time a paraphrase of Hempel's translations of Jahr's work on syphilis ... very freely scattered about Melbourne. The titles of the author, formed into a pyramid of the size of that of Cheops, form the most amusing illustrations of charlatanic fanfaronade in the English language.' Reviewed, in similar terms, in *Melb. med. Record*, 15 May 1875.

Copies: AMAV, BG, CC, EF, KFR, LNSW, NL, SLV, UA, US. 196

Vaccination and its dangers. ... With advice and instruction to parents as to how and when to vaccinate. Melbourne: ... R. N. Henningham ... 1870.

183 × 120. Pp. 14, [ii] (book notice).

Condemns arm to arm vaccination; advocates animal lymph.

Copies: DOS, LNSW, ML, NL, SLV. 197

Spermatorrhoea in its physiological, medical, and legal aspects. ... Melbourne: Walker, May & Co. ... 1870.

221 × 141. Pp. xii, 150. Cloth.

Deplores lack of interest in this condition, and its exploitation by quacks: 'The profession must consider themselves ... responsible for the thousands of wretched sufferers who have drifted into imbecility and the mad-house, and even into the grave, from self-pollution ....'

Copies: BG, CC, DOS, ML, NL, SLS, UA. 198

The Same. 2 ed., 1880. Pp. xvi, 132 (l.b.). Melb., Mason, Firth & McCutcheon.

Copies: BG, CC, EF, KFR, ML, SLV. 199

Constitutional syphilis: being a practical illustration of the disease in its secondary and tertiary phases. ... With twenty coloured plates. Melbourne: F. F. Bailliere ... 1872.

211 × 139. Pp. xii (l.b.), [ii] (v.b.), 470, [2] (book notices). 20 coloured litho. pl. Cloth.

Copies: EF, ML, RACS, UA. 200

The Same. 1872. Pp. xii (l.b.), [iv] (2 blanks), 470, [2]. 20 pl. List of illustrations after contents.

Copies: AMAV, BG, CC, EF, LNSW, NL, SLV. 201

The Same. 3 ed., 1878. Pp. x, [ii] (v.b.), 484. 12 col. pl. Melb., F. F. Bailliere.

Copies: AMAV. 202

The Same. 3 ed., 1880. Melb., McCarron, Bird and Co.

Copies: CC. 203

The Same. 3 ed., 1883. Melb., McCarron, Bird and Co.

Copies: EF. 204

The generative system and its functions in health and disease. ... Melbourne: F. F. Bailliere ... 1872.

210 × 136. Pp. xvi (l.b.), 326, [2] (notice of author's books). Yellow leaf (book notice) inserted. Cloth.

Forerunner in Aust. of popular books on sex, this comprehensive work was widely read, and criticised as pornography. Contraception is commended and introduced without detail.

4 ed. contains 43 pp. of 'Opinions of the press', as 'irrefutable evidence in disproof of the carping criticisms of the envious and the jealous.'

Copies: AMAV, EF, RACP, SLV. 205

The Same. 2 ed., 1875. Pp. xvi, 394, [ii]. Melb.: F. F. Bailliere.

Copies: FF, ML, US. 206

The Same. 3 ed., 1877. With additional chap. on 'Stricture of urethra.' 2 coloured litho. pl. Melb.: F. F. Bailliere.

Copies: AMAV, BG, FF, ML. 207

The Same. 3 ed., 1880. Pp. xvi, 411. Melb.: McCarron, Bird.

Copies: CC. 208

The Same. 4 ed., 1883. Pp. xvi, 480. Syd. & Melb.: Geo. Robertson.

Copies: AMAV, BG, CC, DOS, EF, KFR, ML, RACP, RACS, SLV. 209

[Monogram] Opinions of the press. Constitutional syphilis being a practical illustration of the disease in secondary and tertiary phases . . . [Text begins.]

214 × 142. Pp. 14. ND. [1873.] Purple and gold ornamented borders to each page. Part title and marginal titles in red.

Copies: ML (pp. 3–6 lacking). 210

Children: their treatment in health and disease. . . . Part 1.—Infancy. Melbourne: F. F. Bailliere . . . 1873.

153 × 105. Pp. xvi (ii, l.b.), 253, [3] (book notices). Stiff p. w. (title rptd), or cloth.

Chapters: gestation; lactation; wet nursing; weaning; management when sick; diseases of mouth, eyes, ears, etc.; dentition; brain diseases and convulsions.

Part 11—Childhood, was to follow. No evidence of issue.

Copies: EF, Dr L.J.T. Murphy, Melb., SLT. 211

Lithotomy: its successes and its dangers. Being a verbatim report, from shorthand notes, of an inquest held before the City Coroner. With a preface and commentary by an M.R.C.S.E. Melbourne: F. F. Bailliere . . . 1876.

235 × 154. Pp. xxviii, 132. Pp. iii-x lacking in all copies seen. Usually replaced by un-numbered leaf with 'Sir Astley Cooper . . . on the difficulties of lithotomy', v.b. Litho. frontis. Cloth.

'Report of an inquest, in which Beaney was accused by some fellow practitioners of killing a patient during lithotomy. He was discharged by the coroner with a clean sheet, and this book was his retort . . . he exposes the whole acrimonious and at times libellous discussion.' (Russell, K. F. (1938), *Aust. NZ J. Surg.*, 8 : 17.)

In *The medical embassy*, Bailliere states that of 5,000 copies issued, all were distributed *gratis*. Most copies bear 'With the Publisher's compliments' in rubber stamp.

Copies: AMAV, BG, CC, DOS, EF, FF, KFR, ML, NL, SLV, RACP, RACS, UA, UQ. 212

Doctors differ. A lecture delivered at the Melbourne Athenaeum . . . Melbourne: F. F. Bailliere . . . 1876. . . .

214 × 136. Pp. 24.

Beaney attacks his opponents at the time of criticism associated with incidents noted in *Lithotomy*. Answered in a counterblast: 'Mr. Beaney's doings', *Aust. med. J.*, 1876, 21 : 42.

Copies: DL, DOS, EF, FC, LNSW, ML, NL, SLV. 213

1876. Victoria (1875–6). Robert Berth. Return to an Order of the Legislative Assembly, dated 28th March 1876, for . . . correspondence relating to . . . exhumation of the body of Robert Berth, who died in the Melbourne Hospital . . . after an operation had been performed by one of the honorary surgeons, Mr. J. G. Beaney.

346 × 217. Pp. 2. Colophon—George Skinner, Acting Govt Pr, Melb.

Refers to case described in *Lithotomy*.

Copies: AMAV, LNSW, ML, NL, SLV. 214

The "Argus" & Mr. J. G. Beaney, F.R.C.S.E. [Text begins.]

212 × 129. Single leaf, v.b. NI. (1876.)

'*The Argus* having brought certain accusations, and . . . called upon the persons accused for an explanation, now declines to print that explanation . . .' Leaflet contains two rejected letters.

Copies: SLV. 215

The history and progress of surgery: an address, delivered to the medical students of the Melbourne Hospital, on the occasion of the presentation of the prizes in the class of operative surgery . . . Melbourne: F. F. Bailliere . . . 1877.

198 × 168. Pp. 34. Publisher's slip inserted. Cloth.

The first separate work on med. history published in Australia (Gandevia). For the first Aust. publication on the subject, a journal contribution by Ed. Barker, 1866, see note to No 162.

Copies: CC, EF, FC, LNSW, ML, NL, RACS, SLV, SLW, UA. 216

Surgical diagnosis: a lecture, delivered to the

medical students of the Melbourne Hospital . . . 1877. . . . Melbourne: F. F. Bailliere . . . 1877.

195 × 170. Pp. 32 (2, 4 blank). Paper boards.

Delivered in operating theatre of Melb. Hosp., at the presentation of medals to Beaney's students for proficiency in operative surgery. Criticised in 'Mr. Beaney's medals', *Aust. med. J.*, 1877, 22 : 40. *Aust. med. J.*, 1879, ns 1 : 170, describes publication as 'in showy form, with the freedom of handbills, purely as an advertisement.'

Copies: AMAV, CC, ML, NL, SLV. 217

The Same. 2 ed., 1877. Grey tinted paper.

Copies: ML, NL. 218

Diseases of the hip-joint. . . . Melbourne: F. F. Bailliere, Publisher . . . 1878.

204 × 135. Pp. 20 (last—colophon only). 5 figs (on verso of half title). Paper boards, with cover title. Head of p.1 of text: 'Clinical lecture . . . delivered in the theatre of the Melbourne Hospital.'

Copies: CC, LNSW, ML, SLV. 219

Catalogue of the library of medical works and works of art also, the magnificent and unique collections of surgical instruments, &c., now in the possession of Mr. James George Beaney, F.R.C.S.E. . . . To be sold by auction by R. N. Henningham . . . 29th May, [1878] . . . M'Carron, Bird & Co., Printers . . . Melbourne.

212 × 173. Pp. 54. [1878.] Stiff p. w. (cover title). SLV copy with two following items in fine presentation binding.

Copies: SLV. 220

Catalogue of oil paintings, engravings and oleographs . . . pianofortes, orchestrion, mechanical singing bird . . . Pp. 18 [1878.] Format as above.

Copies: SLV. 221

Catalogue of household furniture & effects, elegant chariot . . . horses . . . Pp. 2, 20. [1878.] Format as above.

Copies: SLV. 222

Clinical lecture on stricture of the urethra, delivered in the theatre of the Melbourne Hospital, March 16th, 1880 . . . [Text begins.]

206 × 134. Pp. [ii] (v.b.), 20 (l.b.). Title from head p.1. Colophon—Mason, Firth & M'Cutcheon . . . Melb.

Also included in *The Generative System*, 4 ed., 1883.

Copies: SLV. 223

The medical embassy to England being a report of the trial Bailliere v. Beaney in the Supreme Court, Melbourne May 1880 (Reprinted from the Argus) with some comments of the Press thereon Melbourne Stillwell and Co. . . . 1880

217 × 137. Pp. 32 (l.b.). Double cols. P. w. (title rptd).

Reports unsuccessful action by Bailliere, Beaney's publisher, for recovery of costs of publishing and for obtaining for him an official appointment from Vic. Govt during a visit to Europe. The latter had been opposed by Med. Soc. of Vic., which publishes this pamphlet. See Nos 1332–3.

Copies: CC, LNSW, ML, SLV. 224

Professional and other testimony in favour of Dr James George Beaney.

NS. Mentioned in *The medical embassy* (1880) as pamphlet distributed to subscribers before Melb. Hosp. staff elections. 225

Clinical lecture on aneurism of the innominate artery, delivered at the Melbourne Hospital . . . [Text begins.]

209 × 140. 46 numbered leaves, printed on recto only. Title from head of p.1. ND. Colophon —Mason, Firth & M'Cutcheon . . . Melb.

Describes two cases of innominate aneurysm, treated by ligation.

Copies: ML. 226

An address introductory to the clinical investigation of disease, delivered at the Melbourne Hospital . . .

254 × 210. Pp. 60 (last 3 blank). Colophon—McCarron, Bird and Co. . . . ND. P. w. (shortened title).

Copies: EF. 227

———

A guide to surgical case taking . . . for the use of his ward clerks and dressers in the surgical wards of the Hospital. Melbourne, Mason, Firth & M'Cutcheon . . .

156 × 110. Pp. [6]. Printed on stiff paper. ND.

For J. G. Beaney (1826–91) MD, FRCSE, MLC, Hon. Surg. Melb. Hosp., see Craig, C. (1950), *Med. J. Aust.*, 1 : 593; Gandevia, B. (1952), *Med. J. Aust.*, 1 : 291; Gandevia, B. (1953), *Med. J. Aust.*, 1 : 614; Murphy, L. (1960), *Med. J. Aust.*, 1 : 313; Ford, E. (1953), *Bibliog. of J.G.B.*, Syd.

Copies: NL. 228

———

See also Reeves, Charles Evans, No 1776.

——— **'A Bystander'**

Melbourne medical morals and British critical opinion. By a Bystander. Melbourne: Fergusson and Moore . . . 1877.

211 × 132. Pp. 20 (l.b.).

Attacks Beaney's opponents in the lithotomy enquiry. Based on *Brit. med. J.* editorial (April 1876), which remarks on the 'sad proof of the length to which medical quarrels are pushed in Australia.'

Copies: FC, NL, SLV. 229

Beard, George M.

A new cyclopaedia of family medicine. Our home physician: a popular guide to the art of preserving health and treating disease; with plain advice for all the emergencies of the family. . . . Revised and enlarged. . . . Sold by subscription. E. B. Treat, Sydney and Melbourne. 1883.

239 × 161. 2 vols. Vol. 1 : pp. (ii) (title, v.b.), xxxii, 33–752. Vol. 2 : pp. 753–1240, 1–104 (Home physician), 1481–1506 (index). Frontis., 63 pl. (many coloured), 150 figs. Title p. tipped in. Further title (N.Y.: E. B. Treat, 1879) appears at p. 461. No title to vol. 2. Leather.

Aust. issue of New York publication. The following, with own title, follows p. 1240 in vol. 2: *Our home physician manual of homoeopathy*, by Samuel Lilienthal. N. Y.: E. B. Treat, 1870.

Copies: EF, KFR. 230

———

The Same. Syd.: McNeil & Coffee, 1885. Single vol., with additional title (lacking imprint) at p. 461.

Copies: LNSW. 231

Bedford, Edward Samuel Picard

Lectures delivered at the Mechanics' Institute, Hobart Town, during . . . 1849. Van Diemen's Land: . . . "Colonial Times" Office, Hobart Town, 1849.

255 × 156. Pp. 48 (l.b.). Double cols.

Includes 'Expression as applied to the fine arts' by E.S.P. Bedford, including anatomy and physiology.

For E.S.P. Bedford (1806–76) FRCS, Asst Col Surg. and founder of St Mary's Hosp., Hobart, and later Hon. Surg. Syd. Infirm., see Crowther, W.E.L.H. (1944), *Med. J. Aust.*, 2 : 25; also Bedford, Ruth, *Think of Stephen*, Syd., 1944.

Copies: ML, NL, SLV. 232

———

St. Mary's Hospital, 5th December, 1859. Gentlemen, The alterations likely to take place at St. Mary's Hospital . . . require that I should lay before you . . . a particular statement of its doings and prospects. [Text continues.]

204 × 130. Pp. [i] (two quotations), 1–11. Colophon—Hobart Town: Printed by Pratt & Son . . . To Com. of Management. Signed: E.S.P. Bedford.

Copies: DL, NL, SLV. 233

———

See also St Mary's Hospital, Hobart; Tas.—Parlt, No 2143.

Beer, Frederick

1861–2. Legislative Assembly. New South Wales. . . . Report from the Select Committee on Dr. F. Beer; . . . with proceedings . . . minutes of evidence, and appendix. . . . Sydney: Thomas Richards, Govt Printer . . . 1862.

333 × 210. Pp. 12 (l.b.), 74.

In 1856 Dr F. Beer, a young Swiss who had lived in Sydney for three years, was sentenced to 10 years imprisonment for procuring abortion by means of belladonna suppositories. Medical evidence at his trial was severely criticised; a petition by citizens to Parliament followed; and Committee above reports that 'belladonna in the mode prescribed could not have procured abortion' and absolved Beer completely. He nevertheless served his sentence.

Copies: LNSW, ML, NL, SLV. 234

The case of Dr. Frederick Beer, with a comment and notes, by J. Sheridan Moore, Principal of Randwick College. Sydney: ... "Guttenberg" Printing Office ... 1868.

178 × 116. Pp. 54, [2]. 1 flg table.

Copies: DL, EF, FC, ML. 235

1868–9. Legislative Assembly. New South Wales. Dr. Frederick Beer. (Petition of.) ... [Text begins.]

232 × 210. Pp. 6 (l.b.).

Beer pleads for redress. He had been released on ticket of leave after serving 4 years hard labour, and after obtaining posts in Shanghai and Calcutta, had been dismissed from each on news of his crime.

Copies: LNSW, ML, NL, SLV. 236

Dr. Beer's case.

212 × 133. Pp. 14. Colophon—Typ., J. Degotardi ... Syd. ND.

Beer protests, with petition to Gov. Gen. (1860), and letter of Sir Benjamin Brodie PRS, Physician to the Queen.

Brodie states: '... both the charge and the verdict are utterly absurd. I can understand that Dr Beer might have prescribed the use of belladonna with a view to prevent premature labour, but I cannot suppose that either he or anyone else should dream of prescribing it for the purpose of procuring abortion.'

Copies: ML. 237

1870–71. Legislative Assembly. New South Wales. Administration of Justice. (Correspondence connected with the case of Dr. Beer.) Ordered ... to be printed, 3 May, 1871. ...

328 × 210. Pp. 18 (l.b.). 2 figs. Colophon—Syd.: Thomas Richards, Govt Pr—1871.

Official papers (1857–1870).

Copies: LNSW, ML, NL, SLV. 238

1873–4. Legislative Assembly. New South Wales. Case of Dr. Frederick Beer. (Recent correspondence respecting.) Ordered ... to be printed, 26 March, 1874. ...

342 × 214. Pp. 14. Colophon—Syd.: Thomas Richards, Govt Pr—1874.

Papers referred to Prof. J. Smith, Dean of Med. Univ. Syd., for opinion on med. evidence. Smith considers that there was 'a very lamentable miscarriage of justice.'

Case is mentioned in Taylor's *Principles and practice of medical jurisprudence*, 3 ed., Lond., 1883 : 190, noting lack of specific action of belladonna on uterus.

Copies: LNSW, ML, NL, SLV. 239

1875. Legislative Assembly. New South Wales. Dr. Frederick Beer. (Opinion of Attorney General respecting case of.) Ordered ... to be printed, 30 April, 1875.

320 × 204. Pp. 4 (l.b.). Signed—William Bede Dalley, Attorney General.

'... I am of opinion that Dr. Beer was wrongfully convicted ... .'

Copies: LNSW, ML, NL, SLV. 240

The whole truth, being still "later papers" in the case of Dr. Frederick Beer, containing a *resumé* of the moral assassination of which he has been a victim for more than twenty-one years.

210 × 134. Pp. 28 (l.b.). Colophon—J. A. Engel ... Syd. (1877.) P. w. (with 'The conspiracy unmasked or still later papers ...').

Copies: DL, FC, ML. 241

1877–8. Legislative Assembly. New South Wales. Beer's Disabilities Bill. (Petition of Frederick Beer, M.D.) ... [Text begins.]

325 × 202. Pp. [2] (v.b.).

Beer pleads to be heard by counsel at the bar of the House.

Copies: LNSW, ML, NL, SLV. 242

The case of Dr. Frederick Beer, MD., ChD., Ob. &c., &c., Univ. Zurich. Speech delivered March, 1878, at the bar of the Legislative Assembly, by Walter H. Cooper, Barrister-at-Law. In advocacy of a Bill to relieve Dr. Beer from all disabilities attaching to him, in consequence of his having been improperly convicted of felony. Sydney: Published by Dr. Beer. 1878.

178 × 117. Pp. iv, 5–36, iv (appendix).

Includes vehement attack on medical witnesses.

Copies: LNSW, ML. 243

Beg, Wazir

Rev. Wazir Beg (1827–85) MD Edin., MRCSE, Presbyterian Minister, though registered and a Director of Syd. Hosp., did not practice medicine here. He was author of works on religious and other subjects.

244

Behrend, Henry

No. 10.] [December, 1882. Health Society of New South Wales. . . . The communicability to man of diseases from animals used as food. By Dr. Henry Behrend. (Two articles from the "Jewish Gazette".) . . . Sydney: . . . Turner & Henderson . . .

201 × 132. Pp. 16.

Copies: ML, NL. 245

Belair Inebriates' Retreat, SA

Inebriates' Retreat. Report of inaugural meeting, held in Adelaide, February 18, 1874, together with articles, letters, &c. Reprinted from South Australian Register. Adelaide: Printed by William Kyffin Thomas . . . 1874.

198 × 130. Pp. 16.

'Asylum for the systematic treatment of dipsomaniacs.'

Copies: SLS. 246

———

Belair Inebriates' Retreat. [Text begins.]

218 × 137. Pp. 4 (l.b.). Colophon— . . . Advertiser Steam Printing Office, Adel.

Annual report for 1879. Shown under above title up to 1885–6 rep., thence Belair Retreat to 1891–2 rep., in 1892–3 termed Hope Lodge.

Copies: SLS (1879–1893). 247

———

Inebriates' Retreat, Belair. by "Vid". . . . Adelaide: W. K. Thomas & Co., Grenfell Street. 1880.

208 × 134. Pp. 12. P. w. (cover title, notice on v. of back wrapper).

Copies: SLS 248

Belfast Hospital and Benevolent Asylum, Vic.

See Port Fairy Hospital.

Bell, Hugh

The dry closet system, after nature; with difficulties in sewerage solved. . . . Brisbane: Printed by Warwick and Sapsford . . . Published by Gordon and Gotch, Brisbane . . . 1881. . . .

214 × 132. Pp. 14. 3 pp. of figs. Stiff p. w. (short title).

Describes author's disposal system, used in Brisbane.

For Hugh Bell (d. 1897) MD Lond., FRCS, Surg. Brisbane Hosp., Member Qd Bd of Health, see obit., *Austsn med. Gaz.*, 1898, 17 : 40; also Jackson, E. S. (1923), *Med. J. Aust.*, 1 : 281.

Copies: DL, ML, NL. 249

Bell, William

On the origin, progress, and treatment of small-pox; with an account of the discovery and advantage of vaccination. . . . Redbank, Picton. . . . Sydney: Clarson, Shallard, & Co. . . .

217 × 140. Pp. 30. ND. (c.1858.) P. w. (title rptd).

Author announces intention of shortly publishing pamphlets 'on other epidemics, such as measles, scarlatina, hooping cough, croup and diphtheria.' NS.

Copies: EF, ML. 250

———

An essay on the wear and tear of human life . . . [Quotation] Sydney: . . . Grocott and Ward . . . 1859.

206 × 130. Pp. vi (ii, iv blank), 20 (l.b.). P. w. (title rptd).

William Bell MRCS, who practised at Picton NSW and was Coroner for Liverpool, later moved to Sydney. He died at Picton, aged 56, in 1871.

Copies: DL, FC, ML, SLV. 251

Bendigo and Northern District Base Hospital

See Bendigo Gold District General Hospital.

Bendigo Benevolent Asylum, Vic.

The Seventh Annual Report of the Committee of Management of the Bendigo Benevolent Asylum . . . for the year ending December 31, 1864. Sandhurst: J. K. Robshaw . . . 1865.

204 × 130. Pp. 26.

Includes rules and regulations. Later called Bendigo Benev. Home.

Copies: SLV. 252

Bendigo Gold District General Hospital Vic.

Eighth Annual Report of the Bendigo Gold District General Hospital, with the rules and regulations ... 1864. Sandhurst: Printed by J. K. Robshaw ... 1865.

204 × 132. Pp. 24 (l.b.).

Re-named Bendigo and Northern District Base Hosp., 1936–7.

See Florance, J. W. (1928), 'A fifty years retrospect ...', *Med. J. Aust.*, 2 : 173 (personal recollections); also Mackay, E. A. (1936), 'Med. practice in the goldfields era in Vic.', *Med. J. Aust.*, 2 : 421.

Copies: SLV (1864–71). 253

The Bendigo Hospital: its rise and progress. Reprinted from the "Bendigo Independent", November, 1865. Sandhurst: Young & Welch ...

204 × 132. Pp. 12.

Early history of hospital.

Copies: SLV. 254

Bendigo United Friendly Societies' Medical Institute & Dispensary, Vic.

Rules and regulations of the Bendigo United Friendly Societies' Medical Institute & Dispensary. 1888. Sandhurst: J. Brockley, Printer ...

178 × 110. Pp. 16. P. w. (title rptd).

Copies: SLV. 255

Benevolent Asylum, Melbourne

See Melbourne Benevolent Asylum.

Benevolent Society, Hobart Town

First Annual Report of the Benevolent Society of Hobart Town, for the year ended 31st December, 1860. Tasmania: John Davies, Printer, Mercury Office ...

204 × 136. Pp. 26. P. w. (title rptd).

Includes rules and regulations.

Copies: ML (1, 1860), SLT (1–29, 1860–1888). 256

Benevolent Society of New South Wales

The Benevolent Society. The Acting Committee of the Benevolent Society have much pleasure in laying before friends of the Institution an abstract of the proceedings of the past year ... [Text continues.]

239 × 188. Pp. 4 (l.b.). (14 Dec. 1819.) Colophon—Sydney: Printed by George Howe. Signed: Richard Hill, Sec.

The first Aust. charity, established in 1818 for the care of the poor blind, aged and infirm, was successor to the NSW Soc. for Promoting Christian Knowledge and Benevolence, formed in 1813. The Benevolent Asylum, built in 1820, provided the earliest hospital accommodation for free persons, and its obstetric wards, named in 1860 the Lying-in Hosp. of NSW, were the first maternity hospital. Society maintains its early functions through its various institutions, including Royal Hosp. for Women.

For Society, see Oliver, T. J. (1870), 'The Benev. Asylum', *NSW med. Gaz.*, 1 : 82; *Austsn med. Gaz.*, 1895, 14 : 499; Peyser, D. (1939), 'Early history of the Benev. Soc.', *JRAHS*, 25 : 89; Cummins, C. J. (1971), *The development of the Benev. Asylum*, Syd.

Copies: Benev. Soc., ML. 257

The Annual Report of the Committee of the New South Wales Benevolent Society: Submitted to the General Meeting held in the Court-Room, at Sydney ... 6th Day of June, 1820. With the Rules of the Society. Also, a list of subscribers, &c. &c. &c. Sydney: Printed by G. Howe, Government Printer, 1820.

174 × 114. Pp. 26. Signed: Lachlan Macquarie, Chairman.

Reports issued annually, June 1819 to date.

Copies: Benev. Soc. (1819/20–), ML (1819/20–), NL (1830/31–1860), SLT (1835), SLV (1826/27–1863). 258

Appeal on behalf of the Benevolent Asylum, Sydney.

193 × 127. Pp. 8. ND. [1842.] NI. Colophon—Printed by Kemp and Fairfax, "Herald" Office.

Copies: NL. 259

1861–2. Legislative Assembly. New South Wales. ... Report from the Select Committee on the Benevolent Asylum, Sydney ... with the proceedings ... evidence and appendix. ... Sydney: Thomas Richards, Govt Printer ... 1862.

333 × 210. Pp. 132. 3 flg plans.

A new institution is urgently required.

Copies: LNSW, ML, NL, SLV. 260

Benevolent Society of New South Wales. The Outdoor Relief Department: Its benefits to the distressed and deserving poor. An appeal to the public. Sydney: W. M. MacLardy, Printer ... 1888.

130 × 100. Pp. 16. P. w. (title rptd).

Copies: ML. 261

Benevolent Society of New South Wales. A plea for the poor. ... [Cut of Benevolent Asylum] ... Sydney: Printed by A. Radcliffe ... 1890.

243 × 167. Pp. 16 (l.b.). 7 figs. P. w. (title rptd).

Copies: ML. 262

Help for the poor and afflicted. The work of the Benevolent Society of New South Wales. Figure and biblical text] ...

280 × 220. Pp. 20. 7 figs. Colophon—Syd.: W. C. Penfold & Co. ... 1891.

Copies: ML. 263

Benevolent Society of New South Wales. Sketches of the poor. By Edward Maxted, Manager. (An appeal for aid for the widow and orphan and the aged and decrepit poor.) Published by authority of the Board of Directors. ... Sydney: W. M. MacLardy Printer ... 1892.

262 × 202. Pp. 24, [28] (advts). Decorated title, 6 pl., figs. P. w. (short title, decorated).

Copies: ML, NL. 264

Benevolent Society of New South Wales. By-laws, and rules and regulations. Revised and approved ... Sydney: Beatty, Richardson & Co., Printers ... 1896.

206 × 132. Pp. 30 (l.b.). P. w. (short title).

Copies: ML. 265

Benham, Agnes

Mental Science Series, No. 1. First steps in mental science. ... Adelaide: Scrymgour and Sons ... 1895.

217 × 140. Pp. 16 (l.b.). P. w. (title rptd, decorated; advt inside back wrapper).

Copies: ML, SLS. 266

Benham, Frederick Lucas—Translator

Death and sudden death. By P. Brouardel ... and F. Lucas Benham ... Second edition London Bailliere, Tindall and Cox ... 1902 ...

214 × 140. Pp. xiv (3 blanks), 330 (l.b.), 4 (book notices). Cloth.

Transl. of *La mort et la mort subite*, Paris, 1895, with additions by translator. 1 Eng. ed., NS. 2 Eng. ed. (above) contains translator's preface dated Dec. 1896.

Univ. Adel. has copy with author's presentation label; also Benham's copy of 1895 French ed. with signature and bookplate.

Paul Camille Hippolyte Brouardel (1837–1906), noted forensic pathologist, was Prof. of Forensic Med. and Dean of Medicine, Paris.

F. L. Benham MD (Lond. & Adel.), MRCP, Asst Phys. Univ. Coll. Hosp. Lond., who qualified in 1877, arrived in SA about 1899 and practised at Exeter SA.

Copies: UA, UM. 267

Benjafield, Harry

The structure of the human body. By Dr. Benjafield, Hobart Town. Hobart Town: Henn & Co., Machine Printers. 1874.

175 × 122. Pp. 14, [ii] (colophon only, r.b.). Printing within frame.

First of a series of lectures to Mercantile Assistants' Assn.

Copies: LNSW, ML, WLC. 268

The nervous system. ... Hobart Town: Henn & Co. ... 1874.

175 × 117. Pp. 14, [ii] (colophon only, r.b.).

Copies: LNSW, ML, WLC. 269

How and why do I breathe? ... Hobart Town: Henn and Co. ... 1874.

175 × 120. Pp. 14, [ii] (colophon only, r.b.).

Copies: LNSW, ML, WLC. 270

The blood and its circulation. ... Hobart Town: Henn & Co. ... 1874.

175 × 117. Pp. 14 (l.b.), [ii] (colophon only, r.b.).

Copies: LNSW, ML, WLC. 271

Food and its forces. ... Hobart Town: Henn & Co. ... 1874.

175 × 110. Pp. 16.

Copies: LNSW, ML, SLT, WLC. 272

Public health. ... Hobart Town: Henn & Co. ... 1874.

175 × 117. Pp. 16.

Contains some discussion of hygiene and living conditions in Hobart.

Copies: LNSW, WLC. 273

The eye. ... Hobart Town: Henn & Co. ... 1874.

175 × 117. Pp. 16.

Copies: LNSW, WLC. 274

A lecture on the mind ... (Reprinted from "The Christian Witness".) ... "Mercury" Steam Press Office, Hobart. 1874.

175 × 117. Pp. 14.

Copies: WLC. 275

A lecture on the human voice. ... Tasmania: L. Henn & Co. ... Hobart Town. 1877.

175 × 117. Pp. 8 (l.b.) P. w. (cover title).

Harry Benjafield (1845–1917) MB, ChM Edin., of Hobart, was a founder of Homoeopathic Hosp., early supplier of calf lymph to various states, and pioneer of Tas. fruit export. See obits, *Tas. Mail*, 14 and 18 June 1917, and *Mercury*, Hobart, 14 June 1917; for vaccination: *Austsn med. Gaz.*, 1882, 1 : 132.

Copies: LNSW, WLC. 276

Bimetallism. The remedy for our depression: Dr. Benjafield, Hobart. ... Published by H. T. Gould ... Tasmania: Cox & Co., Printers ... Hobart. 1895.

210 × 140. Pp. 18. P. w. (cover title, advts other sides).

Copies: SLT. 277

Bennett, C. R.

A treatise on the importance of preserving the teeth, especially the first or milk teeth. Brisbane. [ND.]

NS. Listed in *Cat. Parlt Library of Qd*, 1899.

278

Bennett, George

(From the Magazine of Natural History.) Polynesia. Notices on the native plants of the island of Rotuma, Southern Pacific. [Text continues.]

204 × 132. Pp. 6. (Lond., 5 Dec. 1831.)

Copies: SLV. 279

(From the London Medical and Physical Journal.) An account of the medicinal properties, &c. of the Kava Shrub (Piper Methisticum), Gambir (Nauclea Gambir), and the Ignatia Amara, or St. Ignatius' bean. ... (An abstract of a paper read before the Medico-Botanical Society of London, January 10th, 1832.)

204 × 132. Pp. 8. Plain p. w.

Copies: SLV. 280

Wanderings in New South Wales, Batavia, Pedir Coast, Singapore, and China; being the journal of a naturalist in those countries, during 1832, 1833, and 1834. ... In two volumes. Vol. 1. London: Richard Bentley ... 1834.

214 × 132. 2 vols. Vol. 1 : xvi (l.b.), errata slip, 440, [ii] (v.b.), [2] (advt). Vol. 2 : pp. viii, errata slip, 428, [ii]. Frontis. in each vol.

Facsimile ed., Adel: Libraries Board of SA, 1967.

Describes early Sydney and two long journeys into NSW interior in 1832. Though devoted mainly to natural history, many medical observations occur, including local health, snakebite, ophthalmia, medical properties of flora, and aboriginal medicine and obstetrics. A chapter on a recent small-pox epidemic among aborigines includes discussion with Dr Mair, Asst Surg. 39 Regt and substance of his report to Govt. Chapter reprinted in *NSW med. Gaz.*, 1871, 1 : 215 and J.H.L. Cumpston, *Small-pox in Aust., 1788–1908*, Melb., 1914.

ML copy has ms. letter by author in each vol; UQ copy has author's bookplate and attached ms. biog. by E. A. Vidler.

Copies: AMAV, DL, DOS, EF, FC, ML, NL, OL, SLV, SLW, SPH, UA, UM, UQ, US. 281

Gatherings of a naturalist in Australasia: being observations principally on the animal and vegetable productions of New South Wales, New Zealand, and some of the Austral Islands. ... London: John Van Voorst ... 1860.

220 × 140. Pp. xii, 456. 8 litho pl. (7 hand-coloured), 27 figs.

Includes chapter on snakes and snake-bite treatment.

Copies: AMAV, DL, DOS, EF, FC, ML, NL, OL, SLS, SLT, SLV, SLW, UA, UM, UQ, US. 282

———

Acclimatisation: Its eminent adaptation to Australia. A lecture delivered in Sydney ... Republished by the Acclimatisation Society of Victoria. ... Melbourne: Wm. Goodhugh & Co. ... 1862.

204 × 132. Pp. 40. P. w. (title rptd).

Copies: DL, DOS, LNSW, ML, NL, SLS, SLV, UA, UM. 283

———

The Third Annual Report of the Acclimatisation Society of New South Wales, with an address on the physiology, utility, and importance, of acclimatisation, to Australia. Delivered at the annual meeting of the Society, April 4th, 1864, by George Bennett, M.D. ... Sydney: ... Joseph Cook & Co. ... 1864.

204 × 130. Pp. 44. P. w. (title rptd).

Copies: EF, LNSW, ML, NL, SLV. 284

———

[From the Annals and Magazine of Natural History for April 1872.] A trip to Queensland in search of fossils. ... [Text begins.]

217 × 140. Pp. 8. P. w.

A letter to Richard Owen FRS, London, with his preface: 'I have been favoured by my friend, Dr. George Bennett ... to whom I was indebted for the specimen in my "Memoir on the Pearly Nautilus", and for valuable materials while investigating the generative economy of the Marsupialia and Monotremata.'

Copies: NL, UM. 285

———

Not published. An account of Elau, a Malayan Papuan child, native of the island of Erromanga, one of the New Hebrides Group, Southern Pacific Ocean. ... [Text begins.]

217 × 138. Pp. 10. ND. (c. 1890.) Colophon—F. Cunninghame & Co. ... Syd. 2 ML copies have photo of drawing of native child inserted.

A personal and clinical account of an orphan girl, adopted by Bennett, and brought by him to England, where she died of tuberculosis. Abridged version in *Austsn med. Gaz.*, 1883, 2 : 255.

Copies: DL, ML, NL. 286

———

Private Circulation. George Bennett, M.D., F.R.C.S., F.L.S., F.Z.S., etc.

210 × 147. Pp. 8 (l.b.). ND. NI. [Syd. 1893.] P. w. (cover title).

Biog. memoir, published by Bennett's widow. Two ML copies bear inscriptions by Mrs. G. Bennett.

Copies: FC, ML, NL. 287

———

... Catalogue of a choice portion of the library of the late Dr. Geo. Bennett ... on sale by William Dymock, new and second-hand bookseller ... Sydney. ...

214 × 138. Pp. 66. ND. (Dymock's book list for Aug. 1895 inserted.) P. w. (cover title).

For George Bennett (1804–1893) MD, FRCS, of Sydney, a leader in medicine and science, see *Austsn med. Gaz.*, 1893, 12 : 349; *Proc. Linn Soc. NSW.* 1893, 8 : 542; Plarr, *Lives of the Fellows of the RCS*, 1 : 85; Coppleson, V. M. (1955), 'The life and times of Dr G. B.', *BPCMUS*, 11 : 207 (with bibliog.).

Also published: *Correspondence relating to the cultivation of silk*, Syd., 1870; *On the introduction, cultivation, and economic uses of the orange*, Syd., 1871.

Copies: EF, ML. 288

——— (editor and translator)

Journal of the expedition for the exploration of the Fly River, by L. M. D'Albertis, C.M.Z.S., &c. Printed for the subscribers. Sydney: Printed by Frederick White ... 1877

220 × 138. Pp. 44 (l.b.). 1 flg map. P. w. (title rptd.).

Translated, edited and with preface by Bennett for Committee of the D'Albertis Expedition. Contains appendix on plants by F. von Mueller MD, FRS.

Copies: DL, ML, NL, SLV, US. 289

———, Gibson, Andrew, and Sherwin, William

Reports on the epidemic catarrh or influenza prevailing among the sheep in the Colony of New South Wales, in the year 1835. By George Bennett, Esq., Andrew Gibson, Esq., J. P., and William Sherwin, Esq. Sydney: Printed by Stephens and Stokes, George-Street. 1835.

204 × 124. Pp. [ii] (title, v.b.), [ii] (contents, v.b.), [3], 4–44 (l.b.).

Copies: SLS. 290

Bérengier, Théophile

La Nouvelle-Nursie Histoire d'une Colonie Bénédictine dans l'Australie Occidentale (1846–

1878) . . . Avec gravures & carte [Arms] Librairie Jacques Lecoffre Lecoffre fils et Cie, Successeurs Paris . . . Lyon . . .

8vo. Pp. viii, 386 (l.b.), [2] (errata, v.b.). Frontis., flg map, 33 engravings. ND. [1879.] P. w. (title rptd).

History of New Norcia Mission, WA, with references to Aboriginal food, childbirth, ailments and treatment.

Copies: FC, ML, NL, OL, SLS, SLV, SLW. 291

Berigny, Thiennette Francois

Medical physiology: an appeal to the people of Australia, for the candid investigation of practical medicine. Lectures on homoeopathy . . . Melbourne: Slater, Williams, and Hodgson . . . 1855.

161 × 102. Pp. 32.

T. F. Berigny MD, b. 1792, writer on theology and homoeopathy, practised as a homoeopathic physician in Melb. Also published: *Light for the million. The religion of God not of man*, Melb., 1863; *Light for the million. The education of nature*, Melb., 1863.

Copies: NL, SLV. 292

———

Chaos & order; or the orthodox practice of medicine unveiled, versus the medical heresy! . . . Melbourne: W. Fairfax & Co. . . . 1858.

214 × 138. Pp. viii (l.b.), 9–60. P. w. (title rptd).

Response to newspaper attack on homoeopathy.

Copies: LNSW, ML, NL, SLV, UA. 293

Bernays, Lewis Adolphus

Cultural industries for Queensland. Papers on the cultivation of useful plants suited to the climate of Queensland; their value as food, in the arts, and in medicine; and methods of obtaining their products. First series. . . . Brisbane: . . . James C. Beal, Govt Printer . . . 1883.

214 × 138. Pp. xii, 230. Cloth.

Copies: AMAV, EF, FC, ML, NL, OL, SLS, SLV, SLW, UM, UQ, US. 294

Berncastle, Julius

Australian snake bites: their treatment and cure. The use and abuse of tobacco. . . . Melbourne: Printed by Mason, Firth & Co. . . . 1868.

161 × 105. Pp. 32 (l.b.). Stiff p. w., cloth backstrip; title rptd.

Another issue, 1868. Pp. 32, with advt for Syd. Eye Institution on last p. and continued inside end wrapper.

For snake-bite treatment, author advocates excision, the taking of half to one bottle of brandy, and rest. 'There was nothing so simple as the cure of an Aust. snake's bite; it was almost an insult to the medical profession to ask them to cure it . . . The antidote was spirits . . . .'

'The use and abuse of tobacco' deals with pharmacological action and injurious effects.

Copies: DL, ML, NL, SLS, SLV, UM, WLC. 295

———

The treatment of snake bites. A paper read before the Victorian Medical Association, 12th February, 1869 . . . . Melbourne: Samuel Mullen . . . 1869.

156 × 100. Pp. 16. Repr., *Aust. med. Gaz.*, 1869.

SLV copy has inserted leaf, with author's letter in Melb. *Age*, and druggist's label—'Dr. Berncastle's box for the cure of all Aust. snake bites, with book of directions . . . Price, 10s.' Described in *Aust. med. Gaz.*, 1869, 1 : 176.

Also published: *A voyage to China*, 2 vols, Lond., 1851; *The revolt of the Bengal Sepoys*, Syd., 1857; *The defenceless state of Sydney*, Syd., 1865.

For Julius Berncastle (1819–1870) MRCP, founder and surgeon of the Syd. Ophthalmic Instn, see obits, *Aust. med.* Gaz., 1870, 2 : 119 and *Lancet*, 1871, 1 : 215.

For Syd. Ophthalmic Instn for the Cure of Diseases of the Eye, see advt in *Handbook of Austsia*, by Wm Fairfax, Melb., 1859; also item above.

Copies: SLV, WLC. 296

Berry, Richard James Arthur

The caecal folds and fossae and the topographical anatomy of the vermiform appendix . . . Edinburgh William F. Clay . . . 1897

220 × 140. Pp. x, 11–76 (l.b.). 16 pl. appended, titles on recto of interleaves. Cloth.

"As the vermiform appendix has, within recent years, assumed a clinical importance . . . it has seemed advisable to investigate any anatomical problems which may throw light upon such a treacherous disease as appendicitis.'

Copies: EF, RACS, UM. 297

———

Applied anatomy. Synopsis of demonstrations on applied anatomy . . . Part 1. The upper and lower limbs, and the head and neck. New School, School of Medicine of the Royal Colleges, Edinburgh.

215 × 140. Pp. 30 (l.b.). Interleaved. P. w. (cover title). ND. (c. 1900.)

Copies: KFR. 298

———

Applied anatomy. Synopsis of demonstrations on applied anatomy . . . Part II. The abdomen, pelvis, perineum, and thorax. New School, School of Medicine of the Royal Colleges, Edinburgh.

215 × 140. Pp. 12. Interleaved. P. w. (cover title). ND. (c. 1900.)

Copies: KFR. 299

———

The essentials of regional anatomy. Edinburgh and London: William Green & Sons . . . 1900.

8vo. Pp. x, 484. Cloth.

For R.J.A. Berry (1867–1962) MD Edin. & Melb., FRCSE, Prof. Anat. Univ. Melb. (1905–29), and later Director Burden Inst. Bristol Eng., see obits: *Brit. med. J.*, 1962, 2 : 930; *Lancet*, 1962, 2 : 789; and *Med. J. Aust.*, 1963, 1 : 446.

His extensive later bibliog. includes: *Regional anatomy*, rev. ed., 3 vols, Edin., 1902; *Surface anatomy*, Edin., 1906; *Clinical atlas of sectional and topographical anatomy*, Edin., 1911; *Practical anatomy*, 3 vols, Melb., 1915; 2 ed. 1922; *The modern psychology*, Melb., 1921; *Brain and mind*, N. Y., 1928; *The mental defective* (with R. G. Gordon), Lond., 1931; *Cerebral Atlas*, Lond., 1938; *Your brain and its story*, Oxford, 1939.

Copies: UM. 300

Besant, Annie

The prosecuted work. The law of population: its consequences and its bearing upon human conduct and morals. By Annie Besant. Australian edition. Sydney: Sir Robert Bear, Cheap Book Depot, . . . 1889 . . .

183 × 120. Pp. 56. Advts (9 pp.) interposed from p. 42 to end. P. w. (title rptd).

Advocates and describes contraceptive methods. See Windeyer, William C., for his legal judgement on this work.

Copies: NL. 301

Besomo, Pasquale

The Botany poisoning case [Cut] A brief history of the most famous female poisoners, Borgia family etc. How they killed and what they killed with Symptoms and agonies of arsenic illustrated with photo of Mrs. Chantrelle who was poisoned by her husband With phrenological and physiognomical sketch of Mrs. Louisa Collins the Botany murderess and Kate Cobb the Norwich poisoner. . . . P. Besomo & Co. . . . Sydney: G. Wallace, General Printer . . .

206 × 138. Pp. 16. 3 woodcut figs. ND. P. w. (cover title).

Advertises Signor P. Besomo, phrenologist and homoeopathist, stating that 'the allopathic drugging system murders more infants in one year than they can cure in ten.'

Copies: ML. 302

Best, John

A review of the letter addressed to the householders of Hobart Town by the Reverend H. P. Fry, B.A. By a Member of the Medical Profession. Hobart Town, V. D. Land; Printed at the Advertiser Office, Elizabeth-Street. 1847.

197 × 178. Pp. [ii], ii, 14. P. w. (title rptd).

Attacks Fry's views on the benefits of transportation. Author's name in introduction.

John Best (c. 1809–99) MRCS (1833), practised at Deloraine Tas. for many years. He died at Launceston.

Copies: LNSW, ML, SLV. 303

Bezold, G. M.

The book of charms of simple and sympathetic remedies & divers blessings. Translated from various sources, particularly including those secrets brought by Egyptian Christian Gipsies into Europe, and kept until the present in unpublished concealment. . . . Published by G. M. Bezold. . . . Sydney: Jas. Miller & Co., Printers . . . 1888.

183 × 120. Pp. 88. Cloth.

Sections: 1. Charms against illness, wounds, accidents (many tested and proved by author); 2. Remedies, many with exotic medieval mat. med., e.g. 'when the breasts of a girl are becoming too large, take the testicles of a castrated boar, and grease the right breast with the left testicle, and the left breast with the right one, the breasts will not become any larger . . .'; 3. Blessings.

Copies: BG. 304

Bickle, Leonard Watkins

The early decay of children's teeth with suggestions as to its causes and prevention ... George Robertson and Company Melbourne ... 1897

183 × 122. Pp. 18, [2] (advts). Frontis., 2 figs. P. w. (shortened title).

For L. W. Bickle (1857–1921) FRCSE, Hon. Surg. Adel. Hosp., see obit., *Med. J. Aust.*, 1921, 2 : 130; for his first cholecystectomy reported in Aust., *Austsn med. Gaz.*, 1894, 13 : 147.

Copies: ML. 305

Bigge, John Thomas

Report of the Commissioner of Inquiry into the State of the Colony of New South Wales. Ordered, by the House of Commons, to be printed 5th August, 1822. [448.]

342 × 217. Pp. [iv], 186.

Facsimile ed., Adel.: Libraries Board of SA, 1966.

Bigge's reports of his examination of the convict system in NSW and VDL were made during a visit from 25 Sep. 1819 to 14 Feb. 1821. From their wide terms of reference, these provide valuable and otherwise unobtainable information on life and conditions in the colony.

Includes: condition and treatment of convicts on voyage, employment, rations, clothing, nature of work, discipline and punishments. Refers to individual med. officers, particularly Wm Redfern and D'Arcy Wentworth.

For J. T. Bigge (1780–1843) and his reports, see Dennis, J. (1937), 'Bigge *versus* Macquarie', *JRAHS*, 23 : 411; Ellis, M. H., *Lachlan Macquarie*, Syd., 1947; Ritchie, J. (1974), 'John Thomas Bigge and his reports on NSW', *JRAHS*, 60, (1) : 12.

Copies: DL, FC, ML, NL, SLV. 306

Report of the Commissioner of Inquiry, on the State of Agriculture and Trade in the Colony of New South Wales. Ordered, by the House of Commons, to be printed, 13 March 1823. [136.]

342 × 217. Pp. 112. London, 1823.

Facsimile ed., Adel.: Libraries Bd of SA, 1966.

Section on 'The medical establishments of NSW and VDL' deals with med. personnel and hospitals. Section on 'State and character of the population of NSW and VDL' notes ailments, physique of native born, and charities.

Copies: DL, FC, ML, NL, SLS, SLV. 307

Bilroth, Th.

See Mueller, Sir Ferdinand.

Bird, Frederick Dougan

Remarks upon the radical cure of hernia. ... Reprinted from "The Lancet", Aug. 4th, 1900.

209 × 132. Pp. 8. Colophon—Crawford & Son ... [Melb.]. P. w. (cover title).

For F. D. Bird (1858–1921) MS, Hon. FRCS, son of Samuel Dougan Bird, Hon. Surg. Melb. Hosp., see obit., *Med. J. Aust.*, 1929, 2 : 29.

Copies: ML, NL, SLV. 308

Medical Society of Victoria. President's address. ... (Read ... January 1897.) [Text begins.]

229 × 140. Pp. 12 (l.b.). Colophon—Melbourne: Stillwell and Co. ... Repr. *Intercol med. J. Austsia*, 1897, 2 : 1.

Copies: UM. 308a

Bird, Samuel Dougan

On scurvy, as it appeared in the Allied Armies during the late war with Russia. London: R. Born, 1858.

8vo. Pp. 20.

NS. Listed *SGC*, ser. 1. Mentioned in author's discussion of scurvy in 'On the cases of disease recently arrived by the ship "Dayspring"', *Aust. med. J.*, 1868, 13 : 326.

309

On Australasian climates and their influence in the prevention and arrest of pulmonary consumption. ... London: Longman, Green, Longman, Roberts, & Green. 1863.

224 × 143. Pp. viii (iv, l.b.), [iv] (ii, iv blank), 168, 40 (book advts). Erratum slip. 4 pl., including woodcut view of Melb. (frontis.), 2 colour lithos, and woodcut. Cloth.

Author came to Aust. two years previously, suffering from tuberculosis, and was cured. He claims that the Aust. climate has especially beneficial influence on tuberculosis. Reviewed favourably *Aust. med. J.*, 1864, 9 : 27; severely criticised by W. Thomson (No 2224). For work and its influence, see Thomas, B. and Gandevia, B. (1959), *Med. J. Aust.*, 1 : 1.

Copies: AMAN, AMAV, BG, CC, DOS, EF, KFR, ML, NL, RACP, SLS, SLV, SPH, UA, UM. 310

On the nature and treatment of epidemic cholera, and the influence of quarantine and hygienic precautions in arresting its progress. . . . Re-printed from the *Australian Medical Journal*, together with the discussion . . . before the Medical Society of Victoria.

204 × 135. Pp. 22, [ii] (colophon only, on verso). Colophon—Melbourne: Wilson & Mackinnon . . . 1866.

Cholera had never appeared in Australia. The possibility is discussed and control outlined.

Copies: LNSW, ML, SLV. 311

Climate & consumption. . . . Paper read before the Medical Society of Victoria, April 6th, 1870.

204 × 133. Pp. 14 (l.b.).

Author maintains the views of his *On Australasian climates* (1863) and attacks Wm Thomson, its vigorous assailant.

Copies: LNSW, SLV, UA, UM. 312

On hydatids of the lung their diagnosis, prognosis, and treatment, and observations on their relations to pulmonary consumption, and other diseases of the chest. . . . Melbourne: Samuel Mullen . . . 1874.

209 × 140. Pp. [vi] (iv, vi blank), 7–44. Green paper boards.

Preface to 2 ed. states that the greater part of 1 ed. was lost on its way to Europe.

Original publication of diagnosis of the unbroken cyst, its successful surgical treatment, and radical cure by removal of suppurating intrathoracic cysts. It is stated that 'operative treatment of thoracic hydatid undoubtedly originated in, and is apparently still confined to, this colony.' For review of Aust. hydatid work see Graham, H. B. (1953), *Med. J. Aust.*, 1 : 869.

S. D. Bird (1832–1904) MD St And. and Melb., a distinguished London physician ('having under his care at different times . . . three Prime Ministers . . . Lord Aberdeen, Lord Palmerston and Lord John Russell'), settled in Melb., and was a pioneer of hydatid disease and a local authority on lung ailments. Obits: *Intercol med. J. Austsia*, 1904, 9 : 263; *Austsn med. Gaz.*, 1904, 23 : 310.

Copies: CC, NL, SLV, UA, UM. 313

The Same. 2 ed., 1877, with minor variations in title. Pp. iv, 64. Melb., Geo. Robertson. Fawn paper boards.

Copies: AMAN, AMAV, BG, CC, DOS, EF, KFR, LNSW, ML, NL, RACP, SLV, US. 314

Black, George

Foy and Gibson's The doctor A concise guide to health, and home treatment of diseases. Including advice to mothers on maternal management, and the rearing of infants and children. Edited by Geo. Black, M. B., Edin. . . . Foy and Gibson, Melbourne.

178 × 117. Pp. [2] (advts), [ii] (half title, v.b.). [missing to p. 12], 13–114 (l.b.), [16] (book advts, Ward, Lock & Bowden). Title from front cover. ND. (c. 1894.) Limp cloth.

Copies: BG (incomplete). 315

Black, M. Hume

Queensland. A few facts in connection with the employment of Polynesian labour in Queensland. 1894. By M. Hume Black. Special Agent to the Queensland Government. . . . Westminster, S. W. London Printed by Lake & Sison . . .

217 × 140. Pp. 12. P. w. (cover title). Heading to p. 1—'The Kanaka question in Queensland.' Contradicts statements on abuses in the Queensland labour trade. He admits that the traffic up to ten years previously was 'conducted without supervision, often with great cruelty, and sometimes accompanied by atrocities', but contends that conditions are now rectified. Refers to the health and welfare of native labourers.

Copies: EF, SLV. 316

Blackett, Cuthbert Robert

No. 19. February, 1884. Australian Health Society . . . Disinfection and disinfectants. . . . Melbourne: M'Carron, Bird & Company . . . 1884.

217 × 140. Pp. 8.

Current views on disinfection. Author was Pres. Pharmacy Bd of Vic.

Copies: EF, ML, NL, SLS, SLV. 317

See also No 103.

Blackmore, H. Gairdner

On the value of physical education and its practical introduction into schools. . . . Sydney: Gibbs, Shallard, & Co. . . . 1888.

209 × 135. Pp. 22.
Copies: US. 318

Blair, David

1873. Victoria. Report on the social evil, considered with a view to legislation. ... Presented to both Houses of Parliament. ... John Ferres, Govt Printer, Melbourne.

342 × 217. Pp. 18 (l.b.).

Reprinted, 1878, as paper of Leg. Council, Tas. Pp. 20.

Considers laws for abatement of prostitution valueless, but necessary for controlling venereal diseases. Recommends legislation for compulsory detention and treatment of infected women.

For David Blair (1820–99) MLA, see *Aust. Enc.*

Copies: AMAV, BG, EF, LNSW, ML, NL, RACP, SLV. 319

Blair, John

Remarks on diphtheria. ... Read before the Medical Society of Victoria, June 10, 1868. Melbourne: Stillwell and Knight ...

205 × 130. Pp. 8. 1 fig. P. w. (cover title). Repr., *Aust. med. J.*, 1868.

Copies: LNSW, SLV. 320

———

A case of diphtheria in which the xylostyptic ether was successfully employed. ... (Read before the Medical Society of Victoria on May 6, 1868.)

206 × 127. Pp. 2. 1 fig. Colophon—Stillwell and Knight ... Melb. Repr., *Aust. med. J.*, May 1868.

Copies: SLV. 321

———

On the treatment of diphtheria by tannin. ... [Text begins.]

205 × 130. Pp. 2. Repr., *Aust. med. J.*, Sept. 1870.

Copies: SLV. 322

———

From "The Australian Medical Journal", September 1871. On a case of chronic disease of the knee-joint. [Text begins.]

205 × 130. Pp. 6. Colophon—Stillwell and Knight ... Melbourne.

Includes 'A little about quackery', pp. 3–6, signed 'Scalpel.'

Copies: EF, SLV. 323

———

Address delivered by John Blair ... President of the Medical Society of Victoria ... January 8, 1873. ... Melbourne: Stillwell and Knight ... 1873.

205 × 130. Pp. 20 (l.b.). P. w. (short title).

Includes: living conditions and sanitation in Melb.; eucalyptus oil and other local medical products; medical advances; use and misuse of public hospitals; healing by spiritism.

Copies: CC, EF, SLV. 324

———

Reproduction and extirpation of cancer in the groin, iliac and inguinal regions; and the treatment of diphtheria. ... [Text begins.]

205 × 130. Pp. 6 (misnumbered). 1 litho. pl. Colophon—Stillwell and Knight ... Melb. Repr., *Aust. med. J.*, 1873.

Copies: SLV. 325

———

On a new combination of cod liver oil and iron. ... Melbourne: Stillwell and Knight ... 1874 ...

205 × 130. Pp. 12 (l.b.). P. w. (cover title). Repr., *Aust. med. J.*, 1874.

Preparation criticised by C. R. Blackett (1874), *Aust. med. J.*, 20 : 221. Due to sale under name 'Blair's Compound', author was reproved by Med. Soc. Vic.

Copies: SLV. 326

———

On paying wards in public hospitals. ... Melbourne: F. F. Bailliere, Publisher ... 1877.

214 × 135. Pp. iv, 5–16. Stiff p. w. (title rptd).

Advocates inclusion of ward for paying patients in Alfred Hosp., Melb. Review, *Aust. Practitioner*, 1878, 1 : 115.

Copies: ML, SLT, SLV. 327

———

The Same. 2 ed., 1880, with title *On paying hospitals*. Melb., George Robertson. Pp. 60.

Copies: SLV. 328

———

Opening address to nurses, with notes to nurses and rules for nurses under training added. ... George Robertson ... Melbourne ... 1880.

209 × 140. Pp. 24 (last 2 blank). Stiff p. w. (title rptd).

For John Blair (1835–1887) MD Syd. & Melb., FRCSE, Hon. Surg. Alfred Hosp., see obits, *Austsn med. Gaz.*, 1887, 6 : 150 and *Aust. med. J.*, 1887, ns 9 : 143.

Copies: EF, ML, NL, SLS, US, WLC. 329

The Same. 2 ed., 1883.

Copies: RACS, SLV. 330

Bland, William

Journey of discovery to Port Phillip, New South Wales, by Messrs. W. H. Hovell, and Hamilton Hume: in 1824 and 1825. Sydney: A. Hill, Printer, George Street.

205 × 127. Pp. [iv] (ii, iv blank), viii, 88 (l.b.), [6] (l.b.). ND. [1831.] Dedication to Sir Thomas Brisbane signed W. Bland.

Facsimile ed., Adel.: Libraries Bd of SA, 1965.

The first book on Victoria, compiled by Bland from explorers' journals. Though almost ready for printing in Jan. 1826 and advertised to be issued that year, the work, delayed by Bland's illness and later paper shortage, appeared in Jan. 1831.

SLV copy belonged to Wm Bland; ML copy to W. H. Hovell.

See C. A. McCallum, 'Vic. Historical Collection', in *Across the years*, ed. C. Barrett, Melb., 1948.

Copies: DL, ML, NL, SLV. 331

The Same. 2 ed. Syd., James Tegg, 1837.

Copies: DL, FC, LNSW, ML, NL, SLV. 332

Paper on the present epidemic scarlatina, read to some professional friends. June 19, 1841. Sydney: Printed by James Tegg and Co. George-Street. 1841.

178 × 110. Pp. 14 (l.b.). P. w.

The earliest known contribution to clinical medicine published in Australia. 'The present epidemic is the first instance of scarlatina in any form in the Colony, at least as an epidemic, and infinitely the most frightful in its effects, and the most fatal, if not the most widespread disease with which it has ever been visited. Its fatality has been . . . most appalling, nor less so the rapidly of its ravages . . .' Clinical features and treatment are discussed.

Pamphlet by Little, Robert, 1842, refers to same epidemic. See Ford, E. (1972), 'Some early Aust. med. publications', *Med. History*, 16 : 205.

Copies: FC, LNSW. 333

Suppression of spontaneous combustion in wool ships, &c., &c., &c. By W. Bland. Sydney: Printed by E. Alcock, Observer Office, Jamison Street. 1843.

229 × 143. Pp. 6.

A method for extinguishing fires in ships by filling the holds with carbon dioxide. Casks containing carbonate of lime were to be stowed with cargo, and the gas generated, in case of fire, by introducing acid through pipes from the deck.

Copies: FC, RACP, SLW. 334

The Same. Pp. viii, 8, 2 pl. Plain p. w. Syd., Printed at the 'Australian' (late 'Gazette') Office, Lower George Street, 1843.

Copies: DL, NL. 335

The Same. 2 ed. Pp. x (ii, iv blank), [11]–16. 2 pl. Plain p. w. Syd., D. L. Welch, Printer, Atlas Office, 1845. ML copy has Bland's inscription to Sir John Franklin.

Copies: DL, FC, LNSW, ML, NL, SLV. 336

The Same. 3 ed. Title: Suppression of combustion in wool & other ships, mines, & other confined spaces, invented in 1839, patented in 1867. Pp. x (ii, iv blank), [11]–16. 2 pl. Syd., Printed by J. G. O'Connor, 1867.

Copies: LNSW. 337

Correspondence between Dr. Farquhar M'Crae and Mr. Surgeon Bland, as lately republished by Dr. F. M'Crae, with his comments; and the subsequent correspondence relative to the above between Mr. Bland and the Honorable the Chief Justice. Sydney: Printed by James Reading . . . 1846.

212 × 135. Pp. 42 (l.b.). Plain p. w.

Bland's reply to M'Crae's pamphlet (No 1211).

Copies; DL, FC, LNSW, ML, RACP, SLV. 338

Atmotic ship. Invented by W. Bland.

305 × 193. Pp. [ii] (v.b.), 6 (l.b.), [8] (descriptions of plates, all versos blank). 4 engr. plates by J. Carmichael. Blue tinted paper. NI. At end: Sydney ... October and November, 1855.

Description and plans of a flying boat—a steerable balloon, propelled by steam and sail. It is considered that such craft would shorten the time of passage to London from 2–3 months to 4 or 5 days, and could be used for passanger and mail services, meteorological and other investigation, and exploration.

DL copy in full tooled morocco, lettered in gold: 'Capt. Weston J. P. from the Inventor.'

Copies: DL, FC, ML. 339

Seven views of the atmotic ship consisting of ... [4 lines] Atmotic ship. Invented by William Bland March 10th 1851. Drawn and lithographed by W. L. Hutton, C. E. Sydney

428 × 273. Pp. [4] (title, v.b.; text, v.b.). 7 pl. (hand-coloured). ND.

Notes that plans were sent to England to be registered for patent, 15 April 1851.

Copies: ML. 340

Atmotic ship. By the Hon. W. Bland, M.L.C. [Text begins.]

581 × 459. Single leaf, v. b. 6 cols. Title at head of col. 1. 4 diagrams. ND. Colophon—Syd.: Printed by David Mason, Machine Printers ...

Copies: ML, NL. 341

Sanitary reform of towns and cities. ... Sydney: J. Cox and Co. ... 1857.

215 × 140. Pp. 32. Read at Phil. Soc. NSW, 8 July, 1857. Also with Soc. papers, *Syd. Magazine of Science and Art*, v. 1, 1858.

A public health plan for Sydney, including drainage and filling of waterfront areas, control of harbour pollution, and provision of parks and baths.

ML copy bears author's inscription to Sir Alfred Stephen.

Copies: ML, SLS, SLV. 342

Services rendered to New South Wales by W. Bland. Sydney: Printed and published by Alexander W. Douglas, Atlas Office ... 1862.

214 × 138. Pp. 16 (l.b.).

Copies: DL, FC, ML, NL, RACP. 343

The Same. Services rendered to New South Wales by W. Bland, R. N. 4 ed. Syd., J. G. O'Conner, Printer, 1867. Pp. 16 (l.b.). 2 and 3 eds. NS.

Copies : DL, ML, US. 344

Abstract of some of the services rendered to New South Wales by Dr. W. Bland, R. N. [Text follows.]

236 × 183. Single leaf, v. b. ND. NI. [Syd., c. 1867.]

ML and DL copies are inserted, together with following item, in 'Services rendered to NSW by W. Bland, R. N.', 4 ed., 1867. No 344.) Ferguson, 3 : 3790–1 dates these, from evidence of alterations in Dr Lang's hand in Mackaness copy, as c. 1844, though the date suggested above appears more probable.

Copies: DL, ML, NL. 345

Addendum to the abstract of some of the services rendered to New South Wales, by W. Bland, R. N. [Text follows.]

234 × 185. Single leaf, v.b. ND. NI. [Syd., c. 1867.]

Copies: DL, ML, NL. 346

Sale by auction at the late residence of Dr. Bland, (deceased.) College Street, Hyde Park ... 31st July, 1868. Catalogue. Chandler & Co., Auctioneers ... Caxton Printing Office ... Sydney.

201 × 125. Pp. 16 (last 2 blank).

Copies: ML. 347

Account of the duel between William Bland & Robert Case and the circumstances that led thereto, drawn up for posterity by Dr. William Bland. From the original ms. in Dr. Bland's autograph in the possession of the publishers. To which is appended a report of the trial Rex v. Bland, Randall and Fulton, before the Recorder of Bombay, 14th and 17th April 1813. (Extracted from the Bombay Courier.) Sydney: Angus & Robertson. 1892.

255 × 206. Pp. 118 (all versos blank). 33 numbered copies. DL copy (No 1) has gold stamped leather label: 'To his dear Eliza from

her affectionate husband, William Bland.'

Reprinted by Geo. Mackaness, Syd., 1942. 100 signed copies.

The duel with pistols, in which Bland killed his opponent, resulted in trial for murder and seven years transportation.

William Bland (1789–1868) Surg. RN, convict, and first Aust. full-time private practitioner, at his height regarded as the foremost local surgeon, was a leader in the struggle for representative government in the Colony, and, this achieved, a member of legislature. For biog., see especially McIntosh, A. M. (1954), 'The life and times of W. B.', *BPCMUS*, 10, 109; also Dunlop, N. J. (1924), '... William Bland', *Med. J. Aust.*, 2 : 471; McIntosh, A. M. (1956), 'Surgery in Syd. in the 1830s', *Med. J. Aust.*, 1 : 997. For his extensive political bibliog. see Ferguson.

Copies : DL, FC, ML, NL, SLV, US. 348

Bleasdale, John Ignatius

On colonial wines. ... Read before the Royal Society of Victoria, 13th May, 1867. ... (For private circulation only). Melbourne: Stillwell & Knight ... 1867.

198 × 132. Pp. 24.

Reviews Aust. wines. Warns of mental and physical effects of spirit drinking and advocates use of wines 'in the interest of health and morality.'

Rev. J. I. Bleasdale (1822–83) DD, engaged in histological and chemical work for Melb. Hosp. and Govt Analyst, in addition to clerical duties. He was member of Cent. Bd of Health and Hon. Member of Med. Soc. Vic. For obit.: *Roy. Soc. Vic. Trans*, 1884, 21 : 150.

Copies: LNSW, ML, SLV, SLW, UQ. 349

Bonwick, James

Daily life and origin of the Tasmanians. ... London: Sampson Low, Son, & Marston ... 1870. ...

222 × 143. Pp. viii, [ii] (v.b.), 304, 16 (advts). Coloured frontis., 9 pl., 9 figs, 1 flg map. Cloth.

Includes information on food, childbearing, causes of small population, diseases, physical characters.

For notes on author's works on Tas. aborigines, see Plomley, N.J.B., *An annotated bibliog. of the Tas. aborigines*, Lond., 1969.

Copies: DL, FC, ML, NL, SLT, SLV, UA, UM, US. 350

The Same, 2 ed., Lond., 1898.

Copies: ML, NL, SLT, UQ. 351

Climate and health in South Africa ... Revised by W. C. Burnet, Esq., Cape Government Emigration Agent. London: S. W. Silver & Co. ... 1880.

181 × 125. Pp. [ii], 126. P. w.

Copies: ML. 352

Climate and health in Australasia, to which is added a chapter on the land laws of the colony. New South Wales. Edited by James Bonwick ... With map. London: Street & Co. ... and Street Brothers ... 1886. ...

181 × 120. Pp. viii, 84. 1 flg coloured map.

Series of 7 vols—one for each Aust. colony and NZ. Titles similar except for name of colony. Issued separately; or complete in cloth without inclusive title.

Section on health includes: heat effects, opinions on salubrity, disease statistics, past and present health of Syd., native diseases and medicine, colony as health resort.

Copies: ML, NL, SLS, SLT, SLV. 353

Climate and health in Australasia ... Victoria. ... [As No 353]

181 × 120. Pp. viii, 82 (l.b.). 1 flg coloured map.

Includes: health value of eucalypts, hot winds and sickness, diseases, and consumption in Aust.

Copies: ML, NL, SLS, SLT, SLV. 354

Climate and health in Australasia ... South Australia. ... [As No 353]

181 × 120. Pp. viii, 60 (l.b.). 1 flg coloured map.

Includes: healthiness of NT coast and the dry inland areas, tables of disease and deaths for 5 years, climate and consumption, infant mortality in Adel.

Copies: ML, NL, SLT, SLV. 355

Climate and health in Australasia ... Queensland. ... [As No 353]

181 × 120. Pp. viii, 72 (l.b.). 1 flg coloured map.

Includes: Polynesian deaths, northern fever and ague, coastal climate, Toowoomba for consumption, Brisbane health story, aboriginal medical treatment.

Copies: ML, NL, SLT, SLV. 356

Climate and health in Australasia ... Tasmania. ... [As No 353]

181 × 120. Pp. viii (l.b.), 40. 1 flg coloured map.

Includes conditions on W. Coast, Westbury, Launceston, and Hobart, consumption and sea travel.

Copies: ML, NL, SLT, SLV. 357

Climate and health in Australasia ... Western Australia. ... [As No 353]

181 × 120. Pp. viii (l.b.), 46. 1 flg coloured map.

Includes: mortality of pearl fishers, New Norcia Mission, health in various parts.

For James Bonwick (1817–1906), schoolmaster and prolific author, see *Aust. Enc.*

Copies: ML, NL, SLT, SLV, SLW. 358

Boothby, Josiah

Statistical sketch of South Australia. ... [Royal Arms] Adelaide: ... W. C. Cox, Govt Printer ... 1876.

217 × 127. Pp. [iii], iv-vi (l.b.), 3–66. 2 flg maps, 1 flg table. P. w. (title rptd).

Includes statistics of population, births, marriages, deaths.

Author was Govt Statist, SA.

Copies: EF, FC, ML, NL, SLS, SLV, UM, UQ. 359

The Same. Adel., 1879.

Copies: ML, NL, SLT, SLV, US. 360

The Same. Pp. 86. 2 flg maps, 1 flg table. Cloth. Lond., Sampson Low ..., 1876.

Copies: ML, NL, SLS, SLV, UA, US. 361

Borthwick, Thomas

A contribution to the demography of South Australia (being the thesis presented to the University of Edinburgh for the degree of M. D. ...) ... London: Bailliere, Tindall and Cox ... 1891.

217 × 140. Pp. 68 (l.b.). 3 graphs, blank on verso, numbered 65–67. Cloth.

Statistics, public health progress and difficulties, health legislation, and remarks on some special diseases.

Copies: EF, FC, HDN, ML, NL, SLS, SLV, UA. 362

Tuberculosis and cancer in cattle. Report by Dr. Borthwick. [Reprinted from *S. A. Register*, October 23, 1894.]

264 × 205. Pp. 2. Title at head of p.l. Colophon: W. K. Thomas & Co. ... Adel.

Copies: SLS. 363

Diphtheria and its treatment by anti-toxic serum. ... Sydney: John Sands, Printer ... 1895.

170 × 110. Pp. 24 (v.b.). P. w. (title rptd).

Copies: SLS. 364

Kensington and Norwood Local Board of Health. The science and art of disinfection in relation to the nursing of infectious diseases A lecture to the nurses of the Adelaide Hospital, by the Hon. Bacteriologist Children's Hospital ... Adelaide: Modern Printing Company ... 1896.

206 × 138. Pp. 12. P. w. (cover title).

Copies: SLS. 365

Quarantine. ... Read before the South Australian Branch of B.M.A.

230 × 163. Pp. [ii], 6. (1897.) Colophon—John Sands ... Syd. P. w. (cover title).

The Same, (with appendix), 1901. Adel.: Vardon & Pritchard. (NL, SLS.)

Copies: NL. 366

Notes on the Health Act, 1898. ... Adelaide: W. K. Thomas & Co., Printers ... Adelaide 1899.

182 × 108. Pp. 28.

For Thomas Borthwick (1860–1923) MD Edin. & Adel., MOH Adel., Hon. Bact. Adel. Hosp., whose laboratory, set up in his home for private and public health work, was probably the first of its kind in Aust., see Hone, F. S. (1924) *Health*, 2 : 80.

Copies: SLS. 367

Bosisto, Joseph

Colonial and Indian Exhibition, 1886. The indigenous vegetation of Australia, with special reference to the Eucalypti. A lecture . . . South Kensington. . . . London: William Clowes & Sons . . . 1886.

204 × 135. Pp. 12.

Joseph Bosisto (1827–98) CMG, MLA, of Richmond Vic., performed extensive work on the pharmaceutical properties of Aust. flora, and was mainly responsible for establishment of the eucalyptus oil distillation industry. He was Pres. of first Pharmacy Board, a founder of Melb. Pharmacy College, and hon. member Med. Soc. Vic.

Copies: NL. 368

Bottrell, E.H.T.

At once or never! A pamphlet with a purpose. By Dr. Bottrell . . . Do not delay, and life's line sever! Waste not a day— "At once—or never". . . . Parramatta & Sydney: C. E. Fuller, Printer.

204 × 135. Pp. 12 (l.b.). ND (c. 1885). P. w. (cover title).

Advertises author's treatment for masturbation.

For E.H.T. Bottrell, MD. Edin. Univ. Chicago, see *NSW Leg. Counc. Rep. Sel. Com. on . . . Practice of Med. and Surg.*, 1887. For another pamphlet, *Such things exist* (NS), he was convicted of distributing obscene literature.

Copies: FC. 369

Bowen, Thomas Aubrey

Testimonials in favour of Mr. Thomas Aubrey Bowen, Licentiate of the King and Queen's College of Physicians, Dublin; Member of the Royal College of Surgeons, England; and Licentiate in Midwifery. [Text begins.]

255 × 193. Pp. 4. ND. Colophon—Clarson, Shallard and Co. . . . Syd. Items dated 1862, 1864.

Copies: NL. 370

Some observations on amaurosis, with illustrative cases. . . . being a paper read before the Medical Society of Victoria, November 7, 1866. [Text begins.]

204 × 120. Pp. 10. Colophon—Wilson and Mackinnon . . . Collins Street East.

Copies: AMAV. 371

Ophthalmic testimonials. Dr. Aubrey Bowen . . .

204 × 127. Pp. [8]. ND. [1867.] NI. P. w. (cover title).

Copies: NL, SLV. 372

On the ophthalmia at the Industrial Schools, Prince's Bridge. . . . [Text begins.]

204 × 127. Pp. 10. Repr., *Aust. med. J.*, Sep., 1867.

Copies: CC, EF. 373

Medical Society of Victoria. Some observations on granular lids, with a case illustrative. Melbourne: Stillwell & Knight . . .

217 × 140. Pp. 8. ND.

T. A. Bowen (1843–1893) MRCS, LKQCPI, established the Ophthalmic and Orthopaedic Instn in 1869. This united with the Melb. Instn for the Eye and Ear the following year, and later became the Vic. Eye and Ear Hosp., of which Bowen was Hon. Surg. till death. See *Aust. med. J.*, 1893, ns 15 : 474; *Austsn med. Gaz.*, 1893, 12 : 282; Williams, D. (1947) *Trans Ophth. Soc. Aust.*, 7 : 5.

Copies: AMAV. 374

See also Gunn, William.

Bowes, Arthur

See No 1090 (note).

Bowie, Robert

A short treatise on cholera; with a few remarks on its practical treatment. . . . London: Charles Gilpin . . . H. Armour . . . Edinburgh . . . 1851. . . .

204 × 127. Pp. 8.

Written for use in Jamaica, where cholera was raging. The disease, due to atmospheric causes, is not contagious, but without doubt is spread by foul water.

Copies: EF. 375

A report of the inquiry into the management of the Yarra Bend Lunatic Asylum, as detailed in the nine days' trial of the action for libel Bowie v. Wilson. Held in the Supreme Court, Melbourne, from ... May 28, to ... June 6, 1862. Melbourne: Wilson and Mackinnon ... 1862 ...

212 × 132. Pp. [ii] (v.b.), 120 (l.b.). Double cols. P. w. (title rptd, book notices outside back wrapper).

Account of action brought by Bowie, Surg.-Supt of Asylum, against Wilson of *The Argus*, for publication of statements on his professional fitness and administration. Plaintiff received £100 damages.

Copies: EF, ML, NL, SLV. 376

A companion to the "Argus" report of Bowie against Wilson. Right versus might. ... [Quotation] The mutilated state-supported record; Michie's speech in defence of Dr. Bowie, delivered in the House of Assembly on the 19th January, 1859, and a few remarks on the pleas of justification and the incomprehensible verdict. By An Unbeliever in the "Argus". ... Melbourne: Printed and published by William Robinson. 1862.

204 × 135. Pp. 16.

A trenchant attack. Includes testimonial to Bowie by Melb. doctors.

Copies: SLV. 377

Testimonials, &c. selected from original documents in the possession of Robert Bowie, ... Melbourne: Printed at the Argus Office ... 1865.

204 × 127. Pp. 16. P. w. (title rptd).

Letters and reports (1827–51) and notes on 'my labours in the cholera districts—England, Wales and Scotland', which Gen. Bd of Health, Whitehall (1851), praises.

For Robert Bowie (1788–1869) MRCS, first Med. Supt of Yarra Bend Lun. Asylum (1852–62), and later of Northcote Vic., see obit., *Aust. med. J.*, 1869, 14 : 313; Brothers, C.R.D., *Early Victorian psychiatry, 1835–1905*, Melb., ND; also Yarra Bend Lun. Asylum.

Copies: EF. 378

Bowker, Robert Steer

Operative treatment of oblique inguinal hernia ... Read before the New South Wales Branch of the British Medical Association.

186 × 122. Pp. 12. ND. Colophon—W. E. Smith ... Syd. Cloth.

R. Steer Bowker LRCPE, MRCS, was Hon. Surg. Syd. Hosp. (1897–1911).

Copies: CC. 379

Bowles, Charles

The people and the state. An address for the benefit of the Victorian Trained Nurses' Association, to help stimulate and enlarge the scope of its work, giving some ... points of the Florence Nightingale work and its later outgrowth for the relief of the sick and wounded. ... Melbourne ... 1887. T. Smith & Co. ... Melbourne.

236 × 145. Pp. 16. P. w. (cover title).

Copies: SLV. 380

Bowman, Edward Barons

Testimonials in favour of Edward Barons Bowman, M. D. Edin., M.R.C.S. Eng., &c. ... Melbourne: Printed by Goodhugh & Hough ...

186 × 122. Pp. 16. ND. P. w.

From British teachers (dated 1856).

Copies: ML. 381

Popular medical fallacies, and rational medicine. ... Part 1.—Quacks and quackeries. "Rogues, cozeners, imposters". Sydney: Clarson, Shallard, & Co. ...

217 × 138. Pp. 20. (1864.) P. w. title rptd).

On quack medical practice. Part 1 only seen.

Copies: ML, SLV. 382

Bowman, Robert

Testimonials in favour of Robert Bowman, M.D., Edin., M.R.C.S., Eng. ... [Appointments] Sydney: Waugh and Cox ... 1855.

196 × 127. Pp. 16 P. w. ('Testimonials' on front).

Mainly from Edinburgh and London teachers (1854).

ML copy has pencilled addition to title: FRCSE, late Medical Officer to the Destitute Children's Asylum, Sec. to the Aust. Med. Assn.

R. Bowman, who came to Sydney in 1855 and was Hon. Phys. Syd. Infirm. (1863–5), died in 1872, aged 43.

Copies: DL, ML. 383

Boyce, Rev. Francis Bertie

The drink problem in Australia or the plagues of alcohol and the remedies ... London National Temperance League Publication Depot ... Australia: Edwards Dunlop & Co., Ltd. Sydney and Brisbane. 1893.

184 × 122. Pp. viii (l.b.), 324. Errata slip. Cloth.
Copies: EF, ML, NL, SLS, SLV, UA. 384

The drink bills of New South Wales . . . Sydney: "Christian World" Printing and Publishing House . . . 1898.
177 × 120. Pp. 30. P. w. (shortened title).
Rev. F. B. Boyce (1844–1931) was Rector of St Paul's, Sydney.
Copies: ML. 385

Boyd, Elton

Vitality: how wasted and how preserved. Nervous debility, neurosthenia, &c., diagnosis and treatment. 14th edition of ten thousand. By Elton Boyd, PhD., M. D., Gy. L., &c., &c., . . . Physician in Chief of the Australian Medical and Surgical Infirmary, Sydney . . .
186 × 122. Pp. [vi], 3–112, [4] (advts). ND. (c. 1884.) P. w. (title rptd).
On 'abuses of the sexual function and the horrors which surely result'; advertises Aust. Med. and Surg. Infirmary, Syd.
Authorship noted on title: *Dyspepsia; Nervous diseases of women*; *Pneumonia, its pathology and treatment*; *Diseases of the heart*; *Physical education of women*. NS.
Copies: EF. 386

See also Australian Medical and Surgical Infirmary.

Boyle, Robert

A sanitary crusade through the East and Australasia. Reprinted from "The Building News", September 2nd, 9th & 16th, 1892. [Cut] London: Robert Boyle & Son, Limited, Glasgow. 1892.
178 × 118. Pp. [vi], 44. 7 pl., 3 figs. Paper boards.
Author travelled 'in the interests of sanitary science and of the well-known ventilating and sanitary appliances of which he is the inventor.' Brief notes on sanitation of Bris., Syd. and Melb.
Copies: DL, ML, NL. 387

Bradley, Henry Burton

No. 4.] [Dec., 1877. Health Society of New South Wales. . . . Health: A lecture delivered before the Health Society of New South Wales . . . Sydney: Printed for the Health Society, by John Sands . . .
209 × 135. Pp. 20 (l.b.). P. w. (title rptd).
Copies: FC, ML, NL. 388

No. 7.] [Oct., 1878. Health Society of New South Wales. . . . House poison: A lecture delivered before the Health Society . . . Sydney: printed for the Health Society, by John Sands . . .
214 × 138. Pp. 16. P. w. (title rptd).
On the dangers of bad sanitation in Sydney.
Copies: FC, ML. 389

No. 8.] [Oct., 1879. Health Society of New South Wales. . . . Life & death: A lecture . . . The Hon. Sir Alfred Stephen, C. B., K.C.M.G., in the Chair. Sydney: Printed . . . by John Sands . . .
198 × 132. Pp. 16 (l.b.).
Copies: FC, LNSW, ML, NL. 390

No. 9.] [March, 1881. Health Society of New South Wales. . . . Domestic economy: Sanitary Section. Twelve lectures on the subject of health. . . . Sydney: Printed . . . by Turner & Henderson . . .
216 × 130. Pp. 44.
Lectures on hygiene, personal and environmental, and its application to family health, for domestic economy classes.
H. B. Bradley (1815–94), lawyer, of Sydney, advocate of health reform and sanitation, was Hon. Sec. of the Society from its foundation.
Copies: LNSW, ML, NL. 391

Braemar House, Woodend, Vic.

Braemar House, Woodend, Victoria. A sanitary sanitorium. Reprinted from the *Building, Engineering and Mining Journal* . . . Melbourne.
209 × 135. Pp. 4. 1 pl., 2 flg plans. ND. (?1898). P.w. (cover title).
Copies: SLV. 392

Braim, Thomas Henry

A history of New South Wales, from its settlement to the close of the year 1844. . . . In two volumes. Vol. 1. London: Richard Bentley . . . 1846.
190 × 115. 2 vols. Vol. 1 : pp. vi, 320, frontis., figs; vol. 2 : pp. [ii], 344, frontis., figs. Cloth.
Chapter: 'The climatology and diseases of Aust.', pp. 223–33.

Copies: DL, FC, ML, NL, SLS, SLT, SLV, SLW, UA, UM, UQ, US. 393

Bramwell's Cardiac Tables

Bramwell's Cardiac Tables.

214 × 138. Pp. 12 (last—colophon only). ND. Colophon—W. E. Smith ... Sydney. P. w. (title rptd).

Tables of differential diagnosis.

Copies: EF, WLC. 394

Brandreth, B.

Dr. Brandreth's Almanack for 1859, containing philosophy of the Brandrethian system; together with the mode of curing disease with Brandreth's pills. Certificates of cure; also, valuable receipts ... and much valuable information. [Verse] Melbourne: ... B. Brandreth, M.D. ... No. 160 Great Bourke Street, East.

198 × 140. Pp. 32. 2 figs. P. w. (cover title).

Copies: E. M. Christie, Melb. 395

Brereton, John le Gay

The Turkish bath in health and disease being a lecture delivered ... Sheffield ... December 16th, 1858 ... [Second edition] Sheffield: Reprinted from the "Sheffield Argus", for F. Smith, Proprietor of the Turkish Bath ...

178 × 122. Pp. 14, [2] (advts). ND.

Preface addressed from Bradford; later eds add: 'and now of Sydney.'

3 ed., 1860. Lond., John Lane. 6 ed., ND. Lond., John Lane.

Copies: EF (2, 3 eds), LNSW (6 ed.), WLC (2 ed.). 396

The Turkish bath. A lecture by John Le Gay Brereton, M.D., of Sydney, delivered in ... Hobart Town, on ... 21st December, 1868, His Excellency Col. T. Gore Browne, C. B., in the chair. Tasmania: Published and sold by Messers. J. Walch and Sons. ... 1869.

204 × 127. Pp. 24. P. w. (title rptd).

Author, who introduced the Turkish bath to Sydney, wrote and lectured extensively on this subject. In his press cutting book in ML, 83 pp. are mainly occupied by his articles on Turkish baths, though some are concerned with homoeopathy and cremation.

Copies: ML, NL, SLT, SLV. 397

One teacher: one law With an appendix on the scriptural use of certain anatomical terms ... George Robertson Melbourne, Sydney, and Adelaide 1883

178 × 122. Pp. 68 (l.b.). P. w. (title rptd).

Another ed., 1883. Pp. viii, 68. James Speirs, London.

John le Gay Brereton (1827–86) MD St And., LRCSE, of Bradford, a prolific poet, came to Sydney in 1859 and practised there till his death. Obit., *Austsn med. Gaz.*, 1886, 6 : 53. For poetry, see Miller.

Copies: EF, ML, NL, SLV, UQ, US. 398

Brett, John

... Report on the cultivation of calf lymph. By John Brett, L.R.C.P. Lond., etc. [Text begins.]

342 × 212. Pp. 82–90. 1 fig. (1891.) Colophon —Robt S. Brain, Govt Pr, Melb.

Supt of Calf Lymph Depot, Melb., on overseas methods of vaccine manufacture and local practice.

Copies: NL. 399

Brickfields Invalid Depot, Hobart

(No. 24.) [Royal Arms] 1864. Tasmania. Legislative Council. Brickfields Invalid Depot. Report for 1863. ...

332 × 206. Pp. 4. Colophon—James Barnard, Govt Pr, Tas.

An. rep. for 1863. Reports (1863–83) appear in Parliamentary Papers of Tas. Institution, for male patients, was previously under Hobart Gen. Hosp. Bd.

Copies: LNSW, SLT, SLV. 400

Bright, John

Hand-book for emigrants, and others, being a history of New Zealand, its state and prospects, ... also remarks on the climate and colonies of the Australian Continent. By John Bright, M.R.C.S. Resident for four years in the Southern Hemisphere. ... London: Henry Hooper ... 1841.

186 × 110. Pp. [iv] (l.b.), 212. Errata slip.

General information; slight in regard to climate and health in Aust. colonies.

Copies: ML. 401

The Same. 2 ed., 1841.

Copies: DL, LNSW, ML, NL, SLV, UM. 402

Bright, Richard

An address to the inhabitants of Van Diemen's Land. ... April, 1850. Hobart Town: ... H.

and C. Best, "Courier" Office ... 1850.

191 × 115. Pp. 12 (l.b.).

Author complains of opposition, 'amounting ... to persecution and conspiracy', since his arrival in VDL seven years before. He writes in 'self defence against attacks ... intended to crush me', and gives examples of his successful practice, and of the 'ignorance and neglect of others.' London testimonials dated 1837 included. See also: Ray, James.

Richard Bright (d. 1862) MD, MRCS, came to VDL in 1842 and practised there for 20 years.

Copies: ML, SLV. 403

Brisbane Hospital

Rules and Regulations of the Brisbane Hospital. 1855. Brisbane: ... James Swan, "Courier" Office. 1855.

205 × 132. Pp. 8. P. w. (cover title).

Title became 'Royal Brisbane Hosp.', 1967. For history, see: 'Some old hospitals', *Austsn med. Gaz.*, 1912, 31 : 340; Jackson, E. S., 'Hist. notes from ... the Brisbane Hosp.', *Med. J. Aust.*, 1922, 1 : 685 and 1923, 1 : 281; Powell, O. W. (1967), 'The early development of the Royal Bris. Hosp.: 1848–1867', *Med. J. Aust.*, 1 : 685.

Copies: Roy. Bris. Hosp. 404

———

Seventh Annual Report of the Brisbane Hospital Committee; laid before the Annual General Meeting of Governors 17 January, 1856. Brisbane: James Swan, "Courier Office". 1856.

205 × 133. Pp. 8.

Copies: Roy. Bris. Hosp. (7, 1856–), SLV (47–53, 1895–1900). 405

———

Rules and Regulations of the Brisbane Hospital, together with the Ward Regulations; also, the Benevolent Asylums Act and the Hospitals Act. Brisbane: W. Fairfax, Printer. ... 1862.

205 × 132. Pp. 12.

Copies: Roy. Bris. Hosp. 406

———

Regulations for the Internal Management of the Brisbane Hospital, relating to wardsmen, nurses, servants, patients and visitors. Brisbane: Printed by Belbridge & Atkin ... 1869.

162 × 102. Pp. [ii], 6 (l.b.).

Copies: Roy. Bris. Hosp. 407

———

Rules of the Brisbane Hospital. Brisbane: Printed by Thorne & Greenwell ... 1870.

205 × 133. Pp. 10 (l.b.).

Other editions: 1871, 1873, 1883, 1886, 1896.

Copies: Roy. Bris. Hosp. 408

———

Bye-Laws for the Internal Management of the Brisbane Hospital ... Brisbane: Printed by Thorne & Greenwell ... 1872.

205 × 133. Pp. 12 (l.b.).

Other editions: 1874, 1879, 1886, 1893, 1899.

Copies: Roy. Bris. Hosp. 409

———

The Brisbane Hospital: Facts about its development, management &c. [Views of building and decorations].

168 × 127. Pp. 16. Illustns. P. w. (title rptd, printing all sides). Bris.: Muir and Morcom ... 1892.

Copies: FC. 410

———

The hospital question. Verbatim report of meeting of medical men in Brisbane ... Together with opinions of Professor Anderson Stuart and others. Brisbane: Muir & Morcom ... 1892.

217 × 140. Pp. 28. P. w. (title rptd).

On a dispute between the Hosp. Committee and the hon. med. staff on the status of the latter.

Copies: ML. 411

Brisbane Hospital for Sick Children

See McConnel, Mrs. Mary.

British Medical Association—Ballarat Branch

Proposed by-laws of the Ballarat Branch, British Medical Association.

408 × 357. Single leaf, v.b. 3 cols. ND. NI.

Proof sheet, amended by hand. Laid down with minutes of Ballt Dist Med. Assn of 25 Jan. 1893.

Copies: DOS. 412

British Medical Association—N.S.W. Branch

Proceedings of the New South Wales Branch of the British Medical Association, from February to December, 1880. Sydney: A. W. Beard ... Ben Franklin Printing Office ...

212 × 138. Pp. vi, [ii] (v.b.), 5–64, [ii] (v.b.). P. w. (title rptd).

Copies: LNSW (1880–91), ML (1880). 413

Scale of fees adopted by the New South Wales Branch of the British Medical Association ... 15th Aug., 1883. [Text begins.]

342 × 124. Single leaf, v.b. Decorated heading, capitals and frame in red.

Copies: EF. 414

British Medical Association. Report of the New South Wales Branch for 1883–84. L. Bruck ... Sydney. 1884.

188 × 153. Pp. 16.

Contains list of officers and members.

Copies: ML. 415

British Medical Association. Report of the annual meeting of the New South Wales Branch ... April 6, 1888. Sydney: L. Bruck ... 1888.

178 × 122. Pp. 20.

Includes Pres. Address by J. Mildred Creed, list of members.

Copies: ML. 416

Memorandum and articles of association of the New South Wales Branch of the British Medical Association.

220 × 140. Pp. 18 (l.b.). ND. [1895.] Colophon—W. A. Pepperday & Co. ... P. w. (title rptd).

Copies: ML. 417

British Medical Association—South Australian Branch

Report of the Council of the South Australian Branch of the British Medical Association for 1879–80. Minutes of the Annual Meeting ... June 24, 1880 ... Adelaide: Frearson and Brother ... 1880.

196 × 127. Pp. 8.

Includes by-laws.

Branch founded 1879. For history, see Corbin, J. (1929), *Med. J. Aust.*, 2 : 354.

Copies: AMAV, UA. 418

Proceedings of the South Australian Branch of the British Medical Association, for the year ending 30th June, 1881. Adelaide: Frearson and Brother ... 1881.

200 × 133. Pp. 54.

Reports of monthly meetings, with case reports and papers given (some with litho. plates).

Copies: ML (1890–2), UA (1880–92). 419

British Medical Association—Victorian Branch

British Medical Association. Report of the Victorian Branch. 1879–80. Melbourne: Stillwell and Co. ... 1880.

207 × 127. Pp. 16.

Contains Pres. Address and list of members. Branch founded 1879.

Copies: AMAV (1881/2–1883/4), EF (1881/2, 1882/3), SLV (1879/80, 1881/2). 420

By-Laws of the Victorian Branch of the British Medical Association.

210 × 135. Pp. 6. ND. Colophon—Stillwell and Co. ... P. w. (cover title).

Copies: AMAV, SLV. 421

Broadbent, John

The Australian botanic guide, being a family hand-book of botanic treatment. By John Broadbent, practical medical herbalist. Melbourne: Kemp & Boyce ... 1887. ...

186 × 122. Pp. [vi], 189, [iii]. Errata slip. Woodcut frontis., 11 pl. Cloth.

'... the herbal system has rescued thousands from an early grave ... and thousands who had been given up by doctors owe their present health to Nature's remedies.'

Copies: BG, EF, KFR, ML, RACP, SLV. 422

The Same. 2 ed., 1889. Melb.: Centennial Printing & Publishing Co.

Copies: ML, OL. 423

Botanic multum in parvo being an index of diseases and their treatment with botanic remedies ... Melbourne: ... John Broadbent & Sons ... 1895. Peacock Bros., Printers ...

163 × 110. Pp. 90, (vi) (l.b.). Frontis. portrait.

Copies: SLV. 424

See also *Australian Botanic Practitioner*.

Brodie, Sir Benjamin Collins
See Beer, Frederick; Parton, James.

Brodribb, T. and Springthorpe, John William
Manual of health and temperance by T. Brodribb, M. A., Inspector-General of Schools, Victoria; with appendix on infectious diseases and ambulance work, by J. W. Springthorpe . . . Melbourne: Printed for the Education Department by Robt. S. Brain, Govt Printer. 1891.

196 × 122. Pp. [ii] (v.b.), vi (ii, iv blank), 166 (l.b.), [ii] (l.b.). Cloth.

2 ed., 1901. English ed. (for Sheffield School Board) appeared soon after 1891 ed., and 2 ed. followed. 3 Eng. ed., 1904.

'In 1889 an Amending Education Act . . . provided that in all (Victorian) State Schools lessions should be given on temperance and the laws of health.' Book was designed to provide teaching material for this.

Copies: AMAV, CC, DOS, EF, KFR, LNSW, ML, NL, SLT, SLV, UA, UM, UQ. 425

Brodzky, Maurice
Genius, lunacy, & knavery A story of a colonial physician . . . Melbourne: Walker, May & Co. . . . 1876.

196 × 115. Pp. 30, [2] (book notice, v.b.). P. w. (title rptd, advts both sides of back wrapper).

Life of Dr David Hailprin, a Polish Jew of brilliant scholarship, but apparently unscrupulous and unbalanced. Among the many positions he held in Europe was that of Chief Rabbi of Bukarest. He practised at Sandhurst Vic. in 1860, and died soon after.

EF. copy, formerly in Sir Baldwin Spencer coll., bears author's inscription to Dr Neild, mentioned as having supplied information on Hailprin.

Copies: CC, EF, FC, LNSW, ML, NL, SLV. 426

Bromby, John Edward
No. 17. April, 1883. Australian Health Society, Melbourne. The emunctories . . . A lecture delivered . . . 18th September, 1882. . . . Melbourne: M'Carron, Bird & Co. . . . 1883.

212 × 140. Pp. 16. P. w. (title rptd).

'The meaning of the word "emunctory" is a pocket handkerchief . . . The use of . . . (this) I regard as a token of far advanced civilisation.'

Rev. J. E. Bromby (1809–89) DD, was first Principal, Church of England Grammar School Melb.

Copies: EF, ML, NL, SLS, SLV, UM. 427

———

Second series of lectures under the auspices of the Early Closing Association. Creation versus development. A lecture delivered at . . . Melbourne on August 8, 1870 . . . Melbourne: . . . S. Mullen . . . 1870. Fergusson & Moore, Printers . . .

204 × 132. Pp. 24. P. w. (cover title).

Supports theory of evolution, which is not antagonistic to the idea of a personal creator. *See* Mozley, Ann (1967), 'Evolution and the climate of opinion in Aust., 1840–76', *Victorian Studies*: 428.

Copies: EF, ML, NL, SLS, SLV, SLW, UM, US. 427a

Brook, Maiben
See Knaggs, S. T., No 1101.

Brooks, S. W.
Charity and philanthropy: a prize essay (historical, statistical, and general) on the institutions in Sydney which aim at the diminution of vice, or the alleviation of misery. And are supported wholly, or in part, by the gifts of the charitable. By Rev. S. W. Brooks . . . Published gratis by W. B. Campbell. Sydney: F. Cunninghame & Co. . . . 1878.

212 × 138. Pp. 46, [ii] (l.b.). P. w. (title rptd) or cloth.

A comprehensive survey, includes: Health Soc. of NSW, Syd. Infirm. and Dispens., Prince Alfred Hosp., St Vincent's Hosp., Instn for Deaf, Dumb and Blind, Benev. Soc., and Children's Hosp. (proposed establishment).

Copies: FC, LNSW, ML, NL, SLS, UQ. 428

Brouardel, Paul Camille Hippolyte
See Benham, Frederick L.—Translator.

Brown, Alexander M.
The medical report of the Destitute Children's Asylum. Randwick, 30th April, 1867. [Text begins.]

344 × 217. Pp. 4. Blue paper.

Reports 65 deaths in mixed epidemic from 1 Jan. to 30 April 1867. Main causes of death: measles 25, cancrum oris 8, diarrhoea 7, convulsions 6, typhoid fever 5. Total of inmates not shown, though 660 attended annual picnic on 26th Feb.

Copies: RACP. 429

Wintering at Menton, on the Riviera, a compagnon de voyage, with hints to invalids.

NS. Review, *NSW med. Gaz.*, 1873, 3 : 138.

A. M. Brown MD, left Sydney in 1871, after 17 years practice, during which he was Phys. Syd. Infirm. and Destitute Children's Asylum, Surg. St Vincent's Hosp. 430

Brown, D. Kinnear

Small-pox! A treatise showing the origin of the disease; examining the theory of vaccination; pointing out necessary sanitary regulations and affording a theory of disinfection and deodorization. ... compiled and written with the assistance of the best authorities ... Sydney: J. G. O'Connor ... 1881.

207 × 137. Pp. 16 (l.b.).

Author edited *The history of the year; a record of the chief events ... 1884, Syd.*, 1885; *The history of the year ... 1885*; Syd., 1886.

Copies: ML. 431

Brown, Edwin

Melbourne as it is, and as it should be. A letter addressed to James Butters, Esq., late Mayor of Melbourne, upon the sewage of the city. ... Benalla: John Liston, Printer ... 1868.

220 × 138. Pp. 8.

Describes Melb. drainage and offers scheme for removal of filth, suppression of nausea and effluvium, and relief from Yarra floods. Author was Engineer, Benalla District.

Copies: ML. 432

Brown, Isaac Baker

Australia for the consumptive invalid: the voyage, climates, and prospects for residence ... London: Robert Hardwicke ... 1865.

191 × 127. Pp. viii, 138. Erratum slip. Flg coloured map. Cloth.

Written for invalids, to give author's 'experience of the Australian climate ... and practical directions for the voyage and arrival.' Reviewed, *Aust. med. J.*, 1866, 11 : 155. Author was surg. supt in Emigration Service.

Copies: FC, ML, NL, SLS, SLV. 433

Brown, John Croumbie

African fever and culture of the blue gum-tree to counteract malaria in Italy. ... Aberdeen: ... W. &. W. Lindsay ... 1890.

183 × 122. Pp. 50, iv (advts).

Recommends planting of eucalypts round dwellings as antimalarial measure. Report on culture of *E. globulus* in the Pontine marshes, by A. Vallee, included.

Copies: SLV. 434

Brown, Ralph

A delineation of the character, talents, physiological developments and natural adaptations of M .... By Rev. Ralph Brown. With a table ... naming over 200 pursuits in life, and showing those for which by Nature .... is best adapted. Melbourne: Mason, Firth & M'Cutcheon, General Printers ... 1892.

220 × 138. Pp. 54. Frontis., 68 figs. P. w. (with 'Seventh Edition. Physiological and phrenological chart ...' and phrenological diagram, on front).

Phrenologist's report, in which passages of text, considered applicable to patient, are marked.

Copies: EF, FC. 435

Browne, Hugh Junor

The higher branch of science or materialism refuted by facts. ... read at the Hall of Science, Melbourne, on the 15th August, 1884, which was written with the intention of being read at a meeting of the Royal Society of Victoria, but which was declined by the Council of that conservative association. ... W. H. Terry ... Melbourne.

178 × 125. Pp. 40. ND. P. w. (title, decorated, rptd; author's publications on verso of back wrapper).

'Those who have witnessed ... mesmerism, biology, hypnotism, and clairvoyance, know that the greatest powers of mind are manifested when apparently not one of the physical senses are in use ... (Man) must possess an independent organism ... to account for the phenomena.' This spiritual faculty persists after death. He attacks the conservatism of scientists in regard to spiritualistic investigation, and resigns from Roy. Soc. of Vic. until it 'becomes less illiberal and intolerant.'

Copies: EF, ML, SLV. 436

Browning, Colin Arrott

An address to the prisoners debarked from the "Surry", at Sydney, December 8, 1831;—the

"Arab", at Hobart Town, July 5, 1834;—and the "Elphinstone", at Hobart Town, May 30, 1836. By the Medical Officer, in charge during the voyage. Hobart-Town: Printed by James Ross, 1836.

186 × 107. Pp. [ii], 118 (l.b.), [ii] (errata).

Moral and religious exhortation.

Copies: FC, ML, NL, SLT, SLV, SLW, UM. 437

An address to the women who debarked at Sydney, New South Wales, from the transport ship Margaret, on the 26th August, 1840 ... Sydney: Printed by James Tegg, George Street. 1841.

178 × 107. Pp. vi, 110. Errata slip. Cloth.

Educational and religious instruction. Two ML copies bear author's inscriptions.

Copies: CC, DL, FC, LNSW, ML, NL, SLT, SLV, US, WLC. 438

England's exiles; or, a view of a system of instruction and discipline, as carried into effect during the voyage to the penal colonies of Australia. ... London: Darton and Clark. ... 1842.

188 × 112. Pp. xii, 238. Cloth.

Other editions appeared, with substantial modifications, in combined vol. with *The convict ship* : 2 ed., 1847; 3 ed., 1848; 4 ed., 1849; 5 ed., 1851; 6 ed., 1856.

Describes the system of humane administration and educational and religious instruction developed by author, as surg.-supt of convict ships, for attempted reform during voyage. Appendix on health deals with hygiene, clothing, diet, exercise and diseases. Described by Verso, M. L. (1950), 'A medical account of a voyage on a convict vessel', *Med. J. Aust.*, 1 : 625.

Copies: FC, LNSW, ML, NL, SLT, SLV, SPH, UM. 439

A brief word of advice to the men who disembarked at Hobart Town from the ship "Earl Grey", on the 20th day of January, 1843. ... Van Diemen's Land: James Barnard, Government Printer, Hobart Town. 1843.

212 × 135. Pp. 40. P. w. (title rptd).

Copies: ML, NL, Roy. Soc. Tas. 440

The convict ship; A narrative of the results of scriptural instruction and moral discipline as these appeared on board the "Earl Grey", during the voyage to Tasmania: with brief notices of individual prisoners. ... London: Smith, Elder & Co. ... 1844.

191 × 110. Pp. xvi (ii, xii, xvi blank), 324. Errata slip. Cloth.

Further editions were published, with modifications, in combined vol. with *England's exiles*: 2 ed., 1847; 3 ed., 1848; 4 ed., 1849; 5 ed., 1851; 6 ed., 1856.

US eds, reprinted from 4th Eng. (combined) ed.—Philadelphia: Lindsay & Blakiston, 1850; N. Y.: Robert Craighead, 1855. (Both in FC.)

Supplements author's account of reform measures described in *England's exiles.* These were supported by official instructions, which required surgeons-supt 'to promote a religious and moral disposition in the convicts.' Author suffered severe post-mortem infection during this voyage.

ML copy has author's inscription to Sir George Arthur, 1845.

Copies: BG, DL, FC, ML, NL, SLT, SLV, US. 441

The convict ship, and England's exiles. In two parts. By Colin Arrott Browning, M.D. Surgeon, Royal Navy. Second edition. ... [Biblical quotations] London: Hamilton, Adams & Co. ... 1847.

163 × 102. Pp. xii, 414. Cloth.

The two works combined in this book are condensed, with added communications from prisoners and new matter in appendix. This vol. is referred to as the 2 ed. of each of its component works.

Colin Arrott Browning MD, Surg. RN, served as surg.-supt of convict ships to Australia nine times between 1831 and 1848, with interposed service in war vessels. He was devoted to reform and education, with the organisation of which the greater part of his works are concerned. Few pages are given to health, though his medical efficiency is shown by the exemplary health record of his voyages.

Copies: AMAV, EF, ML, NL, SLT, UA, UQ. 442

The Same. 3 ed. Pp. xii, 352 (l.b.). Lond., Hamilton, Adams, 1848.

Copies: FC, LNSW, SLT, US. 443

———— *The Same*. 4 ed. Pp. xii, 352. Lond., Hamilton, Adams, 1849.
Copies: FC, LNSW, ML, SLV, SLW, US. 444

———— *The Same*. 5 ed. Pp. xvi, 368. Lond., Hamilton, Adams, 1851.
Copies: ML, NL, US. 445

———— *The Same*. 6 ed. Pp. xvi, 276. Lond., Nisbet, 1856.
Copies: SLT. 446

———— **and Willson, Robert William**
Christianity amongst convicts. Reformation and prevention. Dr. Browning and Bishop Willson. (Issued by the Howard Association . . . London, E. C. [Text begins.]
212 × 130. Pp. 4. ND. (1891.)
Brief accounts of life and work of Browning and of Bishop R. W. Willson (*q.v.*).
Copies: ML. 447

Brownless, Sir Anthony Colling
An address delivered in the University of Melbourne, at the annual matriculation of students, on 29th February, 1868. ... Melbourne: Printed at the 'Age' Office . . .
165 × 107. Pp. 24 (l.b.).
Vice Chancellor's address. Notes recognition of recently established Melb. med. course (1862) in Britain, including adoption of certain of its regulations by Univ. Lond.
Copies: EF, ML, SLV, UM. 448

———— An address delivered to the University of Melbourne, at the annual matriculation of students, on March 5th, 1870. . . . Melbourne: Stillwell and Knight . . . 1870.
217 × 132. Pp. 12 (l.b.). P. w.
Copies: ML, SLV, UM. 449

———— An address delivered in the University of Melbourne at the annual matriculation of students, on March 4th, 1871. ... Melbourne: Stillwell and Knight . . . 1871.
186 × 122. Pp. 12 (l.b.).
Includes history of University.
Copies: ML, SLV, UM. 450

———— The University of Melbourne. Chancellor's address at the Annual Commencement, 4th April, 1891. Melbourne: Edgerton & Moore . . . 1891.
207 × 162. Pp. 24 (l.b.). P. w. (title rptd).
Announces recognition of Melb. med. degrees by Gen. Med. Council of Gt Britain.
Chancellor's annual reports signed by Brownless were issued in same format, 1891–96. They contain information on the Melb. Med. School.
For Sir Anthony Colling Brownless (1817–97) MD St And. & Melb., FRCS, founder of the Melb. Med. School (1862), Vice Chancr (1858–87) and Chancr (1887–97) Univ. Melb., Hon. Phys. Melb. Hosp., see obits, *Austsn med. Gaz.*, 1897, 16 : 610, and *Intercol med. J. Austsia*, 1898, 3 : 44; also No 46.
Copies: ML (1891–3, 1895–6), NL (1892–3, 1895, 1896), SLV (1892, 1896–7), UM (1891–7). 451

Bruce, Alexander
Report on pleuro-pneumonia ... Sydney: Thomas Richards, Govt Printer. 1868.
239 × 153. Pp. 24 (l.b.).
History, cause, symptoms, pathology and treatment (including inoculation and preventive measures).
Author was Chief Inspr of Stock, NSW.
Copies: ML, SLS, SLV. 452

———— **and Loir, Adrien**
Les maladies du bétail en Australie par MM. A. Bruce, Inspecteur en chef du bétail, à Sydney et A. Loir, Directeur de l'Institut Pasteur australien. [Text begins.]
229 × 153. Pp. 8 (l.b.). ND. (1891.) Colophon: Sceaux,—Imp. Charaire et fils. Repr., *Ann. Inst Pasteur*, 1891 : 177.
On the Pasteur mission, of which Loir was leader; anthrax and the Pasteur vaccination; pleuropneumonia and Loir's experiments for Qd Govt; scab in sheep; animal quarantine.
For A. Loir and l'Institut Pasteur Australien see No 1171.
Copies: EF, ML, OL. 453

Bruck, Ludwig
A true copy of the depositions taken as evidence at the investigation by the City Coroner of Sydney, relating to a recent case of gastrotomy. ... With appendix. Sydney: L.

Bruck, Medical Publisher ... 1881.

214 × 138. Pp. 48. P. w. ('The case of Susan Nixon ...' on front, publisher's advts all other sides).

A normally pregnant patient dies of peritonitis following operation, under mistaken diagnosis of extra-uterine pregnancy. Includes letters to press from doctors involved. Discussed in *Aust. med. J.*, 1881, ns 3 : 291.

Copies: DL, FC, LNSW, ML, SLV, US. 454

———

Bruck's list of unregistered medical practitioners in Australia and New Zealand. Reprinted from the appendix of the "Australasian Medical Directory and Handbook". ... Sydney: ... "Australasian Medical Gazette" Office (L. Bruck.) 1886.

210 × 138. Pp. 16.

Lists med. colleges of America not recognised in US, and unregistered practitioners for each Aust. state.

Copies: EF, ML, SLS. 455

———

Guide to the health resorts in Australia, Tasmania, and New Zealand. Edited and compiled by Ludwig Bruck ... Centennial edition. Published at the "Australasian Medical Gazette" Office ... Sydney. London: Bailliere, Tindall & Cox ... 1888.

183 × 117. Pp. [2] (advts), viii, 183, xii (advts). Cloth.

Describes over 200 resorts, with analysis and special indications of mineral waters, climatology, and classification according to therapeutic indications.

Copies: AMAV, CC, EF, BG, KFR, ML, NL, OL, RACP, SLS, SLT, SLV, UA, US. 456

———

The mineral springs of Australia. ... Reprinted from "Australasian Medical Gazette" for January, 1891. L. Bruck ... Sydney. 1891.

229 × 178. Pp. 10. P. w. (cover title).

An extension of author's *Guide to the health resorts in Australia*. For later review of subject see Springthorpe, J. W. (1914), *Therapeutics, dietetics and hygiene*, Melb.: 815.

Copies: US. 457

———

The sweating of the medical profession by the friendly societies in Australasia. ... Sydney: L. Bruck ... London: Bailliere, Tindall and Cox.

156 × 90. Pp. [iv], 60. ND. (1896.) P. w. (title rptd).

Copies: ML, NL. 458

———

On the uses and abuses of the public hospitals in Australia, Tasmania, and New Zealand. With thirty-two practical suggestions for reform. ... Sydney: L. Bruck ... 1899.

153 × 102. Pp. 72.

Criticism of Aust. public hospitals, including management, hon. appointments, training, and financial abuses, with suggestions for reform. Review, *Austsn med. Gaz.*, 1899, 18 : 410 (notes gratuitous distribution by author).

L. Bruck (1849–1915), native of Silesia, an enterprising medical publisher of Sydney, came to Australia about 1873. In 1881 he founded *Austsn med. Gaz.*, which he conducted to 1894.

Copies: AMAV, ML, NL, SLV. 459

———

See Australasian Medical Directory and Handbook.

Bryant, James

Observations on the prevailing fever, and on medical ethics. By James Bryant, Fellow of the Medical Society of London, &c.

NS. Announced in *The Tasmanian*, 15 April 1831, as 'to be published next week, in 8vo.' (Note by E. A. Petherick, NL.) 460

Buchanan, David

An evil little thought of and seldom talked of. Reprinted from the *Sydney Morning Herald.* [Text begins.]

217 × 138. Pp. 4. ND. [187–.] Colophon—Lee & Ross ... Syd.

Also appears (abridged) in *The Sydney slang dictionary*, Syd., ND.

Discusses causes of prostitution.

Copies: ML. 461

Bull, Richard Joseph

See Cherry, Thomas, and Bull, R. J.

Bulmer, Thomas Sanderson

Cosmical view of chemistry, and its relations to cholera and other diseases. Montreal: J. Lovell, 1866.

NS. Listed *SGC*, ser. 1. 8vo. Pp. 30. 462

———

Small-pox: its origin, signs, and symptoms; also the germ and contagion theories . . . Part 1. . . . In six parts . . . published by the Author. Melbourne. 1884.

181 × 122. Pp. vi, 112 (l.b.). Cloth.

Another issue, 1884. Small paper. Paper boards.

Preface (from Sanatory Station, Point Nepean) states: 'Under the . . . disorganised, unworkable, and incompetent Board of Health . . . knowledge and experience as regards Small-pox has been diverted . . . reeling like a Bacchanalian through the sloughs and quagmires of error—whilst this fatal disease has been mowing down its myriad of victims.' Bd of Health dispensed with author's services. Part 1 only seen.

T. S. Bulmer MD Toronto (1867) was Supt Quarantine, Wellington NZ and later of Quarantine Stn, Vic. He was in Fitzroy Vic. in 1886 and apparently left Aust. soon after. Publication noted in above: *Physiological chemistry in its relations to anatomy and med.* NS.

Copies: LNSW, SLV. 463

——— **"Nabi Cosmos"**

A series of private notes and memo for thinking men. By "Nabi Cosmos". Belfast [Vic], 1879.

204 × 130. Pp. [50]. Colophon—W. Earle, Belfast, Vic.

Devoted mainly to 'Notes on Darwinism.' Concludes with 'End of Book 1', and notes that following books would shortly appear: 2—Origin of organic matter and world; 3—History and origin of man; 4—Physiological chemistry . . . ; 5—The brain and nerves; 6—Instincts in man and animals; 7—Origin of animal kingdom. Book 1 only seen. Authorship noted in item above.

Copies: LNSW. 464

———

See Headley, Walter Balls–, No 861.

Burdett, Henry Charles

Hospitals and asylums of the world: their origin, history, construction, administration, management, and legislation; with plans of the chief medical institutions accurately drawn . . . In four volumes and portfolio. Volume 1. Asylums—history and administration. London: J. & A. Churchill . . . 1891.

263 × 173. 5 vols. Vol. 1: pp. xvi, 702 (l.b.); vol. 2: pp. xx, 348, [4], 18 plans; vol. 3: pp. xxiv, 944; vol. 4: pp. xlvi, 463; vol. 5 (plans). Vols 1 and 2 published 1891; vols; vols 3 and 4, 1893.

Brief section on Aust. colonies occurs in vol. 3, pp. 383–401. Review, *Austsn med. Gaz.*, 1892, 11 : 299, reasonably describes this as 'scrappy, disjointed, incoherent', and out of date.

Copies: HDN, LNSW, RACP, SLS, SLV. 465

Burgess, Henry Thomas

The fruit of the vine. The £100 prize essay. . . . Published by the South Australian Total Abstinence League and Band of Hope Union. Adelaide: . . . Webb, Vardon, and Pritchard . . . 1878.

208 × 135. Pp. viii (l.b.), 9–138, 6 (l.b., advts). Cloth.

Includes physiological and medical effects of alcohol.

Copies: EF, ML, NL, SLS, SLV, UA, UQ, US. 466

Burnett, Matthew

Lecture . . . on the triumphs of gospel temperance, in the remarkable conversion of the late Dr. Edward Mitchell of Ballarat, Victoria. None need despair.

176 × 124. Pp. 20 (l.b.). ND. NI. Preface addressed: Bourke NSW, 1887. P. w. (title rptd).

On the reform of 'Dr. Mitchell, the clever oculist, the great inventor, the prince of Victorian gamblers, the man who drank two bottles of brandy daily for years.' Author was a Yorkshire evangelist and social reformer.

Copies: ML. 467

Burrangong District Hospital, Young, NSW

Report of the Committee of the Burrangong District Hospital for the year 1891, submitted at the Thirtieth Annual Meeting of subscribers, together with . . . rules, regulations . . . 1892. . . . "Burrangong Argus" Office, Young.

183 × 127. Pp. 10. P. w. (title rptd).

Copies: FC. 468

Butler, Samuel

The hand-book for Australian emigrants; being a descriptive history of Australia, and containing an account of the climate, soil, and natural productions of New South Wales, South Australia, and Swan River Settlement; the facilities they offer . . . Glasgow: W. R. M'Phun . . . Trongate; N. H. Cotes, London;

W. Whyte & Co., Edinburgh. 1839. Second Thousand.

155 × 95. Pp. viii, 240, [4] (advts). Frontis.—flg map. Cloth.

Introduction includes discussion of health of colonists.

Copies: DL, EF, FC, ML, NL, SLS, SLT, SLV, SLW, UA, UM, US. 469

Byrn, Marcus Lafayette

The book of nature. A full and explicit explanation of all that can or ought to be known of the structure and uses of the organs of life and generation in man and woman. Intended especially for the married, or those intending to marry, and who . . . desire to inform themselves upon . . . conjugal pleasures and duties. By Dr. M. Lafayette Byrn, M.D. To which is added a complete medical treatise upon all diseases of the generative organs . . . Fully depicting the mysterious processes of gestation . . . No such complete panorama of the mysteries of human reproduction has ever before been given to the world. Sydney: The Modern Medical Publishing Company . . .

183 × 120. Pp. 224. Frontis., 60 figs. ND. P. w. (title rptd).

Text interspersed with advts of books on sex, contraceptives, and patent remedies.

Many later undated editions issued by same publishers. In one, author's name is shown as 'Byrne.' In Melb. ed., ND., Will Andrade, with similar text, author appears as Thomas Faulkner MD.

Copies: AMAV, DOS, EF, ML. 470

Bystander, A

See Beaney, James George, No 229.

C

Caffyn, Stephen Mannington

Quacks and quackery being a short exposition of homoeopathy, bone-setting, and other anomalies found in these colonies and elsewhere A lecture ... George Robertson Melbourne ... 1883

209 × 127. Pp. 30 (l.b.).

Copies: SLV. 471

———

... How, when, and what to eat. A guide to colonial diet. ... Melbourne: W. H. Williams ... 1883.

214 × 138. Pp. 22. P. w. (title rptd).

Book notices on back wrapper show author's *The mother's guide to the diseases of infancy and childhood* as in press. NS.

Copies: LNSW, ML. 472

———

Eyes their use and abuse with hints on the treatment of colonial eye diseases ... George Robertson Melbourne ... 1883

217 × 140. Pp. 28. P. w. (title rptd).

S. M. Caffyn (1851–96) MRCS, LRCP, who practised in Syd., Wollongong NSW and Melb., published two novels; *Miss Milne and I*, Lond., 1889, and *Poppy's Tears*, Lond., 1890. For personal account see Hugh McCrae, *My father and my father's friends*, Syd., 1935; also *Austsn med. Gaz.*, 1896, 15 : 538.

Copies: EF, FC, ML, SLV, UQ. 473

Callam, James

A letter from Mr. James Callam, surgeon of His Majesty's Ship Supply, to his brother, Mr. Alexander Callam, of East Smithfield, London; containing an account of a voyage from the Cape of Good Hope to Botany Bay, &c. With a short description of the inhabitants, and settlement of the colony.

8vo. Pp. 22 (l.b.). [London, 1789.]

NS. Noted by G. B. Barton, *History of N.S.W. from the Records*, vol. 1., Syd., 1889, p. 583, as a sixpenny pamphlet which the *Monthly Review*, 1 Dec. 1789, describes as: 'Well enough for a private letter; but too crude and trivial for publication; especially after the variety of more important details which have appeared relative to this new and very singular attempt at colonization.'

474

Cameron, Charles

Copy of a letter from Mr. Charles Cameron, a surgeon in His Majesty's Navy, and late Surgeon of the Fergusson convict ship, to the Commissioners for Victualling His Majesty's Navy, and for the Care of Sick and Wounded Seamen.

198 × 125. Pp. 12 (l.b.). ND. NI. Dated 10 Dec. 1829 from London.

Describes voyage from Ireland to NSW in 1828/9. Scurvy, which occurred in Atlantic, was treated with nitre (obtained from gunpowder) in vinegar or lime juice, and health rapidly improved. Nitre is recommended as the best remedy for scurvy, in the absence of fresh vegetables.

Copies: FC. 475

Cameron, Commin and Martin

The septic tank system of sewage treatment. No chemicals. No sludge. Low cost in construction. Nominal annual expenditure.

220 × 136. Pp. 14, [ii] (colophon only, v.b.). ND. (c. 1899.) Colophon—W. Brooks & Co. ... Syd. P. w. (cover title).

Copies: ML. 476

Cameron, S. S.

Report of Mr. S. S. Cameron, M.R.C.V.S., to the Board of Public Health on the results of his use of tuberculin in cattle in Victoria. ... 18 March, 1899.

309 × 204. Pp. 8. Colophon: Robt S. Brain, Govt Pr, Melb.

Tuberculin as a diagnostic aid.

Copies: NL. 477

Campbell, Allan

How to manage a baby. ... A lecture delivered

at the City Mission Hall, Adelaide . . . Adelaide: . . . Advertiser, Chronicle, and Express Office . . . 1878.

212 × 135. Pp. 16.

Copies: ML, SLS. 478

———

The sanitary aspects of the deep-drainage system of Adelaide . . . [Reprinted from the *South Australian Register*.] [Text begins.]

243 × 158. Pp. 10 (l.b.). Double cols. ND. Colophon—W. K. Thomas & Co. . . . Adel.

Copies: ML. 479

———

The people's health. Interesting notes and suggestions. . . . [From the *S. A. Register*, January, 1898.] [Text begins.]

246 × 156. Pp. 10 (l.b.). Double cols. Colophon—W. K. Thomas & Co. . . . Adel.

For Allan Campbell (d. 1898) LRCPE, LFPS Glas., MLC, Hon. Phys. Adel. Children's Hosp., see *Austsn med. Gaz.*, 1898, 17 : 507.

Copies: ML. 480

———

S. A. Institute of Hygiene and Bacteriology. Inaugural address . . . on tuberculosis, 9th August 1898. Adelaide: W. K. Thomas & Co. . . . 1898.

214 × 138. Pp. 14 (l.b.). P. w. (cover title).

Copies: SLS. 481

Cambell, Francis

An abstract of the letters of Iatros, on lunatic asylums, and the treatment of lunatics. By Francis Campbell . . . [Text begins.]

214 × 132. Pp. 16. ND. [1846.]

Circumstances surrounding publication appear in Bostock, J. (1968), *The dawn of Aust. psychiatry*, Syd. In 1846, following public criticism of Tarban Creek Lun. Asylum, five articles by 'Iatros' appeared in *Syd. Morning Herald*, leaving no doubt that it was 'in a bad way, and needed the genius of Dr. Iatros to solve the problem.' Following public enquiry, Campbell became Supt. See also No 1537.

ML copy bears author's inscription to James Mitchell, Esq.

Copies: ML. 482

———

A commentary on the uses and abuses of tobacco, in its effects on the human constitution, in a series of letters: by (Vox E. Deserto,) Francis Campbell, M.D., M.A., &c. [Verse] Sydney: Published for private distribution. 1850.

173 × 102. Pp. viii (ii blank; v, vi lacking), 210 (last—colophon only), [ii] (erratum, v.b.). Colophon—Syd.: Kemp and Fairfax . . .

History and effects of tobacco, 'published in the hope that it may be the means of tempering the insane rage for smoking, so epidemic in this colony . . . I am convinced [smoking] has consigned thousands to the madhouse, and hundreds of thousands to the ever-rankling affliction of incurable diseases of the stomach and associated organs.'

Copies: ML, US, WLC. 483

———

The Same. 2 ed., with title: *A commentary on the influence which the use of tobacco, exerts on the human constitution* . . . Sydney: Published and sold by all the booksellers, 1853. Pp. x (2 blanks), 206. Errata slip. Colophon—Kemp and Fairfax . . . Syd. Dedicated, as 1 ed., to Francis, Archibald, Hugh, Walter, and John Campbell. Cloth, paper label on spine.

DL copy has dedication and pref., loose, in proof, text with ms. amendments.

Copies: DL, EF. 484

———

The Same. 2 ed., 1853. Pp. xii (lacks v, vi; 2 blanks), 206. Errata slip. Dedicated to Robert Lowe, Esq., M.P.; variations in prelim. matter.

Copies: DL, FC, LNSW, ML, NL, SLV, UA. 485

———

A diary of the grumblings of an invalid, on a cruise from Sydney to Manila, in search of the rosy goddess. Printed for private distribution. Sydney: . . . Empire General Steam Printing Office . . . 1855.

235 × 172. Pp. 42. Double cols. Cloth.

Anonymous. Ascribed by ML to Francis Campbell. A health trip on which the ship *Frances Walker* was wrecked (1854).

For Francis Campbell (d. 1877) MD Glas., Med. Supt Lun. Asylum, Tarban Creek NSW, see obit., *Aust. Practitioner*, 1878, 1 : 128; Bostock, J. (1968), *The dawn of Aust. psychiatry*, Syd., (includes case notes of Campbell); Dawson, W. S. (1965), *Annals of psychiatry in NSW. 1850–1900*, Syd., typescript (ML, RACP).

Also published: *An abstract of all the corn*

laws, Syd., 1844 (DL, LNSW, ML); *A treatise on the culture of flax and hemp*, 2 ed. 1845 (DL, ML, NL, SLV); 3 ed., [1864] (EF, FC, ML, NL, US); 4 ed., [1866] (LNSW).

Copies: ML. 486

Campbell, John

Thirty years' experience of a medical officer in the English convict service. ... London: T. Nelson and Sons ... Edinburgh; and New York 1884

181 × 122. Pp. 140 (l.b.), [4] (book advts). Cloth.

In 1850 author (MD, RN), who made a voyage to Hobart as surgeon-supt of the *William Jardine*, describes voyage, duties, and care of convicts.

Copies: CC, FC, LNSW, NL, SLT. 487

Campbell Town Hospital, Tas.

The Campbell Town Hospital, established November, 1855. ... Tasmania: Printed by John Davies, "Mercury" Steam Press Office. 1861.

206 × 136. Pp. 16. P. w. (title rptd).

Includes rules, report.

Copies: SLT. 488

Campbell Town Hospital. [Text begins.]

317 × 198. Single leaf, v.b. Blue paper. ND. At foot: Printed at the ... "Cornwall Chronicle" Newspaper ... Launceston.

Includes revised rules.

Copies: CC. 489

(No. 31.) [Royal Arms] 1864. Tasmania. Legislative Council. Campbell Town Hospital. Statements of receipts and expenditure, and of cases treated. ... ordered by the Council to be printed, July 13, 1864.

332 × 206. Pp. 4 (l.b.). Colophon—James Barnard, Govt Pr, Tas.

An. rep. for 1863. Reports (1863–93) appear in the Parliamentary Papers, Tasmania (1864–94).

Copies: LNSW, SLT, SLV. 490

Candler, Curtis

See Candler, Samuel Curtis.

Candler, Samuel Curtis—"Mucor"

A theory of the causation, and suggestions for the prevention, of dysentery: together with hypotheses on the causation, and views as to the prevention, of typhoid, cholera, yellow-fever, remittent, diphtheria, typhus, and other zymotic diseases in man and animals. By Mucor. Melbourne: Printed by Clarson, Massina, and Co., and published by George Robertson ... 1873.

181 × 125. Pp. xii (l.b.), 336. Cloth.

In *The prevention of measles* (1889) author acknowledges use of pseudonym 'Mucor'.

A speculative hypothesis on the origin of dysentery, and other diseases named, from fungi in human faeces. Review, *Aust. med. J.*, 1873, 18 : 143, extols work as 'the most original book of the day' and expresses confidence in the soundness of the hypothesis.

Copies: BG, CC, EF, LNSW, NL, SLV, SPH. 491

The prevention of consumption. A mode of prevention founded on a new theory of the nature of the tubercle-bacillus. By C. Candler Melbourne, Victoria London: Kegan Paul, Trench & Co ... 1887

224 × 140. Pp. viii (l.b.), 240, 36 (book notices). Cloth.

Author disagrees with Koch's view that the tubercle bacillus is a purely animal parasite. He suggests that a parent form is wide-spread outside the animal body, and lives readily in house dust. Its spores, on inhalation, may develop into bacilli and cause lung disease, and are so profuse that case to case spread is unimportant and segregation of sufferers ineffective. Tuberculosis could be eradicated by the sterilisation of dwellings. Review, *Aust. med. J.*, 1887, ns 9 : 327.

Copies: LNSW, ML, SLV, UA, UM. 492

The prevention of measles. By C. Candler, Melbourne, Victoria. London Kegan Paul, Trench, & Co. ... 1889

191 × 127. Pp. xvi, 382 (last—colophon only), [ii] (blank), 42 (book notices), [4] (book notice). Cloth.

Supports Salisbury's thesis (1862) that 'straw mildew' is the specific cause of measles, and considers that this arises from inhalation of spores of fungi growing on straw mattresses.

Copies: EF, HDN, ML. 493

Koch's proposed cure for consumption with

suggestions on the prevention of consumption By C. Candler ... Reprinted from "The Argus", Melbourne George Robertson and Company Melbourne, Sydney, and Adelaide 1891

220 × 138. Pp. viii, 64.

Author's views are extended in 'The radical error in Koch's view of the causation of phthisis', *Aust. med. J.*, 1892, ns 14 : 366.

Samuel Curtis Candler, (sometimes listed as Stephen Curtis Candler), District Coroner Melb. from (at least) 1869 to 1900, was notable for his studies of infectious diseases during the period of establishment of the germ theory. These had the weaknesses of their hypothetical, non-experimental basis. Though mentioned in the press as 'Dr' Curtis Candler, he was not registered, as noted in an attack in *Aust. med. Gaz.*, 1869, 1 : 70. In 1910 he was Assoc. Member of Med. Soc. Vic.

Copies: SLV. 494

Cannon, Richard

Savage scenes from Australia by Dr. Richard Cannon formerly Surgeon Royal Navy, etc., etc. being a short history of the settlement at Somerset, Cape York, in the form of a lecture delivered for the Young Men's Christian Association of Valparaiso ... with illustrations by Mary D'Arcy Cannon from sketches by the author. ... Sold by J.P.B. Purves & Co. ... Imprenta del Universo de G. Helfmann—Valparaiso 1885.

238 × 162. Pp. 32. Frontis., 16 pl. P. w. (title rptd).

Humourously described and often grim reminiscences of an expedition from Sydney in 1863, in HMS *Salamander*, to establish a settlement on Cape York. Notes on local aborigines include food, infanticide, treatment of wounds and illness.

Copies: ML. 495

Caraman, Ch. Thomas—

Note sur le miel eucalypté naturel sécrété par les abeilles noires sauvages de Tasmanie (Australasie), dans des ruches énormes, construites par elles au sommet d'eucalyptus gigantesques ... Note lue à l'Académie de médicine le 25 janvier 1887. Macon Imprimerie Protat Freres 1887

216 × 140. Pp. 16, 1 fig. P. w. (amended title and forest scene).

Claims that 'eucalyptus honey' is an effective substitute for codliver oil in wasting diseases, acts like digitalis in heart disease, regulates bronchial secretion, cures malaria, has marvellous activity against tubercular, pneumococcal and typhoid infections, and is of value in gonorrhoea.

Criticised by T. P. Anderson Stuart (No 2055), who states that eucalyptol does not appear in the honey of Aust. bees,

Copies: EF, SLV. 496

Carbolic Acid

Carbolic acid. Circular despatch, from the principal Secretary of State for the Colonies, relative to the use of carbolic acid for arresting the spread of fever. ... Sydney: Thomas Richards, Govt Printer. 1869. ...

198 × 132. Pp. 18.

Copies: ML. 497

Carmichael, Jennings

Hospital children Sketches of life and character in the Children's Hospital, Melbourne By Jennings Carmichael ... George Robertson and Company Melbourne ... 1891.

186 × 122. Pp. [viii] (four blanks), 104. Cloth or p. w.

Authoress (Grace Elizabeth Jennings Carmichael, Mrs. Mullis) (1868–1904), who trained as a nurse at Children's Hosp. Melb., achieved local fame for her poems of the bush. For her life and tragic death, see *All about books*, 1937, 9 : 94.

Copies: DOS, EF, FC, KFR, ML, NL, SLV, UQ, US. 498

Caro, Edgar R.

The bubonic plague. ... A pamphlet for the people in language the people can understand ...

163 × 117. Pp. 24. Colophon—Ed. Lee & Co. ... Syd. ND. [?1900] P. w. (cover title).

Published early in the 1900–1909 Aust. epidemic. Contains advts of Med. & Surg. Sanitarium, Summer Hill, Syd., and of Avondale Health Retreat, Cooranbong NSW. E. R. Caro MD was supt of the former, and ed. of *Herald of Health* (q.v.).

Copies: DL. 499

Carr, Rt. Rev. Thomas Joseph

The morality of medical practice. Infanticide. By His Grace the Archbishop of Melbourne. Re-published from the "Austral Light". ...

Central Agency: W. P. Linehan . . . Melbourne.
242 × 153. Pp. 20. (1900.) P. w. (title rptd).
Another ed., 1900, with variation in title. Pp. 20.
A Roman Catholic pronouncement on craniotomy, caesarian section, etc.
Copies: ML, SLV. 500

Carrington Centennial Hospital for Convalescents, Camden, NSW
. . . [Cut of institution] Report of the Carrington Centennial Hospital for Convalescents, Camden, for the year ending December 31, 1891. . . . Sydney: . . . F. Cunninghame & Co. . . . 1892
217 × 140. Pp. 24. P. w. (cover title).
The Hospital, opened 17 months previously, was founded 'for the purpose of restoring bread winners to health, and thus enabling them to resume their occupation, and . . . is not a refuge for persons suffering from incurable disease, destitution, or permanent infirmity.'
Copies: EF, ML. 501

Carter & Werner
Sight, science, and spectacles. Rational treatment of defective vision. Carter & Werner, ophthalmic opticians . . . Ballarat: E. E. Campbell . . . 1898.
186 × 125. Pp. [ii], 32. 16 figs. P. w. (decorated cover title).
Copies: ML. 502

Cascades Contagious Diseases Hospital, Tas.
(No. 7.) [Royal Arms] 1880. Tasmania. House of Assembly. Contagious Diseases Hospital, Cascades: Report for 1879. . . . ordered by the House to be printed, August 10, 1880.
324 × 206. Pp. 4. Colophon—James Barnard, Govt Pr, Tas.
1st an. rep. Hospital was established under Contagious Diseases Act, for the treatment of venereally infected women.
Reports for 1879–90 appear in Parliamentary Papers of Tas. (1880–91), followed by those of Contagious Dis. Hosp., Hobart, 1891–98.
Copies: LNSW, SLT, SLV. 503

Cascades Hospital for Insane, Tas.
(No. 7.) [Royal Arms] 1878. Tasmania. House of Assembly. Hospital for Insane, Cascades: Report for 1877. . . . ordered by the House to be printed, July 16, 1878.
332 × 206. Pp. 4. Colophon—James Barnard, Govt Pr, Tas.
An. reps. (1877–1890) appear in Parliamentary Papers of Tas. (1878–91).
Copies: LNSW, SLT, SLV. 504

Case of Susan Nixon, The
See Bruck, Ludwig.

Catherine Hayes Hospital, Randwick, NSW
See Society for Relief of Destitute Children, Sydney. Hospital was for inmates of Asylum. For account to 1870, see Oliver, T. J. (1871), *NSW med. Gaz.*, 1 : 142.

Cattanach, H.J.G. & Co.
The removal and utilisation of nightsoil considered in relation to public health and agricultural industry. With a subjoined account of Caldwell's system of removal and manufacture of human excrements into a dry and portable guano. Respectfully submitted for the . . . consideration of municipal and sanitary authorities . . . Published by H.J.G. Cattanach & Co., Sydney.
209 × 135. Pp. 30 (l.b.). ND. [c. 1886.]
Copies: DL. 505

———

The Same. 2 ed. ND. Pp. 60 (l.b.), [2] (inserted leaf in red, v.b.). P. w. (cover title).
Copies: ML. 506

Cayley, C. H.
The plague. Its causes, symptoms, diagnosis, and treatment. By C. H. Cayley . . . Divisional Health Officer, Bombay. Edited by C. Reissmann, M.A., M.B., B.C. (Camb.) . . . Published by E. S. Wigg & Son, Adelaide . . .
214 × 135. Pp. 26 (l.b.). (1900.) P. w. (title rptd).
Charles Henry Reissmann (editor), a recent arrival from London, was later Phys., Consumption Dept. Adel. Hosp., and Med. Supt Kalyra Sanitarium, Belair.
Copies: NL, SLS. 507

'Cerimon'
See Thomson, William, No 2248.

Chandler, Charles Walter
. . . Darkest Adelaide and sidelights of city life. . . . Being a similar series of articles for which the author was sent to gaol a few years ago. Printed and published by Charles Walter Chandler, Adelaide.

212 × 144. Pp. [iv], 88. ND. P. w. (title rptd).

Aspects of prostitution in Adelaide, dedicated 'to the Bludgers of this Fair City, with a sincere wish for their speedy extermination.' Recommends a Contagious Diseases Act, enforcing registration, periodic examination and compulsory treatment of prostitutes.

Copies: ML, NL. 508

Charity Organisation Society of Melbourne

A guide to the Melbourne charities giving their objects, management, finances and statistics of relief. Compiled and published by the Charity Organisation Society of Melbourne. Melbourne: Stillwell and Co., Printers 1888. . . .

217 × 138. Pp. 90.

SLV has an. reps, 1887.8–1898.9.

Copies: NL, SLV. 509

———

Proceedings of the Second Australasian Conference on Charity ... Melbourne ... November, 1891. Convened by the Charity Organization Society of Melbourne. ... Robt. S. Brain, Govt Printer, Melbourne.

214 × 138. Pp. xvi (l.b.), 148 (l.b.). P. w. (title rptd).

Contains information on social work and charitable instns. Addresses include: 'Children of the state in NSW', by Dr Arthur Renwick; 'Nursing the sick poor in their homes', by Miss. F. G. Holden; 'Slum life in Melbourne', by Miss Sutherland (refers to foundation of Melb. Dist. Nursing Soc.); 'The Consumptive Sanatorium at Echuca', by Mrs. G. Serjeant.

Proceedings of 1st Austsn Conference, Melb., Govt Pr, appeared in 1890. (NL, SLT, SLV.)

Copies: FC, ML, NL, SLV. 510

Chemist and Druggist of Australasia

The Chemist and Druggist of Australasia. Established in England—1859. Australia—1866. ... Published on the 1st of each Month. ... Melbourne. Vol. 1. No. 1. [Published monthly.] January 1, 1886 ... [Index follows.]

255 × 191. Pp. iv, 22, v-viii. P. w. (cover title).

After 1920, title became *The Chemist and Druggist and Pharmacist of Australasia*; incorporated in *The Australasian Journal of Pharmacy*, 1934.

Copies: See *SSAL*. 511

Chequered Career, A

See [Nesfield, Henry W.]

Cherry, Thomas

Diphtheria antitoxin. By Thomas Cherry, M.D., M. S. Melb. Demonstrator and Assistant Lecturer in Pathology, University of Melbourne. [Text begins.]

204 × 132. Pp. 6. Colophon—Melbourne: Stillwell and Co. Repr., *Aust. med. J.*, 1895.

Thomas Cherry (1861–1945) MD, MS Melb., Prof. Agriculture and later Cancer Research Fellow, Univ. Melb., held the first Univ. classes in bacteriology. He published *A classbook of practical bacteriology*, 2 ed., Melb., 1908; *Bilharziosis*, Melb., 1917. See obit., *Med. J. Aust.*, 1945, 2 : 129; also King, E.S.J. (1951), 'The story of the Melb. School of Pathology', *Med. J. Aust.*, 2 : 101.

Copies: EF. 512

——— **and Bull, Richard Joseph**

Caseous lymphatic glands (pseudo-tuberculosis) in sheep. ... Reprinted from the "Intercolonial Medical Journal of Australasia" for May 20th, 1899. Melbourne: Stillwell and Co. ... 1899.

268 × 153. Pp. 6. 1 pl.

R. J. Bull (1874–1927) MD Melb., a pioneer of bacteriology in Vic., published (with T. Cherry), *A classbook of practical bacteriology*, 2 ed., Melb., 1908; 3 ed., 1913. See obit., *Med. J. Aust.*, 1927, 1 : 838; also King, E.S.J. (1951), 'The story of the Melb. School of Pathology', *Med. J. Aust.*, 2 : 101.

Copies: NL. 513

Children's Hospital, Melbourne

See Melbourne Hospital for Sick Children.

Ching, J. Lionel, & Co.

Halicore Dugong Australis. [Emblem] J. Lionel Ching & Co. from Launceston (Cornwall), England. Sole Proprietors, Dunheved Island, Queensland. Depots at Townsville, Maryborough, Brisbane, Sydney, Melbourne and New Zealand. J. J. Miller, Printer ... Melbourne.

222 × 135. Pp. 8 (l.b.). ND. P. w. (cover title; print on all other sides).

On dugong oil and its medicinal qualities.

Copies: ML. 514

———

See also Faithfull, Paul.

Chirurgeon

See Van Hemart, Francis Thomas.

Citizens' Vigilance Committee of Sydney

A prophetic forecast. The Citizens' Vigilance Committee of Sydney.

229 × 165. Pp. 4 (2, 4 blank). Pink paper. Repr., Editorial, *Austsn med. Gaz.*, 1900, 19 : 206.

Committee was formed early in the 1900–9 plague epidemic 'for combating the plague and influencing the public in the way of cleanliness and sanitary reform.' Supported by health authorities, it had branches throughout the metropolitan area.

Includes poem by James Inglis, MLA. One verse:

Our shores are strewn with garbage,
But our baths are hard to find,
We have 'Widow's carts', and scavengers,
But our roads with filth are lined—
Dead rats in the roads may fester,
And eels in our mains may crawl;
But serene self-satisfaction sits
Supreme in our smug Town Hall.

Copies: US. 515

Civil Ambulance and Transport Brigade of N.S.W.

The Civil Ambulance & Transport Brigade of New South Wales. Annual report ... 1899–1900. ... Headquarters—Sydney. Supported solely by voluntary contributions. Beatty, Richardson & Co., Printers ... Sydney. ...

183 × 120. Pp. 16 (last—colophon only). P. w. (cover title, with badge in red).

Formed 1896. Name changed to Civil Ambulance and Transport Corps of St John Ambulance Brigade, 1903.

Copies: ML (1899–1900). 516

Claridge, R. T.

Hydropathy; or the system of effecting cures by means of cold water: epitomized from the celebrated work of Captain Claridge, F.S.A. Launceston, V. D. Land: Henry Dowling, Printer & Stationer ... 1846.

216 × 138. Pp. iv (ii blank), 24. P. w.

Claridge's *Hydropathy or the cold water cure* was first published in London, 1842.

Copies: ML, NL, SLV. 517

Clark, Charles Dagnall

1883–4. Legislative Assembly. New South Wales. Education. (Report by Dr. Clark on the sanitary condition of the public schools in the City of Sydney and suburbs; also report of Dr. Mackellar.) Ordered ... to be printed, 27 February, 1884. [Text begins.]

320 × 204. Pp. 16. Colophon—Syd.: Thomas Richards, Govt Pr. 1884.

For C. D. Clark (1856–1901) MB Lond., Hon. Phys. Syd. Hosp., who practised at N. Sydney, see obit., *Austsn med. Gaz.*, 1901, 20 : 259.

Copies: LNSW, ML, NL, SLV. 518

Clark, Sir James

The sanative influence of climate: with an account of the best places of resort for invalids in England, the South of Europe, &c. By Sir James Clark, Bart., M.D., F.R.S. Physician in Ordinary to the Queen, and to the Prince Albert. Third edition. London: John Murray ... 1841.

201 × 125. Pp. xxviii, 378, ii (v.b.), 4 (book notices). Cloth.

1 ed., 1829. Pp. xxvii, 328. Lond.: Underwood. (NS.) 4 ed., 1846. Pp. xx (l.b.), 412. Lond: Murray.

Contains 'Aust' climates' (pp. 332–41), with sections on NSW, SA, Swan River, VDL and NZ.

EF copy of 3 ed. is inscribed: 'Presented to the Rev. Dr. Lang by the author in the year 1841.' John Dunmore Lang's *Historical and statistical account of NSW* ... is cited in text.

Copies: EF (3 ed.), SLV (4 ed.) UA (4 ed.). 519

Clark, William

1876–7. Legislative Assembly. New South Wales. Sydney Water Supply. Report to the Government ... on various projects for supplying Sydney with water. ... Sydney: Charles Potter, Acting Govt Printer. 1877.

323 × 212. Pp. 52 (l.b.). 12 plans (8 flg).

W. Clark, hydraulic engineer, was brought from England in 1876 'to decide between conflicting views' on an improved water supply for Sydney, then obtained from Botany and Lachlan swamps. Recommends Upper Nepean scheme.

During this visit author also submitted following reports, all (as above) appearing in NSW. Leg. Assembly, *V&P*, and printed 1877.

1876–7. Supply of water for the town of Bathurst. Pp. 10 (l.b.), 3 plans.

1876–7. Supply of water for the town of Orange. Pp. 10, 10 flg maps.

1876–7. Syd. Water Supply (Letter ...). Pp. 2.

1877. Syd. drainage. ... on interception and disposal of the drainage of Syd. and suburbs. Pp. 38 (l.b.), 9 plans.

1877. Supply of water for the town of Goulburn. Pp. 12 (l.b.), 5 plans.

Copies: LNSW, ML, NL, SLV. 520

Clarke, Alfred

A simple treatise on spectacles and defective vision. ... Sydney: W. C. Penfold & Co. ... 1893. ...

204 × 127. Pp. 22, [ii] (colophon only, v.b.). P. w. (amended title).

Copies: ML. 521

Clarke, Arthur H.

See Harper, Walter R. and Clarke, A. H.

Clarke, William W.

Spiritism unveiled, by William W. Clarke, M.D. Author of "Health in the Heart and Home" ... T. Smith ... Fitzroy.

158 × 102. Pp. 24. (1878.) P. w. (title rptd).

Copies: ML. 522

[Clarkson, Charles Howard]

Exploration of New Guinea. An inland trip. Mackay: H. B. Black & Co., Printers ... 1886.

204 × 138. Pp. 18 (l.b.). P. w. (cover title).

Anonymous account of an expedition which struck inland from the coast at Kapa Kapa, 30m. south of Port Moresby. All suffered malarial attacks. 'The country looks so healthy that the usual precautions seemed superfluous'. For identification of author, see Ferguson, 6 : 13163.

C. H. Clarkson (1842–94) LRCP, LRCSE, was Res. Surg. Hosp. for Pacific Islanders, Mackay Qd at time of expedition. He later moved to Vic. and died at Toorak.

Copies: FC. 522a

Clay, William French

No. 6.] [March, 1878. Health Society of New South Wales. ... Food as connected with public health. A lecture delivered before the Health Society of New South Wales ... 1877 ... By the Rev. William French Clay, M.A., M.D. ... Sydney: ... John Sands ...

206 × 135. Pp. (ii), 16. P. w. (title rptd).

Copies: FC, ML. 523

Cleland, William Lennox

Winegrowing in South Australia. A paper read ... in connection with the Chamber of Manufactures ... Adelaide: ... Andrews, Thomas, & Clark ... 1871.

236 × 153. Pp. 8 (l.b.), double cols.

Copies: ML, UM. 524

———

The Same. 252 × 206. Pp. 4 (l.b.). Treble cols. Colophon: Andrews, Thomas, & Clark, Printers, Adel.

Copies: SLV. 525

———

The Same. 1875. See Adel. Chamber of Manufactures.

———

Some remarks upon wine as a food, and its production. Paper by Dr. S. Cleland, to be read before the Royal Agricultural and Horticultural Society, on Friday, August 27th, 1880.

420 × 309. Single leaf, v.b. Treble columns. NI.

In SLV copy, author's name (in title) is altered in pencil to W. L. Cleland.

Copies: SLV. 526

———

A comparative study of the chronic insane, the habitual offender, and the endemic unemployed, with a view to treatment. ... Delivered before ... the Criminological Society of South Australia, September 30, 1897. Adelaide: Webb & Co. ... 1897.

209 × 132. Pp. 16 (l.b.). P. w. (cover title).

On the possible institutional treatment of 'three classes of society whose care and treatment is one of notorious difficulty.'

For W. L. Cleland (1847–1918) MB, ChM. Edin., Supt Parkside Mental Hosp. and later Col Surg. SA, see obit., *Med. J. Aust.*, 1918, 2 : 481.

Copies: EF, ML, SLS. 527

Clubbe, Sir Charles P.B., and Litchfield, W. F.

A short account of the first one hundred cases of diphtheria treated at the Diphtheria Branch of the Sydney Children's Hospital with anti-toxin, in comparison with the one hundred preceding cases treated without. ... [Text begins.]

229 × 165. Pp. 8 (last 2 blank). P. w. Repr., *Austsn med. Gaz.*, Jan. 1896.

Sir Charles Clubbe (1854–1932), FACS, FRACS, Hon. Surg. Hosp. for Sick Children

Syd., was noted for his contributions to the surgical treatment of intussusception. He published: *Intussusception*, 1 ed., Edin., 1907; 2 ed., Lond., 1921. See obit., *Med. J. Aust.*, 1933, 1 : 70; also Hipsley, P. L. (1952), *The early history of the Roy. Alex. Hosp. for Children*, Syd.
Copies: US. 528

Clunes District Hospital, Vic.

Second Annual Report of the Committee of Management of the Clunes District Hospital ... with the general rules of the institution. Established ... 1871. Ballarat: Charles Evans ... 1872.
204 × 132. Pp. 16.
Copies: SLV. 529

Clutterbuck, James Bennett

Port Phillip in 1849. By James Bennett Clutterbuck, M.D. (Nine years resident in the Colony.) London: John W. Parker, West Strand. 1850.
161 × 97. Pp. [vi] (iv, vi blank), 166, 6 (book advts). Frontis. (flg map). Cloth.
'Climate and diseases' (pp. 18–25). Dysentery and liver inflammation are the chief endemic ailments. Consumption is prevalent, and migration for cure or relief of this is discouraged. 'The most intense cold of England, added ... to a London fog, does not produce such baneful an influence on ... consumption as the sudden vicissitudes of the Australian climate.' On account of the rapid growth of children, he doubts whether they would live 'to a good old age.' Section on aborigines discusses physical and moral degeneration and forecasts extinction in a few years.
Copies: AMAV, DL, ML, NL, SLT, SLV, SLW, UA, UM, WLC. 530

An essay on the nature and treatment of Australian diseases, including, more especially, dysentery and fever. ... Melbourne: Stillwell and Knight ... 1868. Republished from the "Australian Medical Journal".
212 × 132. Pp. [iv] (ii, iv blank), 60, [iv]. Limp cloth.
Serious diseases in Vic. assume a violence and rapidity unknown in England, implying that they differ in nature. Author considers that a specific agent is in operation, 'predisposing, or giving rise to, new forms of disease.' These views are attacked by James Robertson MD, in *Aust. med. J.*, 1868, 13 : 247.
Copies: BG, CC, FC, ML, NL, SLV, UM. 531

Dr. Clutterbuck's reply. To the Editor of the Australian Medical Journal. Melbourne: Stillwell & Knight ... 1868.
204 × 127. Pp. 6 (l.b.). Repr., *Aust. med. J.*, Dec. 1868.
Rejoinder to Robertson's criticism of author's essay on Aust. diseases.
Copies: SLV. 532

Hints on health. A lecture ... at the Mount Barker Institute, on ... October 3rd, 1878, ... [Published by request.] Mount Barker: Printed by C.M.R. Dumas ... 1878.
204 × 140. Pp. 24. P. w. (cover title).
Author was at this time MO, Blinman Hosp., SA.
Copies: NL, SLS. 533

Stray notes on hygiene, and on the prevailing epidemic, influenza. By a member of the old school of medicine (J. B. Clutterbuck), etc. London: Henry Renshaw.
NS. Listed *BMC*. Pp. 69. 1892.
J. B. Clutterbuck MD Erlangen, LSA (1830), a pioneer doctor of early Vic., arrived in 1840, commenced practice in Melb., moved to Kilmore Vic., and later returned to England. In a further Aust. sojourn, he addressed papers from Mt Egerton Vic. (1870), Stanley Vic. (1871) and Blinman SA (1878). The date of final return to Britain is not known.
534

Coast Hospital, Sydney

1885–6. New South Wales. Coast Hospital, Little Bay. (Report on, for 1884.) ... [Text begins.]
336 × 212. Pp. 6. Colophon— Syd.: Thomas Richards, Govt Pr—1886.
Annual from 1884.
In 1934 name was changed to Prince Henry Hosp. despite strong protests. For history, see Boughton, C. R. (1963), *A Coast chronicle. The history of the Prince Henry Hosp.*, Syd.
Copies: HDN, LNSW, ML, NL, SPH, SLV. 535

1887–8. Legislative Assembly. New South Wales.

Treatment of typhoid fever at the Coast Hospital. (Report on.) Ordered . . . to be printed, 17 July, 1888. [Text begins.]

323 × 204. Pp. 4 (l.b.). 1 flg chart. Colophon—Syd.: Charles Potter, Govt Pr—1888.

Report by W. Peirce, Med. Supt, on method of treatment, requested by Bd of Health on account of favourable mortality rate.

Copies: LNSW, ML, NL, SLV. 536

Coats, Joseph

Notes on sea & land being the diary of a journey to New Zealand, Australia, Ceylon and Egypt (October, 1897, till April, 1898) By Joseph Coats M.D. Professor of Pathology in Glasgow University [Vignette] Glasgow Printed for private circulation at the University Press 1898

191 × 127. Pp. xii, 346 (l.b.). Illustns. Cloth.

Visits Hobart, Syd., Melb., Adel. and Albany.

Copies: FC, NL, SLV. 537

Cobb, Nathan Augustus

Department of Agriculture, New South Wales. Miscellaneous Publication, No. 13. Nematodes, mostly Australian and Fijian . . . Sydney: F. Cunninghame & Co., Printers . . . 1893

307 × 242. Pp. 60 (l.b.). 7 litho. pl. Reprint from *Macleay Memorial Vol.*

Copies: UA. 538

———

Department of Agriculture, New South Wales. (Miscellaneous Publication, No. 16.) Host and habitat index of the Australian fungi, 1893. [Royal Arms] Sydney: Charles Potter, Govt Printer . . . 1893

217 × 140. Pp. [iv] (two blanks), 44. P. w. (title rptd).

Copies: UA. 539

———

Department of Agriculture, Sydney . . . Miscellaneous Publication, No. 167. The sheep-fluke: . . . Sydney: William Applegate Gullick, Govt Printer. 1897.

245 × 152. Pp. 32. 1 pl., 29 figs. P. w. (short title and figs on front; author's publications both sides back wrapper).

N. A. Cobb BSc, PhD, was pathologist to NSW Dept of Agriculture.

Copies: ML. 540

Coghlan, Sir Timothy Augustine

Deaths in childbirth in New South Wales. . . . Reprinted from the Journal of the Royal Statistical Society . . . (Printed for private circulation.) 1898.

215 × 140. Pp. 16. 3 graphs. P. w. (cover title).

Copies: ML. 541

———

Childbirth in New South Wales: A study in statistics. Illustrated by eight diagrams. . . . Sydney: William Applegate Gullick, Govt Printer. 1899.

215 × 140. Pp. 68 (l.b.). 8 graphs. P. w. (short title).

Another ed., 1900.

Uses for the first time extensive official figures which included ages of mothers. Similar data was not elsewhere available for many years. A further study followed in 1903: *The decline in the birth-rate of NSW and other phenomena of child-birth*, Syd.

Sir Timothy Coghlan (1856–1926) was NSW Govt Statistician.

Copies: EF, LNSW, ML, NL, OL, SLS, SLV, SLW, US. 542

Cole, Edward William

An essay on the nature of the phenomena called possession by evil spirits. The belief respecting evil spirits, and the various modes practised for casting them out in the different countries of the world. . . . By Edwic *** C. W., M.L.D.A., &c. Melbourne: Robert Bell, Steam Printer . . .

214 × 135. Pp. [ii] (v.b.), 125–172. [?1868.] P. w. (with DEMONS on front).

Reprints chap. 16 of author's *The real place in history of Jesus and Paul*, [1867].

Copies: ML. 543

——— (editor)

Second edition. Enlarged. Advice of ten doctors. . . . Edited by E. W. Cole. . . . Cole's Book Arcade, Melbourne . . .

175 × 127. Pp. 15, 14 (l.b.), 6 (l.b.), 8, 4, 24, 34, 6, 2, 6, 162, 2, 10. ND. (c. 1892.) P. w. (cover title).

Extracts from overseas writers on: enema cure; quacks and quackeries in US; the water cure; sun cure; exercise, pure air and diet; alcohol and tobacco.

Copies: LNSW. 544

———

The pound pamphlet word for word, and other advertised frauds. . . . Cole's Book Arcade, Melbourne.

173 × 122. Pp. [9], 10–126, [2] (advts). Figs. ND. [1892.] P. w. (cover title).

Contains: Dr Jukes on the enema cure; Dr. A. Wilford Hall's hygienic treatment; advertised and peddled wonders sold in US under bond-of-secrecy; cures for drunkenness.

Copies: AMAV, EF, ML, RACP, SLV, UM. 545

The "Dr." Hall cure complete, all about it ... Reader! This book contains directions for the enema cure as given in the pound pamphlet of the so-called "Dr." Hall and also far more complete advice ... E. W. Cole, Book Arcade, Melbourne.

173 × 125. Pp. 48 (includes wrappers). 4 figs. Cover title. ND.

Hall's treatment; also detailed treatise by Dr. Jukes, 'who invented the stomach pump and the enema pump, and also improved the enema fountain 60 years before "Dr Hall" began his fraudulent work ...'

See Hall, A Wilford, for Hall's 'Pound pamphlet.'

Copies: FC. 546

A practical guide to health being a simple manual showing how to cure a number of common disorders of the human body by the use of water and other easily applied remedies. New edition. With a chapter on the common-sense management of children. Melbourne: E. W. Cole ... 1895.

201 × 140. Pp. 64. P. w. (amplified title: Everybody's doctor).

Hydropathy, simple cures, health guide, child care.

Copies: BG. 547

Advice of a hundred doctors on tight-lacing. [2 cuts] ... Edited by E. W. Cole. ... Cole's Book Arcade, Melbourne ...

178 × 127. Pp. 158 (159 on recto end wrapper). ND. (c. 1895.) Stiff p. w.

Publications not seen: *Cole's shilling doctor* and *Child's book of health* (Cole's cat., 1895); *Healthy mothers and sturdy children* (advt, 1895.)

E. W. Cole (1832–1918), bookseller and publisher, was founder of Cole's Book Arcade, Melb.

Copies: AMAV, ML. 548

See Hall, W. W.; also Valentine, Ferdinand C.

Cole, H. S. and Morris, Thomas

The Health Act, the Infant Life Protection Act, the Margarine Act, with regulations, notes of English and Victorian cases, and index. By H. S. Cole, LL.B., Barrister and Solicitor, and Thomas Morris. Melbourne: Charles F. Maxwell (G. Partridge & Co.) ... London: Sweet & Maxwell (Limited). 1894.

214 × 140. Pp. xvi, 358 (l.b.), [ii] (colophon only, v.b.). Cloth.

Copies: EF, ML, SLV. 549

Collingwood Free Medical Mission Dispensary, Vic.

Mission hall & mission work connected with the Collingwood Free Medical Mission Dispensary for the necessitous sick, Wellington Street, Collingwood, which was opened January, 1869. [Text begins.]

208 × 131. Pp. 6. P. w. Colophon—Mason, Firth & M'Cutcheon ... Melb. (1880.)

Contains statement (signed: John Singleton) and 11th an. rep.

Copies: SLV. 550

Collins, David

See No. 2495 (note).

Collins, William

See Hunt, James S., Collins, W., and Wynne, E. T.

Colonial Land and Emigration Commissioners, London

Dietary during the voyage. The passengers are to be in messes of six or more, as the surgeon may determine; and to be victualled according to the following scale ... [Text proceeds.]

331 × 198. Single leaf, v. b. ND. (Dated by hand 1841, 1842.) NI.

Included with reports of Col Surg. (WA) for 1849.

Includes ration lists and med. comforts.

Copies: SLW. 551

Colonists' Handbooks

Colonists' Handbooks. No. 2. Queensland, containing statistical and other information from Government sources, and useful counsels to emigrants ... London: Society for Promoting

Christian Knowledge . . . 1882.

163 × 115. Pp. 48. 1 flg map.

Includes notes on climate, dietary scale on voyage, health. The absence of malaria and the possibility of white labour in the tropics are mentioned.

The series opened with No 1 Canada. Nos 1–4 only seen.

Copies: LNSW, ML. 552

———

Colonists' Handbooks. No. 3. New South Wales, containing statistical and other information from Government sources, and useful counsels to emigrants . . . London: Society for Promoting Christian Knowledge . . . 1882.

163 × 115. Pp. 48. 1 flg map.

Includes notes on climate and health hints.

Copies: LNSW, ML, NL. 553

———

Colonists' Handbooks. No. 4. South Australia, containing statistical and other information from Government sources, and useful counsels to emigrants, with map . . . London: Society for Promoting Christian Knowledge . . . 1883.

163 × 115. Pp. 48. 1 flg map.

Includes notes on: climate, diet on voyage, health hints.

Copies: LNSW, ML, NL. 554

Comettant, Oscar

. . . Au pays des kangourous et des mines d'or Etude des moeurs et coutumes Australiennes Impressions de voyage Paris Librairie Fischbacher Société anonyme . . . 1890 . . .

178 × 117. Pp. [iv] (ii, iv blank), 386, [6] (advts). Cloth.

A French official's visit to Melb. for the International Exhibition, 1888. A chapter (pp. 239–61) is devoted to Melb. med. and. pharm. practice, hospitals and charities. A note: 'Melbourne, though doubtless one of the healthiest places in the world, is perhaps the one where people most frequently consult their doctor. At the least ailment they quickly call him . . . A teething baby has only to be a little irritated; a scratch on an arm or leg . . .'

Copies: EF, ML, NL, SLS, SLT, SLV, SLW, UA, UM, UQ, US. 555

Congreve, G. T.

Consumption and its successful treatment. Showing that direful disease to be curable in all its stages; with observations on asthma, chronic bronchitis etc.

NS. Advt in *Syd. Mail*, 18 June 1887, announces publication by Robertson & Co., Syd. Price 6d.

556

Connell's East Indian Remedies

. . . Connell's East Indian remedies for the relief and cure of liver affections, gout, rheumatism and ague. . . . William Witt & Co., Wholesale Agents . . . Melbourne.

198 × 130. Pp. 58. ND. P. w. (title rptd, decorated with 'the form of an elephant, constituted by nine female forms fully portrayed . . .'

Mainly testimonials of grateful Vic. patients.

Copies: SLV. 557

Consumption

Consumption. From the "Argus" . . . Sept. 18, 1857. [Text begins.]

206 × 127. Pp. 2. NI.

Includes remarks on use of dugong oil in treatment by Moreton Bay doctor (Wm Hobbs, *q.v.*).

Copies: SLV. 558

Consumptive Sanatorium, Echuca, Vic.

See Serjeant, Mrs. G.

Consumptive Voyage to the Medical Society, A

See Thomson, William.

Cook, Edmund Alleyne

A study of homoeopathy . . . Martin & Pleasance . . . and . . . E. G. Owen . . . Melbourne. . . .

183 × 125. Pp. 36 (l.b.). ND. (1895.) P. w. (cover title). Notice for Homoeopathic Hosp. Melb., inside back wrapper.

E. A. Cook, LRCPE, LRCSE, arrived Melb. about 1893, was Hon. Surg. Homoeopathic Hosp. Melb.

Copies: ML, NL, SLV. 559

Cooma Lunatic Asylum (Temporary), NSW

1877. New South Wales. Temporary Lunatic Asylum, Cooma. (Report of Inspector of Insane upon.) . . . [Text begins.]

328 × 208. Pp. [2] (v.b.). Signed: F. Norton Manning.

Copies: LNSW, ML, NL, SLV. 560

Cooper, H. W.

Health and vigor by Dr. H. W. Cooper, M.D., etc. ... Milton House, 267 Elizabeth Street, Hyde Park. Sydney.

181 × 117. Pp. 232. Text figs. ND. Colophon—Printed ... by Arthur Norwood ... Syd. Paper boards.

Later ed., ND. (?1910), has on title: 'by Dr. Percy George Carte, L.R.C.S.I. ... Successor to Dr. H. W. Cooper.' Colophon—Kingston Press ... Syd.

A general medical work, 'as free as possible from technicalities.'

H. W. Cooper appears in Bruck's *List of unregistered practitioners*, Syd., 1886.

Copies: EF, FC, ML, NL. 561

Cooper, Walter H.

See Beer, Frederick.

Corlette, Cyril Ernest

A general account of beri beri as seen in Sydney, based on original observation ...

217 × 138. Pp. 16. (l.b.). (1895.) Colophon—Andrews & Co., Printers ... P. w. (cover title).

A study of 52 cases of beri-beri in Chinese and Japanese at Sydney Hosp., 1892–4.

C. E. Corlette (1868–1960) MD, ChM Syd., DPH Camb., FRACS, Hon. Surg. Syd. Hosp., published extensively, including *Food and nutrition*, Syd., 1921; *A surgeon's guide to local anaesthesia*, Bristol, 1948.

Copies: ML, NL, US. 561a

Cornwall Hospital and Infirmary, Launceston

See Launceston General Hospital.

Cottage Home for Destitute Children, Newtown, NSW

First Report of the Cottage Home for Destitute Children: with remarks on the better methods of dealing with the children of the State. Newtown, 1880. ... Sydney: ... John Woods & Co. ...

209 × 140. Pp. 14. Frontis. P. w. (title rptd).

Official method of child care by the 'boarding out system' is discussed by Mrs M. Jefferis, pioneer of the 'cottage home system' in Sydney, who founded Home in 1879. In 1887 this was moved from Newtown to Burwood.

Copies: FC (1879/80, 1884/5), ML (1879/80–1887/8). 562

Coutts, William Lehman Burdett—

The sick and wounded in South Africa. What I saw and said of them and of the Army medical system ... Cassell and Company, Limited London ... 1900 ...

202 × 136. Pp. xii (l.b.), 260. Stiff p. w. (decorated title).

Criticism of medical arrangements in S. African War. NSW Med. Contingent is described as 'one of the finest specimens of medical service seen in the war.' For Aust. account, which comments on above work, see Skirving, R. S. (1901), *Our army in S. Africa*, Syd.; also *The story of S. Africa*, various authors, 2 vols, Syd., ND. (?1904.)

Copies: EF, LNSW, ML, SLW. 563

Cowan, John

The science of a new life ... Melbourne: Fergusson and Mitchell, Publishers ... 1882.

217 × 130. Pp. 406 (last—colophon only), [2] (advts). 28 figs. Cloth.

First published N. Y., 1874. Reprinted in the Source Library of the Women's Movement, Source Book Press, N. Y., 1970.

On sex and marriage.

Copies: CC, EF, FC, LNSW, NL, SLV, UA. 564

Cox, James Charles

Catalogue of the specimens of the Australian land shells in the collection of James C. Cox, M. D., F.R.C.S. Edin. Sydney: ... John Alex. Engel. 1864.

181 × 110. Pp. 46. P. w. (title rptd).

Author's numerous conchological works include: *A monograph of Aust. land shells*, Syd.: Maddock, 1868; *Distribution of Austsn Volutes*, Syd.: A. W. Douglas, 1872.

Copies: EF, FC, ML, NL, SLV, SLW, UM. 565

———

Presidential address ... Linnean Society of New South Wales, January 31st, 1883 ... Sydney: Frederick White ... 1883.

206 × 127. Pp. 20. P. w. (cover title).

For J. C. Cox (1834–1912) MD, FRCS Edin., Hon. Phys. Syd. Infirm., conchologist, Chairman Aust. Museum, and Pres. NSW Fisheries Commission, see obits, *Austsn med. Gaz.*, 1912, 32 : 370 and *Proc. Linn Soc. NSW*, 1913, 38 : 5; also 'Reminiscences of J. C. Cox', *Old Times*, July 1903.

Copies: ML, SLV. 566

Creed, John Mildred

Extraordinary customs of the aborigines of Central Australia. ... L. Bruck ... Sydney. 1883.

204 × 153. Pp. 4. Repr., *Austsn med. Gaz.*, 1883.

Describes subincision of penis, which is held to render impregnation impossible, from reports of non-scientific observers. Operation for causing sterility in women is also described, on slight evidence. Author was Surg. to SA Govt Exploring Expedition, N. Aust.

Copies: EF. 567

Australian snakebite: fear as a factor in producing many of the alarming symptoms following. ... Reprinted from "The Australasian Medical Gazette" for July, 1884. L. Bruck ... Sydney. 1884.

204 × 127. Pp. 16. P. w. (title rptd).

Recommends trial of prolonged ether anaesthesia for relief of the effects of fright. Warns of dangers of keeping patients awake by forced exercise and other means (mentioning use of a town band for this purpose), and of the hazards of alcohol administration (citing case of a 19 year old girl who was given four bottles of brandy during a 40 mile buggy ride to a doctor).

Copies: ML. 568

The Same. Fear as a factor in producing many of the alarming symptoms following the bite of Australian snakes. Revised ed. Pp. 12 (l.b.). Colophon—Webb, Vardon, & Pritchard ... Adel. ND. (?1887.) Repr., *Trans Intercol Med. Cong. Austsia*, Adel., 1887.

Copies: EF, ML, NL. 569

Cremation Bill. Speech ... on moving the second reading in the Legislative Council of N. S. W., on June 24, 1886. Sydney: L. Bruck ... 1886.

206 × 120. Pp. 12.

Bill to legalise cremation in NSW. See *Austsn med. Gaz.*, 1886, 5 : 228; *ibid*, 1887, 6 : 205.

Copies: ML. 570

Cremation. A lecture delivered by ... President of the Cremation Society of New South Wales. ... Sydney: F. Cunninghame & Co. ... 1890.

217 × 140. Pp. 16.

EF copy bears inscription by author: 'It would be impolitic to make cremation compulsory until the people have been educated to its use by the example of others willing now to make use of it.'

Copies: EF, FC, ML, NL, US. 571

The treatment of diphtheria. Read before the N.S.W. Branch B.M.A. ... Reprinted from the "Australasian Medical Gazette" for December, 1891. L. Bruck ... Sydney. 1891.

186 × 125. Pp. 8 (l.b.). P. w. (title rptd).

Copies: ML. 571a

A case of dipsomania cured under hypnotic suggestion. ... [Text begins.]

186 × 122. Pp. 6. Repr., *Austsn med. Gaz.*, 1893.

Copies: ML. 572

The treatment of drink mania by hypnotic suggestion. Extracted from the paper "Hypnotic suggestion as a therapeutic agent", read before the New South Wales Branch of the British Medical Association on Dec. 23, 1898 ... William Brooks & Co. ... Sydney.

183 × 117. Pp. 8.

Copies: ML. 573

Is the non-ingestion of foods containing starch and sugar necessary for the successful treatment of diabetes and glycosuria? ... [Text begins.]

234 × 158. Pp. 4 (l.b.). ND. Colophon—Melb.: J. Kemp, Govt Pr.

From study of his own case, author concludes that 'the non-ingestion of starch and sugar now insisted on as essential to recovery in cases of glycosuria, including true diabetes, is not only not necessary, but ... even inadvisable.'

Copies: ML. 574

My experience of hypnotic suggestion as a therapeutic agent. ... Reprinted from *The Australasian Medical Gazette*, January 20, 1899. Sydney: L. Bruck ... 1899.

181 × 122. Pp. 40 (l.b.). P. w. (cover title).

For J. M. Creed (1842–1930) MRCS, LRCP, MLC, Hon. Surg. Syd. Hosp., Ed. *Austsn med. Gaz.*, see obit., *Med. J. Aust.*, 1930, 2 : 772; and his own *My recollections of Australia and elsewhere*, Lond., 1916.

Copies: LNSW, ML. 575

See also No 1317.

Cremation

Cremation. From "Iron" of January 3, 1874.

212 × 138. Pp. 12. Colophon—Stillwell and Knight . . . Melb.

Recommends introduction of cremation.

Copies: ML, SLV. 576

Cremation Society of South Australia

See Wylde, R.T.

Cremation Society of Victoria

The Cremation Society of Victoria (Established 26th October, 1892.) . . . [List of office bearers and Council.] 1892.

202 × 125. Pp. 4.

Contains rules of Society.

Copies: ML. 577

Cremation Society of Victoria. Secretary's Report. [Text begins.]

218 × 136. Pp. 8. (1894.) Signed: H. K. Rusden, Sec.

Copies: ML. 578

Cremorne Private Lunatic Asylum, Vic.

See Tucker, George Alfred; also No 1473.

Creswick District Hospital, Vic.

Tenth Annual Report of the Creswick District Hospital, from Jan 1, 1873, to December 31, 1873, with the rules and regulations . . . Creswick: Printed at the "Advertiser" . . . Office . . . 1874.

204 × 132. Pp. 18.

Copies: SLV (1873–93). 579

Creyke, R.

Public health in Brisbane. . . . read before . . . the Philosophical Society of Queensland, at Brisbane . . . [Text begins.]

212 × 138. Pp. 12 (l.b.), flg table. Double cols. Above paper, pp. 1–9. ND. (1861.) Colophon—Fairfax and Belbridge . . . Bris.

Reviews climatic conditions, statistics of births and deaths, and health (in general terms) of Brisbane for 1860, and concludes that the electrical state of the atmosphere is associated with health. Includes discussion of causes of death, infant mortality, and pulmonary disease and the Qd climate.

Copies: FC. 580

'Cringle, Tom'

See [Walker, William], 'Tom Cringle'.

Crivelli, Marcel Urbain

The syphilitic chancre (diagnosis and treatment) . . . Reprinted from the "Intercolonial Quarterly Journal of Medicine and Surgery", May 1894. Melbourne: Stillwell and Co. . . . 1894.

244 × 153. Pp. 16. P. w. (cover title).

Copies: ML. 581

With Dr. Crivelli's compliments. Alcoholism: its pathological physiology and its treatment. . . . Reprinted from the "Intercolonial Medical Journal of Australasia", January 30, 1900. Melbourne: Stillwell and Co. . . . 1900.

214 × 140. Pp. 16. P. w. (title rptd).

M. U. Crivelli (1859–1948) MD Paris & Melb., settled in Vic. about 1887, and practised at Albert Park and Melb. See *Cyclopedia of Vic.*, vol. 1., 1903.

Copies: EF, NL. 582

Croker, Henry Dillon

Quotations on hydropathy, from eminent authors. . . . Melbourne: Mason & Firth . . . 1863

212 × 130. Pp. 16 (l.b.).

H. D. Crocker (1814–87) MRCS came to Aust. about 1853 and practised for 20 years at Beaufort Vic. Obit., *Austsn med. Gaz.*, 1887, 7 : 23.

Copies: ML, SLV. 583

Crowther, Arthur Bingham

The preservation of health: or, everyone his own doctor. A lecture, delivered in the Town Hall, Hobart, on . . . November 17, 1885 . . . Tasmania: Printed at "The Mercury" Office. 1885.

209 × 135. Pp. 12 (l.b.). P. w. (cover title).

Sections on hygiene, housing, clothing, and disposal of the dead. Cremation is advocated, and it is stated that, as drainage from church graveyards in Launceston—closure of which was opposed—was allowed to pollute drinking water, this caused people 'to garnish their tables with a cold and poisonous infusion of their ancestors.'

A. B. Crowther MRCS, LRCP, returned to Tas. after qualification in London in 1874, and practised in Hobart.

Copies: FC. 584

Cullimore, D. H.

The book of climates. Acclimatization; climatic diseases; health resorts and mineral springs; sea sickness; sea voyages; and sea bathing. ... London: Bailliere, Tindall, and Cox ... 1890.

186 × 122. Pp. x, 266. Cloth.

2 ed., 1891.

Climate of Australasia, pp. 242–251.

Copies: AMAQ, LNSW, SLV. 585

Culverwell, E. James

Magnetic hydropathy. A treatise on the beneficial effects of magnetic hydropathy in the care and alleviation of nervous, paralytic, and other painful diseases. By Culverwell & Co. Sydney.

NS. Pp. 37. ND. Written note by E. A. Petherick (NL).

586

When and whom to marry. A popular medical sketch, by E. James Culverwell, M.D., author of "What to eat, drink, and avoid".

NS. Advertised in *Syd. Morning Herald*, 19th Sep. 1850, p. 3. Pp. 50. Price 6d. at Mason's Printing Office, 147 Castlereagh-street.

587

Cumming, Frederick

The Sydney Garden Palace a patriotic and historical poem. ... Published by Stewart & Co. ... Sydney ... 1887.

212 × 135. Pp. 104 (l.b.), [ii] (errata, v.b.). 1 pl. P. w. (title rptd).

Poem, dedicated to the Queen, on the Syd. Garden Palace and its destruction by fire in 1882. Postscript contains testimonial and letters, and notes a warning received against poetry writing, on account of public opinion that this could interfere with professional duties. (Sir Alex. MacCormick later stated that this applied also to music and the arts.) Author adds that such exception did not apply to drinking, sports, and racing.

Frederick Cumming (1808–91) MD Edin. & Melb., Surg. E. India Co's Naval Service, practised at Woollahra, died at Petersham NSW.

Copies: EF, ML, SLV. 588

Cunningham, Peter Miller

Two years in New South Wales; a series of letters, comprising sketches of the actual state of society in that colony; of its peculiar advantages to emigrants; of its topography, natural history, &c., &c. By P. Cunningham, Surgeon, R. N. In two volumes. Vol. 1. London: Henry Colburn ... 1827.

201 × 122. 2 vols. Vol. 1 : pp. xii, 352; vol. 2 : pp. viii, 346, [2] (book notices).

German translations: Leipzig: Hartmann, 1829; Leipzig: Berger, ND (1828); Leipzig: Kayser'sche, 1832. Fascimile ed., Adel., Libraries Bd of SA, 2 vols., 1966. Another ed., Syd., ed. D. S. Macmillan, Angus & Robertson with RAHS, 1966.

Author had made four voyages to NSW as surg.-supt of convict ships and lived there for two years. Notes on health state that fevers (except rum fever) do not occur, 'while measles, hooping cough, small-pox, and all your similar European pests, are alike strangers.' To these are added scarlet fever, intermittent fever and typhus. Dysentery is the most prevalent and fatal disease. Dropsy in the debauched, roundworms in children, phthisis in adolescents, ophthalmia ('the blight'), and an epidemic of influenza, are noted. Syphilis is unknown, gonorrhoea common. A vivid picture is presented of convict transportation, its problems, and his methods.

For appreciation, see Gandevia, B. (1966), 'The contribution of doctors to early Australiana', *J. Amer. med. Ass.*, 196, 1 : 63; Ford, E. (1972), 'Some early Aust. med. publications', *Med. History*, 16 : 205.

Copies: DL, FC, ML, RACP, SLT, SLV, UM, UQ, US. 589

The Same. 2 ed., 1827.

Copies: AMAV, DOS, EF, FC, ML, NL, OL, SLT, SLV, SLW, UM, UQ, US. 590

The Same. 3 ed., 1828.

Copies: FC, ML, NL, OL, SLV, UA, UM, UQ, US. 591

———

Hints for Australian emigrants; with engravings and explanatory descriptions of the water-raising wheels, and modes of irrigating land in Egypt, Syria, South America, &c. ... London: T. and W. Boone ... 1841.

198 × 125. Pp. xii (l.b.), 120 (l.b.). Errata slip. 1 flg plan, 12 figs. Paper boards.

Apart from a chapter on diet, book consists of information on agriculture and husbandry.

Also published: *On the motions of the earth and heavenly bodies ... and the conception, growth, and decay of man, and cause and treatment of his diseases, as referable to galvanic action*, Lond., Cochrane and McCrone, 1834.

Copies: DL, FC, ML, NL, SLV, SLW. 592

Curr, Edward Micklethwaite

The Australian race: its origin, languages, customs, place of landing in Australia, and the routes by which it spread itself over that continent. ... In four volumes. Volume 1. Melbourne: John Ferres, Govt Printer. London: Trübner and Co. ... 1886.

220 × 140. Vol. 1, pp. xx, 426, 17 pl.; vol. 2 (1886), pp. vi, 502 (l.b.), 2 pl.; vol. 3 (1887), pp. viii, 710; vol. 4 (1887), 478 × 343, pp. 46 (l.b.), 1 flg coloured map of Aust. (shows areas of circumcision and subincision). Cloth.

References of medical interest throughout. See particularly vol. 1, pp. 70–76 for infants and children, nutrition, circumcision, subincision and other artificial deformations, infanticide and abortion; pp. 78–83 food; pp. 208–234 diseases and decline.

Author regrets that 'the diseases ... of our aborigines and the peculiarities of their constitutions have hitherto failed to attract the attention of ... the medical profession in these colonies ...'

Copies: DL, EF, FC, KFR, ML, NL, OL, SLT, SLV, SLW, UA, UM, UQ, US. 593

Curtice, Cooper

Australasian edition: abridged and edited, with a preface by F.R.C. Hopkins. The animal parasites of sheep. By Cooper Curtice, D.V.S., M.D. Published by authority of the Secretary ... United States Department of Agriculture ... To which is added ... "Worms in sheep", specially written for Australia. By a Pastoralist. Sydney: Turner and Henderson, 1892.

228 × 147. Pp. [viii] (l.b.), LII (l.b.), [ii] (v.b.), 144, [2]. 24 pl. (4 coloured). Cloth.

Copies: EF, ML, UA, UQ, US. 594

———, **Francis M. and Fuller, Claude**

Department of Agriculture ... New South Wales. Cattle tick. The cattle tick (*Boophilus bovis*, Riley, sp.) Biology by Cooper Curtice, M.D., D.V.S., (Moravia, N. Y.) Preventive measures by Dr. M. Francis, D.V.M. ... Notes on the Queensland tick, by Claude Fuller, ... Department of Agriculture, New South Wales. Sydney: Charles Potter, Govt Printer ... 1896.

247 × 153. Pp. [ii] (v.b.), 18. 3 pl., 2 figs. P. w. (title rptd).

Copies: ML. 595

Cutts, William Henry

Injurious effects of close confinement and overwork. Read before the Victorian Branch of the British Medical Association ... Reprinted from the "Australasian Medical Gazette", for January, 1885. L. Bruck ... Sydney. 1885.

196 × 122. Pp. 16.

For W. H. Cutts (1828–97) MD Edin. & Melb., Hon. Phys. Melb. Hosp., see *Intercol med. J. Austsia*, 1897, 2 : 561; *Austsn med. Gaz.*, 1897, 16 : 363.

Copies: EF, ML, SLV. 596

———

The Same. Reprinted as No 22, Aust. Health Soc. tracts, 1885. Pp. 12. Walker May & Co., Melb.

Copies: ML, NL, SLS, SLV. 597

D

D., W. M.

Instructions for beginners, in the application of the microscope. By a Member of the Royal Society of New South Wales. [Cut of microscope] George Robertson . . . Sydney and Melbourne; and W. MacDonnell & Co., Opticians . . . Sydney.

204 × 132. Pp. 24. 29 figs. (1878.)

Copies: ML. 598

Dahlke's Filter Co.

Dahlke's Filter Co., Limited. Melbourne. Pure water . . . 34 Collins Street West. . . .

175 × 117. Pp. [12]. (1872.)

Advt for locally made earthenware filters.

Copies: SLV. 599

Daish, William Christian

Melbourne to Tokio. Notes by the way. By W. Daish, M.D. . . .

193 × 122. Pp. [viii] (l.b.), 9–104, [ii] (colophon only, v.b.). Frontis. Colophon—C. G. Meehan & Co. . . . South Melbourne. ND. (1900.) Cloth.

Travel notes of voyage as ship's surgeon—Thursday Is., Darwin, Timor, Hong Kong, Japan.

W. Daish MD, Hon. Op Phys. Melb. Hosp. (1885), practised in Melbourne.

Copies: EF, FC, ML, SLV, UQ. 600

D'Albertis, Luigi Maria

See Bennett, George—Editor and Translator.

Dale, John Thomas

Noted by Dr. R. Scot Skirving as author of pamphlet on alcoholism (NS), and while in practice at Balmain was patentee of 'a specific to prevent a desire for, and to cure the deleterious effects of, alcohol when taken to excess.' (*Austsn med. Gaz.*, 1893, 12: 425).

J. T. Dale, LRCP & S. Edin. (1873), who arrived in NSW in 1891 and practised at Tumbarumba and other places, committed suicide in Sydney, 1897 (*Austsn med. Gaz.*, 1897, 16 : 570). 601

Davenport, Arthur Frederick

Notes on the origin of sex. . . . (Read at the Intercolonial Medical Congress . . . Brisbane, September 1899.) [Text begins.]

217 × 140. Pp. 14 (l.b.). Colophon—Melb.: Stillwell and Co. . . .

The sex of a child is determined at the moment of conception, and is the opposite to that of whichever parent is in more vigorous health. The relative health of parents can be adjusted by treatment, so that children of desired sex will be born.

Author (MB Lond., MRCS) practised at St Kilda Vic.

Copies: AMAV, SLV. 602

Davidson, Andrew

Geographical pathology: an inquiry into the geographical distribution of infective and climatic diseases. By Andrew Davidson, M.D., M.R.C.P. Ed. . . . Edinburgh & London: Young J. Pentland. 1892.

229 × 153. 2 vols. Vol. 1 : pp. xiv (l.b.), [ii] (v.b.), 482, [40] (advts, l.b.); vol. 2 : pp. [vi] (l.b.), 483–1006 (l.b.). Cloth.

Sections on Australia and New Guinea (pp. 546–568).

Copies: LNSW, ML, SLV, SPH, UA, UM. 603

Davies, Mrs. Eliza

The story of an earnest life: a woman's adventures in Australia, and in two voyages around the world. . . . Cincinatti: Central Book Concern . . . 1881.

220 × 147. Pp. vi, 7–570. Frontis. Cloth.

Shortly after arrival in Sydney from Scotland in 1838, authoress suffered from an illness ascribed to sunstroke, was attended by Dr (later Sir) Charles Nicholson, and admitted to 'Sydney Hospital'. She vividly describes (pp. 91–8) its prison-like conditions and callous nursing treatment. 'The nurses, both men and women, were, or had been, convicts, and they were drunken, dishonest, and very rough'.

At the time stated the existing 'Sydney

Hospital' was the convict establishment, though her account adds that 'This hospital had been built for convicts, but as free settlers became numerous, they needed another hospital; so another place was provided for the convicts, and ... pay patients admitted ...' However, Sydney Infirmary, replacing the convict hospital, was not opened for patients until 1845.

Copies: FC, ML, NL, SLS, SLV. 604

Davis, Joseph Barnard

Thesaurus craniorum. Catalogue of the skulls of the various races of man, in the collection of Joseph Barnard Davis, M.D., F.S.A. ... [Fig. of skulls] ... London: Printed for the Subscribers. 1867.

220 × 140. Pp. xviii (l.b.), 374, [2]. 2 litho. pl., 1 flg table, text figs. Cloth.

Describes 24 Aust., 12 Tas. skulls.

Copies: LNSW, ML, NL, SLS, SLV, US. 605

———

On the osteology and peculiarities of the Tasmanians, a race of man recently become extinct. ... (Natuurkundige Verhandelingen der Hollandsche Maatschappij der Wetenschappen, 3de Verz. Deel 11, No. 4). Haarlem, De Erven Loosjes. 1874.

295 × 229. Pp. 20. 4 litho. pl. (1 flg).

Includes life and customs of Tasmanians, differences from Australians, and arguments for them being a distinct race. Tas. material in European collections is listed, and measurements of 4 Tas. and 3 Aust. skeletons included.

Copies: LNSW, ML, NL, SLS, SLT, SLV, UA. 606

Day, John

On colour tests as aids to diagnosis. ... A paper read before the Medical Society of Victoria, 6th October. [Text begins.]

215 × 136. Pp. 8. Repr., *Aust. med. J.*, 1869.

On author's development of the guaiacum test for blood, and its extension to pus and saliva.

ML copy inscribed by author to Dr. Neild, Lect. in Forensic Med. Univ. Melb.; SLV copy to Sir Redmond Barry.

Copies: AMAV, ML, SLV. 607

———

Allotropic oxygen in its relations to science and art. A lecture, delivered at the Technological Museum, Melbourne ... on 5th July, 1872. [Text begins.]

208 × 132. Pp. 14 (l.b.). NI.

Discusses guaiacum and hydrogen peroxide test for blood, developed by Day as a medico-legal method. It was first used in 1866, on the washed clothing of a suspected Chinese murderer at Scarsdale Vic., after other tests for blood had failed.

Also mentions peroxide as disinfectant, and ozonic ether 'for destroying the poison of small-pox, scarlet fever and typhoid fever, when used as an atomised spray, or by sponging or inunction.' See also Moffitt, Andrew, for this treatment.

Copies: ML, OL, SLV. 608

———

An attempt to show that the walls and flooring of ordinary hospitals are largely concerned in the production of those septic poisons which give rise to pyaemia, erysipelas, and puerperal fever; with suggestions for remedying the evil. ...

201 × 127. Pp. 8 (l.b.). Colophon: Stillwell and Knight, Printers, Collins Street East. ND. (1875.) Repr., *Aust. med. J.* Nov. 1875.

Copies: NL. 609

———

On the application of nascent oxygen to the disinfection and deodorisation of wounds and ulcerated surfaces. ... [Text begins.]

217 × 147. Pp. 4. Colophon: Stillwell and Knight ... [Melb.] Plain p. w. From *Aust. med. J.*, July 1878.

Claims priority in the introduction of hydrogen peroxide for therapeutic use.

John Day (1816–81) MD, MRCS, of Geelong, one of the ablest doctors in the Colony, an assiduous investigator, worked especially on applications of ozone and hydrogen peroxide, and studied the action of disinfectants. Obit., *Aust. med. J.*, 1881, ns 3 : 78.

Copies: UM. 610

———

See also Industrial and Technological Museum; No 1815.

Dayton, W. T.

See Stuart, Sir Thomas Peter Anderson, No 2053.

Deaf and Dumb Institution of New South Wales

See N.S.W. Instn for the Deaf and Dumb and the Blind.

Dean Case

1895. New South Wales. Regina *versus* George Dean. Report of the Royal Commission, appointed seventh day of May, 1895. Presented to Parliament by Command. Sydney: Charles Potter, Govt Printer . . . 1895. . . .

331 × 212. Pp. 366, 46 (l.b.). Paper boards, cloth spine (title rptd).

Reviews case in which Dean, Sydney ferry-master, had been convicted of attempted poisoning of his wife with arsenic and ? strychnine. The Commission—F. E. Rogers QC (Chairman), Philip Sydney Jones MD, and F. Norton Manning MD—by majority decision of its medical members, Chairman opposing, recommended Dean's release and he received Royal Pardon. Includes medical evidence, and appendix reports animal experiments on dual effects of arsenic and strychnine by C. J. Martin.

For subsequent dramatic events, including Dean's confession and conviction for perjury, and removal of his solicitor from roll of practitioners, see Frank Clune, *Scandals of Sydney Town*, Syd., 1957. *Austsn med. Gaz.*, 1896, 15 : 540 notes article by Havelock Ellis, *J. Mental Science*, Oct. 1896, criticising judgement of med. members of Commission.

Copies: EF, FC, LNSW, ML, NL. 611

De Cosmos, Amor

Twelve hundred valuable secrets Being a compendium of most valuable secrets, processes and recipes, compiled with great care from the latest and most authentic sources . . . Melbourne, C. Smith & Co. Publishers . . .

184 × 123. Pp. 208. ND. P. w. (decorated variation of title).

Includes family and patent medicines and domestic recipes (including insect and vermin poisons, disinfectants and fumigants).

Copies: ML. 612

Dental and Oral Hospital of Victoria

The Dental and Oral Hospital of Victoria. Founded 1895.] [Incorporated 1897. Report and Treasurer's financial statement also by-laws and regulations. July, 1898. Melbourne: D. W. Paterson, Printer . . .

217 × 143. Pp. 16. P. w. (title rptd).

Hosp. founded Jan. 1895, later named Melb. Dental Hosp.

Copies: SLV. 613

See also Aust. College of Dentistry and Melb. Dental Hosp.

Dental Association of Victoria

Useful hints on the care of the teeth, issued by the authority of the Council of the Dental Association of Victoria. June 1893.

150 × 121. Pp. 8. Colophon—C. W. Burford . . . Melb. P. w. (decorated title, list officers on verso).

Copies: SLV. 614

'Deuteronomy Smith'

See Henry, Thomas James.

Devlin, A. A.

See New South Wales—Anthrax Board.

Dewar, James

On the application of sulphurous acid, gaseous and liquid, to the prevention, limitation, and cure of contagious diseases, with cases illustrative of the advantages to be derived from its employment. By James Dewar, M.D., Kirkcaldy. Sydney: John Sands . . . 1868. . . .

212 × 135. Pp. 48. P. w. (title rptd).

Copies: LNSW, ML, SLV. 615

Dick, James Adam

See Tidswell, Frank and Dick, James Adam.

Dick, Report

Hunter River Combined Sanitary District. Report of the Medical Officer for Health for the year 1899. ... to the Local Sanitary Authorities . . . [Text begins.]

323 × 204. Pp. 14. 2 charts. Colophon—Syd.: William Applegate Gullick, Govt Pr—1900. Signed: Robert Dick.

Robert Dick MB, ChM Syd. (1892), DPH Camb., joined NSW Pub. Health Service in 1898 and was GMO Newcastle and MOH Hunter River Dists. He became Pres. NSW Bd Health and Dir Gen. Pub. Health (1924–34).

Copies: EF. 616

See also No 1480.

Diesterweg, Alexander

See Jamieson, James Translator.

Diggles, Silvester

Queensland Philosophical Society. (From the *Queensland Guardian*, September 21, 1864.)

217 × 138. Pp. 4. Double cols.

Contains 'Thoughts suggested by the theory of Mr. Darwin', a lecture by S. Diggles.

Copies: FC. 617

Directions for Restoring the Apparently Drowned

Directions for restoring the apparently drowned. (Vide Government Gazette, 25th November, 1864.) [Text begins.]

216 × 136. Pp. 8. 4 woodcut figs. Colophon—Thomas Richards, Govt Pr . . . 1885. Reprinted from Royal Life-boat Instn Rep., 1864.

Copies: ML. 618

District Trained Nursing Society of South Australia

District Trained Nursing Society. Names of office bearers and general committee. . . . Adelaide: . . . Vardon and Pritchard . . . 1894.

212 × 135. Pp. 8 (l.b.).

Includes constitution and rules.

Copies: SLS. 619

———

District Trained Nursing Society. "Ministering Angels". A graphic narrative. By Seneca. From *S. A. Register*, July 22, 1898. [Text follows.]

340 × 212. Single leaf, v.b. Colophon: W. K. Thomas & Co. . . . Adel.

Copies: SLS. 620

———

District Trained Nursing Society of South Australia. Constitution and rules. Adelaide: . . . Vardon & Pritchard . . . 1899.

212 × 140. Pp. 12. P. w. (title rptd).

Established 1893. For history, see *Nursing in SA*, 2 ed., Adel., 1939.

Copies: ML. 621

Dixson, Thomas (translator)

Elements of pharmacology. By Dr. Oswald Schmiedeberg, Professor of Pharmacology and Director of the Pharmacological Institute University of Strassburg. Translated under the author's supervision. By Thomas Dixson, M.B., Lecturer on Materia Medica, in the University of Sydney, NSW. Edinburgh: Young J. Pentland. 1887.

222 × 140. Pp. xii (l.b.), 222. 7 diagrams. Cloth.

Recognised text book in English speaking medical schools. Translator worked under author at Strassburg for two years. Review, *Aust. med. J.*, 1887, ns 9 : 515.

For Thomas Storie Dixson (1854–1932) MB, ChM Edin., prominent Syd. physician, see obit., *Aust. Museum Magazine*, 1933, 5 : 21.

Copies: EF, SLV, UA, UM, US. 622

Do Not Emigrate Yet

Do not emigrate yet. The writer of this pamphlet having had extended opportunities of judging of the usual conduct of seamen on board of vessels conveying emigrants; and seeing . . . that the better protection of emigrants in general, and of female emigrants in particular, has . . . interested the Upper House of the Legislature; thinks it a duty to give publicity to what he knows on this matter . . . [Text continues.]

209 × 127. Pp. 16, 4. No title-page. ND. (1850.)

Anonymous author attacks conditions of depravity, drunkenness, insanitation and neglect on emigrant ships, stating that 'it is idle for a captain to seek to shelter himself by impugning that frequent and foul pest . . . a drunken or drinking doctor.' He criticises the morality of the Australian colonies, and regards 'Sydney . . . for its population (as) probably the greatest mart for female prostitution in the world . . .' The 'sufferings and murder of the natives, in countries colonized by the British', are also discussed.

Copies: ML, NL. 623

Douglas, Achilles

Devils abroad; and how to fight them. . . . Brisbane: Davison & Metcalf . . . 1888.

186 × 122. Pp. 208. P. w. (shortened title, illustrated).

Attacks vice and depravity (including prostitution, abortion and alcoholism) in Aust. cities. These are 'exposed in repulsive, destroying, fouling, damning ugliness', so that 'several firms were afraid to print and publish these pages.'

Copies: ML, NL, OL. 624

Douglass, Henry Grattan

Hints on the best means of security against the prevailing epidemic. Dublin. 1817.

NS. Discussed in Plomley, N.J.B. (1961), 'Some notes on the life of Dr. Henry Grattan Douglass', *Med. J. Aust.*, 1 : 801.

Typhus, widespread in Ireland, attacked Dublin in Nov. 1817.

625

———

Dissertatio medica inauguralis de origin causis et natura morbi epidemici, qui nuper ir hac insula grassatus est, pro gradu doctoris in medicina, in Collegio Sanctae Individuaeque Trinitatis ... Eblanae [Dublin], 1819.

NS. Thesis on typhus for MD TCD. Noted in Plomley (1961), above. Copy in Library, Roy. Coll. Phys. Ireland. 626

———

Statement, including a correspondence between the Commissioners of the Court of Enquiry, and the Rev. Samuel Marsden, relative to a charge of illegal punishment preferred against Doctor Douglass, held at Parramatta, in July 1825. By order of Lord Bathurst ... Sydney: Printed by Robert Howe, Government Printer. 1828.

212 × 132. Pp. [ii] (half title, v.b.), 54 (l.b.).

For official papers on the bitter, protracted feud between Marsden and Douglass, of which the above charge formed part, see *HRA*, ser. 1, vols 10–15. This resulted in Douglass leaving Sydney in 1828, to return in 1848.

Copies: DL, FC, ML, NL. 627

———

Catalogue of the valuable library and other effects, the property of Henry Grattan Douglass, Esq. which will be sold by auction, by George and John Paul, ... 21st of April, 1828 ... Conditions of sale, prompt payment in sterling money; or dollars at 4s. 4d. each. Sydney: Printed at the Gazette Office. 1828.

12mo. Pp. 16.

Henry Grattan Douglass (1790–1865) MD TCD, MRCS, came to Sydney in 1821 and was in charge of Colonial Hosp., Parramatta. He left Sydney in 1828, practised in France, and returned in 1848. Thereafter he became Hon. Phys. Syd. Infirm. and Benev. Asylum, a mainstay of local charities, and inspirer of foundation of Univ. Syd. See Brown, K. M. (1937), *Med. practice in old Parramatta*, Syd.; Brown, K. M. (1943), *Med. J. Aust.*, 1 : 455; Plomley, N.J.B. (1961), *Med. J. Aust.*, 1 : 801; Noad, K. B. (1962), *BPCMUS* 18 : 125.

Copies: ML. 628

Dovey, William R.

New South Wales as a health resort. ... read before the Insurance Institute of New South Wales on 22nd June, 1899.

161 × 110. Pp. 16. Colophon—McCarron, Stewart & Co. ... Sydney. ND. (1899.) P. w. (cover title).

Directs attention to 'the powerful effects of the Aust. climate in lessening the mortality from respiratory diseases', and purports to prove this by comparative statistics. Author was Actuary, Citizens' Life Assurance Co.

Copies: FC. 629

Doyle, Henry Martin

Voyaging for health.

NS. Noted in *Austsn Med. Directory*, 1892, which shows author, then at Newcastle NSW, as formerly 'MO, invalid sailing-ship *Sabraon*.'

H. M. Doyle MRCS (1886) was Hon. Phys. Newcastle Hosp. ML has collection of press cuttings (c. 1895) on history of Newcastle, compiled and some written by him. Also album of photographs, 'Voyage of the *Sabraon*, 1890–91.' For ship *Sabraon*, see Workman, Francis. 630

Doyne, W. T.

The Turkish bath explained, in a series of letters addressed to the Editor of the "Launceston Examiner" ... Reprinted for Mrs. E. Turnbull ... Launceston. [Text begins.]

211 × 126. Pp. 6. ND. Letters dated 1862. NI.

Mentions Dr. J. le G. Brereton's introduction of Turkish bath to Australia.

Copies: ML. 631

———

The sanitary condition of Melbourne. A series of three letters, by W. T. Doyne, M. Inst. C. E. Reprinted from "The Argus". Melbourne: Sands and McDougall ... 1868.

207 × 135. Pp. 16.

'... the present non-sanitary system costs the people of Melbourne per annum ... 1,500 lives, 30,000 cases of sickness, £70,000, and any quantity of cholera &c., in prospect.'

Copies: ML, NL. 632

Drayton, H. S.

Nervousness: its nature, causes, symptoms and treatment. With notes of cases. ... Illustrated. Sydney: The Modern Publishing Company ... E. T. Radcliffe, Printer ... Sydney

183 × 120. Pp. 64. ND. P. w. (title rptd).

Reprints US publication. Treatment: 'Of hygienic class best adapted for domestic uses.'

Copies: BG, EF, NL, RACP. 633

Dredge, James

Brief notices of the Aborigines of New South

Wales, including Port Phillip in reference to their past history and present condition, and the various schemes hitherto adopted for their benefit with the results and expenses of each, together with a plan for their moral and social improvement. . . . Geelong . . . James Harrison. 1845.

198 × 130. Pp. 46.

Discusses deterioration of physical and moral condition, and depopulation. Author was late Asst Protector of Aborigines.

Copies: SLV. 634

Druitt, Robert

Report on the cheap wines from France, Germany, Italy, Austria, Greece, Hungary, and Australia: their use in diet and medicine. Second edition . . . London: Henry Renshaw . . . 1873.

181 × 122. Pp. xii, 180, [2] (advts). 1 pl. Limp cloth.

1 ed., 1868, was a series of articles from *Med. Times & Gaz.*, 1863–4.

A number of Aust. wines receive high praise, including those of Dr. A. C. Kelly of Tintara.

Copies: ML, SLS. 635

Dückershoff, August

See Hoff, August

Dugong Oil

New therapeutic agent. (Extract from the Moreton Bay Courier, Feb. 5, 1853.) [Text begins.]

255 × 105. Single leaf, v.b. Blue paper.

Notes use of the oil of the dugong as a substitute for cod-liver oil by Mr. Hobbs, Brisbane surgeon, and extols its value in pulmonary and dyspeptic ailments.

See also—Hobbs, Wm, 'Elaiopathy'.

Copies: EF. 636

Sydney International Exhibition of 1879. The Queensland Court. Rise and progress of Queensland industries. Dugong fishery. [Text begins.]

224 × 140. Pp. 4 (l.b.). Colophon—J. H. Reynolds . . . Bris.

Includes note on medicinal use of dugong oil.

Copies: EF. 637

Duncan, Handasyde

The Colony of South Australia. . . . London: T. & W. Boone . . . 1850.

220 × 143. Pp. iv (ii, l.b.), 64, [8] (book notices). Frontis. P. w. (title rptd).

Facsimile ed., Adel.: Libraries Bd of SA, 1962.

Includes chapter on climate and disease, noting advantages of colony for tuberculosis sufferers.

For Handasyde Duncan (1811–78) MD, who came to Adel. in 1839, and later practised in Pt Adel., see Cleland, J. B. (1941), *Pioneer med. men in SA*, Adel.; also biog. and epitome of diary of voyage to SA, by A. A. Lendon, in Archives Dept, Adel.

Copies: ML, NL, SLS, SLV, UA, US. 638

Dunolly District Hospital, Vic.

Report of the Committee of Management of the Dunolly District Hospital . . . together with the rules and regulations . . . Inglewood: Printed by J. Vogel . . . 1861.

204 × 132. Pp. 16. P. w. (cover title).

Opened Nov. 1860. 1st an. rep.

Copies: SLV (1–19; 1861–72). 639

Dunwich Benevolent Asylum, Qd

1885. Queensland. Regulations for the general management of the Benevolent Asylum at Dunwich. Presented to both Houses . . . [Text begins.]

320 × 204. Pp. 4 (l.b.). Colophon—James C. Beal, Govt Pr, Bris.

Copies: LNSW, NL, OL, SLV. 640

1889. Queensland. Report on the Benevolent Asylum, Dunwich, for the year 1888. . . . To the . . . Colonial Secretary. . . .

326 × 204. Pp. 4 (l.b.). Colophon—James C. Beal, Govt Pr . . . Bris.

Reports: 1880–1900.

Copies: LNSW, NL, OL, SLV. 641

Dyring, Carl Peter Wilhelm

Lectures on nursing. . . . [Text begins.]

229 × 150. Pp. 34. Double cols. ND. (1887.) Colophon—'The Reformer' Printing and Publishing Company . . . Brunswick.

General and fever nursing; throat and chest diseases; feeding and management of infants; invalid dietetics.

For C.P.W. Dyring (1860–1931) MB, BS Melb., of Coburg Vic., Anaesthetist to Alfred and Women's Hosps., Melb., see obit., *Med. J. Aust.*, 1931, 2 : 249.

Copies: SLV. 642

E

Eades, Richard

Syllabus of Dr. Eades' lectures on materia medica and therapeutics.

... v. b. ND. (1861.) NI.

...mural lectures, prior ...ed. School. In 1863 ...riginal Univ. Melb.

... (1809–67) MB Dub., ...b. Hosp., MOH and ..., *Aust. med. J.*, 1867,

643

...ge

...rigades for the saving ...colliery explosions & ... the N.S.W. Govern- ...ittee. ... Reprinted ...Medical Gazette ... Sands, Typ.

...cover title).

...t of NSW Med. Corps ...*e story of South Africa*, ..., by various authors.

...956), MB, BCh TCD, ... NSW, served with ...Var and World War 1 ... as Maj Gen. Obit., ...*Med. J. Aust.*, 2 : 209.

644

... invalids and tourists ...ory" Office, 1884. ...

... P. w. (cover title).

...lian voyage for convalescents, and discusses climate and advantages of various colonies.

Copies: LNSW, ML. 645

Echo Farm Home for Male Inebriates, Sydney

"Good Tidings". The first bi-annual report of Echo Farm Home, Middle Harbour, Sydney, established, 1892. ... Hon. Director. ... Courtenay Smith. ... 1892. William Brooks ... Sydney.

209 × 135. Pp. 8.

First NSW inebriate treatment instsn, later called Resthaven. Established 1892.

Copies: ML. 646

An account of Echo Farm for Male Inebriates, Middle Harbour, Sydney ... by A. G. Taylor, entitled: "Intemperance—its ill effects and its cure." [Text begins.]

222 × 135. Pp. 4. ND. (189–.) Colophon—T. B. Perry & Co. ... Syd.

Copies: ML. 647

Eclectic, An

Human life An inquiry touching the duty of the state in relation to pauper children ... George Robertson Melbourne, Sydney, and Adelaide 1877.

210 × 133. Pp. 16. P. w. (title rptd).

Copies: ML, OL, SLV. 648

Edwards, William

Mesmerism: its practice and phenomena: with numerous cases illustrative of sleep walking and clairvoyance. ... Melbourne: Published by John Hunter ... and sold by Harrison, Geelong; Wilkinson, Portland; Piddington, Sydney; Walch, Hobart Town; Dowling, Launceston ... 1850.

186 × 107. Pp. viii, [9]–108. Errata slip. Frontis.—phrenological fig. P. w. (shortened title and cut).

Dedicated to Godfrey Howitt MD, 'the head of the Medical Profession, in this Province.'

Copies: ML, SLV. 649

Edwic * C. W., M.L.D.A.**

See Cole, Edward Wm, No 543.

Electric and Thermopathic Institute, Melbourne

Electric and Thermopathic Institute ... Melbourne. Physician ... G. F. Maberly, M.R.C.S.

. . . Assisted by skilled assistants. [Text begins.]
217 × 135. Pp. 4 (l.b.). ND. [1879.]
Outlines facilities of Institute.
Copies: SLV. 650

Electric and Thermopathic Institute. 98 Collins Street East . . . September 17th, 1879. [Text begins.]
204 × 132. Single leaf, v.b.
Letter, signed G. F. Maberly MRCS, announces opening.
Copies: SLV. 651

Electro-Medical and Surgical Institute, Sydney
See Freeman, Howard and Wallace, Richard.

Ellis, John
The human body described for the instruction of the young of both sexes. In twenty-six lessons. . . . with plates. Melbourne: George Slater, and all booksellers.
163 × 98. Pp. [ii] (v.b.), ii, 34 (l.b.), [ii]. 4 pl. ND. P. w. (variation of title).
Copies: SLV. 652

Elsner, Frederick William—Translator
Hydrotherapeutics, by Dr. W. Winternitz, of Kaltenleutgeben, near Vienna. Translated by F. W. Elsner, F.R.C.S.I. of Melbourne, Victoria.
220 × 140. Pp. 273–624, of vol. 5, von Ziemssen's *Handbook of general therapeutics*, Lond., Smith, Elder, & Co., 1886.
F. W. Elsner FRCSI, Hon. Phys. Alfred Hosp. Melb., was associated with the establishment of a sanatorium for consumptives at Sorrento Vic. (*Austsn med. Gaz.*, 1887, 6 : 173 and 208). He practised at Moree NSW in 1896.
Copies: AMAV. 653

Embley, Edward Henry
Anaesthesia. Extracted from a lecture by E. H. Embley . . . Hon. Anaesthetist to the Melbourne Hospital. [Emblem] Melbourne: The Austral Publishing Co. . . . 1899.
220 × 140. Pp. 12. P. w. (cover title).
Instruction for students.
E. H. Embley (1861–1924) MD Melb., Hon. Anaesth. Melb. Hosp. and Lect. Anaesth. Univ. Melb., was noted for his important scientific studies on the action of anaesthetics, published from 1900 to his death. Univ. Melb. has full set of his papers. See Osborne, W. A. (1924), *Med. J. Aust.*, 2 : 47; also Brown, G., (1939), *Med. J. Aust.*, 1 : 209.
Copies: SLV. 654

Engelmann, Georges J. and Rodet, Paul
La pratique des accouchements chez les peuples primitifs Etude d'ethnographie et d'obstetrique . . . Paris Librairie J.–B. Bailliere et Fils . . . 1886 . . .
230 × 140. Pp. xvi, 388, 8 (book notices). 83 text figs. P. w. (title rptd).
Includes brief notes on pregnancy and parturition in Aust. aborigines. Localities not stated.
Copies: EF. 654a

The Same. Labour among primitive peoples. George Julius Engelmann. 2 ed. St. Louis, Chambers. 1883. NS.
654b

Eskell, Louis
The Australian handbook and guide for the preservation of the teeth. By Louis Eskell, Member of the Royal College of Surgeon-Dentists, London. . . . Sydney: . . . Robert Bone, Phoenix Office . . .
171 × 107. Pp. vi (l.b.), 7–20. Frontis.—head and neck with hinged flap over jaws, covering details of deep structures. (1860.)
Copies: LNSW. 655

Eureka Patent Sanitary Company
The Eureka Patent Sanitary Company, Limited. Newcastle, N.S.W. : Harris & Son . . . "Despatch" Office . . . 1890.
8vo. Pp. 12.
Advertises patent and indicates evils of existing systems of sewage disposal.
Copies: FC. 656

Evans, Fred
Independent slate writing. Biography, testimonials, and press notices of Fred Evans, the world-renowned sensitive for psychography, or independent slate writing. Melbourne: Pater and Knapton . . . 1890.
212 × 135. Pp. 24.
Includes letter from Psychological Soc., Brisbane, stating that 'psychological students have in you superior instruments through which they may obtain phenomena of the greatest importance to mankind', and inviting

acceptance of a purse of sovereigns. Letter from Alfred Russell Wallace states that he had never 'witnessed phenomena of so wonderful a character . . . and so entirely free from suspicion.'

Copies: EF, FC, NL. 657

Evans, Thomas

A new operation for pterygium. . . . Reprinted from the Transactions of the Third Session, Intercolonial Medical Congress of Australasia, Sydney. 1892.

234 × 145. Pp. 4 (2, 4 blank). Syd.: Charles Potter, Govt Pr—1893.

For Thomas Evans (1851–1909), MRCS, Hon. Ophth. Surg. Syd. Hosp., frequently called the first Aust. eye specialist, see *Austsn med. Gaz.*, 1909, 28 : 103; Williams, D. (1947), *Trans Ophth. Soc. Aust.*, 7 : 5.

Copies: ML. 658

Ewing, Rev. Robert Kirkwood

Lecture replying to objections against phrenology delivered . . . by the Reverend R. K. Ewing, of . . . Launceston . . . The third of a course of lectures on phrenology . . . Launceston: Henry Dowling, Printer . . . 1852.

178 × 112. Pp. 52 (l.b.). P. w. (title rptd).

Copies: ML, SLT. 659

Exposition of the State of the Medical Profession

An exposition of the state of the medical profession in the British Dominions; and of the injurious effects of the monopoly, by usurpation, of the Royal College of Physicians in London. . . . [Quotation] London: . . . Longman, Rees, Orme, Brown, and Green . . . 1826.

227 × 138. Pp. [iv] (l.b.), 374 (l.b.). Paper boards, cloth backstrip, paper label on spine.

This attack on the privileges and influence of the Royal College of Physicians was listed, though not seen, by Ferguson (1 : 1070a). It contains no specific reference to Australia.

Copies: EF. 660

Eye and Ear Hospital, Melbourne

See Victorian Eye and Ear Hospital.

F

Faithfull, Paul

... Dunheved Island or, the Dutchman's dream, a tale of submarine squatting ... Printed by M. P. Branston & Co. ... London: Published by John Lionel Ching & Company, Townsville, Queensland, and Sydney ...

212 × 138. Pp. 20. ND.

Includes account of dugong oil as substitute for cod liver oil by Dr. Wm Hobbs, and his lecture on 'elaiopathy' or treatment of chronic diseases with oil. See Hobbs, William.

Copies: NL. 661

Farmer, Paul Ward

The purity and strength of drugs and chemicals. ... Reprinted from the "Intercolonial Medical Journal of Australasia", February 20, 1897. Stillwell and Co. ... Melbourne.

246 × 155. Pp. 10. P. w. (cover title).

Copies: EF. 662

Our duties and responsibilities ... An address to medical students. Reprinted from The Speculum ... July, 1898. Austral Publishing Co. ... Melbourne.

222 × 140. Pp. 8. P. w. (title rptd).

Copies: EF. 663

Three weeks in the Kew Lunatic Asylum by Dr. Paul Ward Farmer (An ex-patient). ... Melbourne: John J. Halligan ... 1900.

214 × 138. Pp. 64. P. w. (title rptd; adds 'Second edition').

Author, a highly esteemed Melb. physician, draws 'attention to the shocking abuse of our present lunacy laws.' Preface mentions 'abortive efforts to block the circulation of the first edition by interested people.'

Copies: DL, EF, ML, NL, SLT, SLV, SLW. 664

Fattorini, Charles Lamonnerie Dictus

To the Legislative Council of New South Wales. The humble petition of Charles Lamonnerie Dictus Fattorini, Doctor of Medicine ... Sydney, respectfully sheweth ... [Text follows.]

220 × 140. Pp. 8. ND. [c 1849.] Colophon: Printed by Kemp and Fairfax ... Syd. Signed by hand, p. 5.

C. L. D. Fattorini, MD Gottingen, petitions against a Bill to regulate the medical profession, which would exclude all but those with British qualifications.

Author came to NSW in 1829, and practised at Pt Macquarie (1836–42).

Copies: DL. 665

Faulding's Medical Journal

Faulding's Medical Journal devoted to medicine, diet and sanitary science. Published by F. H. Faulding & Co., Wholesale Druggists and Manufacturing Chemists, Adelaide, S. A., and Perth, W. A. (Edited by J. P. Giddings.) ... Vol. 1. July 20, 1899. No. 1. [Text begins.]

214 × 138. Pp. 20. Monthly. Distributed free to doctors, nurses and chemists.

In Jan. 1906 title changed to *Faulding's Medical and Home Journal*; in Dec. 1913 to *Faulding's Journal*.

Copies: See *SSAL*. 666

Faulkner, Thomas

See Byrn, Marcus L. (note).

Fawcett, Benjamin

Lecture on the science of medicine, and the doctrine of disease; or, health & how to preserve it, and if lost or injured how to restore it. Delivered at ... Hill End March 20th, 1873 ... Sydney ... F. White ... 1873.

183 × 110. Pp. 44 (l.b.). P. w. (title rptd).

Advocates hygiene and homoeopathy and attacks allopathic medicine.

Copies: ML. 667

Woman, know thyself! An essay on childbirth without danger and nearly painless. Also, ladies' perpetual calendar; with chapter on the qualifications and duties of a good nurse, with advice as to the sure method of raising a healthy family. Respectfully submitted to the perusal of the married ladies of New South Wales. ... Second edition, greatly enlarged. Sydney: F. Cunninghame and Co. ... 1882. ...

183 × 120. Pp. 60. Inserted slip. P. w. (variation of title; advts on other sides).

Deplores ignorance of female diseases by med. profession, by which 'women are drugged into an aggravation of all their evils; outraged by ... useless examinations; ... and leeched and cauterized, until death itself would be a welcome refuge ...'; and recommends his homoeopathic remedies for all female troubles.

Author, who practised in NSW at Hill End, Bathurst, and Ultimo, lacked med. training (*NSW Leg. Council, Rep. Sel. Com. on ... Med. and Surg.*, Syd., 1887); advertised himself as 'Champion healer of cancer' (*Austsn med. Gaz.*, 1889, 8 : 218).

Copies: ML. 668

———

The Same. 3 ed., 1886. Pp. 108.

Copies: EF. 669

Female Friendly Society

Rules of the Female Friendly Society, of the Town of Sydney ... Founded in 1826. Sydney: Printed by R. Howe, Govt Printer. 1827.

181 × 115. Pp. 8.

Founded to provide relief in sickness and old age, Society furnished sickness, accident, maternity and funeral benefits.

Copies: ML. 670

Fiaschi, Thomas

Da cheren a Cassala Note di viaggio del Dott. Tommaso Fiaschi. [Ornament] Firenze, Tipographia di G. Barbera. 1896.

12mo. Pp. 32. P. w. (title rptd).

NS. Formerly in Mackaness coll.

Also published: contribution to *The story of South Africa*, vol. 2, by various authors, Syd., ND (?1904).

For Thomas Fiaschi (1853–1927) MD ChD (Florence & Pisa), Hon. Surg. Syd. Hosp., prominent surgeon and viticulturalist, see obits, *Med. J. Aust.*, 1927, 1 : 732 and J. & P. Roy. Soc. NSW, 1927, 61 : 14; also Aspinall, A. (1933), *Med. J. Aust.*, 2 : 879; for viticulture, Lake M. (1967), *Vine and scalpel*, Bris.

671

'Fiat Justitia'

See Wardley, Edward, No 2448.

Figg, Edward Garland

The rational theory of life, in opposition to Huxley. ... Melbourne: Clarson, Massina, & Co. ... 1869.

192 × 122. Pp. 32.

E. G. Figg (c. 1815–1902) LFPS Glas., Health Officer, Hobson's Bay, relinquished this post in 1890 for practice in Williamstown Vic. He published *Catechism of Irish history*, Melb., 1886, and also poetical and theological works.

Copies: ML, SLV. 672

———

Allopathy vindicated from Dr. Günst's attack. Melbourne: Clarson and Massina. 1870.

NS. Reviewed in *Homoeopathic Progress*, 1870, 1 : 27, and *Aust. med. J.*, 1870, 15 : 255.

673

———

See International Temperance Conference, 1880.

Figgis, R.

A handbook of hydropathy. Water cure for the people. ... E. & P. Traylen, Printers.

165 × 108. Pp. [ii] (v.b.), 70, [2] advts. (Perth, 1895.) P. w. (variation of title).

A hydropathist of Perth describes 'the best processes of water cure for use in the home treatment of diseases ... including typhoid, rheumatism, asthma, &c.'

Copies: ML. 674

Finch's Guide-Book

Finch's guide-book to the squatters' medicine chest, containing directions for the use of the medicines, practical observations on the treatment of diseases and accidents, and a variety of useful prescriptions. Sydney: F. Cunninghame ...

140 × 89. Pp. 52, [20]. ND. (c. 1868.) P. w. (title rptd).

Copies: ML. 675

FitzGerald, Sir Thomas Naghten

A surgeon's visit to the South African battlefields. By Sir T. N. FitzGerald, F.R.C.S.I. Senior Surgeon to the Melbourne Hospital. [Text begins.]

252 × 150. Pp. 12 (3 blanks). P. w. Repr., *Intercol med. J. Austsia*, 1900, 5 : 549.

Report of tour of duty as Cons. Surg. to British Army.

For Sir Thomas FitzGerald (1838–1908) FRCSI, the leading Vic. surgeon of his day, see obit., *Austsn med. Gaz.*, 1908, 27 : 428; also Zwar, B. T. (1932/3), *Aust. NZ J. Surg.*, 2 : 227; Russell, K. F. (1948) 'The Roy. Melb. Hosp. and its early surgeons', *Melb. Hosp. Clin. Rep.*, Centenary Vol.

Copies: EF, UM. 676

Fitzpatrick, Adolphus

A guide to the preservation of health in South Australia. By A. Fitzpatrick, M.D., late Physician-in-Chief to the Polish Army—Physician—Chief to the Foreign Legion of Belgium—Surgeon of the French 6th Hussars . . . Adelaide: Printed and published by Robert Thomas & Co., Hindley Street; sold also by Mr. Platts, Gilles Arcade, and by the author, at his residence, Currie Street.

173 × 106. Pp. viii, 28 (last—colophon). ND. [1841.] P. w. (title rptd).

Pt 1 : 'On the causes of diseases; pt 2 : On the preservation of health. Fewer affections incidental to climate will be found to occur in SA than in any other civilised part of the globe.

Copies: FC, ML. 677

A treatise on the effects of riding on nervous and chronic diseases.

NS. Authorship noted on title of *A guide to the preservation of health* . . .

678

Flett, William Simpson

The order and character of the various dispensations. An address delivered by W. Simpson Flett, M.D., at the Prophetic Conference held at Ballarat, Dec. 1887. [Text begins.]

209 × 138. Pp. 12. Colophon—Watt & Co. . . . Melb.

Copies: EF. 679

The claims of Darwinism rationally and scientifically considered in the light of Darwin's life and letters; being a lecture delivered in Melbourne; 26th July 1888 . . . George Robertson & Co., Melbourne and Sydney, 1888.

220 × 140. Pp. 28 (l.b.). P. w. (title rptd).

'Darwin's System is a reasonless, scienceless and . . . Godless theory.'

Author (MD Edin. & Melb.) arrived in Aust. 1884; practised for many years at Hawthorn and Collins St., Melb.

Copies: CC, EF, KFR, ML, NL, SLV. 680

See Australian Health Society, No 103.

Foord, George

See Industrial and Technological Museum, Melb.

Ford, Frederick Thomas West

The vital statistics of the police force of the colony of Victoria for the past ten years. . . . [Text begins.]

204 × 127. Pp. 4. Colophon—Wilson and MacKinnon . . . Melb. Repr., *Aust. med. J.*, 1866.

For F.T.W. Ford (1821–95) MRCS, Surg. to Vic. Police, see obit., *Austsn med. Gaz.*, 1895, 14 : 509.

Copies: UM. 681

Ford, William

How to develop personal magnetism to strengthen, exercise, and control the will power. By William Ford, A.P.S. Sydney: The Research Publishing Company.

222 × 107. Pp. 16. P. w. (pictorial, with portrait and 'The Power of Will').

Copies: ML. 682

Ford, William, and Co.

William Ford & Co., chemists and druggists, importers and dealers in drugs, chemicals, surgical instruments and appliances, patent medicines . . . Melbourne . . .

122 × 98. Pp. 36. Grey paper. ND. (c. 1875.)

Copies: SLV. 683

Forest, W. E.

Health: the new method; self and home help in certain chronic diseases. By W. E. Forest, B. S., M.D., Member of Y. Y. Academy of Medicine . . . Australasian edition (eighth): edited and published by W. Corrie Johnston . . . "Truth" and "Health" Publication Offices, Melbourne, Adelaide, Sydney and Christchurch . . .

178 × 122. Pp. xii, 13–332, [10] (advts). Christchurch, 1892, on verso of title.

May be bound with No 2437, with covering title: *Health: the new methods . . . and domestic guide to . . . Dr. Schüssler's new remedies.* ND.

Reprints US publication. On treatment by flushing, massage, exercise, diet, deep breathing, etc.

Copies: ML, RACP (NZ issue), SLV. 684

Fowler, Walter

Echuca as a lung resort. By Walter Fowler, M.A., M.B. Camb., F.R.C.S. Eng. [Text begins.]

229 × 140. Pp. 4 (l.b.). Repr., *Intercol med. J. Austsia*, 1900, 5 : 247.

Walter Fowler FRCS, Surg. to Lond. Throat and Ear Hosp. and Seamen's Hosp. Lond., commenced practice in Echuca Vic. about 1892, was at Bendigo in 1911.

Copies: SLV. 685

Fox, William Robert

The bubonic plague; or, the black death. . . . Melbourne: Rae Bros. . . .

242 × 153. Pp. 24. 10 figs. (1900.) P. w. (variation of title).

A popular historical and clinical account.

W. R. Fox (d. 1911) LRCPE (1883), who practised at Fitzroy Vic. and was Hon. Phys. to Benev. Asylum Melb., an early and productive contributor in radiology, died apparently as a result of radiation. Also published: *The urethroscope. Its development and its use*, Melb., 1909. For obit., *Austsn med. Gaz.*, 1911, 30 : 542; for brief appreciation, *Salute to the X-ray pioneers of Aust.*, Syd., 1946.

Copies: ML, NL. 686

Francis, Alexander

Presidential address. Delivered before the Medical Society of Queensland, 4th January, 1898. Sydney: John Sands . . . 1898.

247 × 183. Pp. 6 (l.b.).

Copies: AMAQ. 687

Francis, Henry

The present and future government of the colony of New South Wales, . . . "Kill a man's family and he may brook it, but keep your hands out of his breeches pocket". Sydney: F. Cunninghame & Co. . . . 1869.

210 × 135. Pp. 48.

Criticism of NSW Govt and demand for reform. Mentions insanitary condition of Sydney and poor state of works 'such as cleaning and making sewers, preventing the harbour being converted into a cess-pool, . . . which work is conducted as if it were managed by a lot of Australian blacks.'

Copies: DL, LNSW, ML, NL, SLS. 688

Francis, Henry Alexander

Pregnancy and normal labour. A practical guide for the use of mothers and nurses living in the bush. . . . Brisbane: Pole, Outridge and Co., General Printers . . . 1891.

178 × 122. Pp. 36 (last 2 blank). P. w. (title rptd).

For H. A. Francis MB, BCh Camb., who practised in Barcaldine Qd and Brisbane, see his autobiographical *Then and now. The story of a Queenslander*, Lond., [1935]. Also published: *Asthma in relation to the nose*, Lond., 1903.

Copies: SLV. 689

Francis, M.

See No 595.

Franks, Lizzie

A young Victorian teacher, Lizzie Franks: her trials and triumphs of faith. With preface by Rev. John Thomson . . . and introductory note by Rev. Allen W. Webb, Geelong. . . . The Bible and Tract Repository . . . Melbourne. . . .

180 × 120. Pp. xxiv (last—portrait), 126, [2] (colophon, v.b.). 2 pl., 1 fig. ND. (1897.) Cloth.

Biography and diary of a Ballarat teacher who, during invalidism from tuberculosis which led to her death in 1895, conducted widespread home mission work by correspondence, including printed monthly letter to invalids and prisoners, of which 30,000 were distributed in 2½ years.

Copies: FC, ML, NL, SLV. 690

Lizzie Franks' letters to sufferers and workers. Selected, with preface and concluding remarks on holiness, knowing God, the Lord's leadings, the so-called divine healing, etc., By Rev. John Thomson . . . Melbourne: . . . M. L. Hutchinson . . . and Religious Tract Society of Victoria, . . . Printed by Jas Arbuckle & Co. . . . 1898.

186 × 125. Pp. vi, 130. Frontis. 3 figs. Cloth.

Extracts from correspondence. Editor's notes include sections on her experience of so-called divine or faith healing, and of arguments for and against this.

Copies: EF, ML, NL, SLV. 691

Fraser, Joseph

Physiognomy made easy, or the art of reading faces. ... Melbourne: E. W. Cole ...

181 × 105. Pp. [4] (advts, pink paper), 52, [4] (book notices, pink paper). 46 figs. ND. P. w. (short title with cut of phrenologist's head).

2 ed., 1889.

Prof. Fraser (phrenologist and physiognomist) also published *Hydropathy in the household*. NS.

Copies: ML, SLV. 692

———

Faces and heads or, how to read men as open books. ... Melbourne: E. W. Cole, Book Arcade ... 1894.

183 × 122. Pp. [2] (book notices), 104 (last 3—book notices). Illustrated. P. w. (variation of title).

New ed., ND.; another ed., 1911.

Copies: ML, NL, SLV. 693

Free Hospital for Sick Children, Melbourne

See Melbourne Hospital for Sick Children.

Freeman, Howard and Wallace, Richard

Rescued at last: being clinical experiences on nervous and private diseases, by Sydney's leading specialists, [Emblem] Dr. Howard Freeman, ... and Dr. Wallace ... legally qualified ... in Great Britain, America, and throughout Australasia. 1898.

178 × 120. Pp. xvi, 296 (last—colophon only). 16 coloured litho. pl., 64 figs. Colophon—Turner and Henderson ... Syd. Cloth.

A vividly illustrated treatise on sexual complaints, published by a partnership which later became the Electro-Medical and Surgical Inst., Sydney. Includes such chapters as youthful follies leading to demoralization, nervous debility, masturbation, spermatorrhoea, impotence, venereal diseases.

Howard Freeman, whose qualifications are given as 'M.B.S.A., Prof. of Electricity, Member of Harmon's College, Washington Cor., Cal., U.S.A., legally qualified by med. boards in G. Britain, U.S. and Australasia', an American, conducted the Progressive Remedy Inst. in Brisbane in 1892. He was unregistered in any Aust. state.

Richard Wallace LRCPE, LFPS Glas. (1864), MD Calif., served in the British Army and was on staff of Homoeopathic Hosp., Melb. He apparently joined Freeman about 1898, was deregistered 1904, left Inst. before 1906, and was at New Lambton NSW in 1911. See his *Homoeopathy*.

Copies: EF, KFR, ML. 694

———

Clinical experiences on nervous & private diseases by the Electro-Medical and Surgical Institute [Emblem] Drs. Freeman and Wallace ... 1900.

180 × 118. Pp. xvi, 396 (l.b.). 16 pl., 66 figs. NI. Perforated coloured application slips inserted. Cloth.

Reprints 296 pp. of *Rescued at last*, with added sections, new title and plates.

Withdrawn after enactment of 1900 legislation which gave control of unqualified practice. Replaced by *Clinical experiences of nervous and chronic diseases*, five issues seen, only one dated (1902). This omits all sexual content, and Freeman's medical titles are dropped. Melb. branch added on later titles.

In a successful action by a patient (*Austsn med Gaz.*, 1908, 27 : 568), judge described Inst. as marked by "cruel cunning, unmeasured audacity and hypocritical pretence.' Persons who replied to advertisements were lured on by stock letters to 'arouse their terrors, get them into their clutches, and obtain their money ... He has insanity forecast him, physical decay, ultimately the grave.' In 1908 Post Office stopped delivery of firm's mail and it closed soon after.

Copies: EF, KFR. 695

———

The Same. 1900. Pp. xvi, 398 (l.b.). 29 pl. 66 figs. NI. Notes publication of *Home cures* (NS).

Copies: EF, KFR. 696

———

1897–1898 Souvenir of the English eleven containing photos and performances of each member of the team; also scoring card ...

133 × 108. Pp. 28. 15 figs. P. w. (cover title, advts on other sides).

Advertises "Sydney's leading specialists.'

Copies: ML. 697

Fremantle Hospital, WA

1898. Western Australia. Report of the Board of Management of the Fremantle Hospital.

Presented to both Houses ... Perth: A. Curtis, Acting Govt Printer. 1898.

323 × 198. Pp. 4. (l.b.).

Annual reports. See J. H. Stubbe, *Medical Background ... history of Fremantle Hosp. and doctors*, Perth, 1969.

Copies: SLV, SLW. 698

Fremantle Lunatic Asylum, WA

1878. Western Australia. Report of Lunatic Asylum during year 1877. ... Perth: ... Richard Pether, Govt Printer. 1878.

305 × 191. Pp. 4 (l.b.).

Copies: SLV, SLW (1877, 1879–1900). 699

———

1883. Western Australia. Despatch and correspondence respecting the proposed transfer of the Lunatic Asylum at Fremantle, from the Imperial to the Colonial Government. ... Perth: ... Richard Pether, Govt Printer. 1883.

323 × 204. Pp. 6 (l.b.).

Copies: SLV, SLW. 700

———

1883. Western Australia. Report of the Select Committee of the Legislative Council appointed to inquire into the proposed transfer of the Lunatic Asylum at Fremantle from the Imperial to the Colonial Government. ... Second Session. Perth: ... Richard Pether, Govt Printer. 1883.

323 × 204. Pp. 4 (l.b.).

Copies: SLV, SLW 701

———

1891. Western Australia. Report of the Select Committee of the Legislative Assembly appointed to consider and report as to what is necessary to place the Asylum for the Insane on a satisfactory basis as to accommodation and maintenance ... Perth: ... Richard Pether, Govt Printer. 1891.

326 × 204. Pp. 10.

Copies: SLV, SLW. 702

———

1898. Western Australia. Result of inquiry into alleged ill-treatment of patients at the Fremantle Lunatic Asylum ... Perth: ... Richard Pether, Govt Printer. 1898.

324 × 204. Pp. 4.

Copies: SLV, SLW. 703

——— **and Whitby Falls Lunatic Asylum**

1900. Western Australia. Report of the Select Committee of the Legislative Assembly appointed to inquire into the condition of the Fremantle and Whitby Falls Lunatic Asylums. ... Perth: ... Richard Pether, Govt Printer. 1900.

305 × 204. Pp. 48 (last 2 blank).

Copies: SLV, SLW. 704

Fresh Air League, The

The Fresh Air League for providing the sick and respectable poor with a summer holiday. ... Non-sectarian. Sydney: Batson & Co. ... 1893.

112 × 74. Pp. [8].

Other editions: (? 1898), 1899.

Includes rules.

Copies: ML. 705

———

The Fresh Air League Its object ... [Text continues.]

214 × 130. Pp. [4] (2, 3 blank). ND.

Includes objects, work and methods of League. In later numbers name becomes 'Ministering Children's Fresh Air League.'

Copies: ML (5 numbers, ?1894–1902.) 706

M. C. Fresh Air League. Board of Management ... [Office bearers].

170 × 112. Pp. [8]. 1897. Colophon—Batson & Co., Ltd. ... Syd.

6th an. rep., 1896–7. Includes history of League.

Copies: ML. 707

Fresh Food and Ice Company, Limited, Sydney

Milk. Reports on city dairies taken from the principal newspapers of Sydney, also method adopted by the Fresh Food & Ice Co. ... to ensure the country milk delivered by them being pure and free from infectious germs. H. Solomon, Caxton Printing Office, ... Sydney.

181 × 122. Pp. 20. ND. [c. 1883.] P. w. (cover title).

Includes evidence of insanitary conditions in Sydney dairies.

Copies: FC, ML. 708

Friday Island Lazaret, Qd

1898. Queensland. Legislative Assembly. Report

of the Medical Officer of the Lazaret, Friday Island. Presented to both Houses ... [Text begins.]

342 × 204. Pp. 2. Colophon—Edmund Gregory, Govt Pr ...

Copies: LNSW, NL, OL, SLV. 709

Frith, Henry

Practical palmistry: a treatise on cheirosophy based upon actual experiences. ... With ... illustrations by Edith A. Langdon. E. W. Cole, Book Arcade Melbourne. ... (Printed in England).

186 × 122. Pp. viii, 138. Frontis., 36 figs. ND. (1895.) Cloth.

'... if physicians would devote themselves to the study of Cheirosophy, they would not only vastly increase their own knowledge and reputation, but would confer an inestimable benefit upon mankind.'

Copies: EF, FC. 710

Fuller, Claude

See No 595.

Fullerton, George

The family medical guide; with plain directions for the treatment of every case, and a list of the medicines required for any household. ... Second edition ... Sydney ... Joseph Cook & Co. ...

222 × 127. Pp. xii (viii blank), 550, [ii] (colophon, v.b.). Errata slip. [1875.] Cloth.

A widely used domestic guide, comprising descriptions and treatment of ailments. Preface states author was then an invalid, unable to practice, after 30 years Aust. experience.

1 ed., 1870. NS. (2 ed. notes 5000 copies sold.)

For George Fullerton (1802–1883) MD Edin., ChM Glas., Hon. Phys. Syd. Infirm., see *Aust. med. J.*, 1883, ns 5 : 478; *Austsn med. Gaz.*, 1883, 3 : 24.

Copies: AMAV, EF, ML. 711

The Same. 3 ed., 1878.

Copies: LNSW, SLV. 712

The Same. 4 ed., 1882. Frontis.—signed photo. Syd.: William Maddock, Lond.: Geo. Philip & Son. ML copy has inserted leaf (v.b.), after p. x, on new salicylate treatment.

Copies: BG, EF, ML, NL. 713

The Same. 6 ed., 1884. Frontis. Syd.: William Maddock.

Copies: BG, EF. 714

The Same. 8 ed., ND. Syd.: William Maddock.

Copies: UQ. 715

Testimonials in favour of Doctor George Fullerton. [Text follows.]

8vo. Pp. 36. ND. NI. (c. 1841.)

NS. From ms. note by Sir John Ferguson—though not in Bibliography or FC. 715a

G

Gardner, A. W.

The first few months of infancy: being hints to mothers, with an appendix containing other useful information. [Figure] 2nd edition. Improved and enlarged. Melbourne: Kemp & Boyce . . . 1888.

160 × 103. Pp. 52. P. w. (title rptd).

Preface to 1 ed. (included), signed: 'A. W. Gardner, M.P.S., Eng., Canterbury, Kent, England, 1879'; 2 ed. addressed from Melb.

Copies: ML, SLV. 716

Gardner, William

Paper on treatment of hydatid disease, read before the South Australian Branch of the British Medical Association . . . Adelaide: Frearson's Printing House . . . 1885.

200 × 134. Pp. 20.

Copies: UA. 717

———

The surgical treatment of hydatid disease. By W. Gardner, M.D., Ch.M. Glas. Lecturer on Surgery, Adelaide University, Senior Surgeon to Adelaide Hospital. [Text begins.]

242 × 153. Pp. 8. (l.b.). Repr., *Trans Intercol Med. Cong. Austsia*, 1889 : 345.

Includes recent methods adopted by author.

Copies: KFR, US. 718

———

List of contributions to surgical literature and list of appointments held by William Gardner, M.D., C.M. Glas. . . .

213 × 133. Pp. 12 (three blanks). NI. [Adel., 1895.]

William Gardner (1846–97) MD, ChM Glas., Surg. Adel. Hosp., and later Hon. Surg. Hosp. for Sick Children, Melb., founder of *Intercol Quart. J. Med. & Surg.*, made important contributions in hydatid disease. For obit., see *Intercol med. J. Austsia*, 1897, 2 : 210.

Publications include *MD thesis on hydatid disease*, (Univ. Glas.), 1877, (NS); 'Surgery of hydatid of lung', in Treves' *Manual of operative surgery*, vol. 2, 1891. Univ. Adel. has his case notes on hydatid disease (pp. 42).

Copies: SLS. 719

Garson, J. G.

See Roth, H. Ling.

Geelong District Hospital, Vic.

See Geelong Infirmary and Benevolent Asylum.

Geelong Infirmary and Benevolent Asylum, Vic.

The First Annual Report of the Committee of Management of the Geelong Infirmary, and Benevolent Asylum . . . 1852: also the general rules, and the internal regulations . . . Geelong: Printed by J. Harrison, Advertiser Office.

220 × 132. Pp. 40. P. w. (title rptd).

Founded 1852; became Geelong Dist. Hosp., 1924.

Copies: EF (8, 9; 1859–60), ML (1–5; 1852–6), SLV (1–20; 1852–72). 720

———

Hospital enquiry. The charges against Dr. Reid. From the *Geelong Register*, of 5th, 6th and 7th February, 1868. [Text begins.]

213 × 133. Pp. 24, [ii] (l.b.). Colophon—Wise and Downie . . . Geelong.

Charges against Resident Surg. were not substantiated. For Dr. Reid's justification, see Reid, D. B.

Copies: ML, SLV. 721

———

Geelong Infirmary and Benevolent Asylum. Dietary. [Text begins.]

204 × 127. Single leaf, v.b. ND. (c. 1868.) At foot: Printed by Henry Franks, Geelong.

Copies: SLV. 722

———

Geelong Infirmary & Benevolent Asylum. Bye-Laws. [Text begins.]

204 × 127. Pp. 24. (1872.) Colophon: George Mercer, Printer, Geelong.

Copies: SLV. 723

Gibbons, Charles Samuel

Manhood: a treatise on the nervous system in health and disease, by Dr. Gibbons, M.A., L.R.C.P.E., L.R.C.S.E., L.M., etc. [Picture—'Private ward in the Gibbons Hospital'.] ... Sydney. 2nd edition.

181 × 125. Pp. 12. ND. P. w. (cover title).

On sexual aberrations and diseases.

Copies: CC. 724

Gibbons, Sydney

Air and water poisoning in Melbourne. ... (Read before the Royal Society of Victoria, 22nd November, 1869.) [Text begins.]

217 × 135. Pp. 24 (l.b.). 3 pl. with mounted photographs. Colophon—Stillwell and Knight ... Melb.

On city sewage, and possible pollution of Yan Yean Reservoir by drainage.

Copies: NL, SLV. 725

———

(From the Australian Medical Journal, Sept. 1876.) Kissing and its consequences. ... Delivered before the Australian Health Society. [Text begins.]

214 × 140. Pp. 4. Colophon—Stillwell and Knight ...

On the evils of the promiscuous kissing of children, a pestilent, murderous practice. ('Today a little mound in Greenwood Cemetery is the sole memento of your visit.')

Copies: EF. 726

———

Notes on diet An outline of the philosophy of nutrition ... A lecture ... for the Australian Health Society ... 27th March, 1878. Melbourne: Walker, May & Co. ... 1878.

181 × 125. Pp. 20. Pages framed. Stiff p. w. (title rptd).

Also as 2 ed., A.H.S. pamphlet No 6 (title amended), Pp. 16. Melb.: Walker, May. 1879. The Same, 7th thousand, Melb.: McCarron Bird. 1884.

Copies: EF, ML, NL, SLS, SLV. 727

———

The Melbourne water supply: the causes of its deterioration and the remedy. ... Reprinted ... from the Herald. Published for the Author 1881.

161 × 100. Pp. 16. 2 figs. NI.

Sydney Gibbons FRMS, FCS, of Melb., was a consultant analytical chemist.

Copies: DL, FC, ML, NL, SLV. 727a

Gibson, John

Notes on certain "worm nests" or "worm knots" occurring in the cellular tissue of the brisket in cattle. Read at the Intercolonial Medical Congress, Sydney, 1892.

244 × 147. Pp. 6. 1 pl. Colophon—Syd.: Charles Potter, Govt Pr, 1893.

Description and effects of parasite later named *Onchocerca gibsoni*.

For John Gibson (1857–1910) MD, CM Edin., who practised at Windsor NSW, see obit., *Austsn med. Gaz.*, 1910, 29 : 327.

Copies: SPH. 728

Gilchrist, W. J.

A handy book on the laws relating to public health; containing "The Public Health Statute 1865" ... By W. J. Gilchrist, Barrister-at-Law. ... Evans Brothers, Melbourne ... 1876.

186 × 125. Pp. viii, 128. Limp linen.

Another ed., large paper, 1876.

Copies: EF, ML, SLV. 729

Gillbee, William

To Her Majesty's Land and Emigration Commissioners, are submitted the accompanying testimonials of William Gillbee.

288 × 227. Title p. (v.b.). ND. NI. Precedes coll. of 35 ms. testimonials (dated 1848–52) laid down in scrap-book.

Relate to service on various ships.

For William Gillbee (1825–85) MRCS, a pioneer of Listerian surgery in Vic., see obits, *Aust. med. J.*, 1885, ns 7 : 30, and *Austsn med. Gaz.*, 1885, 4 : 103; also O'Sullivan, D.M. (1966), 'W. G. and the introduction of antiseptic surgery to Aust.', *Med. J. Aust.*, 2 : 871.

Copies: DOS. 730

———

Obituary. William Gillbee, M.R.C.S. Eng. ... From the "Australian Medical Journal", January 1885. Melbourne: Stillwell & Co. ...

212 × 135. Pp. 8. Title in black frame. Author: J. E. Neild.

Copies: UM. 731

Gillen, Frances James

See Horn Scientific Expedition; also Spencer, Baldwin and Gillen, F. J.

Gippsland Hospital, Sale, Vic.

The Seventh Annual Report of the Gippsland Hospital. ... for 1872. Sale: John W. Baker ...

204 × 132. Pp. 16 (l.b.). (1873.)

Copies: SLV (1872–81). 732

Girdlestone, Tharp Mountain

Remarks on modern lithotrity, for the treatment of stone, with notes of a case. ... Reprinted from the Australian Medical Journal for April, 1866.

208 × 135. Pp. 12 (last—colophon only). Colophon—Melb.: Wilson & Mackinnon ...

Copies: SLV. 733

On the causes of our atmospheric impurities. ... [Text begins.]

206 × 138. Pp. 14 (l.b.), [ii] (colophon, v.b.). 3 pl. Colophon—Melb.: Stillwell and Knight ... Repr., *Aust. med. J.*, March 1870.

Air pollution from sewage, associated with deficient health laws and rapid population growth, is 'the greatest enemy to health and life we have ...'

Copies: ML, SLV. 734

No. 4.] [Sept. 1877. Australian Health Society, Melbourne. Under the floor ... A lecture ... for the Australian Society ... September 6, 1876. ... Melbourne: Sands & McDougall, ... 1877.

212 × 138. Pp. 16 (l.b.). P. w. (title rptd).

Reprinted 1883. Revised edition, 1887. Pp. 12. M'Carron, Bird and Co. ... Melb.

A trenchant lecture on Melb. drainage, by the Med. Officer of Health.

T. M. Girdlestone (1823–99) FRCS, was coroner to the goldfields and MLA representing a mining area, and later MOH Melb. and Hon. Surg. Melb. Hosp. He was an early exponent of Lister's technique, and first introduced kangaroo tendon as a suture material. See obit., *Intercol med. J. Austsia*, 1889, 4 : 426; also Russell, K. F. (1948), *Roy. Melb. Hosp. Clin. Rep.*, Centenary Vol. : 15.

Copies: EF, LNSW, ML, NL, SLS, SLV. 735

Gladesville Hospital for the Insane, NSW

1846. New South Wales. Lunatic Asylum, Tarban Creek. Report from the Select Committee on the Lunatic Asylum, Tarban Creek, with appendix to report, minutes of evidence, and appendix ... Ordered, by the Council, to be printed, 21 October, 1846. Sydney, Printed by W. W. Davies, at the Govt Printing Office ...

315 × 197. Pp. [ii], 6, 36, 16. 1 flg plan. Blue tinted paper. From NSW Leg. Council, *V&P*, 1846.

The first comprehensive inquiry into an Australian mental institution. For its initiation, see note to Campbell, F., No 482; also Bostock, J. (1968), *The dawn of Aust. psychiatry*, Syd.; Ireland, A. W. (1964), *Med. J. Aust.*, 1 : 90.

Tarban Creek Lunatic Asylum was renamed Gladesville Hosp. for Insane c. 1868.

Copies: LNSW, ML, NL, SLV. 736

Regulations for the guidance of the officers, attendants, & servants, of the Lunatic Asylum, New South Wales. ... Sydney: Printed by W. W. Davies, at the Government Printing Office ... 1848.

207 × 148. 16 un-numbered leaves (3 printed both sides, remainder v.b.). Interleaved.

Copies: DL. 737

1851. New South Wales. Lunatic Asylum, Tarban Creek. Report of the Board of Enquiry on the Lunatic Asylum, Tarban Creek ... with minutes of evidence and appendix. ... Sydney: Printed by W. W. Davies, at the Govt Printing Office ... 1851.

320 × 198. Pp. [ii] (v.b.), 6 (l.b.), 34 (l.b.). Pale blue paper.

Copies: LNSW, ML, NL, SLV. 738

1865–6. Legislative Assembly. New South Wales. Lunatic Asylums. (Report respecting Asylum at Tarban Creek.) Ordered ... to be printed, 20 March, 1866. Bd of Visitors to Col Sec. [Text begins.]

330 × 206. Pp. 4 (l.b.). Colophon: Thomas Richards, Govt Pr—1866.

Copies: LNSW, ML, NL, SLV. 739

1869. Legislative Assembly. New South Wales. Hospital for the Insane, Tarban Creek. (Reports on general condition, &c., of) ... [Text begins.]

324 × 210. Pp. 12. Colophon—Syd.: Thomas Richards Govt Pr—1869.

Copies: LNSW, ML, NL, SLV. 740

———

1870. Legislative Assembly. New South Wales. Report on the Hospital for the Insane, Gladesville, for the year 1869. ... Sydney: Thomas Richards, Govt Printer. 1870.

222 × 143. Pp. 22. Signed: F. Norton Manning MD, Inspr of the Insane.

An. reps, 1869–78.

Copies: HDN, LNSW, NL, SLV. 741

———

Hospital for Insane, Gladesville. Rules for the attendants, nurses, servants, and others. 1870. N.B.—These rules are to be given up to the Superintendent when the attendant, nurse, or servant leaves the Hospital.

212 × 134. Pp. 36 (l.b.). Signed: F. Norton Manning, Supt.

Copies: LNSW. 742

1875. New South Wales. Hospital for Insane, Gladesville. (Report of proceedings during visit of Inspector to Europe.) Presented to Parliament ... [Text begins.]

323 × 206. Pp. 2. Colophon—Syd.: Thomas Richards, Govt Pr.—1875.

Copies: HDN, LNSW, NL, SLV. 743

———

Catalogue of books in the Library of the Hospital for the Insane, Gladesville, 1882. Sydney: Thomas Richards, Govt Printer. 1882.

214 × 132. Pp. 34 (interleaved with ruled paper). Limp cloth.

Copies: ML. 744

———

See also Manning, Frederick Norton; Nos 1529a,b.

Glass, Charles E.

Drunkenness and the opium habit. Dr. Leslie E. Keeley's system of treatment with the double chloride of gold. The only cure, claiming 95 per cent of patients permanently cured, with over 50,000 drunkards reformed to usefulness. ... Compiled by Chas. E. Glass, 96 Little Collins . Street ... who ... is prepared to supply Dr. Keeley's remedies.

209 × 132. Pp. 48. ND. [1892.] Colophon: Pater & Knapton ... Melb. P. w. (title rptd, print on all sides).

Advertises bichloride of gold treatment for alcoholism and morphine addiction, used by Keeley of Chicago, and solicits investment for a local 'Keeley Instn for Sanitarian Treatment.'

Copies: SLV. 745

Glasson, Henry

Religion in its connection with insanity. By Henry Glasson, B.A. Sydney: L. Bruck, 1884.

NS. Pamphlet. Review, *Austsn med. Gaz.*, 1884, 3 : 211.

Author, chaplain to Hosp. for Insane, Wellington NZ, states that 'whatever doubt may exist as to the relation which religion bears to insanity as an exciting cause, there is none concerning religion as ... ameliorating the condition of sufferers and helping many ...' 746

Gleanings of Gold

... An exhaustive compendium of medical and other recipes for every-day use. ... Gleanings of gold. Containing many simple, yet valuable remedies. Hints on the care of the sick. ... Australian edition; Printed for the American Publishing Co., by A. M. Lewis ... Collingwood.

183 × 122. Pp. 48. ND. P. w. (cover title).

Copies: ML, SLT. 747

Goldsmith, Francis Edward

Northern Territory. Correspondence, relative to Dr. Goldsmith's resignation. Adelaide: Printed by David Gall ... 1865.

202 × 130. Pp. 22.

Official correspondence, published by F. E. Goldsmith MB Lond., Surg. Territory Expedition and Protector of Aborigines, following his threatened dismissal and resignation. The climax to friction with the Govt Resident, his superior, was the punative killing of a native by an armed party sent by the Resident. Goldsmith charged the party with wilful murder, implicating the Resident, though a magisterial inquiry was refused. Testimonial to Goldsmith's service and ability, signed by 48 residents is appended.

Also published: 'Tropical disease in N. Aust.', *Trans Intercol Med. Cong. Austsia*, 1899 : 106.

Copies: SLV. 748

Good Health

Good Health The Australian Hygienic Journal. With which is incorporated "Happy Homes". Edited by Douglas Erle. Vol. 1.—No. 1. Sydney, December 8, 1892. Monthly—Price—3d. [Illustration and advt.]

248 × 188. Pp. [16]. Illustns. Colophon—Printed by E. T. & J. Radcliffe ... Syd.

Domestic hygiene, infant care and home nursing.

Copies: ML (1–4, 1892–3). 749

Goodna and Ipswich Asylums for the Insane, Queensland

1881. Queensland. Asylums for the Insane, Goodna and Ipswich. (Report of the Medical Superintendent for the year 1880.) Presented to both Houses ... [Text begins.]

326 × 204. Pp. 10 (l.b.). 1 flg chart. Colophon—Edmund Gregory, Acting Govt Pr, Bris.

Reports 1880–89.

Goodna Asylum for Insane was previously known as Woogaroo Lunatic Asylum (*q.v.*); Ispwich as Sandy Gallop Lunatic Asylum.

Copies: LNSW, NL, OL, SLV. 750

——— **and Toowoomba Asylum for the Insane**

1891. Queensland. Asylums for the Insane, Goodna and Ipswich, and Toowoomba. (Report of the Superintendent for the year 1890.) Presented to both Houses ... [Text begins.]

326 × 204. Pp. 16 (l.b.). 1 flg chart. Colophon—Govt Pr, Bris.

Reports 1890–97; thence onwards as Reps of Inspr of Hospitals for Insane.

Copies: LNSW, NL, OL, SLV. 751

Goodridge, Charles Medyett

Narrative of a voyage to the South Seas, with the shipwreck of the Princess of Wales cutter, on one of the Crozets, uninhabited islands; with an account of a two years' residence on them by the crew, and their deliverance by an American schooner; to which is added, a further narrative of near eight years' residence in Van Diemen's Land. By Charles Medyett Goodridge, of Paignton, Devon, one of the survivors ... Comprising a statistical view of Van Diemen's Land, giving its geography, geology, climate, health and duration of life ... and other useful information, up to the year 1831, forming a complete emigrant's guide. London: ... Hamilton and Adams ... 1832.

181 × 110. Pp. iv, 5–294. Frontis. and 2 maps (1 coloured, 1 flg). Cloth.

Nine eds appeared from 1832 to 1852. 1 ed., 1832 and 2 ed., 1833 alone include terminal 'Statistical view of V.D.L.' containing section on health.

Health and duration of life (pp. 129–135). Whooping cough, introduced from a female prison ship about three years previously, had spread widely. Small-pox and measles had not appeared. Fever and dysentery were the most frequent ailments, and 'a degree of temporary insanity' affected both male and female prisoners. Goitre had occurred for some years near New Norfolk. There was 'lamentable waste of life' due to alcohol. 'A very large proportion of those who first put a foot on the shores of the Derwent, even ... the more respectable and exemplary class ... were confirmed drunkards, and died in the prime of life.' Excessive eating is considered another potent factor in ill-health and mortality.

Copies: FC, ML, NL, SLS, SLT, WLC. 752

———

The Same. 2 ed.. 1883.

Copies: ML, NL, SLT, SLV. 753

———

Statistical view of Van Diemen's Land, comprising its geography, geology, climate, health and duration of life, divisions of the Island, number of the houses, expenses of the people, manufactures, habits ... nature of plants and animals, price of labour, and other useful information, up to the year 1831, forming a complete emigrant's guide. 1832.

175 × 105. Pp. ii, 105–294. 2 maps (1 flg). Paper boards.

Separate issue of terminal part of author's *Narrative of a voyage*, 1832. Includes sections on health and duration of life.

Copies: ML, NL, WLC. 754

Goodwin, John

Testimonials in favour of John Goodwin, Surgeon and Accoucher ... No. 6, Hunter Street, Sydney.

4to. Pp. 2. Single leaf. Double cols. ND. (c. 1839.) Kemp and Fairfax ... Syd.

Testimonials dated 1837; NSW registration dated 1839. Goodwin practised in Scone NSW, where he suffered great trouble, including trial for manslaughter, with acquittal, following a death in childbirth, and imprisonment for libel in 1844. On these events he based a novel, *Antipodes*, the unpublished ms. of which is in the possession of Mr K. Stewart. The characters are

thinly veiled local figures who conspire to injure him. See *HRA*, ser. 1, 24 : 276–7 and 492.
Copies: K. Stewart, Sydney. 755

Gordon, Patrick Robertson
See Bailey, Frederick Manson and Gordon, P. R.

Gorringe, Thomas F.
Short dissertations on diarrhoea, dysentery, cholera morbus, scarlatina and erysipelas. . . . By Thomas F. Gorringe, Surgeon, Woodville. Hobart Town: H. & C. Best, Printers . . . 1850.
201 × 132. Pp. [ii] (v.b.), 36. P. w. (title rptd).
Copies: ML, SLT, SLV. 756

Scarlatina, more fully described than by the writer in his former short dissertation on that disease. . . . Tasmania: H. and C. Best, Printers . . . Hobart Town. 1853.
206 × 130. Pp. 8.
Includes erysipelatous sore throat; sore throat attended with ulcers. Clinical description and treatment.
Copies: SLT, SLV. 757

Goulburn District Hospital, NSW
The Seventh Annual Report of the Goulburn District Hospital from 1st April 1848, to 1st April, 1849. Names of subscribers,—terms of admission, &c. Goulburn: William Jones, Herald Office.
212 × 140. Pp. 16 (l.b.). ND. (1849). P. w. (title rptd, decorative border).
Copies: DL (7, 1848), ML (10–14, 1851–55). 758

Goulburn Valley Medical Association
See Ballarat and Goulburn Valley Medical Assn.

Gould, James Emery
Homoeopathy and its professors . . . Melbourne: W. L. Ambler, Printer . . . 1873.
217 × 138. Pp. 14 (l.b.), [2] (advts, r.b.). P. w. (title rptd).
For J. E. Gould (1849–83) LRCPE, Phys. Melb. Homoeo. Dispens., who later settled in Wollongong NSW, see obit., *Austsn med. Gaz.*, 1883, 2 : 251.
Copies: EF, ML. 759

Grace, John Frederick
See Hotham and West Melbourne Mutual Aid Society.

Grafton Hospital, NSW
Proposed hospital for the Clarence and Richmond River districts. [Text begins.]
254 × 204. Pp. [4] (2, 4 blank). Blue paper. (1862.) Colophon—R. Stevenson, Printer, 'Examiner' Office.
Prospectus and subscription sheet for building of Grafton Hospital.
Copies: ML. 760

Rules and regulations for the management of the Grafton Hospital, as approved at a meeting of the subscribers, held at Grafton. 21st February, 1864. Grafton: Printed by Richard Stevenson, "Examiner" Office . . .
214 × 140. Pp. 8 (l.b.). P. w. (title rptd).
For Grafton Hosp., see *Austsn med. Gaz.*, 1894, 13 : 318 and 425.
Copies: ML. 761

Graham, George
Address delivered before the Medical Society of Victoria, January 1879. By George Graham . . . President . . .
198 × 127. Pp. 16 (l.b.). Colophon—Stillwell & Co. . . . Melbourne. Repr. *Aust. med. J.*, Jan. 1879.
For George Graham (1828–93) MD, of Richmond, see obit.—*Aust. med. J.*, 1893, ns 15 : 361.
Copies: SLV. 761a

Graham, Sir James
Hydatid disease in its clinical aspects . . . Illustrated with thirty-four coloured plates. Edinburgh & London: Young J. Pentland. 1891.
227 × 145. Pp. xii, 204 (l.b.), 24 (book notices). 35 pl. (31 coloured), with titles on recto of interleaves. Cloth.
Sections on treatment are largely from Aust. experience. 'He denounced all tapping and aspirating operations and gave a clear warning about the danger of puncturing a hydatid cyst except in the course of a planned operation.' (Graham, *infra*). Based on MD thesis, Univ. Edin. Reviewed, *Austsn med. Gaz.*, 1891, 11 : 28; *Aust. med. J.*, ns 13 : 606.
For Sir James Graham MD Edin., Supt Alfred

Hosp., Hon. MO Women's Hosp. Syd., and Lord Mayor of Sydney (1901), see obits, *Austsn med. Gaz.*, 1913, 33 : 245 and *Brit. med. J.*, 1913, 1 : 588; for hydatid work, Graham, H.B. (1953), *Med. J. Aust.*, 1 : 869.

Copies: AMAN, AMAV, BG, CC, EF, KFR, LNSW, ML, NL, RACP, RACS, SLV, UA, UM, UQ, US. 762

Grant, David

On massage. . . . (Reprinted from the Edinburgh Medical Journal for July and August, 1887.) [Text begins.]

206 × 135. Pp. 12 (l.b.). Colophon—Edinburgh: Oliver and Boyd.

'In massage . . . we possess a most powerful therapeutical agent . . . it will probably before long take its proper place as one of our most trusty weapons.' Review, *Aust. med. J.*, 1887, ns 9 : 520 ('this new physical method of treatment').

Copies: SLV, UM. 763

———

On movable kidney. . . . Melbourne: Stillwell and Co. . . . 1887.

209 × 130. Pp. 32. Repr. *Aust. med. J.*

Copies: UM. 764

———

A case of Raynaud's disease. . . . Reprinted from the "Intercolonial Medical Congress of Australasia Transactions". Melbourne: Stillwell and Co. . . . 1889.

209 × 130. Pp. 8. P. w. (cover title).

For David Grant (1854–1931) MD, Hon. Phys. St Vincent's Hosp. Melb., Lect. Mat. Med. Univ. Melb., see obit., *Med. J. Aust.*, 1931, 1 : 766; also *Melb. Hosp. Clin. Rep.*, 1931, 2 : 4.

Copies: UM. 765

Greathead, Robert

Doctors superseded by Greathead's cures for diphtheria and scarlet fevers, &c., &c., giving full description how to mix and use sulphuric acid, &c., and other medicines and ointments . . . Melbourne: Sands and McDougall . . . 1877.

171 × 120. Pp. 36. P. w. (shortened title).

Author divulges his sulphuric acid treatment for diphtheria, scarlet fever and typhoid. In 1873 he offered to disclose his formula to the Vic. Govt for £5000, but this was rejected (*Aust. med. J.*, 1873, 18 : 279). For account of the popular appeal of this remedy, see *Aust. med. J.*, 1874, 19 : 77, 126 and 359.

Copies: ML, SLV. 766

Greenfield, A. P.

The eye, and how to care for it. . . . South Brisbane: . . . "Southern World" Office . . . 1889.

206 × 135. Pp. 16. 1 fig. P. w. (cover title).

Author was Hon. Optician, Brisbane Hosp.

Copies: ML. 767

Greenup, Richard

Vaccination. A letter addressed by Dr. Simon, Medical Officer of the General Board of Health, to the President of the Board, on vaccination. Presented to the Imperial Parliament by command of Her Majesty, 1857. Abridged for the use of the Colony of New South Wales. By Richard Greenup, M.D., Medical Adviser to the Government. Sydney: Thomas Richards, Govt Printer. 1859.

206 × 138. Pp. 36 (l.b.). P. w. (title rptd).

Richard Greenup MD, first Registrar Univ. Syd. (1850), later Member NSW Bd Health and Med. Adviser to Govt, in 1852 became Supt Parramatta Lun. Asylum, where, in 1866, he was killed by a patient. For biog. see Dawson, W. S. (1965), *Annals of psychiatry in NSW 1850–1900*, Syd., typescript (ML, RACP); also Brown, K. M. (1927), *Med. practice in old Parramatta*, Syd.

Copies: EF, LNSW, ML, NL, RACS, SLS, US. 768

Greenway's Patent Earth and Water Closet

May, 1887. A pamphlet on sanitation & sewage. Greenway's patent earth and water closet. P. H. Fisher, Manager, Newcastle. [Ornament] Newcastle: . . . "Herald" Office . . . Newcastle. 1887.

215 × 140. Pp. 8 (last colophon). P. w.

Copies: ML. 769

Gresswell, Dan Astley

Diphtheria as a chronic malady in particular individuals, with liability in them to recrudescence. . . .

210 × 140. Pp. 8. P. w. (cover title). Repr., *Trans Epidem. Soc. Lond.*, 1886.

Copies: EF. 770

———

A contribution to the natural history of scarlatina

Derived from observations on the London epidemic of 1887–1888 Being a dissertation for the degree of Doctor of Medicine in the University of Oxford Printed and published at the expense of the University, as a mark of distinction . . . Oxford At the Clarendon Press 1890 . . .

234 × 150. Pp. viii, 206 (last—colophon), [2] (book notices, v.b.). 1 flg pl. Cloth.

'Clinical observations on scarlatina . . . its variations in relation to season, and . . . suggestions as to the nature of this relation.'

EF copy bears author's incription to Prof. Sir Harry Allen.

Copies: AMAV, EF, HDN, HDV, UM, US. 771

1890. Victoria. Board of Public Health. Report on the sanitary condition and sanitary administration of Melbourne and suburbs. . . . Presented to both Houses of Parliament . . . Robt. S. Brain, Govt Printer, Melbourne.

326 × 204. Pp. 36.

Copies: AMAV, EF, HDV, KFR, LNSW, ML, NL, SLV, UM. 772

Report by Dr. Gresswell on the measures to be adopted with a view to minimising the spread of communicable affections. [Text begins.]

331 × 204. Pp. 12 (l.b.). (1890.) Colophon—Robt S. Brain, Govt Pr, Melb.

Advice to householders and doctors on typhoid, scarlet fever and diphtheria.

Copies: HDV, NL, SLV, UM. 773

Report by Dr. Gresswell on the sanitary condition of the Borough of Ararat and on the prevalence of typhoid fever and fatal throat illness in the Ararat Lunatic Asylum. [Text begins.]

331 × 158. Pp. 16 (l.b.). (1891.) Colophon—Robt S. Brain, Govt Pr, Melb.

Copies: EF, HDV, NL, SLV, UM. 774

1891. Victoria. Report by Dr. Gresswell on the sanitary condition and sanitary administration of the Borough of Clunes. Presented to both Houses of Parliament . . . Robt. S. Brain, Govt Printer, Melbourne.

331 × 158. Pp. 16.

Copies: EF, HDV, LNSW, ML, NL, SLV, UM. 775

Report by Dr. Gresswell on the means of isolation for persons affected with communicable disease in the Metropolitan District. [Text begins.]

331 × 204. Pp. 16 (l.b.). 8 pl. (graphs—annual deaths for various infectious diseases, 1861–90). (1891.) Colophon—Robt S. Brain, Govt Pr, Melb.

Copies: HDV, NL, SLV, UM. 776

Report on typhoid fever in Footscray in the early part of the year 1891. [Text begins.]

331 × 204. Pp. 10 (last 4 flg). (1891.) Colophon—Robt S. Brain, Govt Pr, Melb.

Includes rep. by George Shirres MD, DPH.

Copies: HDV, NL, SLV, UM. 777

Remediable conditions connected with the prevalence of typhoid fever in certain Metropolitan Municipal Districts. [Text begins.]

331 × 204. Pp. 4 (1892.) Colophon—Robt S. Brain, Govt Pr, Melb.

Copies: HDV, NL, SLV, UM. 778

On the scheme adopted by the Melbourne and Metropolitan Board of Works for removing and disposing of the liquid waste and human refuse of the Metropolis. [Text begins.]

331 × 204. Pp. 4 (1892.) Colophon—Robt S. Brain, Govt Pr, Melb.

Copies: HDV, NL, SLV, UM. 779

Report on small-pox and the R.M.S.S. "Oroya" . . . [Text begins.]

331 × 204. Pp. 8. (1892.) Colophon—Robt S. Brain, Govt Pr, Melb.

Copies: HDV, NL, SLV, UM. 780

Report by Dr. Gresswell on Asiatic cholera, and on measures requiring attention in anticipation of, and for the purpose of preventing, its introduction into Victoria. [Text begins.]

331 × 204. Pp. 14. (1892.) Colophon—Robt S. Brain, Govt Pr, Melb.

Includes draft regulations, advice to shipping agents, instructions to port health officers.

Copies: HDV, NL, SLV, UM. 781

Report by Dr. Gresswell on the methods adopted for dealing with the organic waste of the Metropolis. [Text begins.]

331 × 204. Pp. 32 (20, 24 blank; 21–23 flg). (1892.)

Includes tabulated information on current methods and requirements for various districts.

Copies: HDV, NL, SLV, UM. 782

Report by Dr. Gresswell on a localized outbreak of diarrhoea and dysentery in the City of Melbourne. [Text begins.]

323 × 204. Pp. 20. Figs, 2 flg maps. (27 Feb. 1893.) Colophon—Robt S. Brain, Govt Pr, Melb.

Copies: HDV, NL. 783

Milk poisoning in St. Kilda. [Text begins.]

323 × 204. Pp. 8 (l.b.). 1 pl. (maps). (26 Sep. 1893.) Colophon—Robt S. Brain, Govt Pr.

Copies: HDV, NL. 784

Australian Health Society, Melbourne ... President—D. A. Gresswell ... Danger in ice and ice cream. [Text begins.]

212 × 138. Pp. 4 (1, 4 blank). ND. Colophon—Walker, May & Co. ... Melb.

Copies: SLV. 785

1893. Victoria. Charitable institutions of Melbourne ... Ordered by the Legislative Assembly to be printed ... 1893. ... Robt. S. Brain, Govt Printer, Melbourne.

323 × 204. Pp. 20 (l.b.).

Principles of hospital construction, as a guide to Royal Commission in estimating 'the degree of wholesomeness of conditions met with in the hospitals of this metropolis.'

Copies: AMAV, LNSW, ML, NL, SLV. 786

Report on the theatres of Melbourne. [Text begins.]

323 × 204. Pp. 32 (l.b.). (1894.) Colophon—Robt S. Brain, Govt Pr, Melb.

Inspection report; dangers from fires and panic; overseas disasters; recommendation for legislation.

Copies: HDV, NL. 787

Darwinism and the medical profession An address ... Annual Meeting of the Medical Society of Victoria, January 16, 1895. Reprinted from the "Australian Medical Journal". Melbourne: Stillwell and Co. ... 1895.

217 × 140. Pp. 42. Cloth.

Copies: AMAV, CC, NL, SLV, UA, UM, US. 788

1897. Victoria. Report on diphtheria in Hawthorn ... Presented to both Houses of Parliament ... Robt. S. Brain, Govt Printer, Melbourne.

323 × 204. Pp. 24.

Copies: AMAV, HDV, LNSW, ML, NL, SLV, UM. 789

Report by Dr. Gresswell on living forms in air-borne dust in Melbourne. [Text begins.]

323 × 204. Pp. 2. ND. (1 Dec. 1897.) Colophon—Robt S. Brain, Govt Pr, Melb.

Dust cultures by Dr. Thomas Cherry, Univ. Melb.

Copies: ML, NL. 790

Tuberculosis and its prevention. ... [Text begins.]

229 × 140. Pp. 20 (l.b.). (1899.) Colophon—Stillwell and Co. ... Melb. Repr., *Intercol med. J. Austsia*, 1899.

Another ed., 1899, (Board of Public Health), pp. 18, Govt Pr, Melb. Also listed as Aust. Health Soc. pamphlet (1899). NS.

Trathen (*infra*) states that, first published in 1893 as part of author's anti-tuberculosis campaign, further editions appeared in 1894, 1898, 1899 and 1902.

Copies: SLV, UM. 791

Report to the Board of Public Health on communicable diseases and their prevention ... Robt. S. Brain, Govt Printer, Melbourne.

221 × 137. Pp. 28. 2 ed. (1899.)

1 ed., 1890. NS.

Includes advice to householders and doctors on typhoid, scarlet fever and diphtheria.

Copies: HDV, NL, SLV. 792

Board of Public Health. The plague—The black death. Prepared by D. A. Gresswell . . . Chairman. [Text begins.]

390 × 314. Single leaf, v.b. Double cols. Pink paper. 10 Mar. 1900 (at foot). Colophon—Robt S. Brain, Govt Pr, Melb.

A warning of appearance of bubonic plague in rats on Melb. wharves. Includes description, transmission, and prevention by rat control and hygiene.

For D. A. Gresswell (1853–1904) MD Oxon. & Melb., DPH Camb., distinguished health administrator, Chairman of Bd of Health, see *Intercol med. J. Austsia*, 1904, 9 : 613; *Austsn med. Gaz.*, 1904, 23 : 660; Trathen, W. (1924), *Health*, 2 : 1.

Copies: EF. 793

Grierson, Francis Walter

The late Dr. Frank Grierson. From the Dumfries and Galloway Standard, March 11, 1885. [Text begins.]

286 × 224. Single leaf, v.b. Printed within black lines. NI.

F. W. Grierson MB, ChM Edin. came from Scotland in 1883, was RMO Prince Alfred Hosp., Sydney, and died of pulmonary disease in 1885.

Copies: FC. 794

Griffith, Charles J.

Observations on the water supply of Melbourne; by Charles J. Griffith, A. M., President of the Commission of Sewerage and Water Supply. Melbourne: . . . Lucas Brothers . . . 1855.

217 × 141. Pp. 32. P. w. (title rptd).

Official reply to Dr. D. E. Wilkie's published criticism of the Melb. water supply.

Copies: DL, ML, NL, SLV. 795

Guide to Health

The guide to health or private medical friend, a treatise on the causes, symptoms & proper method of cure of nervous, mental and sexual debility, syphilis, gonorrhoea, &c., with cases cured, by a Physician. Published by the Author, at the Medical Depot, 237 Bourke Street East . . . Azzoppardi, Hildreth & Co., Printers . . .

117 × 94. Pp. 14, [2] (advts). ND. [before Nov. 1874.] P. w. (title rptd).

Claims that 'simple, safe and permanent remedies [for ailments above] have been discovered by a Physician and Doctor of Medicine.'

Copies: SLV. 796

Gummow, Benjamin William

Narrative of facts relating to the hospital at Swan Hill, in which Dr. Gummow, J. P., and the Rev. J. Bentley Reid, Presbyterian Minister, are prominently concerned. Melbourne. Fergusson & Moore . . . 1872.

178 × 145. Pp. 16 (l.b.).

Following controversy, Dr. Gummow was dismissed from the post of surg.-supt. Pamphlet gives circumstances and supports his case.

B. W. Gummow (d. 1876), who had practised for 15 years at Swan Hill, now moved to Echuca Vic. See obit., *Aust. med. J.*, 1876, 21 : 143; also Chapman, C. K. (1851), 'Early history of the churches of Swan Hill', *Vic. Hist. Magazine*, 24 : 25.

Copies: SLV. 797

Gunn, J. A.

See Anthrax and Inoculation.

Gunn, William

An interesting case of sympathetic ophthalmia: being a reply to a paper read by Dr. Bowen, Surgeon of the Eye Hospital, Melbourne, with a copy . . . as published in the Australian Medical Journal of June last, by William Gunn, of Kangaroo Flat, Bendigo, in connection with his son, George Gunn's case, who is totally blind through want of proper treatment. Also introductory remarks, and letter by Wm. Gunn to the subscribers of the Victorian Eye and Ear Hospital . . . The correspondence between Mr. Gunn and the Hon. the Treasurer, Royal Humane Society, Medical Society of Victoria, and Eye and Ear Hospital, Melbourne . . . is likewise included . . . The public are respectfully invited to read both sides of this important subject . . . Sandhurst: W. Welch . . . 1885.

210 × 135. Pp. 24. P. w. (cover title).

A bitter attack by the father of a boy, whose case is reported in *Aust. med. J.*, 1884, ns 6 : 252 by Aubrey Bowen, Hon. Surg. Vic. Eye & Ear Hosp.

Copies: SLV. 798

Günst, J. Werner

Diphtheria and its simple treatment. . . . Melbourne: Clarson, Massina, & Co. . . . 1870.

127 × 85. Pp. 16 (last—book notice).

Sulphur by gargling and inhalation, supported by homoeopathic remedies, lowers diphtheria mortality 60 or 70 per cent.

Notifies as 'in press' : *A treatise on the diseases of children peculiar to the Australian colonies*. NS.

Copies: NL. 799

Allopathy versus homoeopathy; in "The Australian Medical Journal"; and homoeopathy versus allopathy; by J. W. Günst, M.D. Knight of the Legion of Honour ... Melbourne. ... Published by Evans Brothers ... Melbourne. 1870.

206 × 130. Pp. 24.

Defends homoeopathy and attacks *Aust. med. J.*, which had criticised a meeting of subscribers of Melb. Homoeopathic Instn.

Jean (or Johannes) Werner Günst (1825–94) MD Leyden, was NSW Govt Analyst, and later a founder of Homoeopathic Hosp. Melb. and ed. *Homoeopathic Progress in Australia*. Obit., *Austsn med. Gaz.*, 1894, 13 : 175.

Copies: EF, ML, NL, SLV. 800

See also *Homoeopathic Progress in Australia*.

Gympie Hospital, Qd

Rules for the management of the Gympie Hospital. As adopted at a public meeting of subscribers, October 26th, 1886. Established 1868. Gympie: ... "Gympie Times" Office ... 1887.

8vo. Pp. 8. P. w. (title rptd).

Copies: OL. 801

H

H., J. B.

A catechism of mesmerism, in which the principles of the science are developed; the popular objections combatted; and examples given illustrative of its power as a curative agent, in most severe disease. Also, directions as to the mode of inducing mesmeric sleep, and the restoration of the patient. Melbourne: Printed and published by S. Goode . . . 1850.

173 × 102. Pp. 20 (l.b.).

Preface signed: J.B.H. Published 'to extend the practice of mesmerism, as a curative agent.'

Copies: SLV. 802

Hagey Institute of New South Wales, The

. . . Hagey Institute bi-chloride of gold treatment. For the permanent cure of liquor, opium, morphine, cocaine & tobacco diseases.

186 × 125. Pp. 12. ND. Colophon—John Sands . . . Syd. P. w. (cover title, gold, decorated).

Copies: ML. 803

Haig, William

The address of the President of the Medical Society of Victoria, delivered . . . on January 14, 1885. . . . Melbourne: Stillwell & Co. . . . 1885.

204 × 127. Pp. 12. P. w. (cover title).

William Haig (1823–93) MD Maryland, practised at Emerald Hill (S. Melb.) and was Hon. Phys. Alfred Hosp. Obits: *Aust. med. J.*, 1893, ns 15 : 361 and *Austsn med. Gaz.*, 1893, 12 : 244.

Copies: AMAV, BG, CC, EF. 804

Hailprin, David

See Brodzky, Maurice.

Halford, George Britton

Experiments and observations on the action and sounds of the heart. Bridgnorth: W. J. Rowley. ND.

NS. Noted in Osborne, W. A. (1929), 'Halford Oration', *Med. J. Aust.*, 1 : 64.

805

———

The action and sounds of the heart; a physiological essay. . . . London: John Churchill . . . 1860.

206 × 127. Pp. 48 (l.b.). 18 figs.

AMAV copy, with author's inscription, has inserted leaf with tracings of diagrams.

Copies: AMAV. 806

———

On the time and manner of closure of the auriculoventricular valves. London: J. Churchill, 1860.

8vo. Pp. 8.

NS. Listed *SGC*; also *BMC* (dated 1861). 807

———

On the use of "magenta" as an aid to investigation and diagnosis. . . . [Text begins.]

205 × 132. Pp. 4 (l.b.). ND. (1863.) NI.

Copies: AMAV. 808

———

Not like man. Bimanous and biped, nor yet quadrumanous, but cheiropodous. . . . Melbourne: Wilson and Mackinnon . . . 1863.

218 × 140. Pp. 18. 4 coloured pl. P. w. (title rptd).

Halford, in his conservative stand in the evolution controversy, challenges statements of Huxley. See Mozley, Ann (1967), 'Evolution and the climate of opinion in Aust.', *Victorian Studies* : 425.

Copies: AMAV, CC, EF, FC, KFR, ML, NL, SLV, UM, US. 809

———

Lectures on the heart, delivered at the Melbourne University . . . during . . . 1864. . . . Reprinted from the "Australian Medical Journal."

206 × 132. Pp. 32. 4 figs. Colophon—Wilson & Mackinnon . . . Collins Street East. Repr., *Aust. med. J.*, 1864, 9 : 225, 257 and 290.

Three lectures, which include Halford's studies on the action of the heart and the heart sounds. H. R. Love considers these the first major contribution to cardiology in Australia. (*Med. J. Aust.*, 1953, I : 169.) G. E. Bauer (*infra*) describes Halford as one of the most gifted physiologists and experimental cardiologists of the mid-19th century.

AMAV copy has author's inscription to Mr Kirkland.

Copies: AMAV. 810

"Lines of demarcation" between man, gorilla, and macaque. Melbourne: Wilson & Mackinnon . . . 1864.

310 × 250. Pp. 22 (l.b.). P. w. (title rptd).

Compares 'in a tabular form some of the most important points in the anatomy of Man, the Gorilla, and Macaque.' Differences are regarded as invalidating evolutionary theory. Review, *Aust. med. J.*, 1864, 9 : 89. For opposing views, see Thomson, Wm.

Copies: EF, KFR, ML, MLWA, SLV. 811

On the skeleton of the gorilla. . . . (Read before the Royal Society, 24th July, 1865.) [Text begins.]

217 × 140. Pp. 16 (l.b.). Colophon—Wilson and Mackinnon . . . Collins Street East. Repr., *Trans Roy. Soc. Vic.*, 7 : 34.

Description and measurements as evidence in the evolution controversy.

Copies: AMAV, ML. 812

Experiments and observations on absorption. (Read before the Royal Society, 11th June, 1866.) [Text begins.]

206 × 134. Pp. 12 (l.b.). Colophon—Wilson and Mackinnon . . . Collins Street East.

Copies: AMAV. 813

On the condition of the blood after death from snakebite, as a probable clue to the further study of zymotic diseases, and of cholera especially. . . . (For private circulation only.) Melbourne: Stillwell & Knight . . . 1867.

211 × 132. Pp. 24. 5 figs. Read before Roy. Soc. Vic. P. w.

For Halford's germ theory of snake poisoning, see Campbell, C. H. (1966), *Med. J. Aust.*, 1 : 552.

ML copy has copious notes in contemporary hand.

Copies: AMAV, ML, SLV. 814

On the injection of ammonia into the circulation. . . . read before the Medical Society of Victoria, April 7th 1869. Reprinted from "The Australian Medical Journal".

204 × 133. Pp. 14. Colophon—Stillwell and Knight . . . Melb.

Introduces author's new treatment of snake bite by intravenous ammonia.

For review of the treatment, and ensuing controversy—one of the most bitter and prolonged in Aust. medical history—ending in its discredit, see Campbell, C.H. (1966), 'Professor Halford's new treatment of snake bite', *Med. J. Aust.*, 1 : 1008.

Copies: AMAV, SLV, WLC. 815

The new treatment of snake-bite, with plain directions for injecting. Melbourne: Stillwell and Knight . . . 1869.

214 × 138. Pp. 16. P. w. (title rptd; Halford's publications listed on verso of back wrapper).

Includes lay instruction on intravenous injection of ammonia and appendix on use in counteracting lethal effects of chloroform. Severely criticised in *Aust. med. Gaz.*, 1869 : 191.

Copies: AMAV, ML, NL, SLV, SLW. 816

The treatment of snake-bite in Victoria. . . . read before the Medical Society of Victoria, June 1st, 1870. Reprinted from "The Australian Medical Journal". Melbourne: Stillwell & Knight . . . 1870.

203 × 132. Pp. 24 (last 2 blank).

Copies: AMAV, ML, NL, SLV, SLW, WLC. 817

On the injection of ammonia into the veins. . . . [Text begins.]

205 × 134. Pp. 8 (l.b.). (1871.) Repr., *Aust. med. J.*, Colophon—Stillwell and Knight . . . Melb.

Copies: SLV. 818

. . . Further observations on the direct injection of ammonia. [Text begins.]

206 × 135. Pp. 8. Repr., *Aust. med. J.*, 1872.

Case histories of snake-bite treated by in-

travenous ammonia.
Copies: NL, SLV. 819

———

Thoughts, observations, and experiments on the action of snake venom on the blood. With an appendix. Melbourne: Stillwell and Co. ... 1894.

217 × 140. Pp. 72 (l.b.). 3 pl. Cloth.

Outlines work of author, C.J. Martin and others. Appendix on experiments with antidotes. Review, *Aust. med. J.*, 1894, ns 16 : 451.

UM copy, with author's inscription, has inserted leaf with original diagrams and 3 photographs of snakes' heads.

G. B. Halford (1824–1910) MD St And., MRCP, distinguished for research on the heart, was first professor and Dean of newly founded Melb. Med. School. See Osborne, W. A. (1929), 'G. B. H. : his life and work', *Med. J. Aust.*, 1 : 64 (with bibliog.); Kenny, A. L. (1941), *Med, J. Aust.*, 1 : 129; Stawell, Sir R. R. (1931), *Med. J. Aust.*, 1 : 1; Bauer, G. E. (1970), 'Four chapters in the history of Aust. cardiology', *Postgrad. med. J.*, 46 : 229.

Copies: AMAN, AMAV, BG, CC, DOS, EF, KFR, ML, NL, RACP, RACS, SLV, SLW, UM. 820

———

See also Industrial and Technological Museum, Melb.; Smyth, Robert Brough.

Hall, A. Wilford

No ... Dr. A. Wilford Hall's hygienic treatment, for the cure of disease, preservation of health and promotion of longevity, without medicine. The exclusive property of [Space for name] who has pledged his honour that the contents of this pamphlet will not be revealed outside his own family ... J. C. Oakman, Proprietor. ... Printed and published by the Proprietor ... Sydney ...

153 × 117. Pp. 48. 1 fig. ND. Plain p. w.

The same, ND. Pp. iv, 52. Proprietor shows as J. Hern, 30 Bourke St, East ... (late ... Fitzroy).

Another ed., 1892. Pp. viii, 76 (l.b.). 7 figs.

See also: Cole, E. W. (ed.) for reprints of 'the pound pamphlet.'

Advocates treatment by profuse 'colon flushing', purported to be a new discovery by author. Price : £1.

Copies: ML, OL, SLV. 821

Hall, Dr.

... Dr. Hall's pocket health guide. Showing how to live long, well & happily. Common-sense hints on dyspepsia, taking cold, sleep, diet, drink, exercise, brain-work, the teeth, the liver, children, accidents and emergencies ... Reprinted from "Health and Home" ... Published for the Health Protection League of Victoria by W. T. Pyke ... Hawthorn. Sold by all respectable booksellers.

158 × 88. Pp. [24]. ND. [?1892.] P. w. (cover title, printed all other sides).

Objects of League: 'to resist the compulsory Vaccination Law and to agitate for its repeal; to disseminate sound hygienic knowledge.'

Copies: SLV. 822

Hall, 'Dr'.

See Cole, E. W.—Editor.

Hall, Edward Swarbreck

Lecture on ozone, delivered at the Hobarton Mechanics' Institute ... 16th July, 1857 ... [Text begins.]

600 × 535. Single sheet, v.b. 8 cols. NI.

Includes plea for better sanitation of Hobart, so that 'the undertaker's office will be more seldom required—more of you will spin out a healthy life to at least the allotted score of three score and ten—not, as now, ... not having a chance of life extending above one third of that period.'

Copies: EF. 823

———

The products and resources of Tasmania, as illustrated in the International Exhibition, 1862. By George Whiting ... Second edition enlarged and corrected. With an appendix ... Hobart Town: ... Daily "Advertiser" Steam Press. 1862.

214 × 140. Op. 50 (l.b.). P. w. (title rptd).

Includes 'Climate and health of Tasmania' (pp. 42–49), by Dr. E. Swarbreck Hall.

Copies: LNSW, ML. 824

———

No. 69. 1869. Tasmania. Legislative Council. Vaccination. Petition of Dr. E. S. Hall. ...

342 × 217. Pp. 4. Colophon—James Barnard, Govt Pr, Tas.

Shows failure of Compulsory Vaccination Act, and recommends amendments.

Copies: BG, ML, NL, SLT, SLV. 825

———

[Royal Arms] Information for the early detection and care of cases of typhoid fever and diphtheria, especially for residents in districts where medical attendance is not immediately available. [Text begins.]

428 × 335. Single leaf, v.b. Hobart Town, 16th July, 1880 (at foot). Signed: E. Swarbreck Hall, Officer of Health.

E. S. Hall (1804–81) MRCS, Asst Col Surg. Hobart, was author of notable publications, of which Cumpston wrote that 'for information on the aetiological factors in diseases during the early period of Aust. history, we are almost entirely indebted to the writings of Hall.' See Cumpston, J.H.L. (1923), 'The first Aust. sanitarian', *Health*, 1 : 89; for med. teaching, Crowther, W.E.L.H. (1952), *Aust. NZ J. Surg.*, 21 : 185.

Also published: *Who translated the Bible?*, Hobart Town, 1875. Pp. xvi, 300.

Copies: EF, SLT, WLC. 826

——— and Abbott, Francis

Results of five years' meteorological observations for Hobart Town; . . . and completing a period of thirty years. . . . by Francis Abbott, F.R.A.S., F.R.M.S. [Royal Arms] Tasmania: James Barnard, Govt Printer, Hobart Town. 1872.

309 × 238. Pp. 38 (l.b.). P. w. (title rptd).

'Climate and vital statistics of Tasmania', by E. Swarbreck Hall, occurs at pp. 9–37.

Copies: ML, NL, SLS, SLT, SLV. 827

Hall, Thomas Sergeant

Catalogue of the scientific and technical periodical literature in the libraries in Melbourne. Compiled by T. S. Hall, M.A. . . . With the assistance of the several librarians. . . . Robt. S. Brain, Govt Printer, Melbourne. 1899.

217 × 138. Pp. viii (l.b.), 226 (l.b.). Cloth.

2 ed. (with E. R. Pitt), 1911.

It is stated: 'The only catalogue of this nature published in Melbourne deals with medical periodicals alone, and was compiled by Prof. H. B. Allen, and issued in 1893.'

Copies: EF, ML, SLV, UM, US. 828

Hall, W. W.

A hundred dozen health maxims by Dr. W. W. Hall. . . . Cole's Book Arcade, Melbourne . . .

175 × 125. Pp. 268, xi. ND. (?1895.) Stiff p. w. (cover title).

Another ed., with variation in title. ND. Cloth.

Copies: EF, ML. 829

Hamilton, A. S.

Science v spiritism, with special reference to the extraordinary pretensions of the trance lecturer, Mr. Thomas Walker . . . and Mrs. Emma Hardinge-Britten, the celebrated inspirational lecturess. By A. S. Hamilton, Professor of Phrenology. The subject is treated purely upon physiological, phrenological, and psychological principles. Sydney: S. Glassop . . . 1878.

210 × 130. Pp. 36. P. w. (title rptd).

Copies: FC, ML. 830

Hamilton, Miss

A course of four lectures delivered to the members of the Clunes Girls' Friendly Society, on sick-nursing, by Miss Hamilton (late nurse of the Clunes Hospital.) Clunes: . . . "Guardian and Gazette" Office . . . 1886.

217 × 140. Pp. 30. P. w. (cover title).

Copies: FC. 831

Hamlet, William Mogford

Anthrax in Australia, with some account of Pasteur's method of vaccination. Demonstration at Junee, N.S.W. by William M. Hamlet . . . Reprinted from the "Intercolonial Medical Congress of Australasia Transactions". Melbourne: Stillwell and Co. . . . 1889.

209 × 135. Pp. 16. P. w. (cover title).

For W. M. Hamlet FIC, FCS, NSW Govt Analyst, member of Anthrax Board which reported on the anthrax vaccine trials by Pasteur's representatives at Junee in 1888, see obit., *J&P Roy. Soc. NSW*, 1932, 66 : 11.

Copies: LNSW, NL. 832

———

See also New South Wales–Anthrax Board.

Hance, J. L.

No. 3, Vol. 1.] [April, 1882. The third number of the Atlas Series of Australian pamphlets, entitled a new era and a new element being a scientific demonstration of the materiality of spirit. . . . Second edition, corrected and revised . . . Published by the Author . . . Glenellen, Kenthurst. . . . Sydney: Edward Lee & Co. . . . 1892.

209 × 132. Pp. 76. P. w. (cover title). Also bound with 6 pamphlets of series in cloth.

Postulates a material system of physical and

spiritual existence, based on three elements—aesthenogen, source of sensation and muscular action; zoogen, of heat and vitality; and einaigen, of separate existence, mind and soul.

Copies: EF, FC, ML, NL, SLV. 833

———

No. 4. Vol. 1.] ... The fourth number of the Atlas Series ... A new era and a new element being a scientific demonstration of the materiality of spirit. Part 11. ... [Imprint as above] 1892.

209 × 132. Pp. 68. P. w. (cover title).

Extends thesis of previous item to the origin of organic life, man and animals, and mind.

Copies: CC, FC, ML, NL, SLV. 834

Hansen, B.

Bacteria and pasteurising ... Reprinted from the "Australian Farm and Home" for March 1899. Tytherleigh & Bayne, 367a Post Office Place West.

217 × 140. Pp. 16. 5 figs. [Melbourne.]

Copies: ML.

Hanson, Sir Richard Davies

Law in nature, &c., &c., &c. Four papers, read before the Adelaide Philosophical Society ... Printed at the request of the Society. Adelaide ... W. K. Thomas, Register and Observer Offices ... 1864.

242 × 183. Pp. vi, 76 (last—colophon only). Stiff p. w. (title rptd).

Critical study of the Darwinian thesis, which 'stands out as a remarkably perceptive and modern comment on evolutionary thought.' See Mozley, Ann (1967), 'Evolution and the climate of opinion in Aust., 1840–76', *Victorian Studies*: 434.

Author (1805–76) was Premier and later Chief Justice of SA.

Copies: EF, FC, ML, SLS, UA. 836

———

The Same, 1865, with additional papers. Title: Law in nature, and other papers. Adel., W. C. Rigby; Melb., Geo. Robertson; Syd., W. Maddock.

Copies: ML, NL, SLV, UA. 837

———

Paper read ... April 9, 1872. Subject—"The theory of evolution." [Text begins.]

255 × 204. Pp. [6]. Colophon—William Kyffin Thomas ... Adel. Read Adel. Phil. Soc.

Copies: ML. 838

Harbury House Retreat for the Insane

See Harcourt, James Thomas.

Harcourt, James Thomas

Private retreat for the insane. Harbury House, Pascoe Vale, near Melbourne. Mr. Harcourt's testimonials. [Text begins.]

247 × 204. Pp. [4]. Double cols. Pale blue paper. NI. [Melb., 1857.]

J. T. Harcourt established above private asylum in 1856; about 1863 transferred this to Richmond Vic. as Cremorne Inebriates and Insane Asylum. See *Aust. med. J.*, 1870, 15 : 350; *Austsn med. Gaz.*, 1884, 4 : 75; also Brothers, C.R.D. *Early Victorian psychiatry, 1835–1905*, Melb., ND.

Copies: LNSW. 839

Hardie, Sir David

Notes on some of the more common diseases in Queensland in relation to atmospheric conditions, 1887–1891. Illustrated by charts prepared from information supplied by the Registrar-General's Department and Chief Weather Bureau, Brisbane, including returns from the hospitals of the Colony. ... Brisbane: James C. Beal, Govt Printer. ... 1893.

220 × 140. Pp. vi, [7]-132, [ii] (v.b.). 1 flg chart. Cloth.

See also author's 'The forecasting of disease', *Austsn med. Gaz.*, 1894, 13 : 45.

For Sir David Hardie (1856–1925), MD, ChM, FRACS, of Brisbane, Hon. Surg. Hosp. for Sick Children, see obit., *Med. J. Aust.*, 1946, 1 :95.

Copies: AMAQ, AMAV, EF, ML, NL, OL, SLV, UA, UM, UQ. 840

Hare, Francis Washington Everard

The cold-bath treatment of typhoid fever. The experience of a consecutive series of nineteen hundred and two cases treated at the Brisbane Hospital ... with illustrations London MacMillan and Co., Limited New York: The MacMillan Company 1898

229 × 145. Pp. xii, 196. Frontis., 3 pl., 1 fig. Cloth.

A study of the hydrotherapy of typhoid, which influenced its adoption as a standard treatment.

A. Jefferis Turner considered this the most

important Aust. medical work published on any subject excepting hydatids (*Intercol med. J. Austsia*, 1898, 3 : 692). It was criticised in a Brisbane pamphlet *Shall they die?* (NS), in yellow wrapper, which created some prejudice among patients (Jackson, *infra*).

For F.W.E. Hare (d. 1929) MD, who was in charge of fever wards, Brisbane Hosp., later in practice at Charters Towers and Brisbane, see Jackson, E. S. (1929), *Med. J. Aust.*, 1 : 365. After return to England, he published *The food factor in health and disease*, Lond., 1905, and *On alcoholism its clinical aspects and treatment*, Lond., 1912.

Copies: BG, EF, KFR, ML, MLWA, NL, RACP, SLV, SPH, UA, UM, UQ, US. 841

Harper, Walter

Simple anthropometrical measurements. ... Ashfield: G. Watson, General Printer ... 1897.

173 × 120. Pp. 8. 1 fig.

For collecting data on aborigines by author's 'out back' correspondents.

Copies: EF, ML. 842

Harper, Walter R. and Clarke, Arthur H.

Notes on the measurements of the Tasmanian crania in the Tasmanian Museum, Hobart ... [Text begins.]

209 × 150. Pp. 14. 6 pl. NI. ND. [?1897.]

Copies: ML. 843

Harris, John

Newcastle Sanitary Association Paper on the pollution of the soil ... under the auspices of the Newcastle Sanitary Association ... Newcastle ... "Herald" Office ... 1887.

217 × 138. Pp. 20 (l.b.). P. w. (title rptd).

On sanitation and waste disposal.

For John Harris (1849–1923) MD, ChM Aberd., Hon. Surg. Newcastle Hosp., see obit., *Med. J. Aust.*, 1923, 1 :540.

Copies: ML. 844

Harrison, George

A word to legislators. Culpable compulsion: a condemnation by competent authorities ... Hobart: Calder, Bowden, & Co., 1889.

204 × 130. Pp. 24 (last 3 blank). P. w. (title rptd).

Vaccination is 'filthy in genesis, dishonored in history, uncertain in operation, false *ex hypothesi*, dangerous in results ... a pretentious superstition that disgraces even this era of mixed science and charlatanism ...'

Copies: FC, LNSW, ML, NL, WLC. 845

———

The Same. ND. (1889 in preface.) Colophon—Whillas & Ormiston, Printers, Adel.

Copies: SLS. 846

Hart, E.

See Australasian Sanitary Conference of Sydney.

Harvie-Linklater, Frederick

See Linklater, Frederick Harvie—.

Haslam, John

Convict-ships. A narrative of a voyage to New South Wales, in the year 1816, in the ship Mariner, describing the nature of the accommodations, stores, diet, &c. together with an account of the medical treatment and religious superintendence of these unfortunate persons. By John Haslam, Junr. Surgeon in the Royal Navy. ... London: ... Taylor and Hessey ... 1819.

212 × 125. Pp. 24 (l.b.).

The earliest of a series of works by surgeons-supt of convict ships. The voyage was healthy and without deaths, a brilliant result of the sweeping reform of the transport service following implementation of a report by William Redfern to Governor Macquarie in 1814. (See note to Surgeons-Supt of Convict Ships, No 2070.)

For John Haslam RN, see Leigh, D., *The historical development of British psychiatry*, vol. 1, Oxford, 1961 : 143. His father was John Haslam MD, of Bethlam Hosp., London, whose writings 'assure him of an important place in the history of psychiatry.'

Copies: ML. 847

Hawker, Thomas D.

A lecture on the small pox, delivered to the members of the Stratton Literary Institution, on ... October 29, 1833, by Mr. T. D. Hawker, Surgeon. Second edition. [Quotation] Adelaide: Printed by Hussey & Shawyer ... 1854.

165 × 105. Pp. 20. P. w. (title rptd).

On small-pox inoculation and cow-pox vaccination. Preface mentions author's use of these during epidemic at Stratton, Cornwall.

Copies: SLS. 848

Hawkesbury Benevolent Society and Hospital, Windsor, NSW

Annual Report of the Hawkesbury Benevolent Society; for the year 1839; . . . Sydney: Printed by James Tegg, George Street . . . 1840.

212 × 132. Pp. 12. Blue paper wrappers.

Now Hawkesbury District Hosp. For history: Bowd, D. G., *History of the Hawkesbury Benev. Soc. and Hosp.*, Windsor, 1947; also Walker, Wm, No 2442.

Copies: ML (various from 1839). 849

Hawkesbury District Hospital, Windsor, NSW

See item above.

Hayter, Henry Heylyn

Crime in New South Wales A paper written for, but rejected by the Royal Society of that Colony . . . Melbourne M'Carron, Bird & Co., Printers . . . 1884.

210 × 138. Pp. 14 (l.b.), [6] (l.b.). P. w. (title rptd).

The 'skeleton in the cupboard' of NSW is excessive criminality compared with other Aust. states and Britain. 'Whether this is due to the convict taint by which portion of her population may . . . be still affected, or to her inhabitants having become demoralised by prosperity' is unknown.

Copies: EF, CC, ML, NL, SLS, SLT, SLV. 850

———

Handbook to the Colony of Victoria, prepared under the direction of the Victorian Government . . . Melbourne . . . John Ferres, Govt Printer. . . .

212 × 132. Pp. 64 (l.b.). 1 coloured flg map. ND. [1884.] P. w. (title rptd).

Includes sections on population, births and deaths, water supply, provident and charitable institutions.

Henry Heylyn Hayter was Govt Statist of Vic.

Copies: EF, ML, NL, SLS, SLV. 851

———

The Same. 2 ed., 1885. Pp. 64. Flg map.

Copies: FC, ML, NL, SLT, SLV, SLW. 852

———

The Same. 3 ed., revised, 1891. Pp. 56. Flg map.

Copies: FC. 853

Hayward, William Thornborough

Septic diseases and antiseptic remedies. . . . President's address at the . . . South Australian Branch of the British Medical Association, . . . June, 1886. Adelaide: Frearson & Brother . . . 1886.

215 × 142. Pp. 14. P. w. (title rptd). Repr., *Proc. SA Branch BMA*.

W. T. Hayward MRCS (1875), LKQCPI, who settled in Adel. after experience in Liverpool, later became Hon. Phys. Adel. and Adel. Children's Hosps.

Copies: ML, NL. 854

Headley, Walter Balls—

On internal tumours. Their characteristic distinctions, and diagnosis. . . . Melbourne: F. F. Bailliere . . . 1876.

191 × 127. Pp. xii, 174, [ii] (book notices). Cloth.

On differential diagnosis of ovarian tumours. The first gynaecology book published in Australia. Review, *Aust. med. J.*, 1876, 21 : 174.

Copies: AMAV, BG, CC, EF, ML, NL, RACS, SLV, UM. 855

———

Dress, with reference to heat . . . Australian Health Society . . . Melbourne: J. & A. M'Kinley . . . 1876.

204 × 132. Pp. 40 (2, 4 blank; last—book notice).

'. . . how we . . . living in a country different in climate from that to which our system has for generations been accustomed, may best dress for the preservation of our health.'

Copies: FC, LNSW, ML, NL, SLV, UM. 856

———

On the use of the medical thermometer. . . . (From the "Melbourne Review".) Melbourne: Alex. M'Kinley & Co. . . . 1877.

236 × 150. Pp. 20 (l.b.). 1 fig.

'. . . about half the members of every family die of acute disease. . . . It becomes then of utmost importance that . . . the people should have a means at hand, by which the first signs of the attack of the enemy may be known.'

Copies: LNSW, ML, SLV, UM. 857

———

Homoeopathy past and present . . . George Robertson, Melbourne . . . 1878.

204 × 132. Pp. 40. P. w. (title rptd).

A vituperative account concludes: 'Homoeopathy was commenced in fraud, continued in slander, and sustained by filching, false-witness, and ignorance; and ... all of Homoeopathic "science" that remains, is its bastard representatives clinging to slander, the last rag of the Homoeopathic skirt.' Review, *Aust. med. J.*, 1878, 23 : 358.

Copies: LNSW, ML, SLV. 858

An account of a case of ovariotomy, in which recovery followed. Melbourne: Stillwell and Co ...

209 × 132. Pp. 4. ND. (1879.)

Copies: SLV. 859

On retroflexion of the uterus. ... Reprinted from "The Australian Medical Journal" for August, 1879.

201 × 130. Pp. 16. 1 pl. Colophon—Stillwell and Co. ...

Copies: SLV, UM. 860

An account of the first case of small-pox in Melbourne in 1882. ... From the Australian Medical Journal, May 1882. Stillwell & Co. ... Melbourne. 1882.

206 × 135. Pp. 28. 1 flg pl.

Includes reports by T. S. Bulmer MD, Quarantine Stn, Sorrento.

Copies: UM. 861

On the treatment of so-called ulceration, with laceration of the cervix uteri, by Emmett's operation of closure. ... (From the Australian Medical Journal of November 1883.)

204 × 135. Pp. 8 (last—emblem). P. w. (cover title). Colophon—Stillwell and Co. ... Melb.

Copies: UM. 862

The natural history of four cases of lacerated cervix uteri. ... Reprinted from the "Australian Medical Journal", May 1884.

204 × 135. Pp. 8. P. w. (cover title). Colophon—Stillwell and Co. ... Melb.

Copies: UM. 863

Seven cases of laparotomy. ... (From the Australian Medical Journal of December 1886.)

209 × 135. Pp. 20 (l.b.). 3 pl., 4 charts (inserted). Colophon—Stillwell and Co. ... Melb. P. w. (cover title).

Copies: UM. 864

Antiseptic midwifery. ... From the "Australian Medical Journal", July 15, 1888. Melbourne: Stillwell and Co. ...

204 × 127. Pp. 8. P. w. (cover title).

Applies Listerian principles to midwifery. Appendix contains: 'Rules for midwifery nurses to be printed on cards and given to them.' See item below.

Copies: CC, EF, UM. 865

Rules for midwifery nurses. [Text begins.]

206 × 132. Card, v.b. Ruled frame with decorated corners. NI. ND. [c. 1888.]

Nine rules of antiseptic practice, for distribution to midwives. Ends: 'These rules being for the purpose of preventing the contamination of the patient, reliance must be placed in the nurse that they are carried out.'

Copies: UM. 866

A second series of seven cases of laparotomy ... From the "Australian Medical Journal", December 15, 1888. Melbourne: Stillwell and Co. ...

209 × 135. Pp. 12 (l.b.).

Copies: UM. 867

Acute peritonitis in women ... From the "Australian Medical Journal", July 15th, 1889. Melbourne: Stillwell and Co. ... 1889.

206 × 135. Pp. 8. P. w. (cover title).

'I desire to show that a large number of women die of peritonitis as a disease consequent on another and original disease and that it may be regarded as a symptom, rather than as the actual cause of death.'

Copies: UM. 868

Conditions warranting removal of the ovaries and tubes. ... Reprinted from the "Intercolonial Medical Congress of Australasia Transactions". Melbourne: Stillwell and Co. ... 1889.

209 × 132. Pp. 8. P. w. (cover title).
Copies: UM. 869

On a case of placenta praevia. ... [Text begins.]
206 × 132. Pp. 12. Repr. *Aust. med. J.*, May 1879. Colophon—Stillwell and Co. ...
Copies: SLV. 869a

From the "Australian Medical Journal" November 15, 1886. Case of chronic puerperal mania—laceration & granular os—trachelorhaphy—immediate recovery. ... [Text begins.]
209 × 135. Pp. [2]. Colophon—Stillwell and Co. ... Melb.
Copies: UM. 869b

Medical Society of Victoria. President's address. ... From the "Australian Medical Journal", January 1890. Melbourne: Stillwell and Co. ... 1890.
206 × 132. Pp. 12.
Copies: UM. 869c

Section of Midwifery. President's address. Also paper on the treatment of the inflammatory diseases of evolution of the uterus and appendages. Read at the Intercolonial Medical Congress, Sydney, 1892.
206 × 132. Pp. 22. Colophon—Syd.: Charles Potter, Govt Pr—1893. P. w. (cover title).
Copies: UM. 870

Intercolonial Medical Congress of Australasia. ... Sydney ... 1892. Section of Obstetrics and Diseases of Women. President's address ... Reprinted from the "Australian Medical Journal", November 15, 1892. Melbourne: Stillwell and Co. ...
206 × 132. Pp. 18. P. w. (cover title).
On the evolution of disease in woman, and the influence exerted by civilisation.
Copies: UM. 871

The evolution of the diseases of women. ... London: Smith, Elder, & Co. ... Melbourne & Sydney: George Robertson & Co. 1894. ...
222 × 140. Pp. xx (3 blanks), 376 (l.b.), [4] (advts). 114 figs. Cloth.
Regarded by local reviewers as the most important medical work by an Aust. doctor up to this time. Review, *Aust. med. J.*, 1895, ns 17 : 187 and *Austsn med. Gaz.*, 1895, 14 : 122.
For Walter Balls-Headley (1842–1918) MD, MS Camb., MD Melb., FRCP, distinguished gynaecologist, Hon. MO Melb. Lying-in Hosp., see *Univ. Melb. Med. School Jubilee*, Melb., 1914; Macdonald, C. (1957), *Med. J. Aust.*, 1 : 25; Forster, F.M.C., *Progress in obst. and gynaec. in Aust.*, Syd., 1967.
Also published: 'The etiology of the diseases of the female genital organs', in Allbutt and Playfair's *System of gynaecology*, pp. 112–151, Lond., 1896.
Copies: AMAN, AMAV, BG, EF, FF, KFR, ML, MLWA, NL, RACS, SLV, UM, US. 872

Health and Home

Health and Home. A magazine of domestic and social improvement. Addressed to parents, politicians, magistrates, clergymen, and other responsible people. No. 2. Melbourne. March, 1892. Price One Penny.
331 × 209. Pp. 8.
Quarterly. Anti-vaccinationist and vegetarian. Ed. and published by W. T. Pyke, Hawthorn Vic. Advertises Health Protection League of Vic. and Vegetarian Soc. of Aust.
Copies: SLV (Nos 2, 3, 1892). 873

Health Protection League of Victoria

See *Health and Home*; also Dr. Hall.

Health Society of New South Wales

No. 1. November, 1876. Health Society of N. S. Wales. Hints for the prevention of scarlet fever. (Abridged from a paper by the Australian Health Society, Melbourne.) ... Sydney: ... John Sands ... 1876.
183 × 122. Pp. 4.
Society was founded for health education, prevention of food adulteration, removal of noxious influences by legislation and pressure on authorities. Its activities appear to have ceased about 1883.
Society's pamphlets were published in numbered series 1–11. Nos. 2 and 3 not seen. For following numbers, see under authors: 4, 7, 8, 9—Bradley, H. B.; 6—Clay, W. F.; 10—Behrend, H.; 11—Moffit, A.
Copies: ML. 874

———

No. 5. March 1878. Health Society of N. S. Wales. Hints on typhoid fever. ... "Prevention is better than cure". Sydney: ... John Sands ... 1878.

173 × 120. Pp. 4. P. w. (cover title).

Copies: FC, ML. 875

Healthy Mothers and Sturdy Children

The Australian wife's advice book on the management of her own health and that of her children, with some words addressed to her husband. Healthy mothers and sturdy children. ... giving the best methods of maintaining health and curing disease, as taught by ... hygienic physicians. ... Melbourne: Pater & Knapton, Printers ... 1893.

161 × 120. Pp. iv, 5–176. Cloth.

Includes sections on: woman in health and sickness, management of children, bathing and hygienic treatment, diet, training of children.

Copies: ML, SLV. 876

Hearne, William Goodall

Treatment of diseases: a short treatise to secure advancement in the science of medicine ... Melbourne: Sands & McDougall ... 1880.

180 × 123. Pp. 48. Cloth.

Apart from initial advt of author, work consists mainly of extracts from various writers. He offers to compete with a doctor, for £1000 a side, in the treatment of 1000 patients.

Copies: AMAV, BG, CC, EF, ML, NL, SLV. 877

Heath, Richard

Deafness: its causes and cure. Being an explanation of the most rational modes of treatment, and an exposition of the fallacies practised ... Geelong: Franks and Jackson ... 1859.

178 × 107. Pp. 48 (l.b.). P. w. (title rptd).

Endorsed 'London, July, 1857' at p. 10; appendix on 'colonial cases.'

Richard Heath (d. 1888) MRCS settled in Geelong in 1858, was later at N. Melb. and Apollo Bay Vic. Obit.: *Austsn med. Gaz.*, 1888, 7 : 153.

Copies: ML, SLV. 878

Heathcote District Hospital, Vic.

Rules of the Heathcote Gold District General Hospital. January, 1859. Heathcote: Printed at "The M'Ivor News" Office. 1859.

150 × 98. Pp. 16. Errata leaf. Printed on blue paper.

Includes report for 1858.

Copies: SLV. 879

———

Eleventh Annual Report of the Committee of Management of the Heathcote District Hospital ... Printed at the "M'Ivor Times" Office ... Heathcote.

204 × 132. Pp. [10]. ND. (1870.)

Report for 1869. Earlier named Heathcote Gold Dist. Hosp.

Copies: SLV (11–15; 1869–73). 880

Hedger, H.

Employment of the blind. Instructions how to work, and information concerning various trades for blind people working in their own homes. ... Sydney: S. E. Lees ... 1899.

183 × 125. Pp. 40. P. w. (title rptd).

Author was manager, Syd. Industrial Blind Instn.

Copies: ML. 881

Helidon Spa Water Co.

A natural mineral water of absolute purity. [Fig., within red circle: Helidon Spa Water Co. Ltd.] Brisbane, ... Watson, Ferguson & Co. ...

165 × 102. Pp. [12]. ND.

Includes report by Prof. Anderson Stuart (1899) with constitution and probable medical value of water.

Copies: ML. 882

Henderson, Andrew

Scraps and facts of convict ships ... April 2nd, 1845. Devonport: Printed by J. Heydon ...

237 × 148. Pp. [ii] (v.b.), 26 (l.b.). Errata slip. Cloth.

Andrew Henderson MD, FRCPE, Surg. RN, who made nine voyages to Australia as surg.-supt of convict ships (1829–42), describes his system of convict education, with observations on *Hindostan* voyage made to VDL with 200 boys without serious illness.

ML copy inscribed by author to Duke of Wellington.

Copies: ML. 883

Henderson, John

Observations on the colonies of New South Wales and Van Diemen's Land. ... Calcutta: ... Baptist Mission Press ... 1832.

209 × 135. Pp. xxvi (l.b.), [ii] (v.b.), 180.

Frontis., 2 pl. Cloth. Paper label.

Facsimile ed., Adel.: Libraries Bd of SA, 1965.

Dr. John Henderson, Bengal Med. Service, visited VDL in 1829 and explored parts from Hobart to Oyster Bay and on E. Coast. Later, from Sydney, he made a journey to Wellington NSW and beyond in search of a supposed inland sea. The book includes sections on the economy and natural history of the colonies.

ML copy has inserted obit. from *The Agra Ukhbar*, 19 March 1836, announcing author's death following a journey to Little Thibet and the Indian Caucasus, on which he suffered extreme privation, wounds and injuries.

Copies: DL, FC, ML, NL, SLS, SLT, SLV, SLW, UA, UQ. 884

Henry, Louis

Massage. ... From the Australian Medical Journal, August 15th, 1884. Melbourne: Stillwell & Co. ...

220 × 135. Pp. 12. P. w. (cover title).

Copies: NL, UM. 885

———

Some aspects of the pathology & treatment of typhoid fever. ... Reprinted from "The Australasian Medical Gazette", August 20, 1900. Sydney: John Sands ... 1900.

180 × 120. Pp. 8 (l.b.).

Louis Henry (d. 1924) MD Wurzburg and Melb., came to Australia in 1879 and practised at Brunswick Vic. He was Hon. Phys. Alfred Hosp.

Copies: SLV. 886

[Henry, Thomas James]

The awful and ethical allegory of [Cut] Deuteronomy Smith. Edinburgh: E. & S. Livingstone.

209 × 165. Pp. 68. Decorated title in red frame. Figs. ND. [?1891.] Cloth, with amended title and fig. on front, including: '... or the life history of a student of medicine ...'

Written 1881, first published by Geo. Dryden, Edin. (NS). Student's ed. (15th), ND, pp. 32, Edin.: Livingstone (NS). Another ed., 1909.

A humourous account of student life in Edinburgh.

EF copy bears author's inscription to Dr. A. A. Brodziak, dated 1895.

Copies: AMAN, EF, US. 887

———

Claude Garton: A story of Dunburgh University. ... Edinburgh: E. & S. Livingstone, 1897.

183 × 122. Pp. [viii]. [5]–411. Cloth.

Aust. ed. published by Geo. Robertson in conjunction with Livingstone.

Fictional tale of Edinburgh medical student. EF copy inscribed to Dr. A. A. Brodziak.

T. J. Henry (1860–1940) FRCSE, who practised at Grafton and Warialda NSW, later lived at Manly NSW till his death.

Copies: EF. 888

Hepburn Mineral Spring Water

Medical opinions on the Hepburn Mineral Spring Water. Melbourne: 1872.

153 × 102. Pp. 12.

Testimonials from Vic. doctors.

Copies: SLV. 889

Herald of Health

Herald of Health. An advocate of Sound Living. E. R. Caro, M. D., Editor. Vol. 1. No. 1. Melb., Jan. 1898.

209 × 178. Pp. 16.

A popular health journal. Vols 1–4, Melb. and Syd., 1898–1901.

Advertises Med. and Surg. Sanitarium Summer Hill NSW, of which editor was Med. Supt.

Copies: ML (vol. 2), SLV (all pub.). 890

Hermes Medical Supplement

See *Sydney University Med. Society, Journal of the*

Hern, John

Advanced hygiene; or, how to cure disease without recourse to drugs or medicines of any kind. A practical treatise on the value of hygiene in preventing and curing disease and promoting longevity ... The most valuable book in the world except the Bible. Melbourne: Mason, Firth & M'Cutcheon ... 1892.

214 × 140. Pp. viii, 328. Cloth.

On self-treatment by enemas, baths and vegetarian diet.

The book was later taken over by Cole's Book Arcade. In some copies a slip is inserted, reducing price from £1 to 3s.6d; others have half title inserted, with 'Explanation' of altered price on verso.

Copies: AMAV, BG, CC, DOS, EF, KFR, ML, NL, RACP, SLV. 891

John Hern's new book on hygiene and hygienic treatment for the cure of all diseases. Melbourne: Spectator Publishing Company ... 1892.

186 × 120. Pp. 304. Stiff p. w. with 'John Hern's new book Advice of sixteen doctors ...' on front.

Reprints passages from writers on health, diet, hydropathy, nature healing, etc.

Copies: ML, OL. 892

Hickson, John Bell

Medical reform. Homoeopathy vindicated, as a necessary and scientific reform in medical practice ... Slater, Williams, and Hodgson ... Melbourne; and ... Castlemaine. 1856.

209 × 132. Pp. 62 (l.b.). P. w. (title rptd).

Copies: LNSW, ML, SLV, WLC. 893

He will not drink wine: or, alcoholic beverages, considered socially and physiologically ... Melbourne—George Robertson, Gordon & Gotch. London—Gordon & Gotch ... Sydney—W. Maddock. Adelaide— W. A. Cawthorne. Brisbane—G. Slater. Hobart Town—Walch & Son. Launceston—Walch Bros. & Burchall. 1869.

212 × 140. Pp. 46, [2] advts.

An anti-liquor pamphlet.

J. B. Hickson MD Homoeo. Coll. Penn. USA practised as a homoeopath in Melb., S. Yarra, Ballarat. For claims of *Melb. Med. Record* that he was the writer of four of Beaney's major works, see Gandevia, B. (1952), 'Review of Victoria's early med. journals', *Med. J. Aust.*, 2 : 184; Gandevia, B. (1953), 'Some aspects of ... Beaney', *Med. J. Aust.*, 1 : 614.

Copies: LNSW, ML, SLV. 894

Hickson, Robert R. P.

Sewage purification and disposal. Being a digest of the evidence ... and reports submitted to, the Parliamentary Standing Committee on Public Works during their inquiry into the sewerage schemes for Manly, North Shore, the Western Suburbs of Sydney, and Parramatta. ... Sydney: Charles Potter, Govt Printer ... 1895. ...

250 × 156. Pp. [ii] (v.b.), 72. P. w. (title rptd).

On the efficiency of various disposal methods. Author was Chief Engineer for Pub. Works., NSW.

Copies: EF, ML. 895

Higginbottom, John

The non-alcoholic treatment of disease ... Sydney: Hanson and Bennett ... 1863.

173 × 120. Pp. 14. P. w. (title rptd).

Copies: ML, SLV. 896

Hill, Rosamond and Florence

What we saw in Australia ... London: Macmillan and Co., 1875 ...

186 × 125. Pp. xii, 438. Frontis. Cloth.

Account of tour by two philanthropic nieces of Sir Rowland Hill, who reviewed charitable and reform services, and inspected main institutions.

Copies: FC, ML, NL, SLS, SLT, SLV, SLW, UA, UQ, US. 897

Hiller, F.

Consumption and its prevention, with remarks on koumiss, as a hygienic remedy for debilitating, nervous & wasting diseases. ... Sydney: W. E. Smith ... 1879.

212 × 143. Pp. 12. P. w. (cover title).

Koumiss—a fermented drink prepared from milk.

Copies: LNSW, ML, NL. 898

Koumiss. The great dietetic and hygienic remedy for debilitating, nervous, and wasting diseases. Salisbury & Co., Manufactory, 30 Campbell St., Sydney. Sydney: W. E. Smith ... 1879.

204 × 132. Pp. 16. P. w. (cover title).

Manufacturer states that author, F. Hiller MD, 'undertakes the direct supervision and responsibility' of manufacture.

Copies: ML. 899

Koumiss, great dietetic and hygienic remedy for debilitating, nervous, and wasting diseases. Koumiss Manufacturing Company, Sydney, Melbourne, Queensland and Tasmania. Office: —Phillip Street ... Sydney.

196 × 132. Pp. 14, 2. 1 flg leaf. Pink slip (v.b.) inserted. ND. (?1882.) Signed: F. Hiller, M.D. ... Sydney.

Copies: LNSW. 900

Hirsch, August

Handbook of geographical and historical pathology. By Dr. August Hirsch, Professor of Medicine in the University of Berlin. Volume 1.—Acute infectious diseases. Translated from the Second German edition by Charles Creighton, M.D. London: The New Sydenham Society. 1883.

214 × 138. 3 vols. Vol. 1, 1883: pp. xviii (l.b.), 710; vol. 2, 1885: pp. xii, 682 (l.b.); vol. 3, 1886: pp. xvi (l.b.), 780. Cloth.

1 ed., 1860—*Handbuch der historisch-geographischen Pathologie*, 2 vols, Erlangen. 2 ed., 1881–86, 3 vols, Stuttgart.

Australian references included.

Copies: AMAV, EF, KFR, RACS, SLV, SPH, UA, UM, UQ, US. 901

Hitchman, W.

The connexion between medical reform and spiritualism. An address delivered before the British Medical Reform Association, by W. Hitchman, M.D., D.C.L., F.R.S. W. H. Terry ... Melbourne. 1880.

181 × 120. Pp. 32. P. w. (title rptd).

Copies: ML, SLV. 902

Hobart General Hospital

(No. 10.) [Royal Arms] 1861. Tasmania. General Hospital. Report of Board of Management. ... Ordered by the House to be printed, 20 August, 1861.

330 × 205. Pp. 8. Colophon—James Barnard, Govt Pr, Tas.

1st an. rep. (1860) of Hosp. Board, appointed Jan., 1859, on transfer of control from Imperial Govt to Colony. Board was also responsible for Brickfields Invalid Depot.

An. reps (1860–) appear in Parliamentary Papers, Tas.

For history, see P. S. Seager (1921), *Hobart Gen. Hosp. ... epitome of its history*, Hobart; Hume, A. W. (c. 1920), *Hobart Gen. Hosp.*; *Its early history*, Hobart. Now named Royal Hobart Hosp.

Copies: LNSW, NL, SLT, SLV. 903

Rules and regulations of the General Hospital and Dispensary, Hobart Town. Approved February 4, 1871. [Royal Arms] Tasmania: James Barnard, Govt Printer, Hobart Town. 1871.

214 × 140. Pp. 12 (last 2 blank). P. w. (title rptd). Other eds: 1877, pp. 24; 1897, pp. 40.

Copies: ML (1877), SLT (1871), WLC (1877, 1897). 904

No. 40. 1873. Tasmania. Legislative Council. Tuition at General Hospital, Hobart Town. ... Return to an order ... (Mr. Crowther.) ...

339 × 217. Pp. 4 (2, l.b.). Colophon—James Barnard, Govt Pr ...

Hosp. Bd answers questions on tuition for students, of which 8 were admitted from 1869–79. Attendance shortened study period at a British school by one year.

Copies: BG, LNSW, NL, SLT, SLV. 905

(No. 4.) [Royal Arms] 1877. Tasmania. House of Assembly. General Hospital, Hobart Town; Report of Commission, with evidence. ...

344 × 212. Pp. ii (v.b.), viii (l.b.), 40 (l.b.). Colophon—James Barnard, Govt Pr, Tas.

On general condition and management.

Copies: LNSW, NL, SLT, SLV. 906

Hobart Nurses' Home

Report of the Nurses' Home, (instituted 1882), under the Ladies' Christian Association, Hobart. Hobart: J. Burnet, Printer ...

180 × 120. Pp. 8. P. w. (cover title, decorative frame).

Report for 1884. Named Hobart Nurses' Home in short title. Founded as home 'from which general and monthly nurses can be obtained at any time.'

Copies: SLT (1884, 1885). 907

Hobart Town General Dispensary and Humane Society

The Hobart Town General Dispensary and Humane Society; for providing medical attendance, medicine, and other aid for the indigent sick, free of expense. ... Established 1847. Hobart Town: Printed by William Gore Elliston ... 1847.

135 × 98. Pp. 8. Plain p. w.

Copies: ML, NL, SLT. 908

Hobart Town Water Supply

Memorial to His Excellency Sir William T. Denison, Knt., Lieutenant Governor of Van Diemen's Land and its dependencies, praying him to assert and maintain the rights of the inhabitants of Hobart Town to an independent supply of pure water. Printed by William Pratt ... Hobart Town.

293 × 193. Pp. 8 (last—title rptd without imprint). ND.

Copies: ML. 909

The right of the inhabitants of Hobart Town to an independent supply of pure water. Hobart Town: . . . William Pratt . . .

220 × 138. Pp. [iv], 76. 1 flg plan. ND. [1847.] P. w. (title rptd).

Memorial to Governor complaining of encroachment, by owner of water mills and breweries, on the people's rights in water flowing from Mt Wellington.

Copies: FC, ML, SLT, SLV. 910

(No. 22.) 1896. Session 11. Parliament of Tasmania. Hobart Water Supply and river pollution: correspondence. Presented at both Houses . . .

344 × 217. Pp. 8. William Grahame, Govt Pr . . .

Copies: LNSW, NL, SLT, SLV. 911

Hobbs, W.

Pocket guide of hygienic medication for the million. By Dr. W. Hobbs, M.D., M.R.C.S., M.R.C.P. Graduate of the Hygieo-Therapeutic College, New York. Fourth Edition. Sydney: Printed for the author by G. R. Addison . . .

120 × 72. Pp. 64, 2 inserted flg leaves. ND. P. w. (title rptd).

Includes advt for author's Kingston Hygieo Therapeutic Establishment, Newtown NSW.

Copies: ML. 912

Hobbs, William

Elaiopathy; the administration of the oil of the dugong (Halicore Australis), as a curative agent in chronic disease. A lecture . . . Melbourne: W. Fairfax & Co. . . . 1857.

222 × 145. Pp. 12 (l.b.). P. w. (cover title). Introduction (p. 1) headed: Consumption. From the 'Argus', Sept. 18, 1857.

Introduces dugong oil as substitute for cod-liver oil in treatment of chronic ailments. The term 'elaiopathy' is coined to indicate the 'systematic use of oil as a curative agent.'

For William Hobbs (1822–90) MRCS, MLC, first Health Officer and GMO for Moreton Bay, see *Austsn med. Gaz.*, 1891, 10 : 125; Jackson E. S. (1923), *Med. J. Aust.*, 1 : 281; McCallum F. (1927), 'Physician and health officer : A Brisbane pioneer', *Health*, 5 : 98.

Copies: ML, SLV. 913

See also Consumption; Dugong Oil; Faithfull, Paul.

Hodgson, Ralph

Cycling for ladies. Contains elementary anatomy and physiology for cyclists, medical effects of cycling on the body, on muscle, in heart disease and consumption. Advice for lady cyclists. . . . By Dr. Hodgson. . . . Being as far as the lecturer now remembers the words delivered by him to an audience of 1,500 people in the Protestant Hall, Sydney, on 10th May, 1897. . . . First Edition. . . .

178 × 116. Pp. 24. P. w. (title rptd). Colophon—William Andrews & Co. . . . Syd.

Copies: LNSW, ML. 914

Hodgson's tales of medical students . . . London: John Bale, Sons & Danielsson Ltd. . . . 1899. . . .

178 × 123. Pp. viii (l.b.), 418 (l.b.). Cloth.

Copies: EF, ML, OL, RACP, UQ. 915

Look under your nose. A realism . . . A. D. 1900.

185 × 124. Pp. 136. Colophon—J. W. Eedy . . . Syd. Paper boards.

'A short novel, . . . mainly in the form of dry medical discussions' (Miller).

For Ralph Hodgson (1855–1905) LRCP, MRCS, of Croydon NSW, who wrote profusely for newspapers and engaged in public advocacy of a meat diet, see obits, *Austsn med. Gaz.*, 1905, 24 : 96; *Evening News*, Syd., 19 Jan. 1905; and *Daily Telegraph*, Syd., 19 Jan. 1905.

Copies: EF, ML, SLT, UQ, US. 916

Hodson, Francis Octavius

A "bush doctor's" journey. By the late F. O. Hodson, L.K.Q.C.P., Irel., late of Walgett, N.S.W. Written three days before his death.

204 × 163. Pp. 4. Cover title, black edged, fig. of horseman. ND. NI. Repr., *Austsn med. Gaz.*, 1886.

Account of a 42 mile ride to a murder inquest. Ends: '. . . Three months ago I went 22 miles to find a poor unknown man dying; held the p.m., and the magisterial inquiry; improvised a corrugated iron coffin, and then read the burial service over him; for which services I have never yet had the slightest acknowledgement. Now let those benighted individuals, who think a . . . medical man can make money easier here than at home, try a "bush practice ..."'

F. O. Hodson (1859–86) practised at Hillston NSW, Mackay Qd and Walgett NSW, where he died from an accidental revolver wound, self inflicted. Author of *Within sound of the surf* and *From the Great Bear to the Southern Cross*. NS. Obit.: *Austsn med. Gaz.*, 1886, 5 : 266.

UM copy bears rubber stamp of L. Bruck, Medical Publisher.

Copies: UM. 917

Hoff [Dückershoff], August

The skin in health and disease. ... Sydney: L. Bruck ... 1884.

190 × 124. Pp. 64 (l.b.). 1 fig. Cloth.

A. Dückershoff (generally known as Hoff) MD Leipzig, of Sydney, devoted himself entirely to diseases of skin and larynx, and was described as 'the only pure specialist in such diseases throughout the Aust. Colonies.' He died of phthisis in 1887, aged 44. For note see *Austsn med. Gaz.*, 1887, 6 : 317.

Copies: AMAV, BG, CC, DOS, EF, KFR, ML, NL, SLV, US. 918

Hogg, Jabez

The domestic medical and surgical guide, for the nursery, the cottage, and the bush; giving the best advice, in the absence of a physician or surgeon, in cases of accident or illness ... The Government medical chest explained, as to the properties of the medicines and the quantity to be taken. Written at the request of Mrs. Caroline Chisholm, by Jabez Hogg ... To which is appended ... preservation of health at sea ... London: Ingram, Cooke, and Co. 1853.

185 × 120. Pp. viii, 152. Figs. Cloth.

Sections on hygiene and diet, medicines and instruments, family medicine chest, med. and surg. ailments. Health at sea refers especially to the Aust. voyage.

Copies: CC, NL, UA. 919

———

The Same. Pp. viii, 156. Minor amendments to text and figs, added index.

Copies: EF (lacks title p.). 920

Holbrook, Martin Luther

How to strengthen the memory; or, natural and scientific methods of never forgetting. By M. L. Holbrook, M.D. ... Melbourne: E. W. Cole ...

185 × 120. Pp. [vi], [7]–82, [2] (book advts). ND. (c. 1887).

Reprints US ed.—N. Y., Holbrook & Co., 1886. Another ed., Melb., 1920.

Sections on physiology; results of fatigue, illness and narcotics; training methods.

Copies: EF, ML, SLV, WLC. 921

Holcombe, William Henry

Lazarus of Bethany The story of his life in both worlds. By W. H. Holcombe, M.D. ... Melbourne George Robertson ... 1872.

168 × 110. Pp. iv, 5–212 (l.b.). Paper boards. 2 ed., 1872.

A novel, opening with discussion on preservation of human bodies and the discovery of an ancient manuscript, on which the narrative is based.

W. H. Holcombe (1825–93) MD, US homoeopathist, published extensively, particularly on homoeopathy.

Copies: EF, LNSW, ML, SLV, SLT, UQ. 922

Holden, Miss Frances Gillam

Trained nursing: a paper read at the late Victorian Social Science Congress; together with the root of hospital reform ... Sydney: F. Cunninghame & Co. ... 1882.

183 × 122. Pp. 40. P. w. (title rptd).

Copies: ML. 923

———

Women's ignorance and the world's need. A plea for physiology ... George Robertson: Melbourne ... 1883.

217 × 135. Pp. 16. P. w. (title rptd).

'... if women ... had a sound knowledge of physiology, infinite suffering and disease would be prevented.'

Copies: FC, ML. 924

———

Plain words to mothers and temperance reformers on food and health ... Sydney: George Robertson ... 1883.

217 × 135. Pp. 16 (l.b.). P. w. (title rptd).

Copies: ML. 925

———

The travels of red-jacket & white-cap or a history of the circulation of the blood ... Sydney: George Robertson & Co. ...

156 × 102. Pp. 28 (l.b.). 1 pl. ND. (1884.) Cloth.

An allegorical story for children. Preface by Andrew Ross MD.

Copies: LNSW, ML. 926

Her father's darling, and other child pictures . . . Sydney: Turner and Henderson. 1887.

161 × 107. Pp. 96. Cloth.

Verse and essays. The latter mainly relate to the Children's Hospital, Sydney.

Copies: LNSW, ML, UQ, US. 927

What typhoid is, and how to nurse it. Words of cheer for women, showing how much is in their own power. . . . Sydney: Turner & Henderson. 1887.

175 × 117. Pp. 24 (l.b.). P. w. (title rptd).

Advice on nursing and hygiene, in Nightingale manner.

Copies: EF, LNSW. 928

The Same. 3 ed., 1888. Pp. 42. Title includes: 'Its simple and effective treatment.'

Copies: BG, ML. 929

The Same. 7th thousand, 1889. Pp. 54.

Copies: NL. 930

The Same. 1890.

Copies: US. 931

The Children's Hospital. Memo. re Mr. Mitchell's (the President) official letter to Mr. Whittingdale Johnson, S. M. [Text begins.]

313 × 206. Pp. 4 (Aug. 30 1887.)

Reply to statements of Hosp. Pres. (J. S. Mitchell) during controversy which led to Miss Holden's dismissal. Severely criticises hon. med. staff.

Copies: EF. 932

The Glebe, 19th September, 1887. To the benefactors and subscribers of the Hospital for Sick Children. [Text begins.]

260 × 209. Pp. [4] (2, 4 blank).

A 'concluding contribution to the history of the recent unhappy episode at the Children's Hospital', following differences with med. staff and dismissal by Hosp. Board. Miss Holden was Lady Supt, 1880–87. See Hipsley, P. L. (1952), *The early history of the Roy. Alex. Hosp. for Children, Syd.*; also Syd. Hosp. for Sick Children, No 2120.

Copies: EF. 933

See also No 510.

Hollick, F.

The male generative organs, in health and disease, from infancy to old age. A complete, practical, and popular treatise on the anatomy and physiology of the male system. . . . Illustrated by numerous engravings and colored plates. Australian edition, revised and with additions. Sydney: The Modern Medical Publishing Company . . .

163 × 102. Pp. xviii, [iv] (l.b.), 31–370, [12] (advts). Frontis., 12 pl., figs. ND. Colophon— . . . A. Radcliffe . . . Ultimo, Syd. Cloth.

Advertises as available from Sir Robert Bear, Book Depot, Syd., new Aust. eds, uniform with above, of following works by F. Hollick MD: *The marriage guide: or, natural history of generation; A popular treatise on venereal diseases in all their forms; The diseases of women, their causes and cure familiarly explained; The matron's manual of midwifery, and the diseases of women during pregnancy and childbirth*. NS.

Copies: AMAV. 934

Holroyd, Arthur Todd

Dissertatio medica inauguralis de homoeopathia . . . pro gradu doctoris, summis in medicina . . . Arthur Todd Holroyd, Anglus . . . Edinburgi: Excudabat Jacobus Walker. 1830.

231 × 138. Pp. [vi]. 28.

Dissertation for MD Edin.

Copies: ML. 935

The quarantine laws, their abuses and inconsistencies. A letter, addressed to the Rt. Hon. Sir John Cam Hobhouse . . . London: Simpkin, Marshall & Co. . . . and W. Tait, Edinburgh. 1839.

204 × 132. Pp. 66 (last—notices of author's books).

Discusses plague in Egypt, and states that in two years author had not met a single fact to warrant a belief in its contagious nature. Quarantine practice, based on this, is therefore useless and oppressive.

Copies: ML. 936

———

Prickly Comfrey: its history, cultivation, extraordinary production, and uses ... Sydney: F. Cunninghame & Co. ...

206 × 140. Pp. 16 (l.b.). 2 figs. [1876.]

On the introduced fodder plant *Symphytum asperrimum*, with notes on medicinal properties.

Copies: FC, ML, NL, SLS, SLV. 937

———

Suakim and the country of Soudan. ... Written expressly for the information of the New South Wales Military Contingent bound for service in Africa. [Royal Arms] ... Sydney: Thomas Richards, Govt Printer. 1885.

216 × 137. Pp. iv, 26 (l.b.). 1 flg map. P. w. (title rptd).

Official guide-book from notes of early travels, with many medical references.

Also published: *Egypt and Mahomed Ali Pacha, 1837*, Lond., 1838; *Notes on a journey to Kordofan in 1836–7*, Lond., 1839; *Bowls and bowling with the laws and rules of the game*, Syd., A. W. Beard, 1874.

A. T. Holroyd (1806–87) MD Edin., MB Camb., who travelled widely in the Middle East and subsequently abandoned medicine for law, later came to Sydney and was distinguished in politics and law. See Jervis, J. (1933), *JRAHS*, 19 : 129.

Copies: EF, FC, ML, NL, SLV, SLW, UM, US. 938

Holtermann, Bernard Otto

See No 108 (note).

Home and Training School for Nurses, Sydney

Sydney, August 1882. Proposed Sydney Home & Training School for Nurses. [Text begins.]

204 × 130. Pp. 4.

Copies: ML. 939

———

First Annual Report of the Home and Training School for Nurses for the Sick, 52 Phillip-St., Sydney ... Presented at the annual meeting of subscribers held in December, 1883 ... Sydney: F. White ... 1883.

178 × 117. Pp. 16. P. w. (title rptd).

Copies: FC, ML (1–8, 1883–90). 940

Home for Incurables, Adelaide

Regulations for Home for Incurables. Adelaide: ... R. K. Thomas ... 1879.

165 × 117. Pp. 4. P. w. (cover title).

Copies: SLS. 941

———

Home for Incurables South Australia. Incorporated 1879. Seventh annual report. Adelaide: W. K. Thomas & Co. ... 1886.

209 × 132. Pp. 14.

Copies: ML. 942

———

Rules and regulations of the Home for Incurables Incorporated 23rd October, 1879. Adelaide: Printed by J. H. Sherring & Co. ... 1897.

206 × 137. Pp. 12 (v.b.). P. w. (title rptd).

Copies: SLS. 943

Home Training School and Lying-in Hospital, Newtown, NSW

Home Training School and Lying-in Hospital, Stanley Street, Newtown. Report for the year ended 28th February, 1900.

224 × 140. Pp. 8. 3 figs (portraits). P. w. (cover title, decorated; letterpress other sides).

Includes: lecture syllabus, rules for trainees, midwifery training.

Copies: ML. 944

Homoeopathic Association, Sydney

Proposed Homoeopathic Association, Sydney. [Text begins.]

204 × 132. Pp. 4 (2, 4 blank). ND. [c. 1880.]

An appeal for subscribers.

Copies: ML. 945

Homoeopathic Dispensary, Melbourne

The First Annual Report and Rules of the Melbourne Homoeopathic Dispensary (Established October 1869), 153 Collins Street East. ... Melbourne. Printed by Mason, Firth, & M'Cutcheon ... 1870.

153 × 130. Pp. 16.

In 1875 Dispensary became Homoeopathic Hosp. and Dispensary.

Copies: ML (1869/70, 1872/3), SLV (1869/70–1873/4). 946

———

Rules of the Melbourne Homoeopathic Dispensary. Melbourne: Fergusson and Moore ... 1870.

178 × 120. Pp. 8.

Copies: SLV. 947

Homoeopathic Hospital and Dispensary, Melbourne

Annual Report of the Homoeopathic Hospital and Dispensary, 17 Spring Street, Melbourne, for the year ending 30th June, 1877. Incorporated 1877. Melbourne: Fergusson and Moore, Printers . . . 1877.

200 × 127. Pp. 16 (l.b.).

Melb. Homoeopathic Dispensary became Homoeopathic Hosp. and Dispensary, 1875; name changed to Prince Henry's Hosp., 1934. For history, see Templeton, J. (1969), *Prince Henry's; the evolution of a Melb. hospital*, Melb.

Copies: EF (1882), ML (1893–), SLV (1875–84). 948

Homoeopathic Pharmacy, Launceston, Tas.

The medical telephone containing hints on the preservation of health. Notes on nursing and feeding. Plain directions for treating diseases. Ambulance lectures on wounds and fractures. Price sixpence. Published by the Homoeopathic Pharmacy, Hobart. 1883.

123 × 82. Pp. viii, 116. P. w. (title rptd).

Copies: CC, SLT, WLC. 949

Homoeopathic Progress in Australia

Homoeopathic Progress in Australia; Monthly Journal of Record and Domestic Practice, edited by J. W. Günst, M.D. Vol. 1. Melbourne: Printed by E. Purton & Co., 106 Elizabeth Street.

214 × 135. Pp. x (ii, iv blank), 372. Woodcut pictorial frontis. precedes title p. ND. (Preface dated Aug., 1870.)

Vol. 1, 1870–1, only. 12 unnumbered, undated issues, with running pagination, each titled 'Australian Homeopathic (or Homoeopathic) Progress.'

Copies: CC (no 4), EF, LNSW, ML, NL, SLV. 950

Hone, Frank Sandland

The Christian attitude towards scientific research. A paper read by Dr. Frank Hone, B.A., before the Annual Meeting of the Baptist Union, September 13, 1900. [Text begins.]

208 × 140. Pp. 8. Title at head of p. 1. Double cols. Colophon: W. K. Thomas & Co., Printers, Adel.

F. S. Hone (1871–1951) CMG, MB, BS Adel., Hon. Phys. Adel. Hosp. and Chief Quarantine Officer (SA), an ardent advocate of preventive medicine and med. research, influenced the development of Aust. health services. He was original discoverer of a form of endemic typhus not associated with human lice or past history of louse-borne typhus (*Med. J. Aust.* papers, 1922, 1923, 1927). Obit., *Med. J. Aust.*, 1951, 1 : 919; and see also *The Review*, Adel. Med. Students' Soc., Diamond Jubilee ed., 1949 (dedicated to him).

Copies: SLS. 951

Hope Lodge

See Belair Inebriates' Retreat, S. A.

Horn Scientific Expedition to Central Australia

Report of the work of the Horn Scientific Expedition to Central Australia. Part IV.—Anthropology. Edited by Baldwin Spencer . . . London Dulau and Co. . . . Melbourne Melville, Mullen and Slade. . . . 1896.

255 × 191. Pp. [vi] (l.b.), 200. 20 pl. (2 flg, 4 coloured flg).

Anthropology (pp. 1–157), by E. C. Stirling, includes physical and personal features of Aborigines, congenital and artificial deformities, circumcision and subincision, mental attributes, native foods, venesection, diseases, native therapeutics, making of medicine men, pathological conditions affecting white settlers in Central Aust. Appendices on measurements, human crania (Prof. Watson), and a human skeleton (Prof. Watson and author).

Notes on some manners and customs of the Aborigines of the McDonnell Ranges (pp. 159–180) by F. J. Gillen includes birth, infanticide, circumcision and subincision, making of medicine-men, blood as a therapeutic agent.

Copies: ML, NL, SLS, SLV, SPH, UA, UM, UQ, US, WLC. 952

Hospital Saturday and Sunday, Melbourne

Hospital Saturday and Sunday, Melbourne. September 26th and 27th 1873. First Annual Report of the Committee . . . Statement of monies received and distributed to the respective charities. Melbourne: Stillwell and Knight, Printers . . . 1875.

196 × 160. Pp. 12 (l.b.).

Annual appeal for Melbourne hospitals.

Copies: SLV (1, 1873–25, 1897). 952a

Hospital Saturday Fund of New South Wales

The Hospital Saturday Fund of New South

Wales. Memorandum and articles of association. Incorporated the twelfth day of September, 1894. . . . Sydney: Samuel E. Lees . . . 1894.

214 × 138. Pp. 32 (l.b.). P. w. (title rptd).

This method of fund collection was criticised in *Austsn med. Gaz.*, 1898, 17 : 363.

Copies: ML. 952b

———

Hospital Saturday Fund of New South Wales. (Incorporated . . . 1894.) Fifth Annual Report, 1899. [Text begins.]

265 × 214. Pp. 4 (l.b.).

Copies: ML. 952c

Hotham and West Melbourne Mutual Medical Aid Society

Hotham and West Melbourne Mutual Medical Aid Society, Victoria Street, Hotham, for providing medical or surgical attendance, and the supply of medicines, &c., to subscribers. Physician and Surgeon, Dr. Grace, M.D. . . . Melbourne: J. & A. McKinley . . . 1875 . . .

138 × 110. Pp. [8] (l.b.). P. w. (title rptd).

John Frederick Grace MD, MRCS, came to Vic. about 1856 and practised in Geelong, later in W. Melb., where he died in 1884, aged 63.

Copies: AMAV. 953

———

Hotham and West Melbourne Mutual Medical Aid Society . . . Prospectus.

209 × 130. Single leaf, v.b. ND. NI.

Copies: AMAV. 954

Houison, Andrew

Some reminiscences of the early days of Parramatta. By Andrew Houison, B.A., M.B., C.M. . . . Sydney, 1889.

229 × 150. Pp. [iv] (ii, iv blank).

Title p. and preface for 20 numbered articles from *Cumberland Mercury*.

A. Houison (1850–1912) MB, ChM Edin., Hon., Phys. Syd. Infirm., Sec. NSW Med. Bd, Pres. Roy. Aust. Hist. Soc. and ed. of Society's *Journal*, wrote widely on NSW history and philately. Published: *History of the Post Office . . . with an historical account . . . of postage stamps in NSW*, Syd., 1890, Obit.: *Austsn med. Gaz.*, 1912, 32 : 235.

Copies: ML, SLV. 955

Howard, George Thomas

Inaugural address to students. . . . Delivered at the Melbourne Hospital, March 23, 1900. [Text begins.]

236 × 147. Pp. 14 (l.b.). From *Intercol med. J. Austsia*, 1900, 5 : 133.

Medical curriculum, advice to students.

For G. T. Howard (1857–1934) MD Melb., Hon., Phys. Melb. Hosp., see obits, *Med. J. Aust.*, 1934, 2 : 403 and *Melb. Hosp. Clin. Rep.*, 1934, 5 : 57. At his death Howard was writing, with Felix Meyer, the early history of the profession in Vic., of which extracts were published by Graham, H. B. (1954), *Med. J. Aust.*, 1 : 971.

Copies: US. 956

Howchin, Stella

Notes on physiology. . . . For use in the Unley Park School. Adelaide: Sands & McDougall . . . 1900.

217 × 135. Pp. [ii] (v.b.), 68. Interleaved with plain paper. Paper boards.

Another ed., 1902. References to Unley Park School omitted.

Copies: EF, ML, NL, SLS. 957

Howitt, Alfred William

On Australian medicine men; or doctors and wizards of some Australian tribes. By A. W. Howitt, Esq., F.G.S. . . . London: Harrison and Sons . . . 1886.

214 × 135. Pp. 60 (l.b.). P. w. (cover title). Repr., *J. Anthrop. Inst.*, Aug. 1886.

ML copy has inserted letter from author to W. E. Hearn.

Copies: FC, ML. 958

Howlett, Henry

Lecture delivered by Henry Howlett, Esq., Member of the Royal College of Surgeons, England . . . Subject: "The moral, social, and physical evils of drunkenness . . ." Melbourne: Printed by Benjamin Lucas . . .

217 × 130. Pp. iv, [5]–24 (l.b.). (1853.) P. w. (title rptd).

Copies: ML. 959

Hoyle, William E.

Letter of application of William E. Hoyle M.A. (Oxon.), M.R.C.S. Eng., F.R.S.E.; candidate for the Chair of Biology in the University of Melbourne.

220 × 140. Pp. 12. ND. (1886.) NI.

Copies: NL. 960

Hudson, Robert Fawell

On aortic insufficiency and on sudden death arising therefrom; with cases illustrative of the causes, pathology, and treatment of aortic diseases in general, as observed in Australia. . . . [Text begins.]

224 × 147. Pp. 14. (1861.)

R. F. Hudson (1834–98) MD St And. & Melb., of Ballarat, was a leading authority on hydatid disease in Vic. in the pre-Listerian period. See obit., *Austsn med. Gaz.*, 1898, 17 : 182; for hydatid work—Graham, H. B. (1953), *Med. J. Aust.*, 1 : 869.

Copies: EF. 961

Huet, Frank A.

A few general remarks on the importance of preserving the teeth, especially children's. Frank A. Huet and Son, Dental Surgeons, Brisbane, 1891.

NS. Listed, *Cat. Parlt Library of Qd*, 1899. 962

[Hughes, J. Vaughan], 'A Physician'

Seventy years of life in the Victorian era Embracing a travelling record in Australia, New Zealand, and America, &c. By a Physician London T. Fisher Unwin . . . 1893.

190 × 130. Pp. [vi] (l.b.), 284 (last—colophon), 24 (book notices). Frontis., 16 illustns. Cloth.

An English doctor's travels in 1889–90, including visits to Albany, Adel., Syd., Launceston and Hobart.

Copies: EF, FC, ML, SLT, SLV, UA. 963

Hughes, Wilfred Kent

Congenital talipes equino-varus. (With photographs.) . . . Reprinted from the "Intercolonial Medical Journal of Australasia", March 20, 1896. Melbourne: Stillwell and Co., Printers . . . 1896.

245 × 156. Pp. 12. 1 flg pl. P. w. (cover title).

On anatomy and treatment.

Copies: SLV. 964

No. 23. Unabridged. Published by the Board of Public Health, Victoria, on behalf of the Australian Health Society. . . . The human foot: its use and abuse. A lecture . . . Robt S. Brain, Govt Printer, Melbourne.

217 × 135. Pp. 16. 4 figs. ND. (1898.)

A popular account: anatomy, physiology, functions, and remarks on footwear.

Wilfred Kent Hughes (1865–1942) MB Lond., was ENT Surg. Melb. Hosp. and Orthopaedic Surg. Children's Hosp. He devised an operation for congenital club foot. Obit.: *Med. J. Aust.*, 1942, 1 : 122.

Also published: *The stupidity of removing tonsils for catarrh*, Melb., 1933; 2 ed., 1938.

Copies: ML, SLV. 965

——— **and Walsham, W. J.**

The deformities of the human foot: with their treatment. . . . London: Bailliere, Tindall and Cox . . . 1895.

212 × 135. Pp. viii (l.b.), 550, [2], 42 (book advts). 301 figs. Cloth.

A comprehensive work based on experience at St Bart's Orthopaedic Dept, of which senior author, W. J. Walsham FRCS, was in charge, W. Kent Hughes, Clin. Asst. Review, *Aust. med. J.*, 1895, ns 17 : 426.

Copies: AMAV, BG, DOS, EF, KFR, RACP, SLV, UA, UM. 966

[Hugo, William Marks]

Inebriate asylums. Valuable information relative to inebriate asylums, obtained from various sources. . . . Adelaide: Printed at the Advertiser and Chronicle Offices. 1873.

200 × 135. Pp. 10 (l.b.).

Copies: SLS. 967

'Humanity'

Sketches of Chinese character, illustrative of their moral and physical effect on the rising generation of Victoria. By Humanity. Castlemaine F. Y. Benham . . . 1878.

186 × 112. Pp. 12. P. w. (title rptd).

Attacks vice and insanitation of Chinese quarters of Castlemaine, Maryborough, Golden Point (Ballarat) and Melbourne. These are described as 'nurseries of fevers, leprosy, black fever, and ulcerous skin eruptions' as well as of 'fiery evils, wickedness, idolatry, gaming, lasciviousness, murder, and all other deadly sins.' Writers of opposing view exhibited the Chinese as industrious, law-abiding citizens.

Copies: FC, ML, NL. 968

Hume, James H.

Phrenologist Hume [3 heads] reads characters correctly, . . . Melbourne. Hume's mental figure gallery No. 1.—Education. Parents should bring their children, business men, everybody, should avail themselves of his undoubted skill in pointing out the most suitable occupations, and the natural bent of their minds. Fitzroy Steam Printing Works . . .

8vo. Pp. 4. P. w. (cover title). ND. (1878.)

See *NSW med. Gaz.*, 1875, 5 : 330 for changing attitude to phrenology.

Copies: NL. 969

———

Thought reading and kindred subjects divested of their mystery and explained by Professor Hume. . . . Melbourne: William Inglis and Co. . . . 1886.

183 × 125. Pp. [2] (advts), [vi], 96, iv (advts). P. w. (short title, litho. portrait and figs).

A Collingwood 'professor of phrenology' deals with clairvoyance, somnambulism, mesmerism, animal magnetism as an anaesthetic and healing agent, and phrenology.

Copies: EF, ML, SLV. 970

Hunt, J. Sidney

See Tidswell, Frank, No 2269.

———, Collins, W., and Wynne, E. T.

Queensland. Report on tick fever by Dr. J. Sidney Hunt and Mr. William Collins, Special Commissioners of the Government of Queensland to the United States of America; also, report of investigations at Hughenden on Texas or tick fever . . . 1896, by Dr. Wynne. . . . Brisbane: . . . Edmund Gregory, Govt Printer . . . 1896.

247 × 158. Pp. 44 (l.b.). 1 flg map, 1 flg coloured pl., 9 pl. P. w. (title rptd).

Report by E. T. Wynne MB includes notes on parasite, ticks, and preliminary observation on serum prophylaxis.

Copies: LNSW, ML, OL. 971

Hunter, Charles Deavie

No. 7.] [Sept. 1878. Australian Health Society, Melbourne. "What kills our babies." . . . Copyright presented to the Australian Health Society by Dr. Hunter on the occasion of his leaving Victoria. . . . Melbourne: Mason, Firth & M'Cutcheon . . . 1878.

217 × 140. Pp. 24 (l.b.). P. w. (title rptd).

Reprinted 1883.

Advice to mothers on infant feeding and management. Author was first RMO appointed to Melb. Hosp. for Sick Children.

Copies: CC, EF, LNSW, ML, NL, RACP, SLS, SLV. 972

Hunter, John (Captain)

See No 2495 (note).

Hunter, John (Palmer, James Frederick, Editor.)

The works of John Hunter, F.R.S. with notes. Edited by James F. Palmer, Senior Surgeon to the St. George's and St. James's Dispensary . . . In four volumes, illustrated by a volume of plates, in quarto. Vol. 1. London . . . Longman, Rees, Orme, Brown, Green, and Longman . . . 1835.

Text—4 vols. 224 × 138. Plates—1 vol. 288 × 222. Vol. 1: pp. xxiv, 644, engr. frontis. and facsimile letter, folded; vol. 2: pp. xvi, 488; vol. 3: pp. xx, 686 (l.b.); vol. 4: pp. xii, xl, 506; vol. 5: pp. 28, frontis., 60 engr. pl. (7 flg). Cloth, paper label on spine.

'Descriptions of some animals from New South Wales' (vol. 4) forms part of appendix to White's *Journal of a Voyage to New South Wales*.

Editor, Sir James Palmer (1804–71), who settled in Melbourne in 1840 and was distinguished in medical, political and business circles, was Mayor of Melb., Speaker of 1st Vic. Parlt, and a founder and Pres. Melb. Hosp. See obit., *Aust. med. J.*, 1871, 16 : 156; Russell, K. F. (1948). *Roy. Melb. Hosp. Clin. Rep.*, Centenary Vol.

Copies: AMAV, EF, KFR, MLWA, RACP, RACS, SLV, UA, UM, US. 973

Huxley, Thomas

Protoplasm: The physical basis of life. By Professor Huxley. (Reprinted from the Fortnightly Review.) . . . Melbourne: . . . Peter C. Alcock . . . 1869.

204 × 132. Pp. 16.

The subject was hotly discussed in the evolution arguments of the time. In the year of issue of above pamphlet, Melb. Univ. Council refused to permit Prof. Halford to lecture in public on protoplasm (*Aust. med. J.*, 1869, 14 : 259), presumably as provocatively entering the conflict between churches and Darwinians. See note to Nayler, B. S.

Copies: ML, NL, OL, SLV. 974

Huxtable, Louis Ralston

Snake-bite in Australia. Recent statistics and a review of recent observations. Read at the Intercolonial Medical Congress, Sydney, 1892.

247 × 153. Pp. [ii] (v.b.), 18 (l.b.). Colophon—Syd.: Charles Potter, Govt Pr—1893. P. w. (title rptd).

Appraisal of Mueller's strychnine treatment. Suggests death rate is higher in cases so treated than with other methods.

For L. R. Huxtable (1856–95) MB, ChM Edin., Hon. Phys. Syd. Hosp. and Hosp. for Sick Children, see obit., *Austsn med. Gaz.*, 1895, 14 : 346; Hipsley, P. L. (1952), *The early history of the Roy. Alex. Hosp. for Children*, Syd.

Copies: ML. 975

Hygienic Messenger of Health

The Hygienic Messenger of Health. A Monthly Magazine for the Promotion of Health and Longevity.

NS. Notice in John Hern's *Advanced Hygiene*, 1892, announces issue on 1 Feb. 1893; annual subscription, 4s. 976

Hyndman, John L.

A paper on sewage and sewerage. Adelaide: Printed by J. H. Sherring . . . 1867.

210 × 138. Pp. 18. Plain p. w. Author's name in dedication to Mayor and Councillors of Adelaide.

Copies: SLS. 977

I

Iliffe, John

Odontological Society of Victoria. Dental education. (The aim of the Society). Its progress and prospects in the Colony of Victoria. A paper, read ... by Mr. J. Iliffe, President ... Melbourne: Pater & Knapton ... 1893.

204 × 132. Pp. 12. P. w. (cover title).

Reviews dental education and legislation in Vic. from the foundation of the Soc. in 1884.

John Iliffe, 'father of dentistry in Vic.', Surg. to the first Dental Hosp., was a founder and Pres. of Odontological Soc. and Dental Assn Vic., and ed. *Aust. J. Dentistry*.

Copies: SLV. 978

Imlay, Alexander

See James, T. Horton; also Jameson, R. G.

Immigration Hospital, Melb.

See No 2372.

Impartial Observer, An

See [Lhotsky, John].

Independent Order of Odd Fellows

Laws for the government of the Medical Institute of the Independent Order of Odd Fellows, Manchester Unity, Friendly Society ... Sydney. Established A. D. 1847. Revised ... Sydney: F. W. White ... 1890.

209 × 135. Pp. 14, [2]. P. w. (title rptd).

Copies: ML. 979

Indian Snake-Poisoning Commission

Report of the effects on artificial respiration, intravenous injection of ammonia, and administration of various drugs, &c. in Indian and Australian snake-poisoning; and the physiological, chemical, and microscopical nature of snake-poisons. By the Commission appointed to investigate the subject. Calcutta: ... Bengal Secretariat Press. 1874.

247 × 165. Pp. [ii] (v.b.), 78 (l.b.), [2], lxxvii (l.b.). 4 pl., 1 fig. Cloth. Signed: J. Ewart MD (Pres.), V. Richards MRCS, S. Coull Mackenzie MD.

Includes experimental proof of ineffectiveness of Halford's ammonia treatment.

Russell copy has inserted cuttings (undated) from 'Daily Telegraph', Melb., containing two letters from V. Richards (of the Commission) criticising Halford's methods and approving report of Med. Soc. Vic. (No 1330) on his treatment.

Copies: KFR, UM. 980

Industrial and Technological Museum, Melbourne

Industrial and Technological Museum. Lectures delivered ... during the Spring Session of 1870. ... Melbourne: Samuel Mullen ... 1871. ...

209 × 135. Pp. xii, 206 (l.b.), [ii] (v.b.). P. w. (title rptd) or cloth.

Includes: 'Notes ... on the circulation of the blood', by G. B. Halford; 'On food preservation', by George Foord.

Copies: EF, ML, NL, SLS, SLV. 981

Industrial and Technological Museum, Melbourne. Lectures delivered ... during the Autumn Session of 1871 ... Melbourne: Samuel Mullen ... 1871

201 × 135. Pp. vi, 200 (l.b.). P. w. (title rptd).

Some copies erroneously show 'Autumn Session of 1870' on title, which was later corrected. ML has both issues.

Includes 'Respiration' by G. B. Halford.

Copies: ML, SLS, SLV. 982

Industrial and Technological Museum, Melbourne. Lectures delivered ... during the First Session of 1872. ... Melbourne: Samuel Mullen ... 1873. ...

214 × 132. Pp. [vi] (ii blank), 136. Colophon—Mason, Firth, and M'Cutcheon ... Melb. P. w. (title rptd).

Includes: 'Allotrophic oxygen in its relations to science and art', by John Day MD; 'Dirt and

disease', by James Edward Neild MD.
Copies: ML, SLV. 983

Industrial Blind Institution, Sydney
The First Report of the Committee of the Industrial Blind Institution, presented to the subscribers ... to 5th May, 1881. Sydney: ... Robert Bone, "Phoenix" Office ... 1881.
212 × 135. Pp. 12, [2] (v.b.).
Includes office bearers and rules.
Later named Royal Blind Society of NSW.
Copies: EF (1890), ML (1881–). 984

———

Rules of the Industrial Blind Institution, Boomerang Street, Woolloomooloo. [Text begins.]
212 × 138. Pp. 4. ND. [c. 1881.] Colophon—R. Bone, Machine Printer ... Syd.
Copies: ML. 985

———

Industrial Blind Institution, Boomerang Street, Woolloomooloo, Sydney, N.S.W. [Cut of building] Photographs illustrating the work carried on by the inmates. Sydney, July, 1892.
255 × 186. 5 pl. P. w. (cover title).
Copies: ML. 986

Industrial Home for Blind Women
See NSW Home Teaching Soc. for the Blind.

Industrial School for the Blind, North Adelaide
Report of the opening ceremony of the Industrial School for the Blind ... North Adelaide. Thursday, April 30, 1885. Adelaide: W. K. Thomas & Co., Printers ... 1885.
203 × 132. Pp. 14 (two blanks). P. w. (title rptd).
Renamed Royal Industrial School for the Blind, 1903.
Copies: SLS 987

———

Industrial School for the Blind, North Adelaide, S. A. First Annual Report, together with ... constitution, regulations, &c. May, 1886. Adelaide: Scrymgour and Sons, Printers ... 1886.
195 × 130. Pp. 22 (2 blanks). P. w. (title rptd).
Copies: ML (13th, 1898), SLS (1–, 1886–). 988

Inebriate Retreat, Northcote
See Melbourne Retreat for Cure of Inebriates.

Infants' Home, Gorton, Ashfield, NSW
See Sydney Foundling Hospital.

Infirmary for Diseases of the Throat, Chest, Eye & Ear, Melb.
The Self Supporting Infirmary for Diseases of the Throat, Chest, Eye & Ear 39 Russell Street South was established and opened Septr. 13th. 1871 wholly free from State aid ... [Text continues.]
Manuscript. 204 × 127. Pp. 4 (last 2 blank). Blue paper. (Oct. 18, 1872—at foot.)
1st an. rep. John Wilkins FRCS, Hon. Surg. Opening noted in *Aust. med. J.*, 1871, 16 : 288.
Copies: SLV. 989

Iniquities of Lunacycraft
See [R., C. F.].

Institut Pasteur Australien
See Loir, Adrien, No 1171 (note).

Institute of Hygiene and Bact., Adel.
See No 2504.

Intercolonial Medical Congress of Australasia
Transactions of the Intercolonial Medical Congress of Australasia, First session ... Adelaide ... August-September, 1887. ... Adelaide: ... Vardon and Pritchard ... 1888.
227 × 147. Pp. xiv, 304 (last—colophon). 6 pl., errata slip. P. w. (title rptd).
Copies: See *SSAL*. 990

———

Intercolonial Medical Congress of Australasia. Transactions of Second Session, held in Melbourne, Victoria, January, 1889. ... Melbourne: Stillwell and Co., Printers ... 1889.
234 × 153. Pp. [ii] (title, v.b.), [iii]-xxxvi, 1030 (l.b.). 19 pl., 2 flg tables. Cloth.
Copies: See *SSAL*. 991

———

Intercolonial Medical Congress of Australasia. Transactions of the Third Session, held in Sydney ... September, 1892. Edited ... by L. Ralston Huxtable, M.B. Sydney: Charles Potter, Govt Printer. 1893.
235 × 152. Pp. [ii] (title, v.b.), [ii] (v.b.),

[v]-xiv (l.b.), 752. 42 pl., 2 flg charts. Cloth.
Copies: See *SSAL*. 992

———

Intercolonial Medical Congress of Australasia. Transactions of the Fourth Session, held in Dunedin, New Zealand, February, 1896. ... Dunedin: The Otago Daily Times and Witness Newspapers Company, Limited. 1897.

242 × 153. Pp. xxxii (3 blanks), 400. 10 pl. Cloth.

Copies: See *SSAL*. 993

———

Intercolonial Medical Congress of Australasia. 5th Session. Brisbane, Queensland, September 18 to 23, 1899. Brisbane: Watson, Ferguson and Co. ...

180 × 132. Pp. 24. (1899.) P. w. (variation of title, multicoloured and highly decorated, on front; coloured emblem on back wrapper).

Includes programme, officers, and papers.

Transactions of this Congress were published in 1901.

Copies: UM. 994

Intercolonial Medical Journal of Australasia

Intercolonial Medical Journal of Australasia for 1896. Volume 1. Melbourne: Stillwell and Co. ... 1896.

236 × 153. Pp. 728.

Vols 1–14; Jan. 1896-Dec. 1909. Monthly.

Journal was established in 1896 by amalgamation of *Australian Medical Journal* and *Intercolonial Quarterly Journal of Medicine and Surgery*.

Copies: See *SSAL*. 995

Intercolonial Quarterly Journal of Medicine and Surgery

Intercolonial Quarterly Journal of Medicine and Surgery for 1894–5. Volume 1. Melbourne: Stillwell and Co. ... 1895.

236 × 147. Pp. 408.

Vols 1–2, 1894/5–1895/6 only published.

Founded in 1894, *Journal* in 1896 merged with the *Australian Medical Journal* (1856–95) to form the *Intercolonial Medical Journal of Australia*.

Copies: See *SSAL*. 996

International Temperance Conference, 1880

International Temperance Conference Melbourne, 1880. Papers, debates, and general proceedings. Edited by H. G. Rudd and H.T.C. Cox. Melbourne ... 1880.

181 × 117. Pp. viii, [iv], 266. Colophon—Bones & Watt ... Melb. Cloth.

Med. Section includes: 'The relation of the temperance movement to science', Norman Kerr MD; 'Does alcohol give strength, or is it a food', Dr. J. P. Lucas [probably T. P. Lucas]; 'Alcohol on the human subject', Dr. E. G. Figg.

Copies: ML, SLV. 997

International Temperance Convention, 1888

Temperance in Australia The memorial volume of the International Temperance Convention Melbourne 1888. Containing the papers and correspondence and full reports ... Illustrated with portraits of Australian temperance reformers ... Melbourne: Temperance Book Depot ... 1889.

217 × 140. Pp. xxiv, 408, [8] (advts). 71 woodcut pl. Cloth.

Med. Section includes: 'Physiological effects of alcohol', S. J. Magarey MD; and 'Sixty years' med. experience', John Singleton MD.

Copies: EF, ML, SLS, SLV. 998

Ipswich Asylum for the Insane, Qd

See Goodna and Ipswich Asylums.

Iredell, Charles Lesingham Maynard

Ten years' practice in Australia. ... Melbourne: Published for the author by A. H. Massina & Co. ... 1896.

186 × 147. Pp. [iv], [9]–104. P. w. (variation of title).

Essays on health and practice.

Author (LRCPE, MRCS) practised in Melb. 1886–1925. Also published *Something about voice*, Melb., Geo. Robertson, 1902.

Copies: AMAV, BG, EF, KFR, ML, NL, SLS, SLT, SLV, US, WLC. 999

Isaacs, George

Rhyme and prose; and, a burlesque, and its history. ... Melbourne: Clarson, Shallard, & Co. ... 1865.

181 × 122. Pp. viii, 9–128. Cloth.

Includes 'The burlesque of Frankenstein or the man gorilla', which refers to the evolution controversy waged in Melb. between Prof. Halford (Alferd here), who opposed the thesis, and others, notably William Thomson FRCSE, who supported it. Halford's views are given in the following extract:

Ah! Doctor Waldman comes: the sceptic donkey,
Who would have man to be the heir to monkey;
Who bones the foot of finger-footed apes,
And at the foetid members cuts and scrapes
To prove a foot's a hand, as if when proved,
A man would be a monkey once removed.
The infidel! the devil!

... Firm like a column,
Amidst inferior animals Man stands,
And walks upon his feet and not his hands.
There are some scoffers say the Gorilla,
Between the man and smaller monkeys fill a
Long missing link—but this is humbug—rot!
I, Alferd, say it.

Author complains of failure to have the piece played in Melbourne.

Copies: BG, ML, NL, OL, SLV, SLW. 1000

J

Jackson, Henry Willan

Contagious Diseases Acts as measures of social reform. A public lecture . . . at the request of . . . the New South Wales Social Purity Society . . . Sydney: F. Cunninghame & Co. . . . 1882.

217 × 140. Pp. [6], 7–30 (l.b.). P. w. (title rptd).

Attacks proposed Contagious Diseases Act for prevention of venereal disease, providing for compulsory examination of prostitutes and detention for treatment. Similar legislation had failed elsewhere and was oppressive, immoral and futile.

Copies: ML, NL, OL, SLS. 1001

———

New South Wales Social Purity Society The social evil: its nature, causes, and remedies. A public lecture . . . Sydney: J. L. Holmes & Co. . . . 1883.

204 × 135. Pp. 30.

H. W. Jackson (1842–1902) MRCS, LRCP, practised in Sydney from 1871 to 1889. He engaged in religious and philanthropic work and as lecturer on social questions. See *Aust. men of mark.*, Syd., 1889, 2 : 121.

Copies: ML. 1002

Jackson, J. F.

The science of health; being a treatise on some of the most important elements which regulate and govern the well-being of the human system; together with a few plain instructions how to act in many cases of emergency . . . Melbourne: Printed by Azzoppardi, Hildreth and Co. . . . 1874.

180 × 107. Pp. 48. P. w. (title rptd).

Popular hygiene and treatment of a few common ailments. Author appears on title as 'Professor Jackson, Lecturer in Anatomy and Physiology, late of Guy's Hosp.'

Copies: SLV. 1003

Jackson, M. E.

See No 2424.

Jackson, R. E. Scoresby—

Medical climatology: or, a topographical and meteorological description of the localities resorted to in winter and summer by invalids of various classes, both at home and abroad. By R. E. Scoresby-Jackson, M.D., F.R.S.E. . . . London: John Churchill . . . 1862.

193 × 120. Pp. xii (l.b.), 510 (l.b.). Frontis., 1 flg map. Cloth.

Climate of Aust. and NZ discussed at pp. 140–165.

Copies: EF, LNSW, SLV, UA. 1004

James, George Lacon

Shall I try Australia? or health, business and pleasure in New Wales forming a guide to the Australian Colonies the emigrant settler and business man . . . Liverpool Edward Howell . . . London Simpkin Marshall Hamilton Kent & Co 1892

183 × 120. Pp. [iv] (l.b.), iv, 290, [6] (advts). Frontis., 1 pl. Cloth.

The same, 1892. London: L. Upcott Gill.

Author made two visits, with two years residence. Includes ocean travel, food, climate and health resorts of NSW. Deals superficially with health and epidemics of NSW.

Copies: FC, ML, NL, OL, SLV. 1005

[James, Stanley], 'The Vagabond', 'Julian Thomas'

The Vagabond papers Sketches of Melbourne life, in light and shade First series George Robertson Melbourne, Sydney, and Adelaide 1877.

183 × 125. Pp. [2] (advts) viii (l.b.), 9–206 (l.b.), 8 (book advts). Paper boards.

Articles on Melb. institutions, including Melb. Hosp. ('A morning at the Hospital'); the Benev. Asylum ('Three days at the Benevolent Asylum'); Kew and Yarra Bend Lunatic Asylums ('Our lunatic asylums').

The Vagabond Papers were published in 5 series: 1st-4th, 1877; 5th, 1878. Abridged ed., Melb., M.U.P., 1969.

For Stanley James (c. 1840–1896), known in

Australia as Julian Thomas, see *Aust. Enc.*

Copies: AMAV, DL, EF, FC, KFR, ML, NL, SLS, SLT, SLV, SLW, UA, UM, UQ, US. 1006

———

The Vagabond papers Sketches of Melbourne life, in light & shade Second series George Robertson Melbourne, Sydney, and Adelaide 1877.

183 × 125. Pp. [2] (book notice, v.b.), viii (l.b.), 9–204 (l.b.), 10 (book advts). Paper boards.

Includes article on Alfred Hosp. ('Three weeks in the Alfred Hospital'), where author spent three weeks as hall porter.

Copies: AMAV, DL, EF, FC, KFR, LNSW, ML, NL, SLS, SLV, SLW, UA, UM, UQ, US. 1007

———

See Knaggs, S. T., and Others.

James, T. Horton

Six months in South Australia; with some account of Port Philip and Portland Bay, in Australia Felix; with advice to emigrants ... London: J. Cross ... and Simpkin and Marshall ... 1838.

171 × 110. Pp. viii (l.b.), 296 (l.b.), [4] (book notices). 1 flg map. Cloth.

Facsimile ed., Adel.: Libraries Bd of SA, 1966.

Descriptive of SA. Includes as appendix (pp. 229–37), Dr. Alexander Imlay's diary of an exploring journey from Adelaide to the River Murray in 1838. This also appears, abridged, in Jameson, R. G. (below).

Alexander Imlay (d. 1847), army surgeon, arrived in NSW in 1829, served as asst surg., Sydney (1830–33), and took up land at Twofold Bay. For biog., see Lendon, A. A. (1931), 'Dr. Alexander Imlay', *JRAHS*, 17 : 206; Mackay, E. A. (1934), 'Med. men as pastoral pioneers', *Med. J. Aust.*, 2 : 476.

Work is severely criticised by Stephens, John, in *South Australia. An exposure of the absurd, unfounded, and contradictory statements in James's 'Six Months in SA'*, Lond., 1839; 2 ed., 1839.

Copies: FC, ML, NL, SLS, SLT, UA, US. 1008

———

The Same. 2 ed., [1839]. No date on title.

Copies: FC, UA. 1009

Jameson, R. G.

New Zealand, South Australia, and New South Wales: a record of recent travels in these colonies, with especial reference to emigration and the advantageous employment of labour and capital. By R. G. Jameson, Esq. late surgeon superintendent of emigrants to South Australia. ... London: Smith, Elder, and Co. ...

204 × 122. Pp. xii, 372. 2 pl., 2 flg maps. ND. [1841.] Cloth.

R. G. Jameson MRCSE came to SA in 1838 as surg.-supt of emigrant ship *Surrey*, and was two years resident in Australia. An abridgement of Dr. Alexander Imlay's diary of his exploring journey from Adel. to R. Murray in 1838 is included at pp. 34–6. For this, see also James, T. Horton.

Copies: ML, SLV. 1010

———

The Same. Another ed., 1842.

Copies; DL, FC, LNSW, ML, NL, SLS, SLT, SLW, UA, UM, US. 1011

———

Australia and her gold regions: a full description of its geology, climate, products, natives, agriculture, mineral resources, society, and principal cities ... The whole forming a complete guide-book to the gold mines. ... New York: Cornish, Lamport & Co. ... 1852.

186 × 117. Pp. viii (l.b.), 5–160 (l.b.). (6) (advts). Coloured flg map. Cloth. 2 ed. (noted in preface).

Includes notes on climate, prevalent diseases, hygiene and health on voyage.

Copies: LNSW, ML, NL, SLV, UA. 1012

Jamieson, James

How to feed infants. A manual of diet and digestion. With remarks on infant mortality ... Melbourne: Stillwell and Knight ... 1871.

161 × 102. Pp. 48. P. w. (title rptd).

A guide for mothers and nurses. Preface addressed from Warrnambool Vic. Review, *Aust. med. J.*, 1871, 16 : 314.

Copies: LNSW, NL, SLV, UM. 1013

———

Homoeopathy: its claims and its fallacies. ... Melbourne: Stillwell and Knight ... 1874.

212 × 135. Pp. 20 Repr., *Aust. med. J.*

Copies: ML, SLV, UM. 1014

On the parasite theory of disease. ... [Text begins.]

212 × 135. Pp. 20 Colophon—Stillwell and Knight ... Repr., *Aust. med. J.*, 1876.

Copies: UM. 1015

Experiments on the comparative power of some disinfectants. ... [Text begins.]

201 × 127. Pp. 12 (l.b.). ND. Colophon—Mason, Firth & M'Cutcheon ... Melb. Read Roy. Soc. Vic., 11 Oct. 1877.

Copies: SLV. 1016

On the chief cause of convulsions in children. ... [Text begins.]

209 × 138. Pp. 12. Colophon—Stillwell and Co., Printers ... Repr., *Aust. med. J.*, 1878.

Copies: NL, UM. 1017

Royal Society of Victoria. The perception of colour. ... Price, 6d.

207 × 136. Pp. 8. (l.b.). (1878.) Colophon—Mason, Firth & M'Cutcheon ... Melb. P. w. (cover title).

Copies: ML, NL, UM. 1018

Royal Society of Victoria. Photographs on the retina. ... [Text begins.]

207 × 136. Pp. 4. (1878.) Colophon—Mason, Firth & M'Cutcheon .. Melb. P. w. (cover title).

Reviews work on retinal physiology.

Copies: ML, UM. 1019

Royal Society of Victoria. A new point of resemblance in the respiration of plants and animals ... Price, 6d.

208 × 136. Pp. 8 (l.b.). (1878.) Colophon—Mason, Firth & M'Cutcheon ... P. w. (cover title).

Copies: ML, NL, SLV, UM. 1020

Diseases which should be prevented. A lecture ... of the Australian Health Society. ... Melbourne: Stillwell and Co. ... 1879.

214 × 140. Pp. 16. P. w. (cover title).

Another issue, June 1879. Melb: Sands & McDougall. No 8 in Aust. Health Soc. pamphlets. Reissued 1882, 1889, 1890.

Discusses reduction of Melb. death rate from infectious diseases by improvement of sanitation, water and milk supplies, and infant care.

Copies: EF, ML, NL, SLS, SLV, UM. 1021

Experiments on the range of action of the digestive ferments. ... [Text begins.]

208 × 136. Pp. 8 (l.b.). ND. (c. 1879.) Colophon—Melb.: Stillwell and Co. ...

Copies: NL, UM. 1022

Introductory lecture to the course on obstetrics at the University of Melbourne. ... Delivered March 24, 1879. [Text begins.]

209 × 138. Pp. 20. Colophon—Stillwell and Co. ... P. w. (cover title).

Author was Lect. in Obstetrics and Diseases of Women and Children, Melb. Univ.

Copies: UM. 1023

Puerperal fever: its causes, prevalence, and prevention ... [Text begins.]

204 × 156. Pp. 20 (l.b.). Colophon—Stillwell and Co. ... Repr., *Aust. med. J.*, 1879; ns 1 : 1.

'In lying in hospitals ... evidence enough of the good effects of the antiseptic method has been supplied to make its use obligatory.' Controversy arose from author's statement that Melb. Hosp. 'had been for some time a nursery of surgical fever, and presumably a cause of puerperal fever having become firmly rooted in our midst.' Correspondence is reprinted in *Aust. med. J.*, 1879, ns 1 : 133.

Copies: ML, NL, SLV, UM. 1024

Medical education. An introductory lecture. ... [Text begins.]

209 × 138. Pp. 12. ND. [188–.] Colophon—Stillwell and Co.

Copies: SLV, UM. 1025

Royal Society of Victoria. The influence of light on the development of bacteria. ... Price, 6d.

208 × 136. Pp. 10 (l.b.). (1882.) Colophon—Mason, Firth & M'Cutcheon ... Melb. P. w. (cover title).
Copies: NL, UM. 1026

Royal Society of Victoria. The influence of light on bacteria. ... Price, 6d.
212 × 138. Pp. 6 (l.b.). (1883.) Colophon—Mason, Firth & M'Cutcheon ... Melb. P. w. (cover title).
Copies: NL, ML, UM. 1027

The present state of the puerperal fever question. ... From the "Australian Medical Journal", June 15, 1884. Melbourne: Stillwell & Co. ...
270 × 137. Pp. 12 (l.b.).
Copies: NL, UM. 1028

A sketch of the history of midwifery. ... Melbourne: Stillwell & Co. ... 1885.
209 × 138. Pp. 16.
Introductory lecture of obstetrics course, Univ. Melb., 1885.
Copies: SLV, UM. 1029

The influence of sex in health and disease. An introductory lecture. ... Melbourne: Stillwell and Co. ... 1887.
209 × 138. Pp. 16. P. w. (title rptd). Repr., *Aust. med. J.*, 1887.
Copies: NL, SLV, UM. 1030

Contributions to the vital statistics of Australia. ... L. Bruck ... Sydney. 1882.
183 × 156. Pp. [ii] (v.b.), 30. P. w. (title rptd). Repr. *Austsn med. Gaz.*, 1882.
Contains: On the frequency of abortion in Victoria; Puerperal fever, its prevalence and pathological affinities; Infant mortality.
Copies: NL, SLV, UM. 1030a

Two cases of cardiac disease. ... From the "Australian Medical Journal", July 15, 1888. Melbourne: Stillwell and Co. ...
209 × 138. Pp. 12 (l.b.). P. w. (cover title).
Copies: NL, UM. 1030b

Typhoid fever in Melbourne: its prevalence and causation. ... Medical Society of Victoria, 12th January, 1887. ... Melbourne: Stillwell and Co. ... 1887.
214 × 132. Pp. 16. P. w. (cover title).
An appeal for improved sanitation. Includes notes of investigations, as MOH for Melbourne, on water and milk supplies, night-soil disposal, and drainage.
Copies: NL, SLV, UM. 1031

The drainage of Adelaide and its influence on the death-rate. ... (Read November 1st, 1887.) [Text begins.]
209 × 138. Pp. 8. NI. P. w. (cover title).
Paper to Roy. Soc. SA., which relates fall in mortality rate of Adelaide, especially from typhoid and dysentery, to improved sanitation.
Copies: NL, UM. 1032

On want of proportion in the signs and symptoms of diseases of the heart and great vessels. ... Reprinted from the "Intercolonial Medical Congress of Australasia Transactions". Melbourne: Stillwell and Co. ... 1889.
208 × 136. Pp. 8. P. w. (cover title).
Copies: NL, UM. 1033

On the nature & causes of diphtheria and its relation to croup. ... Reprinted from the "Intercolonial Medical Congress of Australasia Transactions". Melbourne: Stillwell and Co. ... 1889.
209 × 138. Pp. 8. P. w. (cover title).
Copies: UM. 1034

The influence of meteorological conditions on the prevalence of typhoid fever ... Melbourne: Stillwell and Co. ... 1890.
214 × 135. Pp. 16. 2 charts. P. w. (title rptd). Repr., *Aust. med. J.*, 15 Mar. 1890.
Copies: NL, UM. 1035

The diagnostic significance of alterations of the reflexes. ... Melbourne: Stillwell and Co. ...
209 × 135. Pp. 16 (l.b.). P. w. (cover title). Repr., *Aust. med. J.*, 15 Nov. 1891.
Copies: NL, UM. 1036

———

No. 5. ... Australian Health Society ... Hereditary disease. A lecture ... Melbourne: Walker, May & Co. ... 1895.

209 × 135. Pp. 16. Number duplicated in series.

Copies: NL, SLV. 1037

———

Tuberculosis and its prevention. ... [Text begins.]

250 × 158. Pp. 8. Repr., *Intercol med. J. Austsia*, 1898.

Copies: NL. 1038

———

The crusade against consumption: hints on its prevention and cure. Aust. Widows' Fund Life Assurance.

NS. (? 1898.)

James Jamieson (1840–1916) MD Glas. & Melb., was Lect. in Obst. & Dis. of Women & Children (later in Med.) Univ. Melb., Hon. Phys. Alfred Hosp. MOH Melb. (1885–1912), ed., *Aust. med. J.*, His numerous works, published separately after 1900, are in NL (Cumpston coll.). See obit., *Med. J. Aust.*, 1916, 2 : 218; also *Unive. Melb. Med. School Jubilee*, Melb., 1914.

1039

———

See also Aust. Health Society, No 103; Rudall, J. T., and Jamieson, J.

——— (translator)

The doctrine of the unity of man's being, and the contradictions in modern physiology in connection with the changes occurring in the child after birth. By Professor Alexander Diesterweg (of the University of Berlin). Translated by James Jamieson, M.D. Warrnambool ... Fairfax and Laurie. 1871.

207 × 133. Pp. 20 (l.b.). Double cols. P. w. (abbrev. title).

Translator's preface addressed from Warrnambool Vic. Published for private circulation. Contains two series of physiological propositions, compared in double columns: Views of the physico-chemical school, the neuropathologists, and the humoral pathologists; Views of the cellular pathologists.

Copies: ML, UM. 1040

Jamison, Sir John

See Australian Chivalry.

Jeanneret, Henry

Hints for the preservation of the teeth, by Henry Jeanneret, M.D. Etc. Etc. Etc. Surgeon and Dentist. Sydney: Printed by R. Mansfield, for the Executors of R. Howe; Published and Sold by W. M'Garvie ... George-Street, 1830.

204 × 127. Pp. xii, 13–34.

The first work on dentistry published in Australia. Review, *Syd. Gazette*, 8 May 1830. For account, see Ford, E. (1952), *Dental J. Aust.*, 24 : 113; Levine, S. (1967), *Ann. Aust. Coll. Dent. Surg.*, 1 : 19.

Copies: ML. 1041

———

Dr. Jeanneret possesses, and will be happy to shew, certificates of attendance upon the following institutions:- In Oxford—the Radcliffe Infirmary ... In London—The London Hospital as Dresser ... In Edinburgh—The Royal Infirmary ... [Text continues in 2 cols].

222 × 155. Single leaf, v.b. ND. (c. 1844.) NI.

Includes testimonials, three only dated (Edin., 1827); also letter from J. F. Clarke, MD, PMO, re Jeanneret's unsuccessful application for position of Col Surg., dated 1840. Tas. State Archives copy bound with correspondence dated 1844.

Copies: Tas. State Archives GO 33/50/p. 798). 1042

———

A letter to the Right Hon. Earl Grey, Secretary of State for the Colonies ... being a short explanatory appeal, &c. ... By Henry Jeanneret, M.D., late Superintendent of Flinders' Island. London: Hope and Co. ... 1851.

193 × 127. Pp. 12.

Includes outline of his troubles in NSW, and the difficulties and opposition encountered in his official VDL post.

Copies: DL. 1043

———

The vindication of a colonial magistrate from the aspersions of His Grace the Duke of Newcastle, by official documents and attestations, with a remonstrance; and exposure of colonial conspiracy, whereby Her Majesty the Queen has been imposed upon in a petition against Henry Jeanneret, M.D., late Superintendent of the Aborigines of Van Diemen's Land. London: Hope and Co. . . . 1854.

209 × 127. Pp. 66.

Describes author's troubles in Australia from 1829 to 1851, with years of disappointing negotiations for an expected land grant, subsequent difficulties in his post in charge of Aborigines' Establishment, Flinders Is., and dismissal after 10 years service. In 1853 his petition for compensation for losses was rejected and he accuses Newcastle, Col Sec., of countenancing his persecution, confiscation of property, defamation of character, and loss of livelihood.

ML copy has author's inscription to Ed., Launceston *Examiner*.

Copies: ML, SLT, WLC. 1044

———

Epidemic cholera diarrhoea and dysentery. Pointing out an effectual and expeditious method of cure. With cases submitted to the Medical Council of the Board of Health, during the epidemic of 1854. . . . London. George Philip & Son . . . and . . . Liverpool. 1857.

204 × 130. Pp. [ii] (v.b.), 34.

Announces the value of camphor in the treatment of cholera. The severe 1854 epidemic in Britain referred to was Asiatic cholera. Author also mentions, as cholera, diarrhoeal disease in Tasmania in 1849, which was less severe and less fatal. In Sydney, in 1830–1, 'it took the type of dysentery and, as usual with that disease in Australia, was often metastatic with rheumatism.' No valid evidence exists for the presence of true cholera in Australia at any time.

ML copy bears author's inscription to Sir Alfred Stephen.

Copies: ML. 1045

———

De la guérison prompte et facile du choléra asiatique par la méthode de . . . Cheltenham, 1865.

NS. Listed *SGC*, ser. 1. 8vo. Pp. 11.

1046

[Jenkins, Edward Johnstone]

Case taking card for the use of students of medicine at the Prince Alfred Hospital . . . Compiled by the Clinical Medical Tutor. Second edition. Sydney: Angus and Robertson . . . 1894.

122 × 90. Pp. 8, interleaved. P. w. (cover title).

Inscribed note in ML copy identifies author.

For E. J. Jenkins (1855–1940) MD, FRCP, Hon. Phys. Syd. Hosp. and Syd. Hosp. for Sick Children, see Skirving, R. S. (1940), *Med. J. Aust.*, 2 : 392; Hipsley, P. L. (1952), *The early history of the Roy. Alex. Hosp. for Children*, Syd.

Copies: ML. 1047

Jenkins, Henry C.

1900. Victoria. Department of Mines. Instruction to miners. No. 2. Testing mine gases for carbon dioxide. By Henry C. Jenkins, A.R.S.M., Govt Metallurgist. . . . Robt. S. Brain, Govt Printer, Melbourne.

268 × 180. Pp. 8 (3 blanks). 1 fig.

Copies: ML, SLV. 1048

Jenkins, William Henry

The family medical index or, what to do in cases of emergency. Written expressly for the Colonies. . . . Melbourne: F. F. Bailliere, Publisher, 1874.

214 × 138. Pp. xvi, 228 (l.b.). Cloth.

Ailments are dealt with alphabetically, with emphasis on local interest, and reference to local authors and practice. First published as weekly supplement to Hamilton *Spectator*, commencing April 1873.

William Jenkins (1831–75) MRCS practised at Inverleigh, Hamilton, and in latter days in Melb., where he died. He was a local pioneer of Listerian surgery. See obit., *Aust. med. J.*, 1875, 20 : 61; also Power, Sir D'A. (1935), *Aust. NZ J. Surg.*, 4 : 368; Forster, F. (1965), *Med. J. Aust.*, 2 : 1047; Thompson, B. E. (1968), *Med. J. Aust.*, 1 : 365.

Copies: AMAV, DOS, EF, ML, SLV. 1049

———

The Same. 2 ed., 1874.

Copies: ML. 1050

Jenner, A. J. B.

A lecture on homoeopathy, delivered at the Mechanics' Institute, Launceston . . . Launceston: Robert Harris, 1867.

161 × 102. Pp. 44. P. w.

Copies: SLV 1051

Jenner, Edward

An inquiry into the causes and effects of the variolae vaccinae, a disease discovered in some of the western counties of England, particularly Gloucestershire, and known by the name of the cow pox. . . . Second edition. London: Printed, for the Author, by Sampson Low, No. 7, Berwick Street, Soho: and Sold by Law, Ave-Maria Lane; and Murray and Highley, Fleet Street. 1800. 3a 134–84

263 × 209. Pp. [ii] (title, verso—Syd. imprint), [ii] (preface, v.b.), [iii]-vi (dedication, l.b.), 184. 4 coloured litho. pl. Reprinted by Authority: Thomas Richards, Govt Printer, Sydney, 1884. Half calf, marbled paper.

Facsimile reprint, published by NSW Govt following 1881–2 epidemic of smallpox, the most serious ever reported in Australia.

Though preface describes book as a perfect facsimile, many differences occur. For these, see Ford, E. (1951), 'The Sydney reprint of Jenner's Inquiry', *Med. J. Aust.*, 2 : 320; W. R. Le Fanu, *A bio-bibliography of Edward Jenner*, London, 1951.

Copies AMAQ, AMAV, BG, EF, KFR, ML, MLWA, NL, SLV, SPH, UA, UM, US. 1052

Jobson, David Wemyss

Prize Essay. An essay on pleuro-pneumonia, its symptoms and treatment . . . Melbourne: . . . John Ferres, Govt Printer. F. F. Bailliere . . .

217 × 140. Pp. 72 (l.b.). ND. [?1865.] P. w. (title rptd).

Author (MRCSE) is described on title as 'formerly Surgeon-Dentist to Her Majesty, the late King, and H.R.H. the Duke of Sussex.' Mitchell (*Cumberland Disease*), on this essay, states that after its publication author stated he had never seen a case of the disease, and adds that this is fully borne out by his treatise.

Copies: EF, ML, NL, SLS, SLV. 1053

———

A metrical version of the Sermon on the Mount . . . [Royal Arms] Melbourne: H. T. Dwight . . . Clarson, Shallard, & Co., Sydney; Trubner . . . London; and Tichnor & Fields, Boston. 1884.

220 × 138. Pp. [viii] (l.b.), 9–29, [2] (author's book notices). All pp. in frames.

Preface states that work forms part of Biblical versification made by author during two years imprisonment with hard labour, for 'writing a few verses (construed as libellous) . . . on a Scottish baronet, who chanced to be the grand-nephew of the Duke of Wellington . . .' He attributes his punishment to the perjury of 'The Right Honorable Benjamin Disraeli, whose contempt of the truth is proverbial', and states that he 'was obnoxious for having, as a member of the Queen's household, in the . . . affair of Lady Flora Hastings, refused to assist in hurrying to the grave a lady who had no protection but her innocence.'

Title shows authorship of: *History of the French Revolution*, *Memoirs of Louis Philippe*, *Metternich*, *Garibaldi*, &c., of which the first three titles appear in *BMC*, together with *A metrical version* . . . by D.W.J., 1864.

Advt lists 15 books as 'ready for publication as soon as subscriptions for 1000 are received', and 15 others 'preparing for publication.' The latter include *The teeth; their disease and treatment*, 3 ed., of which two earlier eds., 1834, 1844, appear in *SGC*, ser. 1.

Copies: ML, NL, SLV. 1054

Johnson, Edward Angas

Ein Beitrag zu den klinischen und therapeutischen Erfahrungen über die multiple tuberculöse Darmstrictur. Inaugural-Dissertation zur Erlangung der Doctorwürde in der Medizin, Chirurgie und Geburtshülfe der Hohen medizinischen Fakultät der Georg-Augusts-Universität zu Göttingen vorgelegt von E. Angas. Johnson, approb. Arzt aus Adelaide, Süd-Australien. Göttingen 1899. Druck der Dieterich'schen Univ.-Buchdruckerei. . . .

229 × 145. Pp. 28.

On multiple tubercular strictures of bowel. MD Göttingen thesis. Dedicated to Prof. Watson MD, FRCS, Adel.

Copies: ML, NL. 1055

———

Copy of testimonials received by Edward Angas Johnson, M.B., B. S., Melbourne . . .

197 × 127. 18 leaves, numbered 1–18 on recto, all versos blank. ND. NI. Stiff p. w. (cover title).

Letters, mainly from Melb. teachers, dated 1897.

E. A. Johnson, MD (Göttingen & Adel.) MB, BS Melb., FRSanI, was Hon. Phys. Adel. Hosp. MOH Adel., Memb. Med. Bd and Bd of Health SA.

Copies: SLS. 1056

Johnson, J. B.

Lecture to men, of vital importance . . . as delivered to large audiences in various parts of the colony. . . . Melbourne: Varley Bros. . . .

1892.

188 × 143. Pp. 40 Frontis. P. w. ('Startling Revelations! . . . men only . . .' on front).

On venereal diseases and sexual irregularities.

Copies: ML. 1057

Johnson, William

On the correlation, conversion, or allotropism, of the physical and vital forces. . . . Melbourne: F. F. Bailliere . . . 1864.

207 × 127. Pp. 52, [4] (book advts). 1 fig.

Author, Govt Analyst, was Pres. Pharmaceutical Soc. of Vic.

Copies: EF, ML, NL, SLV. 1058

Johnston, Robert Mackenzie

How far can the general death-rate for all ages be relied upon as a comparative index of the health or sanitary condition of any community? . . . [Text begins.]

209 × 135. Pp. 24 (l.b.). ND. (?1887.) Colophon— . . . 'The Mercury' Office. [Hobart.]

Copies: FC, NL, SLT. 1059

———

The health of Hobart . . . Paper (with diagrams) read at . . . Royal Society of Tasmania . . . 28th May, 1896 . . . William Grahame, Jun., Govt Printer, Hobart. 1896.

220 × 140. Pp. 22 (l.b.). 4 graphs. P. w. (cover title).

R. M. Johnston FLS was Reg. Gen. and Govt Statistician, Tas.

Copies: ML, NL, SLT. 1060

Jonasson, Hermann

Remarks on a case of morbus addisonii, with fatty degeneration of the heart. . . . read before the Medical Society of Victoria, October 4, 1865. . . . Reprinted from the "Australian Medical Journal".

212 × 130. Pp. 14, [ii] (colophon, v.b.).

Copies: SLV. 1061

———

Valedictory address of the President of the Medical Society of Victoria for the year 1870. . . . [Text begins.]

204 × 127. Pp. 12. Colophon—Stillwell and Knight . . . Melbourne.

H. Jonasson (1825–95) MD Wurzburg & Melb., Hon. Phys. Melb. Hosp., was MO to Vic. Railways. Obits, *Austsn med. Gaz.*, 1895, 14 : 469 and *Intercol med. J. Austsia*, 1896, 1 : 45.

Copies: CC, EF, SLV. 1062

Jones, Henry

Human science essays (No. 1.) on noses [5 faces in circular cut] . . . Syd. D. Smith, Printer . . . Sydney . . .

163 × 102. Pp. 16. 8 figs. ND. P. w. (cover title).

Character estimation (by consulting phrenologist) from nose shape, with note on proper breathing.

Copies: ML. 1063

Jones, Sir Philip Sydney

The open-air treatment for consumption. A lecture . . . under the auspices of the Sydney Ladies' Sanitary Association. . . . Sydney: . . . "Christian World" Office . . . 1900.

171 × 122. Pp. 25, [7] (advts). P. w. (short title).

Copies: EF, ML, NL. 1064

———

Report on the open-air treatment of consumption. (Tuberculosis of the lungs). . . . Sydney: Merchant's City Printing Press . . . 1900.

222 × 140. Pp. 24 (l.b.). P. w. (cover title).

Report on the sanatorium, or open air treatment of tuberculosis in Europe.

Sir Philip Sydney Jones (1836–1918) MD, FRCS, Hon. Surg. Syd. Hosp., Vice-Chancr Univ. Syd. (1904–6), was a local pioneer of ovariotomy, lithotrity and the sanatorium treatment of tuberculosis. See *Med. J. Aust.*, 1918, 2 : 272; Skirving, R. S. (1926), 'Surgery and surgeons in Edin. and Syd.', *Med. J. Aust.*, 1 : 290.

Copies: ML. 1065

———

See also Dean Case.

Jones, Richard

Small pox & vaccination. . . . Published and distributed at the request of the Board of Public Health, Melbourne. . . .

234 × 150. Pp. 12. 2 figs. ND. Colophon—McCutchan & Co. . . . Richmond. P. w. (cover title).

Richard Jones LKQCPI, LRCSI (1887), was Med. Inspr of Lepers in Hawaii and later practised at Hamilton, Tas. About 1897 he settled in Eaglehawk Vic. and was Hon. Phys.

Bendigo Hosp., subsequently moving to Hawthorn.

Copies: NL. 1065a

Jones, Robert

Vegetarianism, with special reference to its connection with temperance in drinking ... Lecture ... before the Melbourne Total Abstinence Society ... Second edition. Edited Joseph Knight ... Melbourne and Sydney: George Robertson & Co. ... 1889.

182 × 128. Pp. 32. P. w. (cover title).

Includes advt of Vegetarian Soc. of Aust.

Copies: ML, NL, SLT. 1066

Jordain's Dental Journal

Jordain's Dental Journal; or information for the people. [Motto.] Vol. 3] [Melbourne, 1858. [No. 1.

191 × 127. Pp. 4. Colophon—Abbott & Co., Printers, Melb., Beechworth and Yackandandah.

Advertises Melb. practice of Mr. Jordain, Surgeon Dentist, who has practised in the Vic. diggings for the past five years.

Copies: NL. 1067

Jordan and Beck, Drs.

Catalogue of the Anthropological Museum, at the Gallery of Illustrations, ... Melbourne, Australia. Principals: Drs. Jordan & Beck. 51, Latrobe St. East, Melbourne, and 40, Bond Street, New York, U.S.A. Open daily for gentlemen only from 10 a.m. till 10 p.m. Stillwell & Knight, Printers ... Melbourne. 1867.

161 × 107. Pp. 30, [4] (advts).

Lists 1000 anatomical and pathological preparations, models and diagrams 'mostly on subjects ... such as the functions and derangements of the generative organs, reproduction, marriage, the way to preserve health and chastity ...' Practice of Jordan and Beck is advertised, though Beck, who conducted a similar museum in New York, was never in Australia.

Henry Jacob Jordan, then registered in Vic., had conducted a museum in London, and was deregistered there in 1863.

After two years display in Melbourne, the Museum, in an unsuccessful action against attacking Melb. newspapers, was described 'as a means of frightening patients, and extorting from them fees of a magnitude to which the most eminent members of the profession would lay no claim.' See Robertson, E. G. (1956), 'Melbourne's public anatomical and anthropological museums, and the Jordans', *Med. J. Aust.*, 1: 164; *Aust. med. J.*, 1869, 14 : 275 and 283.

Copies: SLV. 1068

———

An address, &c. [Text begins.]

217 × 143. Pp. 8. ND. [c. 1867.] Colophon—Stillwell and Knight, Printers ...

Advertised in Museum cat.: *On the functions and disorders of the nervous system and reproductive organs*, pp. 168; *Nervous debility* (lecture); *Marriage, its obligations and impediments; The philosophy of marriage*. NS.

Copies: ML. 1069

Joseph, Robert E.

Royal Society of Victoria. Incandescent lamps for surgical and microscopical purposes ... [Read 10th May, 1883.] [Text begins.]

214 × 127. Pp. 4. Colophon—Mason, Firth and M'Cutcheon ... P. w. (cover title).

Copies: ML. 1070

Joske and Morton

A sketch of mineral springs and their uses, with references to the properties of the Ballan selters water. Melbourne: Joske and Morton, Proprietors ...

156 × 96. Pp. 36. Cover title.

Copies: SLV. 1071

Joyce, John F.

A popular treatise on the symptoms and treatment of sunstroke. By John F. Joyce, L.R.C.P., &c. Adelaide: George Robertson, 1879.

NS. Noted in Gill, T., *Bibliog. of S.A.*, Adel., 1885. 1072

K

Keck, Thomas
Anatomy of the voice. A simple and comprehensive treatise, dealing with the principal physiological parts of our organism which are called into requisition in the art of voice production; also, an explanation of the uses of the laryngoscope. . . .
168 × 102. Pp. 26. Pink paper. ND. George Whitehurst, Printer . . . Richmond [Vic.]. P. w. (variation of title, framed).
For teachers and students of singing and voice production.
Copies: EF. 1073

Keene, James
On the use of pulverised liquids in the treatment of affections of the air passages. By James Keene, M.R.C.S., Eng., Editor of the "Medical and Surgical Review" (Australasian) . . . [Text begins.]
203 × 127. Pp. 4. ND. Colophon—Fergusson & Moore, Printers . . . Melb.
Atomised fluids in respiratory affections.
Copies: SLV. 1074

———

Practical observations on the treatment of stricture, with a description of some new instruments used for that purpose. . . . Reprinted from the "Medical and Surgical Review" (Australasian) October, 1863. Melbourne: Fergusson and Moore, Printers . . . 1863.
204 × 132. Pp. 8.
James Keene MRCS, late Surg. W. Lond. Hosp., was ed. of the short-lived *Med. & Surg. Rev.* (*Austsn*), which commenced in Melb. March 1863.
Copies: SLV. 1075

Kelly, Alexander Charles
The vine in Australia. By A. C. Kelly, M.D. Melbourne: Sands, Kenny and Co. Sydney: Sands & Kenny. 1861.
212 × 135. Pp. x (l.b.), [ii] (v.b.), 216 (l.b.), 8 (advts). Cloth.
Copies: BG, EF, ML, NL, SLT, SLV, UM. 1076

———

The Same. 2 ed., 1862, with title: *The vine in Australia; its culture and management*. Melb.: Sands & McDougall, Syd.: John Sands. Paper boards, cloth backstrip, paper label.
Copies: ML, SLS, SLV, UQ. 1077

———

Wine-growing in Australia, and the teachings of modern writers on vine-culture and wine-making. . . . Adelaide: . . . E. S. Wigg . . . 1867.
212 × 138. Pp. viii, 234. 8 figs. Cloth.
For A. C. Kelly MD Edin., MRCSE, founder of the Tintara vineyards, see Cleland, J. B. (1938), 'The first 52 names in the Med. Register of SA', *Med. J. Aust.*, 2 : 732; Lake, M., *Vine and scalpel*, Bris., 1967.
Copies: EF, FC, ML, NL, SLS, SLV, UQ. 1078

———

See also Adelaide Chamber of Manufactures.

Kelly, William
Life in Victoria or Victoria in 1853, and Victoria in 1858 showing the march of improvement made by the colony within those periods, in town and country, cities and diggings. . . . In two volumes. . . . London: Chapman and Hall . . . 1859.
191 × 120. 2 Vols. 1: pp. xvi, 382 (l.b.); vol. 2: pp. x, 360. 1 flg map. Cloth.
A vivid account; includes notes on irregular medical practice, and section (1 : 288–94) on climate, health and current diseases.
Copies: FC, ML, NL, SLS, SLV, SLW, UA, UM. 1079

———

The Same. Another ed., 1860. Lond.: Chapman & Hall; Melb.: George Robertson.
Copies: LNSW, OL, SLT, UM, UQ. 1080

Kelly, William Henry

The sexual system in health and disease. New edition. Illustrated by 19 wood engravings. Sydney: W. H. Kelly.

8vo. Pp. xvi, 161. ND. [?189–.]

NS. Formerly in Cumpston coll., Canberra. 1081

Kelsh, Rev. Thomas

"Personal recollections' of the Right Reverend Robert William Willson, D. D. (First Bishop of Hobart Town) ... Hobart: Davies Bros. ... 1882.

183 × 120. Pp. xiv, [ii] (v.b.), 158 (l.b.). Frontis.—mounted photograph. Cloth.

Bishop Willson (1794–1866) was intensely interested in the treatment of the insane. At Nottingham in 1839, prior to VDL service, he registered his house as a private lunatic asylum, and had people treated under his care. Includes account of his Aust. associations. See Willson, Robert William.

Copies: FC, ML, NL, SLT, SLV, WLC. 1082

Kerr, Norman

See International Temperance Conference, 1880.

Kesteven, Leighton

Typhoid fever treated antiseptically by the use of eucalyptus ... Second edition. Melbourne: Paul & Hewitt, Printers ... 1895.

222 × 145. Pp. 16. P. w. (title rptd).

Reprints two papers from *Practitioner* (1885, 1887), with preface. Eucalyptus oil 'comes in contact with the ulcerated Peyerian patches, and by virtue of its powerful healing properties counteracts the local mischief ... I can claim as low a mortality as has been recorded for this disease.'

Author (MRCS 1873), of Bourke NSW, was formerly Surg. Supt NZ Emigration Service, GMO Fiji, Med. Supt Brisbane Hosp.

Copies: EF, ML. 1083

Kew Lunatic Asylum, Victoria

1876. Victoria. Report from the Board appointed to inquire into matters relating to the Kew Lunatic Asylum; ... with the minutes of evidence and appendix. Presented to both Houses ... John Ferress, Govt Printer, Melbourne.

342 × 215. Pp. 128 (l.b.) (report), 352 (evdence).

Inquiry into alleged neglect and ill-treatment of patients, and the general management and treatment. Severely criticised in *Aust. med. J.*, 1876, 21 : 398 ('will hardly be read by anyone anxious for the preservation of his reason ...').

Copies: AMAV, LNSW, ML, NL, SLV, UM. 1084

Kiama Cottage Hospital, NSW

Kiama Cottage Hospital. Rules & regulations for the general administration and management of the institution. ... Kiama: ... Independent Steam Machine Printing Office ... 1887.

191 × 135. Pp. 16. P. w. (title rptd).

See also Thompson, J. A., No 2200.

Copies: FC. 1085

Kilgour, James

Effect of the climate of Australia upon the European constitution, in health and disease. ... Geelong: William Vale ... 1855. ...

224 × 135. Pp. 42 (l.b.). P. w. (title rptd).

The Australian climate has a bad effect on European colonists, shown especially in loss of weight, muscular power, and vital energy. Other results include an increase in miscarriage and accidents of pregnancy, mental and cerebral disease, and infant mortality. The current opinion that the climate is suitable for tuberculous patients should be viewed critically. These opinions are refuted by Mingay Syder (No 2094.).

James Kilgour (d. 1897) MD Edin., arrived in Melbourne in 1839, later practised at Geelong. Prior to 1883 he moved to Auckland NZ and was Hon. Phys. Thames Hosp. (*Austsn med. Gaz.*, 1897, 16 : 529).

Copies: EF, KFR, ML, NL, SLV, RACP. 1086

Kingston Hygieo-Therapeutic Establishment

See Hobbs, W.

Kirby, Joseph Coles

Three lectures concerning the social evil: its causes, effects, & remedies. ... Port Adelaide: E. H. Derrington ... August, 1882.

204 × 127. Pp. 46 (l.b.).

Discusses state regulation of prostitution, its failure from hygienic standpoint, venereal diseases, contagious disease legislation, and suggestions for abatement.

Copies: CC, FC, ML, OL, SLS. 1087

———

Remedies for the great evil which injures social purity. ... second and revised edition of the third of three lectures ... Port Adelaide: E. H. Derrington ... 1883.

204 × 140. Pp. 20.

Discusses legislative and philanthropic measures for the control of prostitution, seduction and exploitation of women for immoral purposes.

For author (1837–1924), see Kiek, E. S., *An apostle in Aust., the life & reminiscences of Joseph Coles Kirby, Christian pioneer & social reformer*, Lond., 1927.

Copies: ML, NL, SLS, SLV. 1088

Kirkland, John Drummond

Introductory lecture on organic chemistry, delivered at the Medical School, Melbourne University, October term 1865. ... From the "Australian Medical Journal" of November, 1865. Melbourne: Wilson & Mackinnon ... 1865.

212 × 132. Pp. 12 (l.b.). P. w. (title rptd).

For author (MB Melb. 1872), first Prof. Chem. Univ. Melb., see obit., *Aust. med. J.*, 1885, ns 7 : 512.

Copies: AMAV, ML, NL, SLV, UM. 1089

Kite, Charles

Essays and observations, physiological and medical, on the submersion of animals, and on the resin of the Acoroides Resinifera, or yellow resin from Botany Bay. To which are added, select histories of diseases; with remarks. ... London: Printed by G. Woodfall, for C. Dilly, in the Poultry. 1795.

227 × 145. Pp. viii (l.b.), 434, [ii] (v.b.). 10 flg tables. Paper boards, label on spine.

Describes chemical and clinical tests on resin of grass-tree, known as 'Botany Bay gum' (pp. 141–210). Includes use in gastrointestinal ailments, by Arthur Bowes, surgeon of *Lady Penrhyn* (of First Fleet). Author concludes that the gum has value in ailments of stomach and intestines, and various other conditions. Large stocks, held by druggists, were available at 3s 6d a pound. The resin, used and noted by White (*Journal*, 1790), was subsequently listed with Kino, as having special properties, in various pharmacopoeias.

Charles Kite (d. 1811) Assn of Surgeons, Lond., practised at Gravesend.

Copies: EF, ML, NL, SLV, UA. 1090

Knaggs, Samuel Thomas

Contributions to operative surgery. ... Printed for the Author. By John Falconer ... Dublin. 1873.

204 × 135. Pp. 14. Repr., *Dublin J. Med. Science*, Feb. 1873.

Observations on ovariotomy.

Copies: US. 1091

———

Lessons from general practice ... Printed for the Author by John Falconer ... Dublin. 1873.

204 × 135. Pp. 12. Repr., *Dublin J. Med. Science*, July 1873.

Retention of urine; hydatids of liver.

Copies: US. 1092

———

Lessons from general practice. Reprinted from the Dublin Journal of Medical Science—January, 1874. Dublin: ... John Falconer ... 1874.

204 × 135. Pp. 8. Frontis.

On fracture of femur treated by extension.

Copies: US. 1093

———

Tea poisoning. A pamphlet shewing some of the deleterious effects produced by the excessive use of tea. ... Reprinted from the "New South Wales Medical Gazette", April, 1874. Sydney: Gibbs, Shallard & Co. ... 1874.

209 × 137. Pp. 18.

'It is as ... detrimental to health to indulge in excess of tea as in tobacco, opium, or alcohol.' Immoderate or continuous use by those for whom it is unsuitable produces a poisonous effect, and excessive abuse has serious results. Case histories purport to indicate physiological reactions and effects on nerve centres, and a basis for diagnosis and treatment.

Copies: ML, US. 1094

———

An analysis of the mechanism of producing flexion of the human fingers considered as an illustration of the sagacity of nature's plan as exhibited in the arrangement of the flexor tendons of the digits of vertebrate animals. ... Sydney: Gibbs, Shallard & Co. ... 1875.

212 × 140. Pp. 22 (l.b.), [ii]. 9 litho. pl., hand-coloured, descriptions on verso. Repr., *NSW med. Gaz.*, 1874.

Copies: LNSW, ML, UM, US. 1095

———

Phrenology. The claims of phrenology to be classed as a science scientifically considered. . . . Reprinted from the "New South Wales Medical Gazette", September, 1875. Sydney: Gibbs, Shallard & Co. . . . 1876. . . .

206 × 138. Pp. 8. P. w. (title rptd).

Copies: ML, US. 1096

———

Contributions to medical and surgical science. By Samuel T. Knaggs, M.B., Ch.M. . . . 1878.

224 × 135. Title page for 6 pamphlets, each with own pagination.

Copies: RACS, UM. 1097

———

Report of 660 cases of midwifery in Australia. . . . Reprinted from the Dublin Journal of Medical Science—May, 1881. Dublin: . . . John Falconer . . . 1881.

224 × 140. Pp. 20 (l.b.). P. w. (title rptd).

Author's experience in Newcastle NSW from 1871 to 1880.

Copies: EF, ML. 1098

———

Recreations of an Australian surgeon . . . Sydney: . . . W. M. Maclardy . . . 1888.

212 × 125. Pp. 156. Cloth.

Collected essays, papers and addresses.

Copies: AMAV, DOS, EF, ML, NL, OL, SLV, UA, UQ, US. 1099

———

Some observations on medical ethics. An address to the . . . Sydney University Medical Society . . . Sydney W. M. Maclardy . . . 1890.

217 × 135. Pp. 22. P. w. (title rptd).

Copies: EF, LNSW, ML. 1100

———

. . . Dr. De Lion, clairvoyant. Confessions of a vagabond life in Australia, as narrated by Maiben Brook. Sydney: Angus & Robertson. London & Edinburgh: Young J. Pentland. 1895. . . .

175 × 92. Pp. 200. Stiff p. w. (shortened title).

A novel, said to be based on fact, dealing with 'medical clairvoyance and quackery as a pernicious outcome of certain defects in legislation in NSW.' Review, *Austsn med. Gaz.*, 1895, 14 : 299.

Copies: AMAN, BG, DOS, EF, FC, ML, NL, RACP, SLV, UA, UQ, US. 1101

———

. . . Human fads, foibles, fallacies, fallibilities, &c. Sydney: Angus & Robertson. London & Edinburgh: Young J. Pentland. 1898. . . .

175 × 98. Pp. [viii] (3 blanks), 5–109, [7] (advts). Stiff p. w. (title rptd).

Essays. Includes: The psychological aspect of spiritualism; minor forms of hypnotic suggestion; the rationale of miraculous cures in modern days; Dr. Koch's reputed cure for consumption; poisons and poisoners. EF and ML copies bear author's inscriptions.

Copies: DOS, EF, ML, NL, UQ. 1102

———

Human fallibility and its relation to accidents by railway and on sea. . . . [Text begins.]

247 × 184. Pp. [6] (all v.b.). Double cols. ND.

Recommends periodical examination of persons responsible for the safety of passengers.

S. T. Knaggs (1842–1921) MD Aberd. & Syd., ChM, FRCSI, after practice in Newcastle NSW, moved to Sydney and was Hon. Surg. St Vincent's and Roy. Prince Alfred Hosps, member NSW Bd of Health. At various times he was ed. *NSW med. Gaz.*, *Aust. Practitioner*, and *Austsn med. Gaz.* Obits, *Med. J. Aust.*, 1921, 1 : 320, and *J. & P. Roy. Soc. NSW*, 1921, 55 : 1.

Also published: *Common complaints and simple remedies*, Syd., 1906.

Copies: ML. 1103

———

Mediums and their dupes. A complete exposure of the chicaneries of professional mediums, and explanation of so-called spiritual phenomena. . . . Sydney: Greville's Telegram Company . . . 1879.

217 × 135. Pp. 52 (last 3—advts). P. w. (short title).

2 ed., 1879; 3 ed., 1879.

Papers by 'The Vagabond', T. T. Wilton, 'Maori', and Knaggs, the latter contributing 'Dr. Slade and the spirits', and 'Spiritualism considered as an infections mental disease.' Answered in *Spirits and their friends, being an appeal to reason and justice* by E. C. Haviland, Syd., 1879; and also in *Vagabonds and their dupes*, by H.W.H. Stephen, Syd., 1879. The latter contains 'Maunderings by Dr. Knaggs.'

Copies: EF, FC, ML, NL. 1104

Knight, Charles

By Royal [Royal Arms] Letters Patent. Mr. Charles Knight's Electro-Chemical Baths ... Melbourne ... For the extraction of mercury and other metallic or extraneous substances, which by impairing the vital functions, become the ... [Text continues.]

178 × 115. Pp. 24. ND. Colophon—R. T. Clarke ... Collingwood. P. w.

Includes testimonials from Vic. and Tas. doctors (1855–59). 'Caution' on back wrapper states: '... if I do no good, I promise not to injure the patient. Not so with the Medical Profession,—they hold a license to kill or cure—I have only permission to cure.'

Copies: ML. 1105

———

Mr. Charles Knight is the only practical medical galvanist in Victoria ... Galvanism cures ... [List of diseases—12 lines] Galvanic and medicated hot baths for extracting mercury and metallic medicines from the body ... No charge for advice. R. T. Clarke ... Collingwood.

204 × 127. Pp. 8. ND. P. w. (decorated title).

Includes list of Melb. doctors who have referred patients, and testimonials dated 1857–8.

Copies: ML, SLV. 1106

———

Electro galvanism. [Cut] Ought not galvanism to be more generally resorted to in various diseases, instead of so much poisonous medicines? especially in the undermentioned complaints: [List of diseases—7 lines.] This is no quackery. The following are a few more extraordinary cures, effected by Mr. Charles Knight, the only practical medical galvanist in Victoria. ... [Text begins.]

188 × 130. Pp. 4. ND.

Copies: ML. 1107

Knowlton, Charles

Australasian Edition. Fruits of philosophy, or the private companion of young married people. By Charles Knowlton, M.D. ... Melbourne: Printed for the Publisher by A. Asher ... Richmond. 1878.

204 × 132. Pp. viii (ii blank), 9–34. P. w. (title rptd).

Contains preface signed 'Melbourne Editor' —since attributed to Henry Keylock Rusden—followed by preface to prosecuted London ed. of 1877, signed by Charles Bradlaugh and Annie Besant. Footnote on contraceptive publications by anonymous Melb. publisher (p. 29). Numerous Aust. eds were published, a Sydney printing appearing as late as 1935.

The fore-runner of modern contraceptive practice first published N. Y., 1832, by a Massachussetts physician. Eng. ed. appeared in 1834 and others followed without restraint. In 1876, its London publisher was found guilty of circulating an obscene work. Chas. Bradlaugh and Mrs. Besant, contesting the suppression of important information, then republished the work, were found guilty, and the verdict quashed on appeal. For trial, see *Queen v Charles Bradlaugh and Annie Besant*, Lond., ND; for official attempts to suppress the work in Aust.—Coleman, P., *Obscenity, blasphemy, sedition*, Bris., 1962.

Copies: DL, EF, FC, ML. 1108

———

The fruits of philosophy. The private companion for young married people Melbourne: Will Andrade ... McCutchan and Co., Printers, Richmond.

178 × 127. Pp. 64 (54–56, illust. cat. of contraceptives). ND. P. w. (title rptd, adds: 'Genuine edition of the work published by Charles Bradlaugh and Annie Besant').

Includes anatomy and physiology of generative organs, conception, pregnancy, parturition, and methods of contraception, of which douching is preferred.

Copies: NL. 1109

Koch, Robert

See Laycock, George Lockwood—Translator.

Kolk, J.L.C. Schroeder van der

See Schroeder van der Kolk, J.L.C.

Krefft, Gerard

Two papers on the vertebrata of the Lower Murray and Darling; and on the snakes of Sydney, read before the Philosophical Society of New South Wales, 10th September, 1862 ... Sydney: Reading and Wellbank, Printers ... 1865.

220 × 135. Pp. 60. P. w. (cover title).

Includes observations on toxicity of bites.

For Johann Ludwig Gerard Krefft (1830–81), Curator Aust. Museum, see Whitley, G. P. (1961), *Proc. Roy. Zool. Soc. NSW*, 28 Feb.

Copies: ML, NL, SLS, SLV, SLW. 1110

———

The snakes of Australia; an illustrated and descriptive catalogue of all the known species. . . . Sydney: Thomas Richards, Govt Printer . . . 1869.

260 × 198. Pp. xxvi (4 blanks), 100. 12 litho pl. (coloured or plain). Stiff p. w., linen backstrip.

Includes characters of venomous species, snake poisons, treatment (pp. 10–16).

Copies: DL, FC, ML, NL, OL, SLS, SLT, SLV, SLW, UA, UM, US. 1111

Kreitmayer and Wiseheart's Grand Anatomical Museum

Catalogue of Messrs. Kreitmayer and Wiseheart's Grand Anatomical Museum Only adults admitted. Melbourne: Charlwood & Son . . . 1861.

204 × 135. Pp. iv, 5–20. P. w.

Museum contained anatomical models, including embryological and obstetrical preparations and a series on venereal disease, 'illustrative of the results of vicious indulgence.' See Robertson, E. G. (1956), 'Melbourne's public anatomical and anthropological museums', *Med. J. Aust.*, 1 : 164.

Though elsewhere shown as 'Kreitmeyer', name appears herein, as above, throughout.

Copies: ML. 1112

———

See also Baume and Kreitmayer's Grand Anatomical Museum.

Kreitmeyer's Waxworks Exhibition

Kreitmeyer's Waxworks Exhibition, 99 Bourke Street East . . . Catalogue. . . . [Text begins.]

204 × 132. Pp. 24. ND. Colophon—Clarson, Massina, & Co. . . .

Item 259: 'Dr. James Patrick Murray, owner of the notorious "Carl" . . . chief instigator of the cruelties committed on the poor islanders, who were enticed by all cowardly means on board . . . were shot down, and the dead and wounded thrown in the sea. Of all the cruel wretches in this chamber of horrors Dr. Murray will not find his equal in atrocity.' See No 1438.

Copies: ML (incomplete), SLV. 1113

Kress, Lauretta

The experiences of two mothers [Cut of mother and infant] By Lauretta Kress, M.D. . . . Published by the Australasian Good Health, Cooranbong, N.S.W.

175 × 122. Pp. 16 (l.b.). 3 figs. ND. P. w. (shortened title).

A story on infant management, with appended notes.

Copies: ML. 1114

Krosse, Nurse

. . . Nurse Krosse's little doctor. Simple and effective remedies for common complaints, and useful hints to those who may have to attend the sick. . . . E. T. Radcliffe Printer . . . Sydney.

156 × 107. Pp. 20. ND.

Copies: BG, EF, RACP. 1115

Kugelmann, H. E.

. . . Medical despotism or liberty Which? The science of medicine is founded on conjecture and improved by murder.—Sir Astley Cooper. Melbourne: H. E. Kugelmann & Co. . . . 1888.

212 × 138. Pp. 56. P. w. (title rptd).

Counterblast to newspaper attack on a 'consulting herbalist.' 'I shall ever protest against those medical bigots and croakers who rejoice in the fact they are "legally licensed" to kill and experiment upon their suffering fellows . . . constantly clamoring for further State enactments, so that they may protect their craft from the competition of more successful men than themselves.'

Author appears in Bruck's *List of Unregistered Med. Practitioners* (1886) as styling himself 'Professor of natural science and organic medication', and 'the most skilled diagnostist, and only successful consulting and curativė herbalist in the present age.'

Copies: ML. 1116

Kyneton Hospital, Vic.

Annual Report of the . . . Kyneton Hospital for 1871. With the bye-laws and rules . . . Kyneton: G. W. Sands, "Observer" Office . . .

204 × 132. Pp. 16.

Copies: SLV (1870, 1871). 1117

———

Pharmacopoeia compiled for use in the Kyneton Hospital. First edition. 1896. Kyneton: M. K. Armstrong, Printer . . .

127 × 84. Pp. [x], 81. Cloth.

Inserted note by Dr. J. H. Downing states no further issue made.

Copies: UM. 1118

L

Lachlan Park Mental Hospital, Tas.
See New Norfolk Lunatic Asylum.

'Lacon'
The coming plague. By "Lacon" ... Melbourne: Samuel Mullen ... 1872.
212 × 132. Pp. 12.
A vehement appeal for Melbourne sewerage.
Copies: ML. 1119

Lacy, George
Vaccination in the light of modern enquiry ... Sydney: City of Sydney Printing & Publishing Co. ... 1881.
220 × 145. Pp. 16. P. w. (title rptd).
2 ed., 1881. Pp. 24 (l.b.).
Anti-vaccination pamphlet.
Copies: DL, FC, LNSW, ML. 1120

Laing, Edward
See Trotter, Thomas.

Lake, Joshua
See Melbourne Hospital for Sick Children.

Lamartine, E. A.
Dr. Lamartine's physiology and marriage guide, containing a complete description of the human system, both male and female, and full particulars of the diseases to which each is subject, with remedies for the same ... Reproduction thoroughly explained. By E. A. Lamartine, M.D. ... Sydney: The Modern Medical Publishing Company ... E. T. Radcliffe, Printer ... Sydney.
165 × 102. Pp. viii, 9–304. Figs. ND. P. w. (title rptd, with 'Dr. Lamartine's silent friend'; advts all other sides).
Copies: AMAV, BG. 1121

Lamert, Lima and Lamert, Samuel
The science of life; or, self-preservation: a guide to health, strength, and vigorous old age, and what to eat, drink and avoid: including the treatment of nervous and other disorders resulting from the loss of nervous and physical force. By Lima Lamert, M.D. ... and Samuel Lamert, M.D. ... Melbourne: W. H. Williams ... Printer ...
163 × 98. Pp. 156, [4] (advts, l.b.). ND. P. w. (title rptd).
Emphasises sexual ailments; advertises Melb. practice. *NSW med. Gaz.*, 1871, 1 : 245, citing *Lancet*, 10 July and 30 Oct. 1869, identifies authors with Samuel La Mert, who was 'struck off' in Lond. for infamous conduct in 1863, and Lima Abraham La Mert, whose qualifications LRCP and MRCS were cancelled in 1868 and 1869, and who 'descend to tricks of charlatans and imposters of the lowest stamp.'
Lima Abraham La Mert MD Erlangen, LSA (1862) was registered in Vic. prior to 1883, and died at St Kilda in 1891. It appears that Samuel La Mert was not in Australia. He is named by Courtenay, F. B., *On spermatorrhoea and ... debilities of the generative system*, 12 ed., Lond., 1882, as the villain in a cautionary tale—of wealth extracted from inexperienced youths by terror and wickedness.
Copies: ML. 1122

La Moile, F.
Victoria Water-Cure Establishment, Malvern Hill, near Toorak. Conducted by M. La Moile. Melbourne ... Clarson, Shallard, & Co. ... 1861.
210 × 130. Pp. 8.
Announces opening of hydropathic establishment and claims that '... all diseases curable and many incurable by any previous known means can be ... successfully treated.'
Copies: SLV. 1123

Lancelott, F.
Australia as it is : its settlements, farms and gold fields. ... In two volumes. ... London: Colburn & Co. ... 1852.
196 × 120. 2 vols. Vol. 1 : pp. xii, 318 (l.b.), 16 (book advts), frontis.; vol. 2 : pp. vi, 304, 16 (book advts), frontis. (plan).
Vol. 1 includes climate, its effect on health, and advice on preservation of health.

Copies: DL, ML, NL, OL, SLV, SLW, UA, WLC. 1124

The Same. 2 ed., revised, 1853.
Copies: FC, ML, OL, SLS, SLV. 1125

Lang, John Dunmore

An historical and statistical account of New South Wales, both as a penal settlement and as a British Colony. ... In two volumes. Vol. 1. [Biblical text] London: Cochrane and M'Crone ... 1834.

2 vols. 200 × 122. Vol. 1 : pp. xiv, 402; vol. 2, pp. iv, 444 (l.b.). Map.

An account of climate, health, and disease occurs in vol. 2, pp. 184–94, and is repeated with amendments in subsequent editions. Ophthalmia, dysentery, and influenza or catarrh are regarded as the most frequent ailments.

Later editions have variations in titles.
Copies: FC, ML, NL, US. 1126

The Same. 2 ed. Lond., A. J. Valpy; Edin., Bell & Bradfute, 1837.
Copies: ML, NL, US. 1127

The Same. 3 ed. Lond., Longman, Brown, Green, & Longmans, 1852.
Copies: FC, ML, NL, OL, SLV, UQ, US. 1128

The Same. 4 ed. Lond., Sampson Low ..., 1875.
Copies: DL, EF, FC, ML, NL, SLS, SLT, SLV, SLW. 1129

Langdon, John Arthur

Copy of letter sent. Mr. "Gill" alias "Dr. R. Royston Russell". Sir,—1. ... I have nade certain inquiries concerning you. 2. As a result I am now in a position to be able to denounce you as an unmitigated imposter. ... 7. I have already sent reports to the Police in Lismore, Casino, Woodburn and Coraki; and ... communicated with the Deans of ... Arts and Medicine, Trinity College, Dublin, with reference to the "Diploma" (?) bearing the name of "R. Royston Russell" in your possession. ... [Text continues.]

201 × 132. Single leaf, v.b. Coraki (NSW), 28th July, 1890. NI. Signed at foot.

Original NS. Photograph from late Dr. R. E. Longworth, Lismore NSW.
1130

Langford, William

This deadly blot ... Remington & Co., Limited London & Sydney 1893

181 × 117. Pp. viii, 312, 8 (book notices). Cloth.

William Langford MRCS (1854) practised at Kyneton Vic. He published another novel, *Tifana's Revenge*, with same imprint, 1893 (NS).
Copies: ML. 1131

Langston, William

Varicocele and its cure without operation by Surgeon Langston, M.R.C.S., Eng. ...

105 × 69. Pp. 8. ND. (c. 1900.) Colophon—Rae Brothers, Printers ... Melb. P. w. (cover title).

Advertises Langston's Irresistable binder and support.
Copies: SLV. 1132

Langtree, C. W.

The mineral springs of Victoria. Extract from the annual report of the Secretary for Mines ... for 1887. ... Robt. S. Brain, Govt Printer, Melbourne. 1889.

163 × 102. Pp. 28. P. w. (title rptd).
Copies: ML. 1133

Launceston Benevolent Society, Tas.

The Second Annual Report of the Launceston Benevolent Society, established Oct. 1835. Patron, His Excellency the Lieutenant-Governor, Launceston, V. D. Land; printed by H. Dowling ... Brisbane St. 1836.

8vo. Pp. 18 (l.b.). P. w.
Copies: SLT. 1134

Launceston General Hospital, Tas.

Cornwall Free Hospital and Infirmary. The Government having decided that the hospital hitherto open to the public shall be closed at the termination of the present year, the duty has devolved on this community, of making adequate provision to meet those emergencies ... [Text continues.]

250 × 198. Pp. [4] (last 3 blank). Blue tinted paper. ND. (1854.) NI. P. w.

Appeal for funds to establish public hospital.
Copies: CC. 1135

———

Cornwall Hospital and Infirmary. Established July 1, 1854. Rules, regulations, report ... Launceston: Printed by Charles Wilson ... 1854.

204 × 130. Pp. 16.

Copies: SLT, SLV. 1136

———

First Annual Report of the Cornwall Hospital and Infirmary. Established July 1, 1854. Together with the rules, regulations ... Launceston: Printed by Charles Wilson ... 1855.

204 × 130. Pp. 24 (last—colophon).

An. reps, 1859–62, appear in Parliamentary Papers of Tas., 1860–63.

Copies: CC (4, 1858), ML (2–6, 1856–60), SLT (2–4, 1856–8; 7, 1861), SLV (1–6, 1855–60). 1137

———

(No. 22.) [Royal Arms] 1864. Tasmania. Legislative Council. Launceston General Hospital. Report for 1863. ...

332 × 206. Pp. 6 (l.b.). Colophon—James Barnard, Govt Pr, Tas.

In 1863 the Cornwall Hospital, removed to a new building, assumed the name of Launceston General Hospital. An. reps, from 1863 onwards, appear in Parliamentary Papers of Tas. (1864–).

For history see Craig, C. C. (1963), *Med. J. Aust.*, 1 : 328.

Copies: LNSW, SLT, SLV. 1138

———

Rules and regulations of the General Hospital, Launceston. January, 1879. [Arms] Tasmania: James Barnard, Govt Printer, Hobart Town. 1879.

8vo. Pp. [iv], 5–22 (l.b.). P. w. (title rptd).

Copies: CC (1879, 1883, 1890). 1139

Lauterer, Joseph

Australien und Tasmanien. Nach eigener Anschauung und Forschung wissenschaftlich und praktisch geschildert von Dr. Joseph Lauterer ... Freiburg im Breisgau. Herdersche Verlagshandlung. 1900. ...

236 × 163. Pp. [viii], 482. Coloured frontis., 1 map, 158 figs. Cloth.

Joseph Lauterer (1848–1911) MD Freiburg, of S. Brisbane, wrote on native medicinal plants, scorpions, leprosy and aboriginal languages. Also published: *Excursions Flora von Freiburg* ..., Freiburg, 1874. See Maiden, J. H. (1921), 'Records of Aust. botanists', *J. & P. Roy. Soc. NSW*, 55 : 163; *Austsn med. Gaz.*, 1911, 30 : 480.

Copies: ML, NL, OL, SLS, SLT, SLV, UA, UM, UQ, US. 1140

Lavers, Josiah Vincent

Testimonials as to the efficacy of Mr. J. T. Laver's patented process for preserving, in a fresh condition, the flesh of animals recently killed. ... Sydney: ... J. G. O'Connor, for the Publisher, J. V. Lavers ... 1870.

206 × 130. Pp. [10] (advts), iv, [5]–14, [20] (advts). P. w. (title rptd, advts both sides back wrapper).

Sodium sulphite as preservative.

Copies: DL, ML. 1141

Law, Hartland and Law, Herbert E.

Viavi hygiene for women, men and children ... Australian Viavi Co. Melbourne ... Sydney ... Adelaide ... British Viavi Co. Ltd. ... London W. ...

190 × 140. Pp. 610. Title p. tipped in. Frontis. (1899.) Cloth.

Another issue, 1899, has imprint: San Francisco ... The Viavi Company. Australia Viavi Co. ... Sydney. Other Aust. eds—1902, 1909.

Treatment, especially of diseases of female generative system, by Viavi remedies and system of hygiene. According to Oleson, C. W. (1903), *Secret nostrums & systems of medicine*, 10 ed., Chicago, Viavi was 'a mixture of tannin, opium and cacao butter in capsules.'

Copies: EF, UA. 1142

Law, William George Lemuel

Testimonials in favour of William George Lemuel Law, Licentiate King and Queen's College of Physicians, Ireland. Licentiate Royal College of Surgeons, Edinburgh. ...

8vo. Pp. 20 (l.b.). ND. (1874.) Colophon: Asher and Co. ... 'Kew and Hawthorn Express' Office.

Copies: CC. 1143

Lawrence, Herman Fermor

The toilet by Herman Lawrence ... George Robertson and Company Melbourne ... 1892

181 × 122. Pp. viii, 54 (l.b.). P. w. (title rptd).

Sections on skin, hair, nails, complexion,

baths, clothing and exercise; also teeth, by E. L. Oldfield.

Also published: *Radium: how & when to use*, Melb., 1911; section on 'Radiotherapy' in J. W. Springthorpe's *Therapeutics, dietetics, and hygiene*, vol. 2, Melb., 1914.

For H. F. Lawrence (1863–1936) MRCPE, Hon. Derm. Melb. and St Vincent's Hosps, a pioneer of radiotherapy, see Kenny, A. L. (1937), *Med. J. Aust.*, 1 : 270; Lempriere, W. W (1953), 'H. L., Doyen of Dermatology', *Aust. J. Derm.* 2 : 99; Johnson, A. (1954), *Aust. J. Derm.*, 2 : 149.

Copies: SLV. 1144

Laycock, George Lockwood (translator)

The etiology of cholera. By Dr. Robert Koch. Translated by George Lockwood Laycock, M. B. . . .

214 × 138. Pp. 325–384. *In Recent essays . . . on bacteria in relation to disease*, ed. W. Watson Cheyne, Lond., New Sydenham Soc., 1886.

G. L. Laycock MB, ChM Edin. (d. 1926) practised at Windsor Vic. and was Hon. Phys. Children's Hosp. and Hon. Med. Electrician, Melb. Hosp. He published chapter 'Electrotherapy' in J. W. Springthorpe's *Therapeutics, dietetics, and hygiene*, Melb., 1914.

Copies: EF, RACP, SLV, UM, US. 1145

Laycock, Thomas

The social and political relations of drunkenness: two lectures. By Thomas Laycock, M.D., F.R.S.E., &c. Professor of the Practice of Medicine . . . in the University of Edinburgh. Tasmania: Printed by H. and C. Best, "Courier" Office, Hobart Town. 1857. . . .

212 × 130. Pp. 38, [ii] (colophon, v.b.).

Copies: ML, NL, SLV. 1146

Leach, Harry

The ship captain's medical guide. Compiled by Harry Leach, Resident Medical Officer, Hospital-ship "Dreadnought". Second edition. By authority: reprinted by Thomas Richards, Govt Printer, Sydney . . . 1869. . . .

214 × 140. Pp. [iv], 80. Paper boards, cloth backstrip.

NSW Govt reprint of British Board of Trade handbook for vessels at sea.

Copies: ML, NL, SLV. 1147

Lee, William

Brandy and salt; being an effectual remedy for most of the diseases which afflict humanity By William Lee, Esq. Sydney: Printed and sold by James Tegg George-street. 1842.

153 × 98. Pp. 24. P. w. (title rptd, book list on verso of back wrapper).

Reprints English work advocating use of brandy and salt, internally or externally, for treatment of practically all ailments. *The Australian*, Sydney, 21 April 1839, has announcement (reprinted in *Med. J. Aust.*, 1955, 1 : 22) of an earlier edition by Tegg (NS), together with warning that pure French brandy was essential, and offer to publicise cures.

Copies: LNSW, ML. 1148

The use of brandy and salt, as a remedy for inflammation, illustrated and explained by the discoverer William Lee, Esq. Fifth edition. Tasmania: Charles Wilson, Printer . . . Launceston. 1863.

178 × 115. Pp. 36. P. w. (title rptd).

Reprint, with parts addressed from Leeds, dated 1835, 1836, 1839 and 1840.

Remedy noted in Bell and Redwood, *Hist. sketch of the progress of pharmacy*, Lond., 1880 : 124.

Copies: ML, SLV. 1149

Leigh, W. H.

Reconnoitering voyages and travels, with adventures in the new colonies of South Australia; a particular description of the town of Adelaide, and Kangaroo Island; and an account of the present state of Sydney and parts adjacent, including visits to the Nicobar and other islands of the Indian Seas, Calcutta, the Cape of Good Hope, and St. Helena, during the years 1836, 1837, 1838. By W. H. Leigh, Esq. late Surgeon of the Australia Company's Ship "South Australian". Embellished by numerous engravings. London: Smith Elder and Co. . . . 1839.

214 × 134. Pp. xiv, [ii] (v.b.). 292 (l.b.). 8 pl. incl. frontis. and vignette title. Cloth.

Author, who arrived in Adelaide in 1837, hopes that his book will 'have the effect of deterring even one individual from embarking on a rash and untried venture . . .'

Copies: DL, ML, NL, SLS, SLV, UM, US. 1150

The Same. 2 ed., 1840.

Copies: ML, SLT, US. 1151

Plate 1

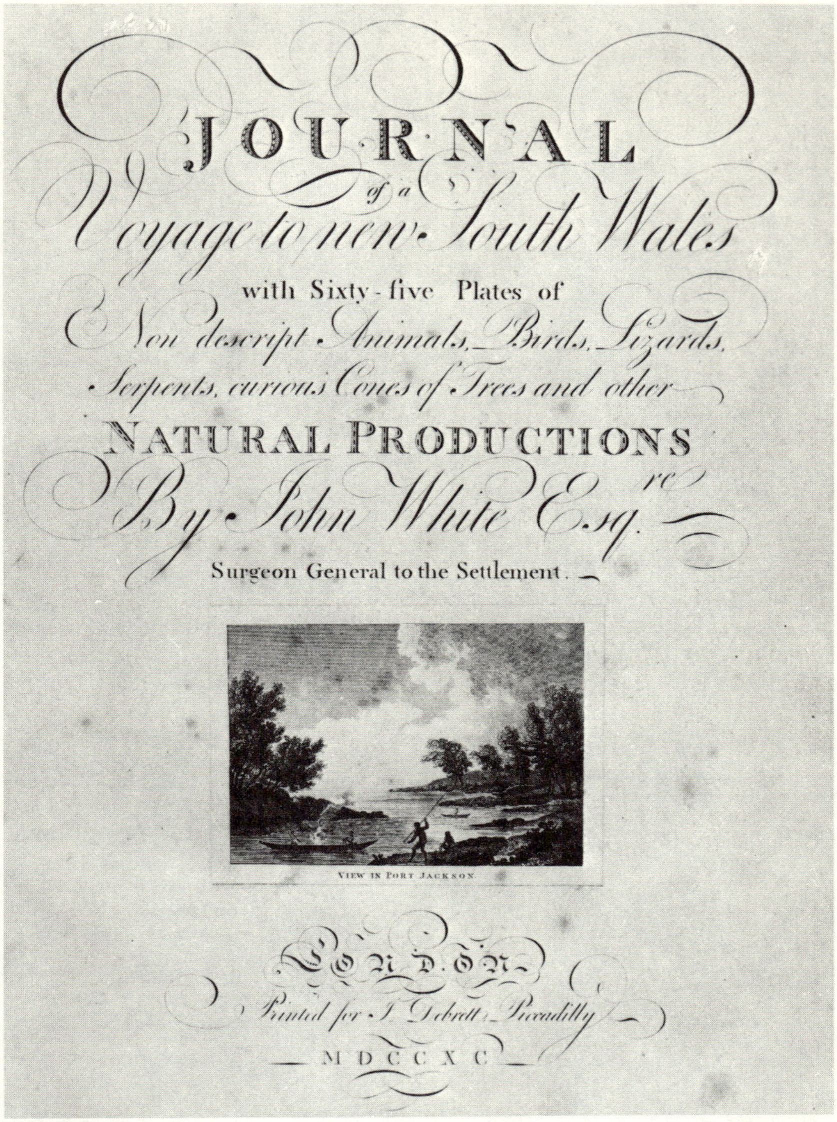
JOURNAL
of a
Voyage to new South Wales
with Sixty-five Plates of
Non descript Animals, Birds, Lizards,
Serpents, curious Cones of Trees and other
NATURAL PRODUCTIONS
By John White Esq.[re]
Surgeon General to the Settlement.

VIEW IN PORT JACKSON

LONDON
Printed for J. Debrett Piccadilly
MDCCXC

[2495] John White's *Journal of a voyage to new South Wales*, 1790. *Copy*: UM

Plate 2

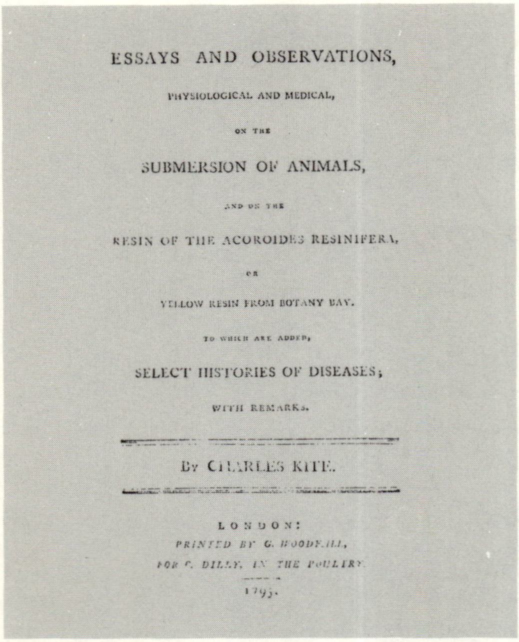

ESSAYS AND OBSERVATIONS,

PHYSIOLOGICAL AND MEDICAL,

ON THE

SUBMERSION OF ANIMALS,

AND ON THE

RESIN OF THE ACOROIDES RESINIFERA,

OR

YELLOW RESIN FROM BOTANY BAY.

TO WHICH ARE ADDED,

SELECT HISTORIES OF DISEASES;

WITH REMARKS.

BY CHARLES KITE.

LONDON:
PRINTED BY G. WOODFALL,
FOR C. DILLY, IN THE POULTRY.
1795.

[1090] Charles Kite's *Essays and observations*, 1795. *Copy*: EF

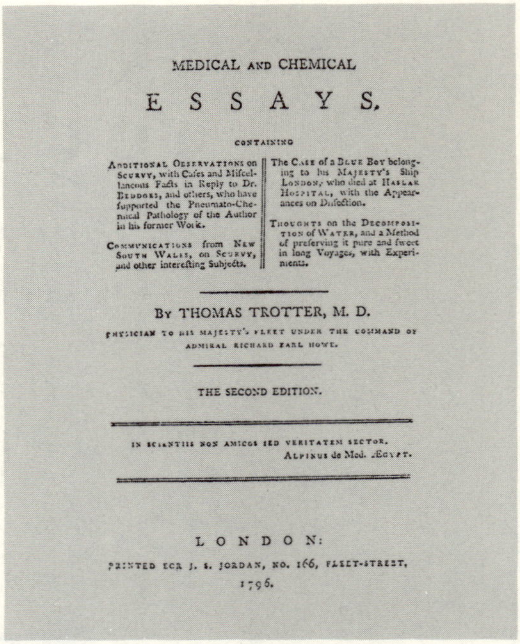

MEDICAL AND CHEMICAL

E S S A Y S,

CONTAINING

ADDITIONAL OBSERVATIONS on SCURVY, with Cases and Miscellaneous Facts in Reply to Dr. BEDDOES, and others, who have supported the Pneumato-Chemical Pathology of the Author in his former Work.

COMMUNICATIONS from NEW SOUTH WALES, on SCURVY, and other interesting Subjects.

The CASE of a BLUE BOY belonging to his MAJESTY's Ship LONDON, who died at HASLAR HOSPITAL, with the Appearances on Dissection.

THOUGHTS on the DECOMPOSITION of WATER, and a Method of preserving it pure and sweet in long Voyages, with Experiments.

BY THOMAS TROTTER, M. D.

PHYSICIAN TO HIS MAJESTY'S FLEET UNDER THE COMMAND OF ADMIRAL RICHARD EARL HOWE.

THE SECOND EDITION.

IN SCIENTIIS NON AMICOS SED VERITATEM SECTOR.
ALPINUS de Med. ÆGYPT.

LONDON:
PRINTED FOR J. S. JORDAN, NO. 166, FLEET-STREET,
1796.

[2283] Thomas Trotter's *Medical and chemical essays*, 1796. *Copy*: ML

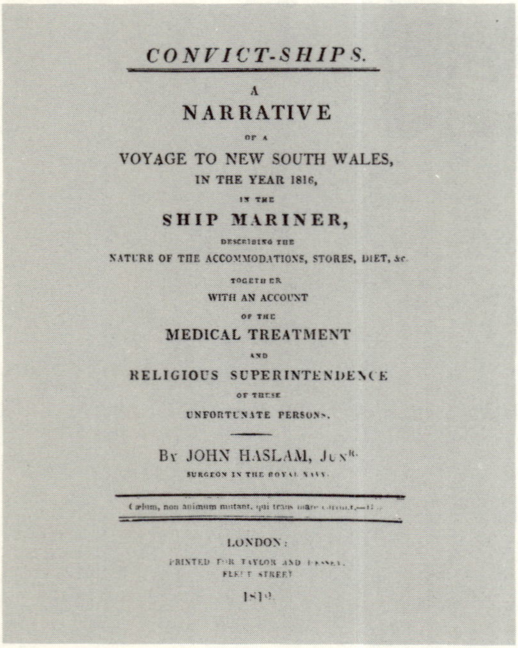

CONVICT-SHIPS.

A
NARRATIVE
OF A
VOYAGE TO NEW SOUTH WALES,
IN THE YEAR 1816,
IN THE
SHIP MARINER,
DESCRIBING THE
NATURE OF THE ACCOMMODATIONS, STORES, DIET, &c.
TOGETHER
WITH AN ACCOUNT
OF THE
MEDICAL TREATMENT
AND
RELIGIOUS SUPERINTENDENCE
OF THESE
UNFORTUNATE PERSONS.

BY JOHN HASLAM, JUN[R].
SURGEON IN THE ROYAL NAVY.

Cælum, non animum mutant, qui trans mare currunt.—

LONDON:
PRINTED FOR TAYLOR AND HESSEY,
FLEET STREET
1819.

[847] John Haslam's *Convict-ships*, 1819. *Copy*: ML

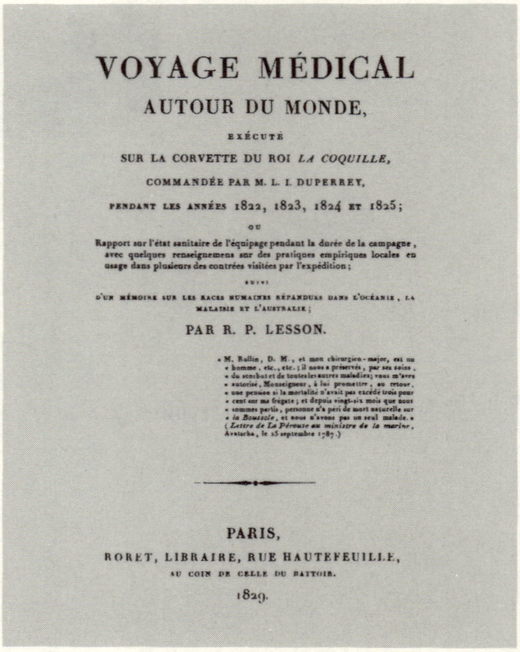

VOYAGE MÉDICAL
AUTOUR DU MONDE,
EXÉCUTÉ
SUR LA CORVETTE DU ROI *LA COQUILLE*,
COMMANDÉE PAR M. L. I. DUPERREY,
PENDANT LES ANNÉES 1822, 1823, 1824 ET 1825;
OU
Rapport sur l'état sanitaire de l'équipage pendant la durée de la campagne, avec quelques renseignemens sur des pratiques empiriques locales en usage dans plusieurs des contrées visitées par l'expédition;
SUIVI
D'UN MÉMOIRE SUR LES RACES HUMAINES RÉPANDUES DANS L'OCÉANIE, LA MALAISIE ET L'AUSTRALIE;

PAR R. P. LESSON.

« M. Rollin, D. M., et mon chirurgien-major, est un « homme, etc., etc.; il nous a préservés, par ses soins, « du scorbut et de toutes les autres maladies; vous m'avez « autorisé, Monseigneur, à lui promettre, au retour, « une pension si la mortalité n'avait pas excédé trois pour « cent sur ma frégate; et depuis vingt-six mois que nous « sommes partis, personne n'a péri de mort naturelle sur « *la Boussole*, et nous n'avons pas un seul malade. » (*Lettre de La Pérouse au ministre de la marine*, Avatscha, le 25 septembre 1787.)

PARIS,
RORET, LIBRAIRE, RUE HAUTEFEUILLE,
AU COIN DE CELLE DU BATTOIR.
1829.

[1157] R. P. Lesson's *Voyage médical autour du monde*, 1829. *Copy*: EF

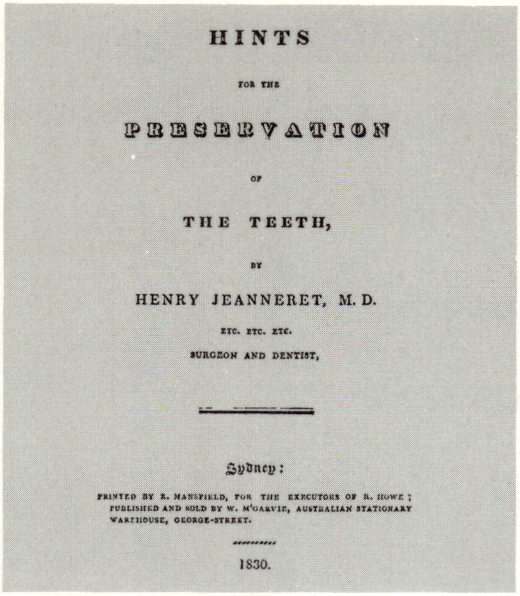
HINTS
FOR THE
PRESERVATION
OF
THE TEETH,
BY
HENRY JEANNERET, M. D.
ETC. ETC. ETC.
SURGEON AND DENTIST,

Sydney:
PRINTED BY R. MANSFIELD, FOR THE EXECUTORS OF R. HOWE; PUBLISHED AND SOLD BY W. M'GARVIE, AUSTRALIAN STATIONARY WAREHOUSE, GEORGE-STREET.
1830.

[1041] Henry Jeanneret's *Preservation of the teeth*, 1830—the first Australian dental publication. *Copy*: ML

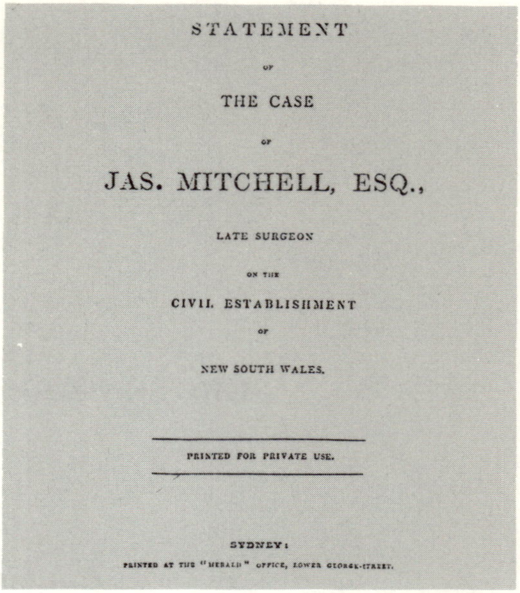
STATEMENT
OF
THE CASE
OF
JAS. MITCHELL, ESQ.,
LATE SURGEON
ON THE
CIVIL ESTABLISHMENT
OF
NEW SOUTH WALES.

PRINTED FOR PRIVATE USE.

SYDNEY:
PRINTED AT THE "HERALD" OFFICE, LOWER GEORGE-STREET.

[1393] *Statement of the case of Jas. Mitchell*, (1838). *Copy*: ML

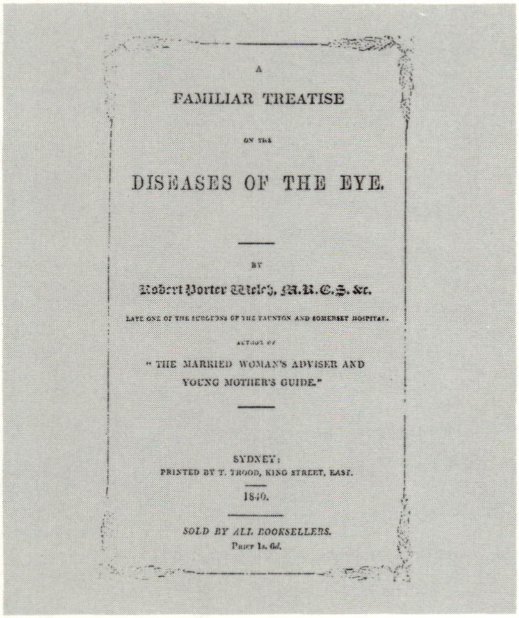
A
FAMILIAR TREATISE
ON THE
DISEASES OF THE EYE.
BY
Robert Porter Welch, M.R.C.S. &c.
LATE ONE OF THE SURGEONS OF THE TAUNTON AND SOMERSET HOSPITAL.
AUTHOR OF
"THE MARRIED WOMAN'S ADVISER AND YOUNG MOTHER'S GUIDE."

SYDNEY:
PRINTED BY T. TROOD, KING STREET, EAST.
1840.
SOLD BY ALL BOOKSELLERS.
Price 1s. 6d.

[2466] Robert Porter Welch's *Diseases of the eye*, 1840—the first medical work separately published in Australia. *Copy*: ML

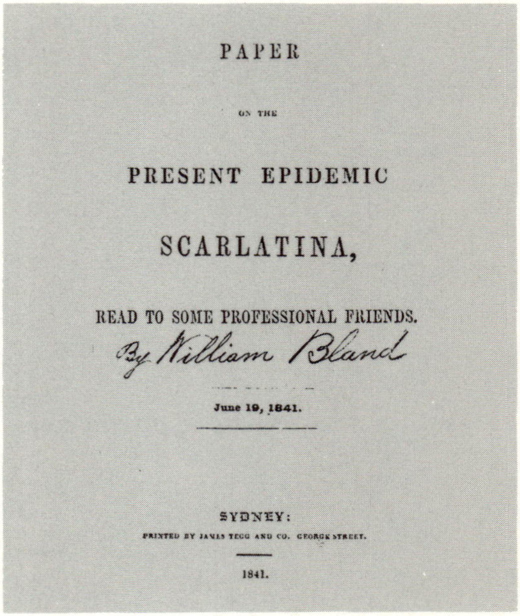
PAPER
ON THE
PRESENT EPIDEMIC
SCARLATINA,
READ TO SOME PROFESSIONAL FRIENDS.
By William Bland
June 19, 1841.

SYDNEY:
PRINTED BY JAMES TEGG AND CO. GEORGE STREET.
1841.

[333] Williams Bland's *Epidemic scarlatina*, 1841—earliest contribution to clinical medicine published in Australia. *Copy*: LNSW

Plate 4

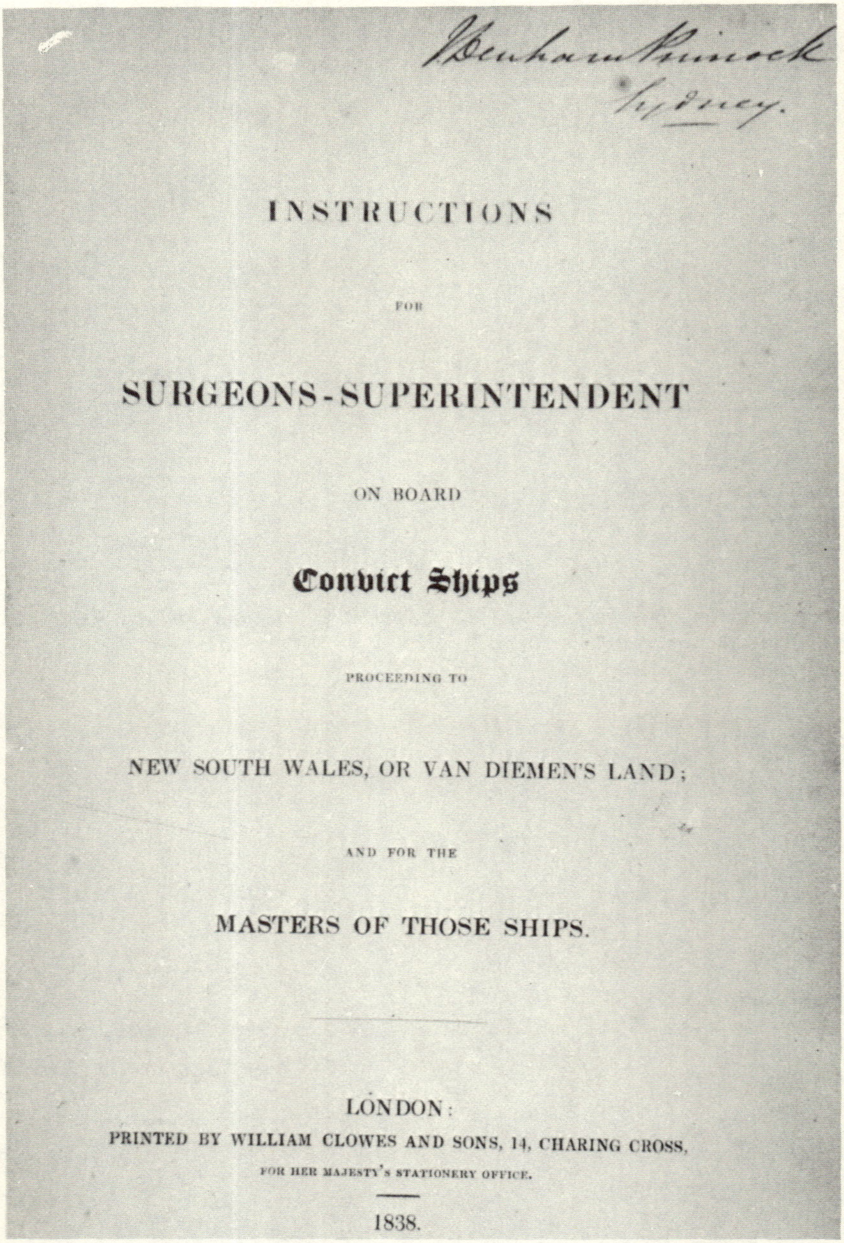

INSTRUCTIONS

FOR

SURGEONS-SUPERINTENDENT

ON BOARD

Convict Ships

PROCEEDING TO

NEW SOUTH WALES, OR VAN DIEMEN'S LAND;

AND FOR THE

MASTERS OF THOSE SHIPS.

LONDON:
PRINTED BY WILLIAM CLOWES AND SONS, 14, CHARING CROSS,
FOR HER MAJESTY'S STATIONERY OFFICE.

1838.

[2071] *Instructions for Surgeons-Superintendent on board convict ships*, 1838. *Copy*: ML

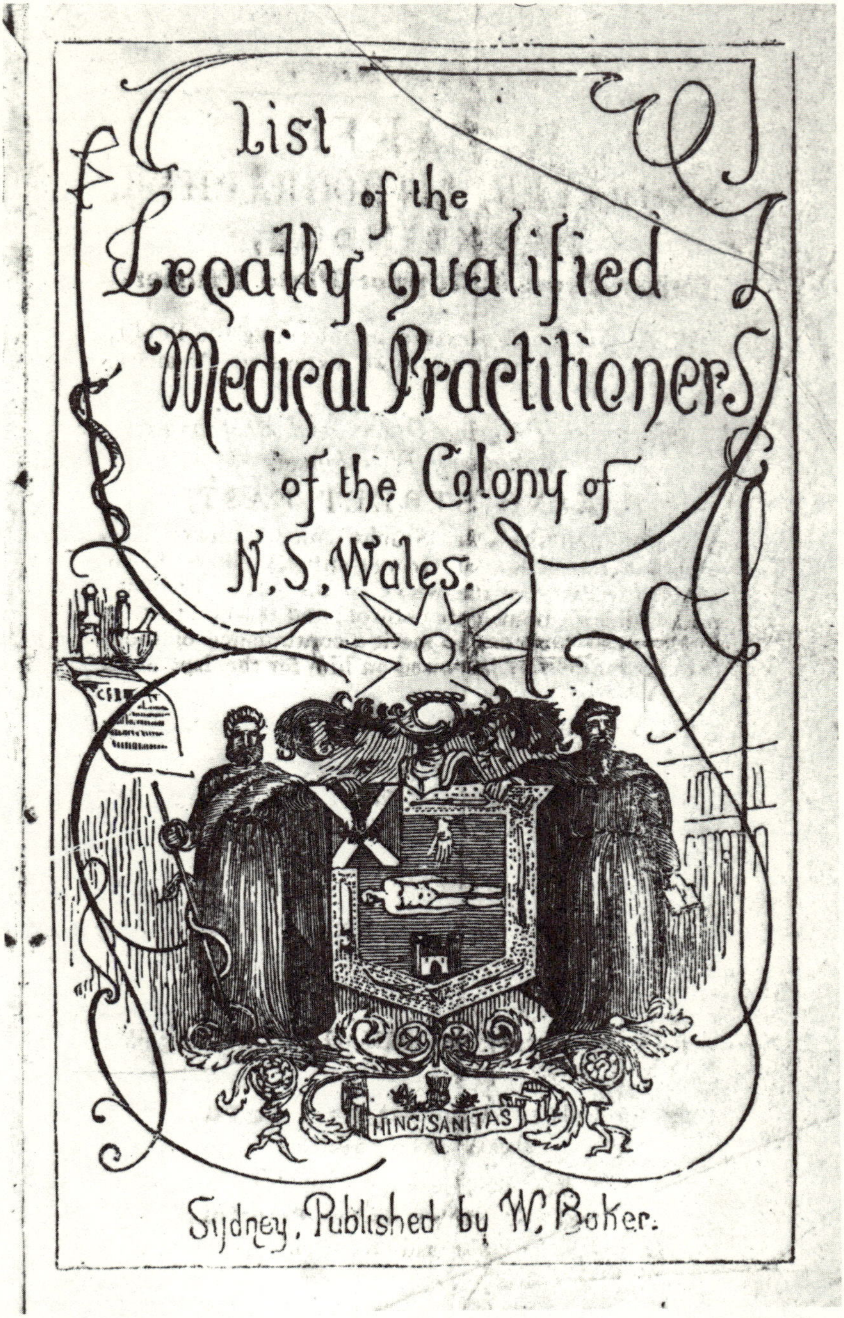

[126] Frontispiece of W. Baker's *The New South Wales Medical Act*, 1842, which includes the first Australian medical directory. *Copy*: AMAV

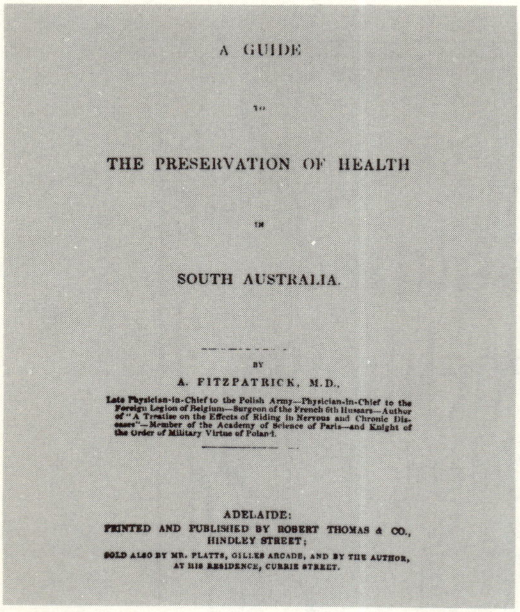

A GUIDE

TO

THE PRESERVATION OF HEALTH

IN

SOUTH AUSTRALIA.

BY

A. FITZPATRICK, M.D.,

Late Physician-in-Chief to the Polish Army—Physician-in-Chief to the Foreign Legion of Belgium—Surgeon of the French 6th Hussars—Author of "A Treatise on the Effects of Riding in Nervous and Chronic Diseases"—Member of the Academy of Science of Paris—and Knight of the Order of Military Virtue of Poland.

ADELAIDE:
PRINTED AND PUBLISHED BY ROBERT THOMAS & CO.,
HINDLEY STREET;
SOLD ALSO BY MR. PLATTS, GILLES ARCADE, AND BY THE AUTHOR,
AT HIS RESIDENCE, CURRIE STREET.

[677] Adolphus Fitzpatrick's *A guide to the preservation of health in South Australia*, [1841]. *Copy*: ML

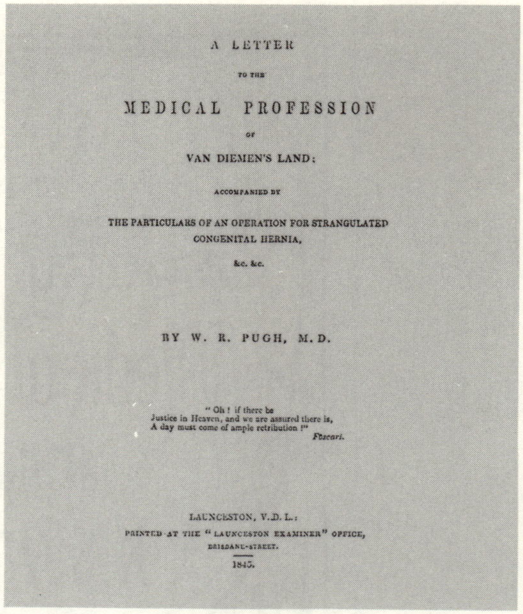

A LETTER

TO THE

MEDICAL PROFESSION

OF

VAN DIEMEN'S LAND;

ACCOMPANIED BY

THE PARTICULARS OF AN OPERATION FOR STRANGULATED
CONGENITAL HERNIA,

&c. &c.

BY W. R. PUGH, M.D.

"Oh! if there be
Justice in Heaven, and we are assured there is,
A day must come of ample retribution!"
Foscari.

LAUNCESTON, V.D.L.:
PRINTED AT THE "LAUNCESTON EXAMINER" OFFICE,
BRISBANE-STREET.
1845.

[1718] W. R. Pugh's *A letter to the medical profession of Van Diemen's Land*, 1845—first Australian publication on a surgical subject. *Copy*: ML

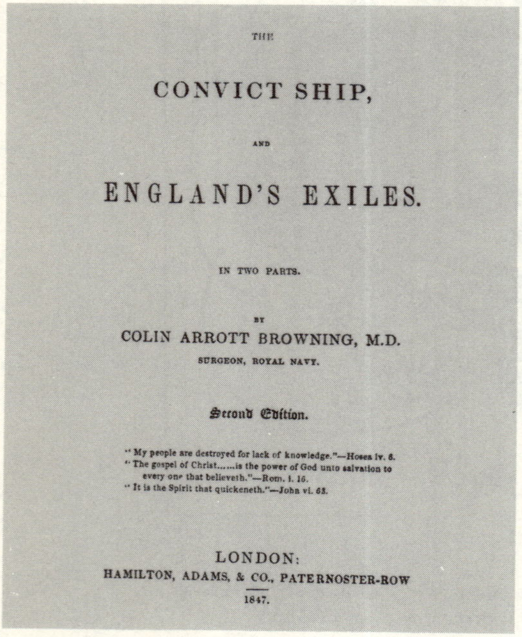

THE

CONVICT SHIP,

AND

ENGLAND'S EXILES.

IN TWO PARTS.

BY

COLIN ARROTT BROWNING, M.D.
SURGEON, ROYAL NAVY.

Second Edition.

"My people are destroyed for lack of knowledge."—Hosea iv. 6.
"The gospel of Christ......is the power of God unto salvation to every one that believeth."—Rom. i. 16.
"It is the Spirit that quickeneth."—John vi. 63.

LONDON:
HAMILTON, ADAMS, & CO., PATERNOSTER-ROW
1847.

[442] Colin Arrott Browning's *The convict ship, and England's exiles*, 1847. *Copy*: EF

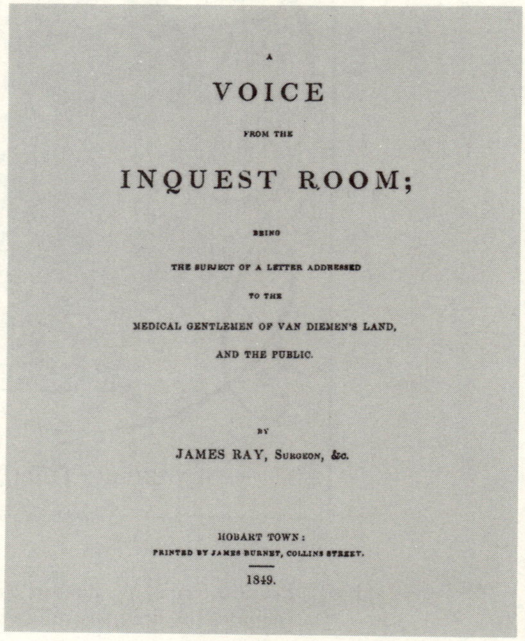

A

VOICE

FROM THE

INQUEST ROOM;

BEING

THE SUBJECT OF A LETTER ADDRESSED

TO THE

MEDICAL GENTLEMEN OF VAN DIEMEN'S LAND,

AND THE PUBLIC.

BY

JAMES RAY, SURGEON, &c.

HOBART TOWN:
PRINTED BY JAMES BURNET, COLLINS STREET.
1849.

[1767] James Ray's *A voice from the inquest room*, 1849. *Copy*: SLT

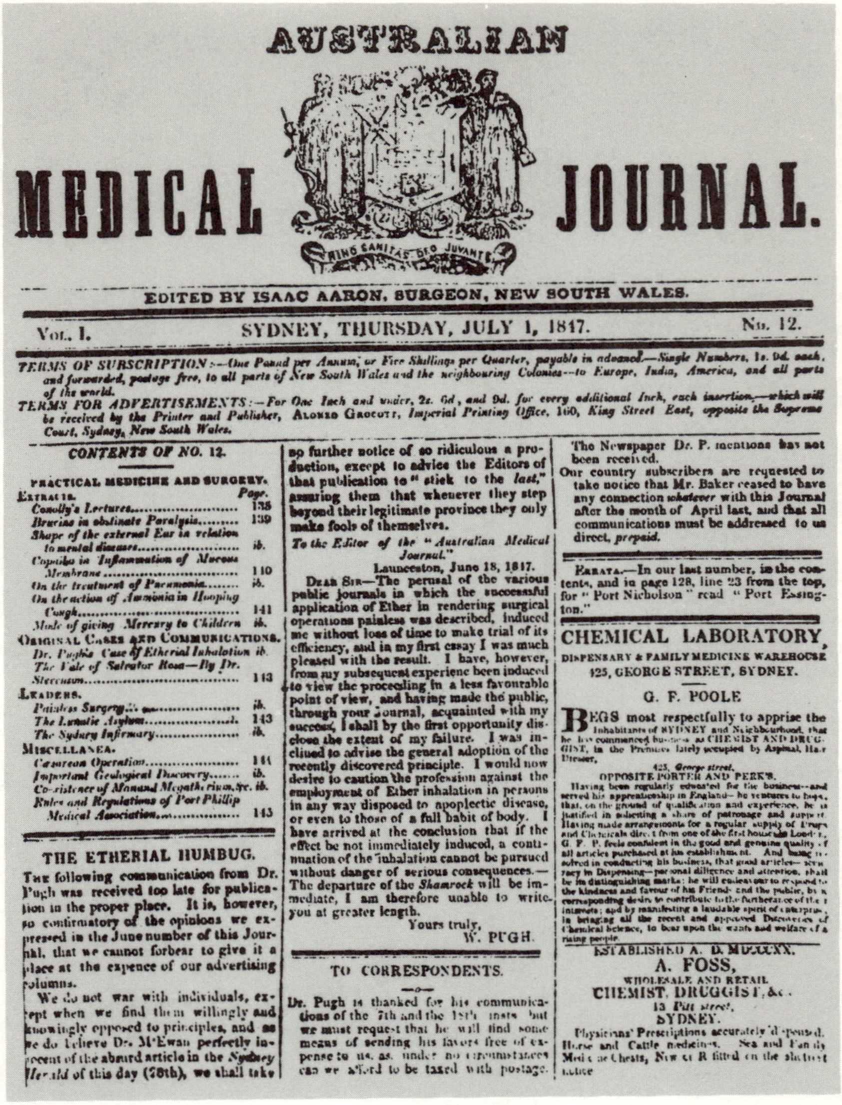

AUSTRALIAN MEDICAL JOURNAL.

RINO SANITAS DEO JUVANTE

EDITED BY ISAAC AARON, SURGEON, NEW SOUTH WALES.

Vol. I. SYDNEY, THURSDAY, JULY 1, 1847. No. 12.

TERMS OF SUBSCRIPTION:—One Pound per Annum, or Five Shillings per Quarter, payable in advance.—Single Numbers, 1s. 9d. each, and forwarded, postage free, to all parts of New South Wales and the neighbouring Colonies—to Europe, India, America, and all parts of the world.

TERMS FOR ADVERTISEMENTS:—For One Inch and under, 2s. 6d., and 9d. for every additional Inch, each insertion,—which will be received by the Printer and Publisher, Alonzo Grocott, *Imperial Printing Office, 160, King Street East, opposite the Supreme Court, Sydney, New South Wales.*

CONTENTS OF NO. 12.

THE ETHERIAL HUMBUG.

The following communication from Dr. Pugh was received too late for publication in the proper place. It is, however, so confirmatory of the opinions we expressed in the June number of this Journal, that we cannot forbear to give it a place at the expence of our advertising columns.

We do not war with individuals, except when we find them willingly and knowingly opposed to principles, and as we do believe Dr. M'Ewan perfectly innocent of the absurd article in the *Sydney Herald* of this day (28th), we shall take no further notice of so ridiculous a production, except to advice the Editors of that publication to " stick to the *last*," assuring them that whenever they step beyond their legitimate province they only make fools of themselves.

To the Editor of the "Australian Medical Journal."

Launceston, June 18, 1847.

Dear Sir—The perusal of the various public journals in which the successful application of Ether in rendering surgical operations painless was described, induced me without loss of time to make trial of its efficiency, and in my first essay I was much pleased with the result. I have, however, from my subsequent experienc been induced to view the proceeding in a less favourable point of view, and having made the public, through your Journal, acquainted with my success, I shall by the first opportunity disclose the extent of my failure. I was inclined to advise the general adoption of the recently discovered principle. I would now desire to caution the profession against the employment of Ether inhalation in persons in any way disposed to apoplectic disease, or even to those of a full habit of body. I have arrived at the conclusion that if the effect be not immediately induced, a continuation of the inhalation cannot be pursued without danger of serious consequences.—The departure of the *Shamrock* will be immediate, I am therefore unable to write you at greater length.

Yours truly,
W. PUGH.

TO CORRESPONDENTS.

Dr. Pugh is thanked for his communications of the 7th and the 18th insts. but we must request that he will find some means of sending his favors free of expense to us, as, under no circumstances can we afford to be taxed with postage.

The Newspaper Dr. P. mentions has not been received.

Our country subscribers are requested to take notice that Mr. Baker ceased to have any connection *whatever* with this Journal after the month of April last, and that all communications must be addressed to us direct, *prepaid*.

Errata.—In our last number, in the contents, and in page 128, line 23 from the top, for " Port Nicholson " read " Port Essington."

[114] *Australian Medical Journal*, published in Sydney, 1846–7—the first Australian medical periodical. *Copy*: ML

Plate 8

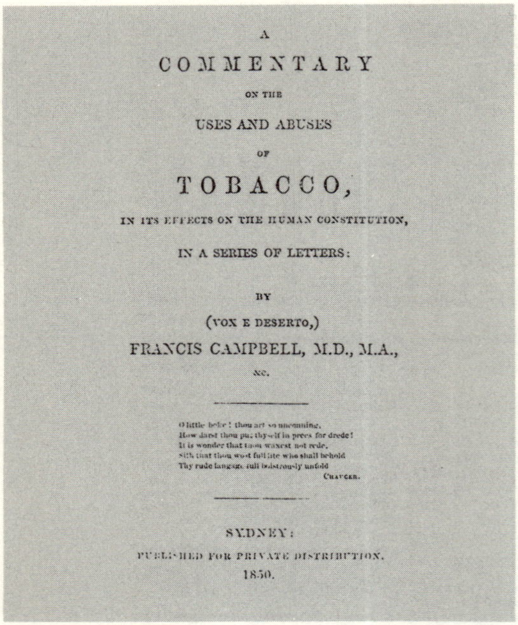

A

COMMENTARY

ON THE

USES AND ABUSES

OF

TOBACCO,

IN ITS EFFECTS ON THE HUMAN CONSTITUTION,

IN A SERIES OF LETTERS:

BY

(VOX E DESERTO,)

FRANCIS CAMPBELL, M.D., M.A.,

&c.

O little boke! thou art so unconning,
How darst thou put thyself in prees for drede!
It is wonder that thou waxest not rede,
Sith that thou wost full lite who shall behold
Thy rude language full boistously unfold

CHAUCER.

SYDNEY:

PUBLISHED FOR PRIVATE DISTRIBUTION.

1850.

[483] Francis Campbell's *Commentary on . . . tobacco*, 1850. *Copy*: ML

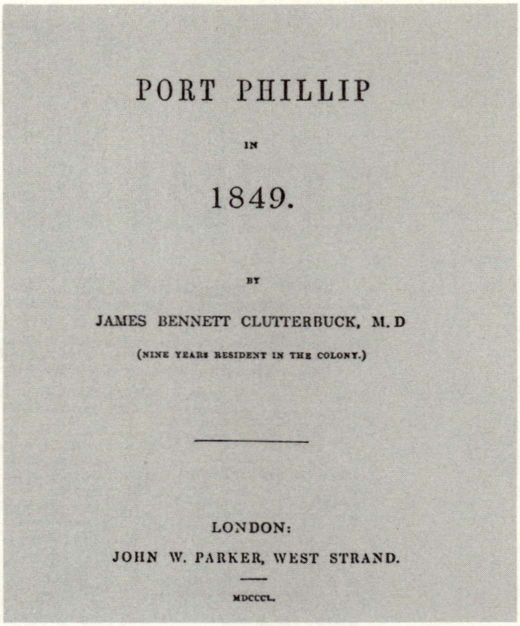

PORT PHILLIP

IN

1849.

BY

JAMES BENNETT CLUTTERBUCK, M. D

(NINE YEARS RESIDENT IN THE COLONY.)

LONDON:

JOHN W. PARKER, WEST STRAND.

MDCCCL.

[530] James Bennett Clutterbuck's *Port Phillip in 1849*, 1850. *Copy*: ML

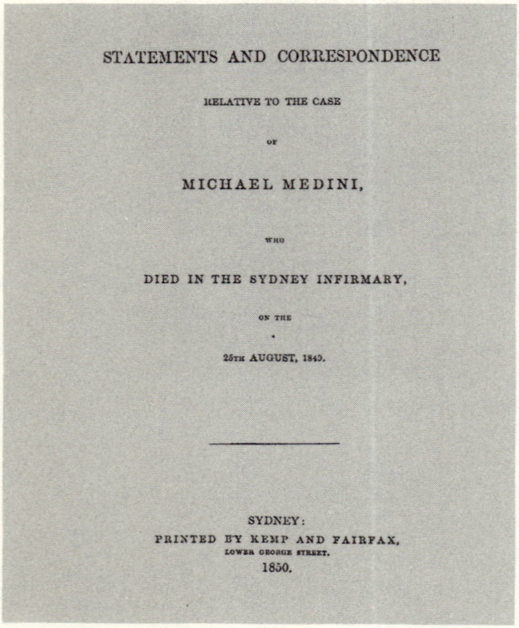

STATEMENTS AND CORRESPONDENCE

RELATIVE TO THE CASE

OF

MICHAEL MEDINI,

WHO

DIED IN THE SYDNEY INFIRMARY,

ON THE

25TH AUGUST, 1849.

SYDNEY:

PRINTED BY KEMP AND FAIRFAX,

LOWER GEORGE STREET.

1850.

[1337] *The case of Michael Medini*, 1850. *Copy*: ML

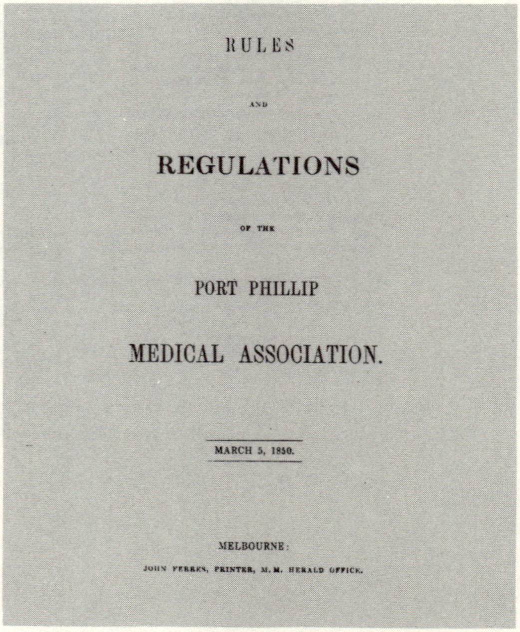

RULES

AND

REGULATIONS

OF THE

PORT PHILLIP

MEDICAL ASSOCIATION.

MARCH 5, 1850.

MELBOURNE:

JOHN FERRES, PRINTER, M.M. HERALD OFFICE.

[1684] *Rules and regulations of the Port Phillip Medical Association*—earliest Australian medical society, 1850. *Copy*: AMAV

Plate 9

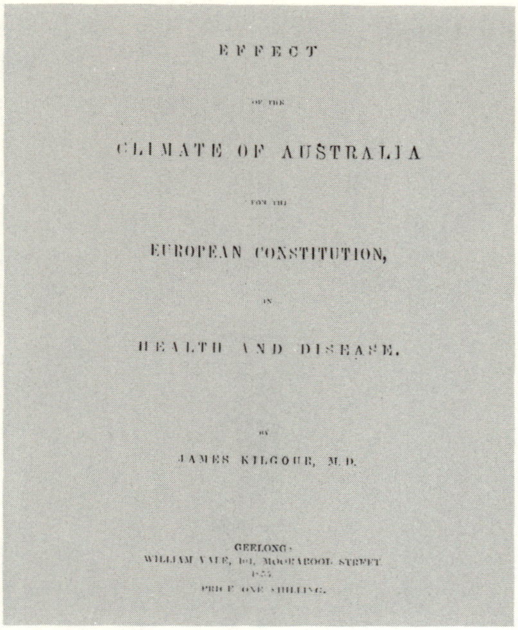

EFFECT

OF THE

CLIMATE OF AUSTRALIA

UPON THE

EUROPEAN CONSTITUTION,

IN

HEALTH AND DISEASE.

BY

JAMES KILGOUR, M.D.

GEELONG:

WILLIAM VALE, 101, MOORABOOL STREET.

1855.

PRICE ONE SHILLING.

[1086] James Kilgour's *Effect of the climate of Australia upon the European constitution*, 1855. *Copy*: EF

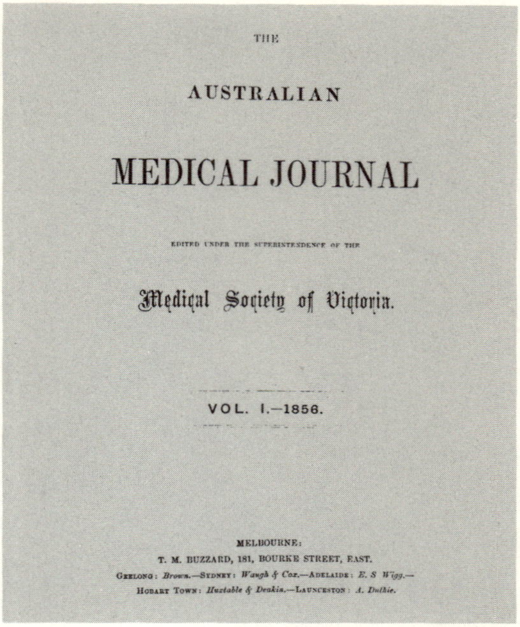

THE

AUSTRALIAN

MEDICAL JOURNAL

EDITED UNDER THE SUPERINTENDENCE OF THE

Medical Society of Victoria.

VOL. I.—1856.

MELBOURNE:

T. M. BUZZARD, 181, BOURKE STREET, EAST.

GEELONG: *Brown*.—SYDNEY: *Waugh & Cox*.—ADELAIDE: *E. S. Wigg*.—

HOBART TOWN: *Huxtable & Deakin*.—LAUNCESTON: *A. Duthie*.

[115] *Australian Medical Journal*, published in Melbourne, 1856–95. *Copy*: UM

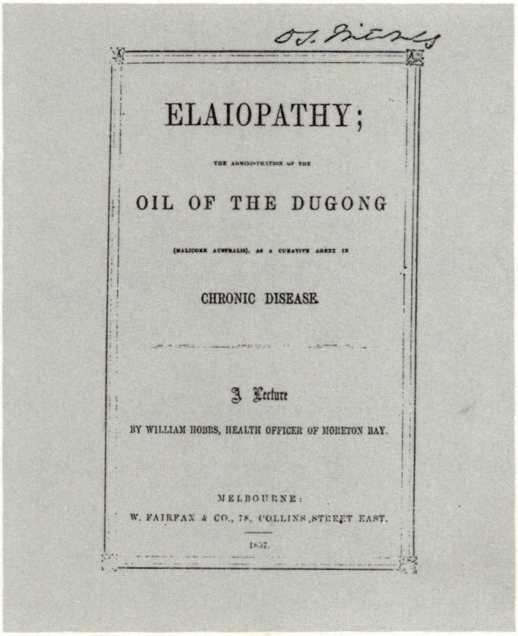

ELAIOPATHY;

THE ADMINISTRATION OF THE

OIL OF THE DUGONG

(HALICORE AUSTRALIS), AS A CURATIVE AGENT IN

CHRONIC DISEASE.

A Lecture

BY WILLIAM HOBBS, HEALTH OFFICER OF MORETON BAY.

MELBOURNE:

W. FAIRFAX & CO., 78, COLLINS STREET EAST.

1857.

[913] William Hobbs's *Elaiopathy*, 1857. *Copy*: ML

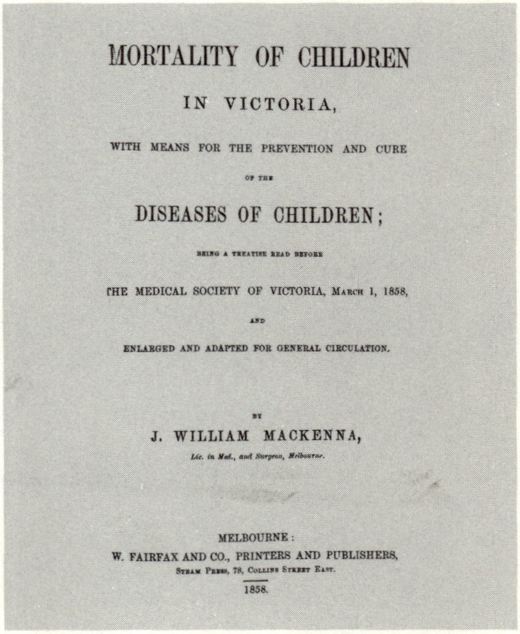

MORTALITY OF CHILDREN

IN VICTORIA,

WITH MEANS FOR THE PREVENTION AND CURE

OF THE

DISEASES OF CHILDREN;

BEING A TREATISE READ BEFORE

THE MEDICAL SOCIETY OF VICTORIA, MARCH 1, 1858,

AND

ENLARGED AND ADAPTED FOR GENERAL CIRCULATION.

BY

J. WILLIAM MACKENNA,

Lic. in Med., and Surgeon, Melbourne.

MELBOURNE:

W. FAIRFAX AND CO., PRINTERS AND PUBLISHERS,

STEAM PRESS, 78, COLLINS STREET EAST.

1858.

[1232] J. William Mackenna's *Mortality of children in Victoria*, 1858. *Copy*: AMAV

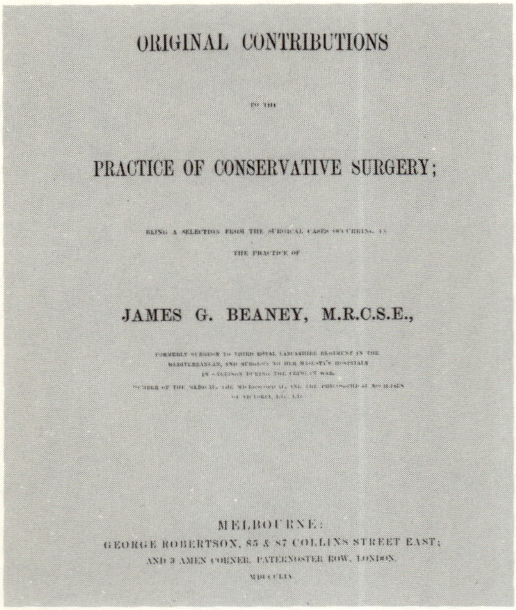

ORIGINAL CONTRIBUTIONS

TO THE

PRACTICE OF CONSERVATIVE SURGERY;

BEING A SELECTION FROM THE SURGICAL CASES OCCURRING IN

THE PRACTICE OF

JAMES G. BEANEY, M.R.C.S.E.,

FORMERLY SURGEON TO THIRD ROYAL LANCASHIRE REGIMENT IN THE MEDITERRANEAN, AND SURGEON TO HER MAJESTY'S HOSPITALS IN GARRISON DURING THE CRIMEAN WAR.

MEMBER OF THE MEDICAL, THE MICROSCOPICAL, AND THE PHILOSOPHICAL SOCIETIES OF VICTORIA, ETC. ETC.

MELBOURNE:
GEORGE ROBERTSON, 85 & 87 COLLINS STREET EAST;
AND 3 AMEN CORNER, PATERNOSTER ROW, LONDON.
MDCCCLIX.

[191] J. G. Beaney's *Practice of conservative surgery*, 1859—the first surgery book published in Australia. *Copy*: KFR

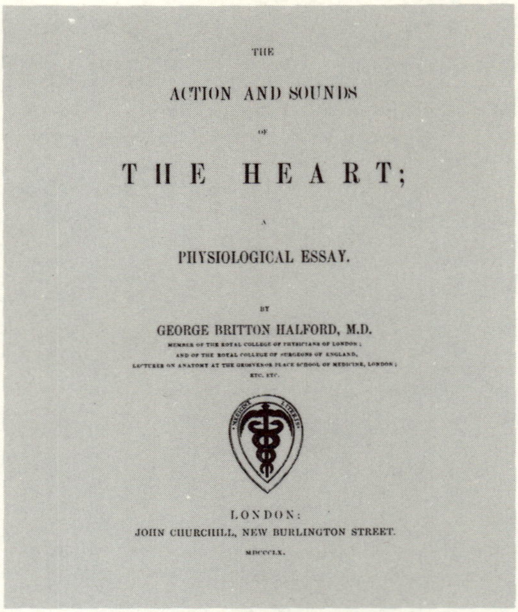

THE

ACTION AND SOUNDS

OF

THE HEART;

A

PHYSIOLOGICAL ESSAY.

BY

GEORGE BRITTON HALFORD, M.D.

MEMBER OF THE ROYAL COLLEGE OF PHYSICIANS OF LONDON;
AND OF THE ROYAL COLLEGE OF SURGEONS OF ENGLAND,
LECTURER ON ANATOMY AT THE GROSVENOR PLACE SCHOOL OF MEDICINE, LONDON;
ETC. ETC.

LONDON:
JOHN CHURCHILL, NEW BURLINGTON STREET.
MDCCCLX.

[806] George Britton Halford's *The action and sounds of the heart*, 1860. *Copy*: AMAV

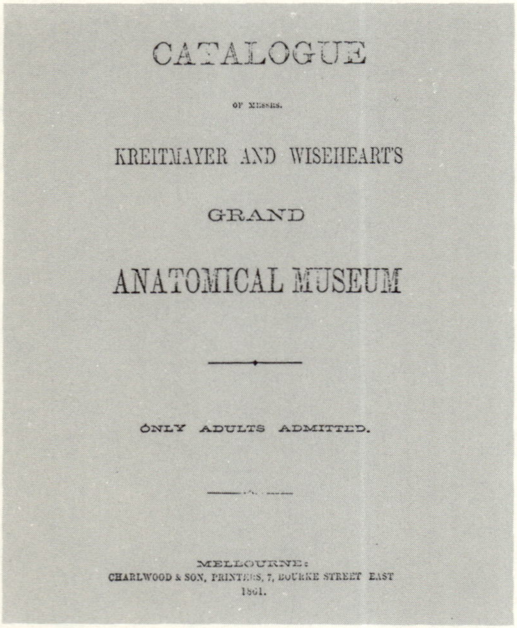

CATALOGUE

OF MESSRS.

KREITMAYER AND WISEHEART'S

GRAND

ANATOMICAL MUSEUM

ONLY ADULTS ADMITTED.

MELBOURNE:
CHARLWOOD & SON, PRINTERS, 7, BOURKE STREET EAST
1861.

[1112] *Catalogue of Kreitmayer and Wiseheart's Grand Anatomical Museum*, Melbourne, 1861. *Copy*: ML

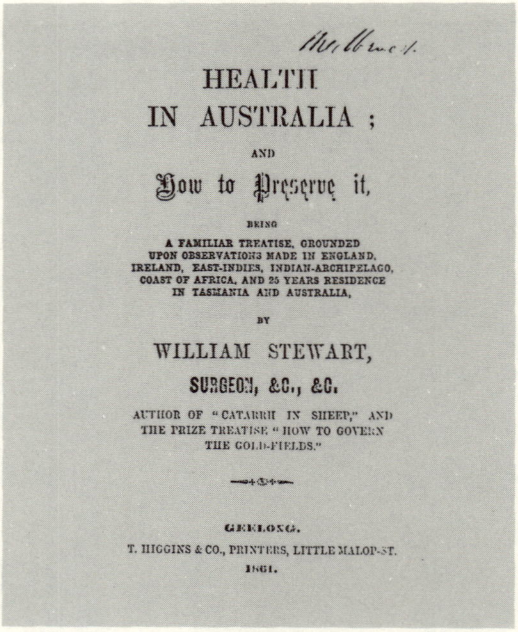

HEALTH
IN AUSTRALIA;

AND

How to Preserve it,

BEING

A FAMILIAR TREATISE, GROUNDED UPON OBSERVATIONS MADE IN ENGLAND, IRELAND, EAST-INDIES, INDIAN-ARCHIPELAGO, COAST OF AFRICA, AND 25 YEARS RESIDENCE IN TASMANIA AND AUSTRALIA,

BY

WILLIAM STEWART,

SURGEON, &C., &C.

AUTHOR OF "CATARRH IN SHEEP," AND THE PRIZE TREATISE "HOW TO GOVERN THE GOLD-FIELDS."

GEELONG.
T. HIGGINS & CO., PRINTERS, LITTLE MALOP-ST.
1861.

[2037] William Stewart's *Health in Australia*, 1861. *Copy*: ML

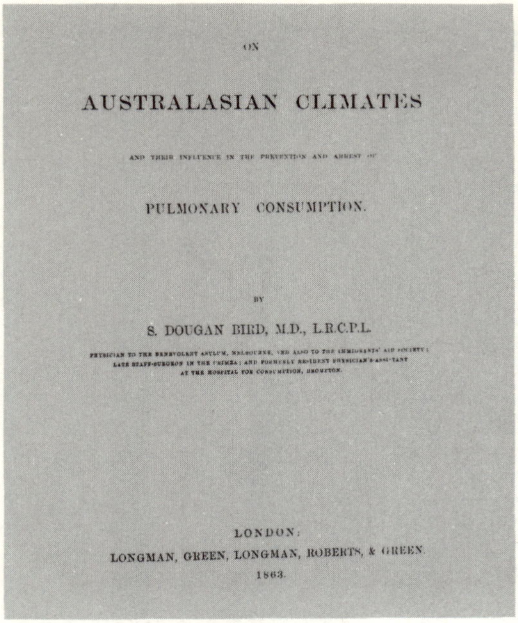
ON

AUSTRALASIAN CLIMATES

AND THEIR INFLUENCE IN THE PREVENTION AND ARREST OF

PULMONARY CONSUMPTION.

BY

S. DOUGAN BIRD, M.D., L.R.C.P.L.

LONDON:
LONGMAN, GREEN, LONGMAN, ROBERTS, & GREEN.
1863.

[310] Samuel Dougan Bird's *On Australasian climates*, 1863. *Copy*: KFR

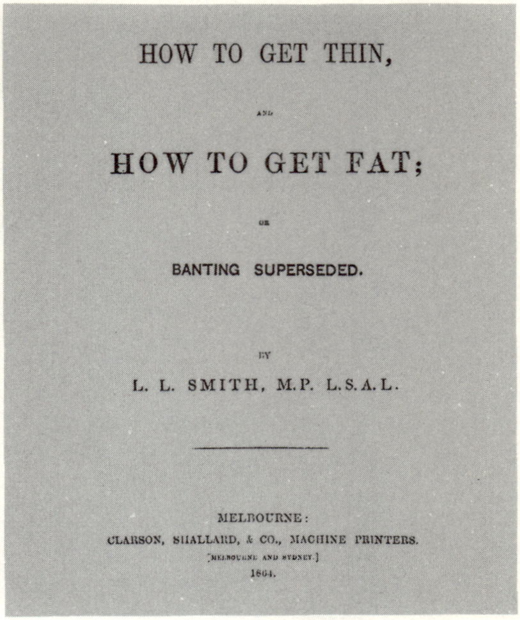
HOW TO GET THIN,

AND

HOW TO GET FAT;

OR

BANTING SUPERSEDED.

BY

L. L. SMITH, M.P. L.S.A.L.

MELBOURNE:
CLARSON, SHALLARD, & CO., MACHINE PRINTERS.
[MELBOURNE AND SYDNEY.]
1864.

[1935] L. L. Smith's *How to get thin, and how to get fat*, 1864. *Copy*: LNSW

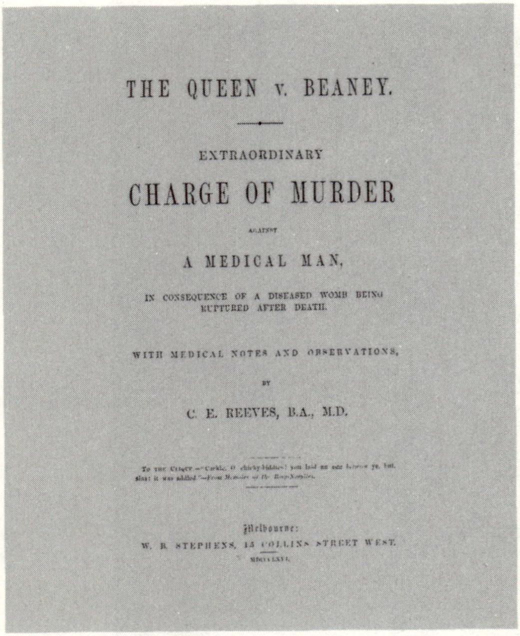
THE QUEEN v. BEANEY.

EXTRAORDINARY

CHARGE OF MURDER

AGAINST

A MEDICAL MAN,

IN CONSEQUENCE OF A DISEASED WOMB BEING RUPTURED AFTER DEATH.

WITH MEDICAL NOTES AND OBSERVATIONS,

BY

C. E. REEVES, B.A., M.D.

Melbourne:
W. B. STEPHENS, 15 COLLINS STREET WEST.
MDCCCLXVI.

[1776] C. E. Reeves' *The Queen v. Beaney*, 1866. *Copy*: KFR

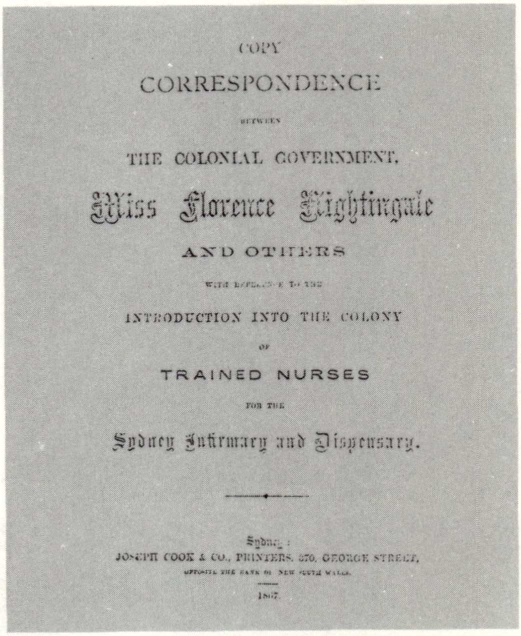
COPY

CORRESPONDENCE

BETWEEN

THE COLONIAL GOVERNMENT,

Miss Florence Nightingale

AND OTHERS

INTRODUCTION INTO THE COLONY

OF

TRAINED NURSES

FOR THE

Sydney Infirmary and Dispensary.

Sydney:
JOSEPH COOK & CO., PRINTERS, 370, GEORGE STREET,
OPPOSITE THE BANK OF NEW SOUTH WALES.
1867.

[1604] *Correspondence between the Colonial Government, Miss Florence Nightingale and others*, 1867. *Copy*: ML

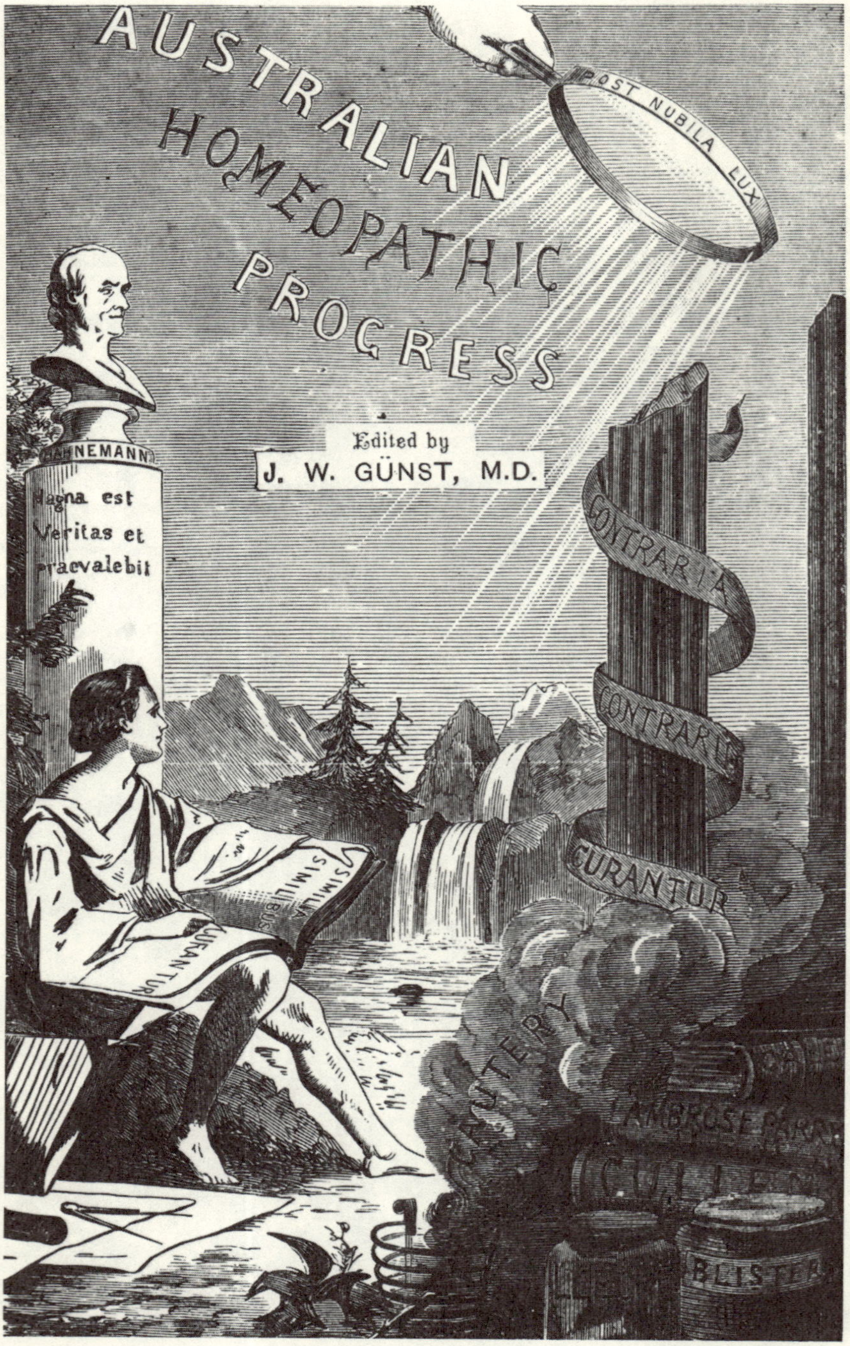
AUSTRALIAN HOMEOPATHIC PROGRESS
POST NUBILA LUX
Edited by
J. W. GÜNST, M.D.
HAHNEMANN
Magna est Veritas et praevalebit
CONTRARIA
CONTRARIIS
CURANTUR
SIMILIA SIMILIBUS CURANTUR
AMBROSE PARRE
BLISTER

[950] Frontispiece to *Homoeopathic Progress in Australia*, Vol. 1, 1870–1. *Copy*: EF

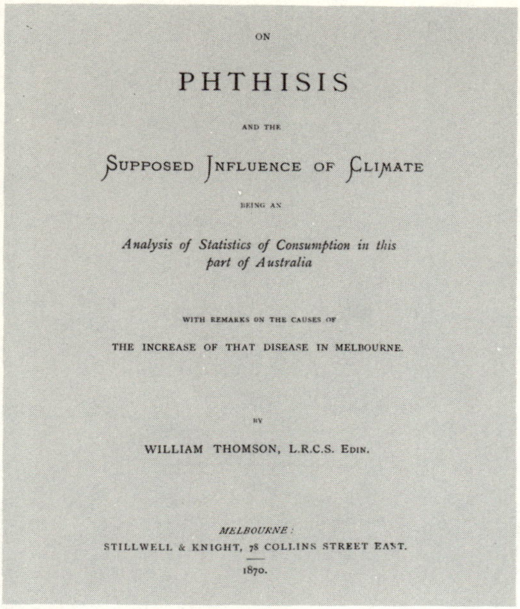

ON

PHTHISIS

AND THE

SUPPOSED INFLUENCE OF CLIMATE

BEING AN

Analysis of Statistics of Consumption in this part of Australia

WITH REMARKS ON THE CAUSES OF

THE INCREASE OF THAT DISEASE IN MELBOURNE.

BY

WILLIAM THOMSON, L.R.C.S. EDIN.

MELBOURNE:
STILLWELL & KNIGHT, 78 COLLINS STREET EAST.
1870.

[2225] William Thomson's *On phthisis and the supposed influence of climate*, 1870. *Copy*: UM

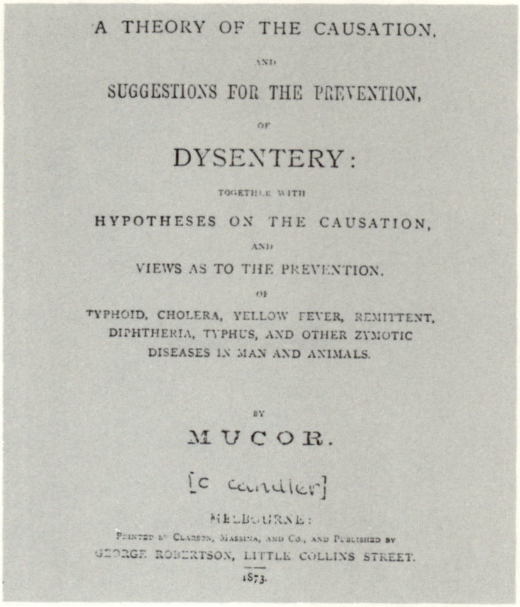

A THEORY OF THE CAUSATION,

AND

SUGGESTIONS FOR THE PREVENTION,

OF

DYSENTERY:

TOGETHER WITH

HYPOTHESES ON THE CAUSATION,

AND

VIEWS AS TO THE PREVENTION,

OF

TYPHOID, CHOLERA, YELLOW FEVER, REMITTENT, DIPHTHERIA, TYPHUS, AND OTHER ZYMOTIC DISEASES IN MAN AND ANIMALS.

BY

MUCOR.

[C Candler]

MELBOURNE:
PRINTED BY CLARSON, MASSINA, AND CO., AND PUBLISHED BY
GEORGE ROBERTSON, LITTLE COLLINS STREET.
1873.

[491] Samuel Curtis Candler's pseudonymous *A theory of the causation . . . of dysentery*, 1873. *Copy*: EF

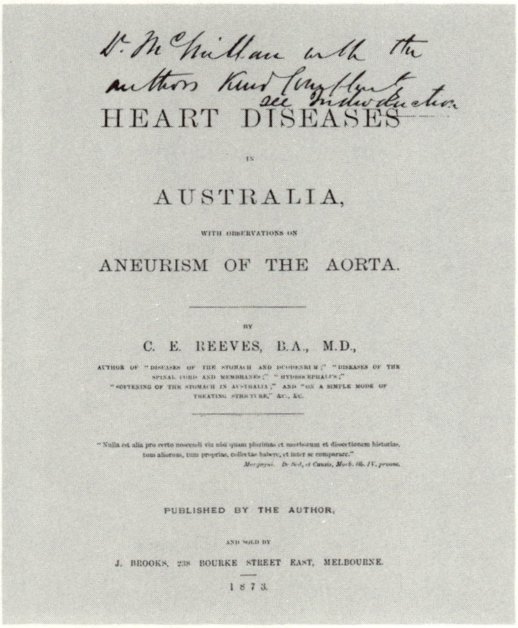

Dr McMillan with the authors kind compliments
see introduction

HEART DISEASES

IN

AUSTRALIA,

WITH OBSERVATIONS ON

ANEURISM OF THE AORTA.

BY

C. E. REEVES, B.A., M.D.,

AUTHOR OF "DISEASES OF THE STOMACH AND DUODENUM;" "DISEASES OF THE SPINAL CORD AND MEMBRANES;" "HYDROCEPHALUS;" "SOFTENING OF THE STOMACH IN AUSTRALIA;" AND "ON A SIMPLE MODE OF TREATING STRICTURE," &C., &C.

"Nulla est alia pro certo noscendi via nisi quam plurimas et morborum et dissectionem historias, tum aliorum, tum proprias, collectas habere, et inter se comparare."
Morgagni. De Sed. et Causis, Morb. lib. IV. proem.

PUBLISHED BY THE AUTHOR,

AND SOLD BY

J. BROOKS, 238 BOURKE STREET EAST, MELBOURNE.

1873.

[1780] C. E. Reeves' *Heart diseases in Australia*, 1873. *Copy*: KFR

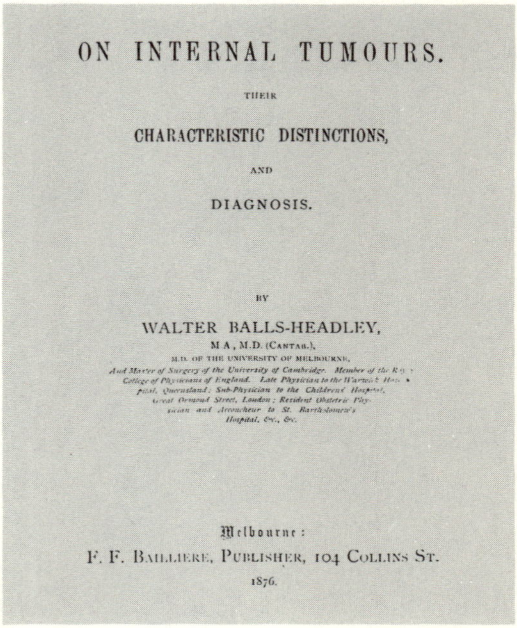

ON INTERNAL TUMOURS.

THEIR

CHARACTERISTIC DISTINCTIONS,

AND

DIAGNOSIS.

BY

WALTER BALLS-HEADLEY,

M.A., M.D. (CANTAB.),

M.D. OF THE UNIVERSITY OF MELBOURNE,

And Master of Surgery of the University of Cambridge. Member of the Royal College of Physicians of England. Late Physician to the Warwick Hospital, Queensland; Sub-Physician to the Children's Hospital, Great Ormond Street, London; Resident Obstetric Physician and Accoucheur to St. Bartholomew's Hospital, &c., &c.

Melbourne:
F. F. BAILLIERE, PUBLISHER, 104 COLLINS ST.
1876.

[855] Walter Balls-Headley's *On internal tumours*, 1876—the first gynaecology book published in Australia. *Copy*: EF

Plate 14

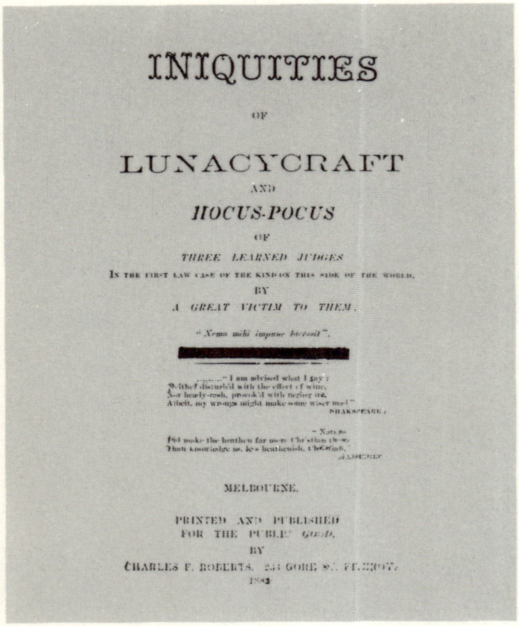

INIQUITIES

OF

LUNACYCRAFT

AND

HOCUS-POCUS

OF

THREE LEARNED JUDGES

IN THE FIRST LAW CASE OF THE KIND ON THIS SIDE OF THE WORLD,

BY

A GREAT VICTIM TO THEM.

"Nemo mihi impune lacessit".

........"I am advised what I say:
Neither disturb'd with the effect of wine,
Nor heady-rash, provok'd with raging ire,
Albeit, my wrongs might make some wiser mad."

SHAKESPEARE.

[illegible]

MELBOURNE.

PRINTED AND PUBLISHED
FOR THE PUBLIC *GOOD,*
BY
CHARLES F. ROBERTS, [illegible] GORE ST., FITZROY.
1883.

[1805] C. R. Roberts' *Iniquities of Lunacycraft*, 1883. *Copy*: SLV

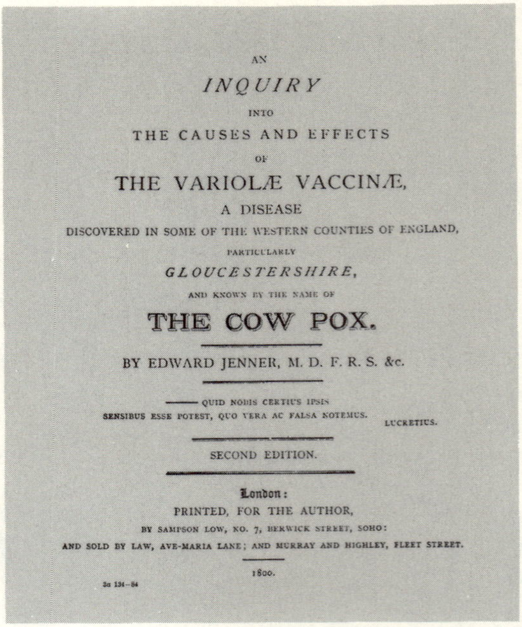

AN

INQUIRY

INTO

THE CAUSES AND EFFECTS

OF

THE VARIOLÆ VACCINÆ,

A DISEASE

DISCOVERED IN SOME OF THE WESTERN COUNTIES OF ENGLAND,

PARTICULARLY

GLOUCESTERSHIRE,

AND KNOWN BY THE NAME OF

THE COW POX.

BY EDWARD JENNER, M. D. F. R. S. &c.

—— QUID NOBIS CERTIUS IPSIS
SENSIBUS ESSE POTEST, QUO VERA AC FALSA NOTEMUS.
LUCRETIUS.

SECOND EDITION.

London:
PRINTED, FOR THE AUTHOR,
BY SAMPSON LOW, NO. 7, BERWICK STREET, SOHO:
AND SOLD BY LAW, AVE-MARIA LANE; AND MURRAY AND HIGHLEY, FLEET STREET.

1800.

3a 134-84

[1052] The Sydney republication of Edward Jenner's *Inquiry*, 1884. *Copy*: KFR

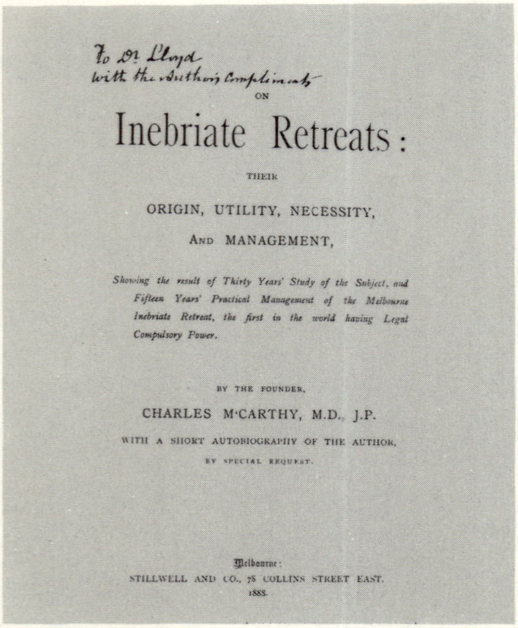

To Dr Lloyd
with the Author's Compliments

ON

Inebriate Retreats:

THEIR

ORIGIN, UTILITY, NECESSITY,

AND MANAGEMENT,

Showing the result of Thirty Years' Study of the Subject, and Fifteen Years' Practical Management of the Melbourne Inebriate Retreat, the first in the world having Legal Compulsory Power.

BY THE FOUNDER,

CHARLES McCARTHY, M.D., J.P.

WITH A SHORT AUTOBIOGRAPHY OF THE AUTHOR,

BY SPECIAL REQUEST.

Melbourne:
STILLWELL AND CO., 78 COLLINS STREET EAST.
1888.

[1205] Charles McCarthy's *On inebriate retreats*, 1888. *Copy*: EF

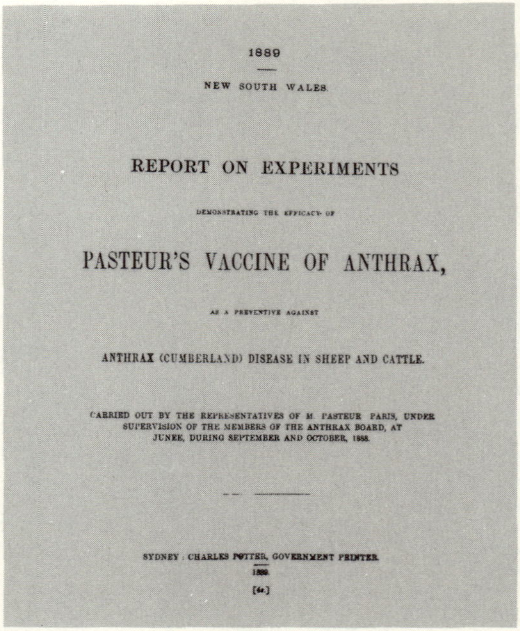

1889

NEW SOUTH WALES.

REPORT ON EXPERIMENTS

DEMONSTRATING THE EFFICACY OF

PASTEUR'S VACCINE OF ANTHRAX,

AS A PREVENTIVE AGAINST

ANTHRAX (CUMBERLAND) DISEASE IN SHEEP AND CATTLE.

CARRIED OUT BY THE REPRESENTATIVES OF M. PASTEUR, PARIS, UNDER SUPERVISION OF THE MEMBERS OF THE ANTHRAX BOARD, AT JUNEE, DURING SEPTEMBER AND OCTOBER, 1888.

SYDNEY: CHARLES POTTER, GOVERNMENT PRINTER.
1889.
[illegible]

[1483] New South Wales Anthrax Board's *Report on . . . Pasteur's vaccine of anthrax*, 1889. *Copy*: ML

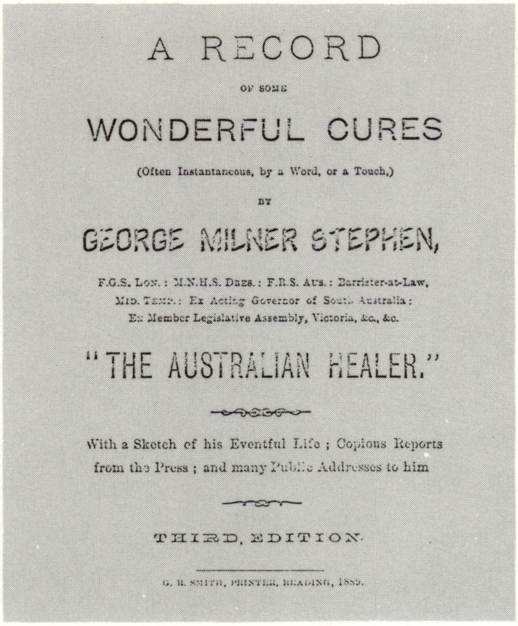

A RECORD

OF SOME

WONDERFUL CURES

(Often Instantaneous, by a Word, or a Touch,)

BY

GEORGE MILNER STEPHEN,

F.G.S. Lon.: M.N.H.S. Dres.: F.R.S. Aus.: Barrister-at-Law, Mid. Temp.: Ex Acting Governor of South Australia: Ex Member Legislative Assembly, Victoria, &c., &c.

"THE AUSTRALIAN HEALER."

With a Sketch of his Eventful Life; Copious Reports from the Press; and many Public Addresses to him

THIRD EDITION.

G. R. SMITH, PRINTER, READING, 1889.

[2032] *Some wonderful cures . . . by George Milner Stephen*, 1889. *Copy*: ML

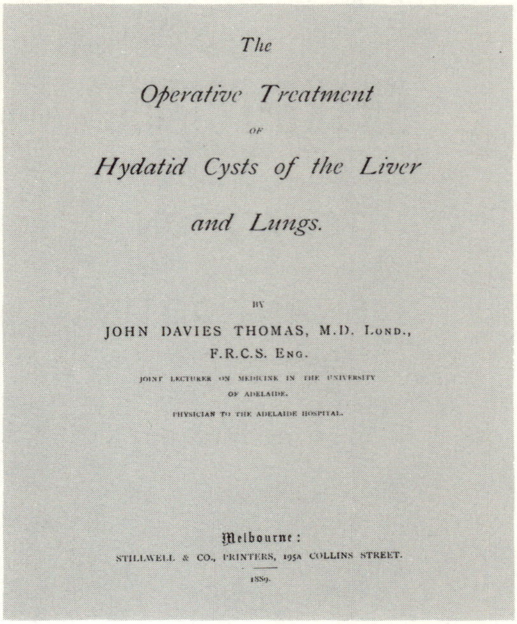

The

Operative Treatment

OF

Hydatid Cysts of the Liver

and Lungs.

BY

JOHN DAVIES THOMAS, M.D. Lond.,

F.R.C.S. Eng.

JOINT LECTURER ON MEDICINE IN THE UNIVERSITY OF ADELAIDE.

PHYSICIAN TO THE ADELAIDE HOSPITAL.

Melbourne:

STILLWELL & CO., PRINTERS, 195A COLLINS STREET.

1889.

[2185] John Davies Thomas's *Operative treatment of hydatid cysts of the liver and lungs*, 1889. *Copy*: AMAV

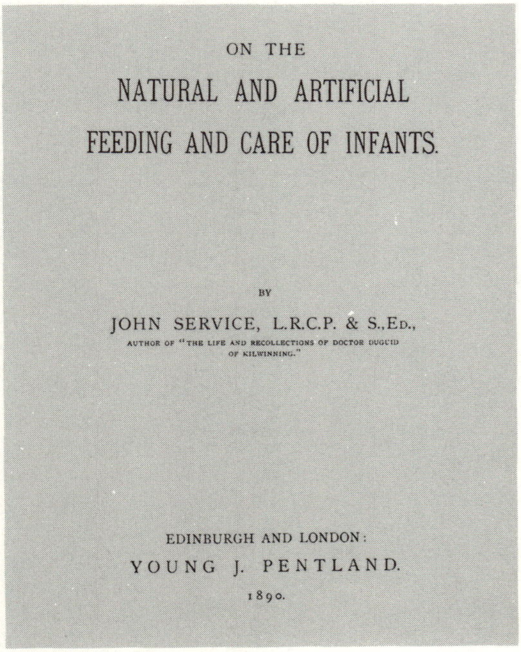

ON THE

NATURAL AND ARTIFICIAL

FEEDING AND CARE OF INFANTS.

BY

JOHN SERVICE, L.R.C.P. & S.Ed.,

AUTHOR OF "THE LIFE AND RECOLLECTIONS OF DOCTOR DUGUID OF KILWINNING."

EDINBURGH AND LONDON:

YOUNG J. PENTLAND.

1890.

[1894] John Service's *On the . . . feeding and care of infants*, 1890. *Copy*: EF

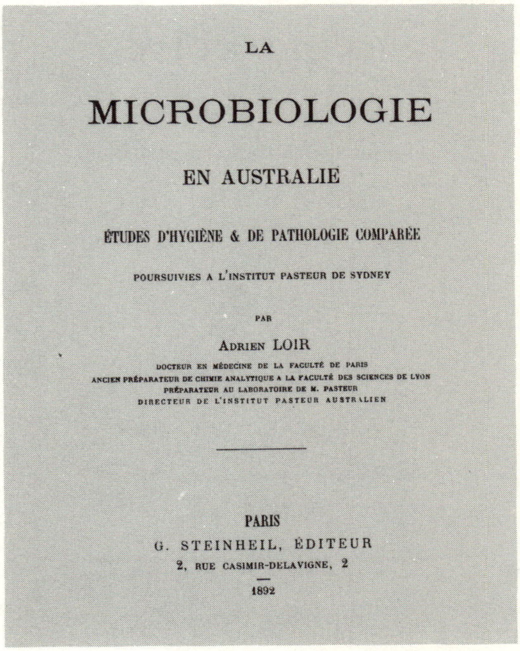

LA

MICROBIOLOGIE

EN AUSTRALIE

ÉTUDES D'HYGIÈNE & DE PATHOLOGIE COMPARÉE

POURSUIVIES A L'INSTITUT PASTEUR DE SYDNEY

PAR

Adrien LOIR

DOCTEUR EN MÉDECINE DE LA FACULTÉ DE PARIS

ANCIEN PRÉPARATEUR DE CHIMIE ANALYTIQUE A LA FACULTÉ DES SCIENCES DE LYON

PRÉPARATEUR AU LABORATOIRE DE M. PASTEUR

DIRECTEUR DE L'INSTITUT PASTEUR AUSTRALIEN

PARIS

G. STEINHEIL, ÉDITEUR

2, RUE CASIMIR-DELAVIGNE, 2

1892

[1171] Adrien Loir's *La microbiologie en Australie*, 1892. *Copy*: EF

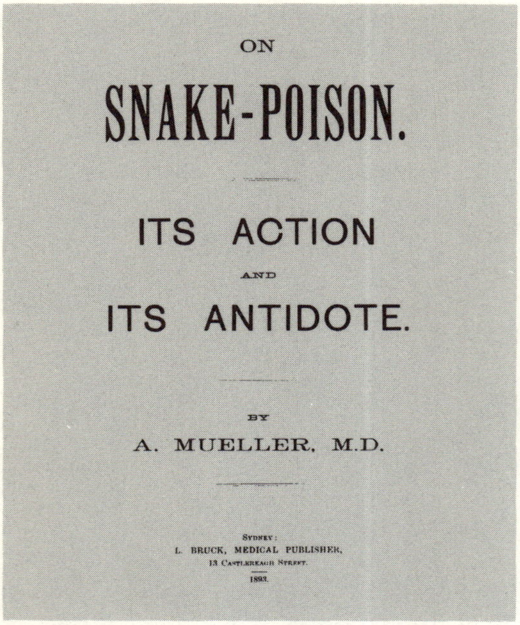

ON

SNAKE-POISON.

ITS ACTION

AND

ITS ANTIDOTE.

BY

A. MUELLER, M.D.

SYDNEY:
L. BRUCK, MEDICAL PUBLISHER,
13 CASTLEREAGH STREET.
1893.

[1420] Augustus Mueller's *On snake poison*, 1893. *Copy*: KFR

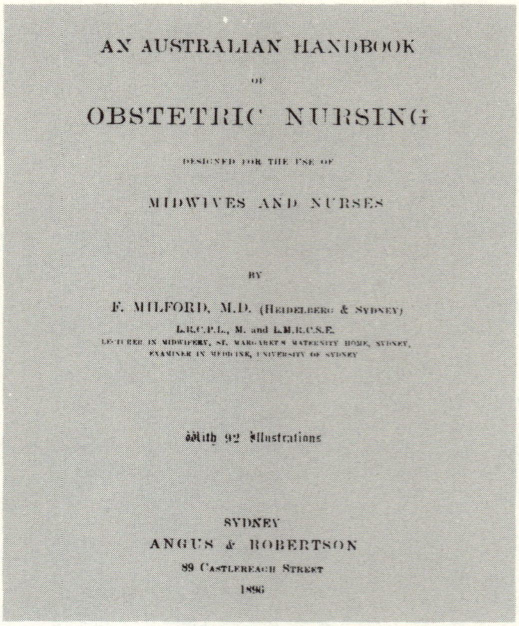

AN AUSTRALIAN HANDBOOK

OF

OBSTETRIC NURSING

DESIGNED FOR THE USE OF

MIDWIVES AND NURSES

BY

F. MILFORD, M.D. (HEIDELBERG & SYDNEY)
L.R.C.P.L., M. and L.M.R.C.S.E.
LECTURER IN MIDWIFERY, ST. MARGARET'S MATERNITY HOME, SYDNEY,
EXAMINER IN MEDICINE, UNIVERSITY OF SYDNEY

With 92 Illustrations

SYDNEY
ANGUS & ROBERTSON
89 CASTLEREAGH STREET
1896

[1338] Frederick Milford's *Australian handbook of obstetric nursing*, 1896—earliest local manual on its subject. *Copy*: EF

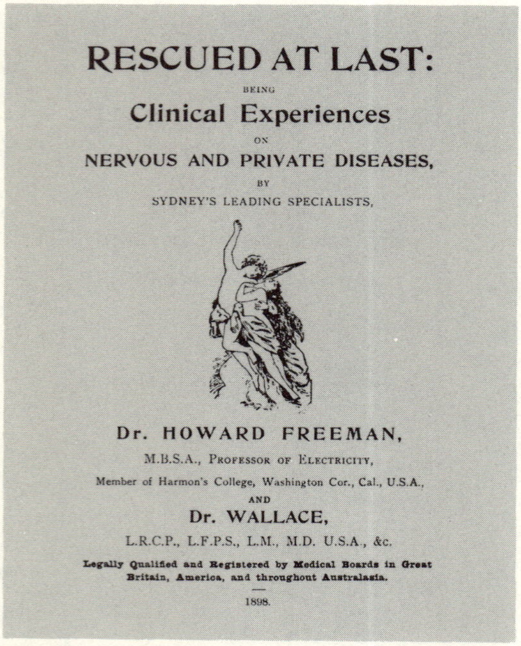

RESCUED AT LAST:

BEING

Clinical Experiences

ON

NERVOUS AND PRIVATE DISEASES,

BY

SYDNEY'S LEADING SPECIALISTS,

Dr. HOWARD FREEMAN,
M.B.S.A., PROFESSOR OF ELECTRICITY,
Member of Harmon's College, Washington Cor., Cal., U.S.A.,
AND
Dr. WALLACE,
L.R.C.P., L.F.P.S., L.M., M.D. U.S.A., &c.
Legally Qualified and Registered by Medical Boards in Great Britain, America, and throughout Australasia.
1898.

[694] Howard Freeman and Richard Wallace, *Rescued at last*, 1898. *Copy*: KFR

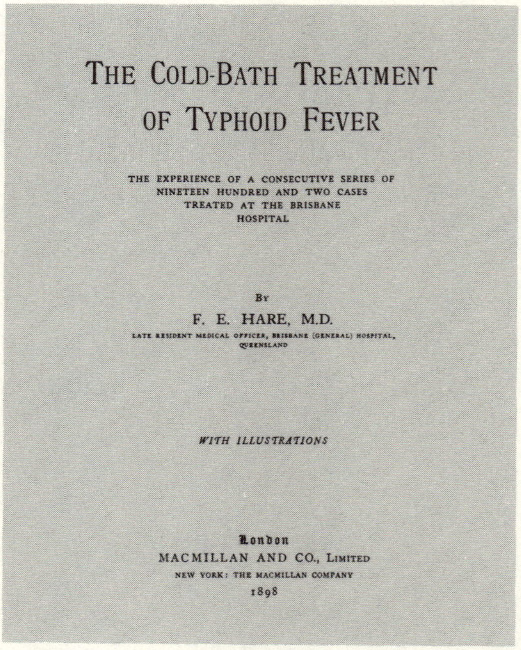

THE COLD-BATH TREATMENT
OF TYPHOID FEVER

THE EXPERIENCE OF A CONSECUTIVE SERIES OF
NINETEEN HUNDRED AND TWO CASES
TREATED AT THE BRISBANE
HOSPITAL

BY

F. E. HARE, M.D.
LATE RESIDENT MEDICAL OFFICER, BRISBANE (GENERAL) HOSPITAL,
QUEENSLAND

WITH ILLUSTRATIONS

London
MACMILLAN AND CO., LIMITED
NEW YORK: THE MACMILLAN COMPANY
1898

[1841] Francis E. Hare's *The cold-bath treatment of typhoid fever*, 1898. *Copy*: UM

———

The Emigrant: A tale of Australia. ... London: ... Simmonds and Ward ... Bucklersbury. 1847.

224 × 138. Pp. [iv], 228, [iv] (book notices, l.b.). Cloth.

The first novel associated with SA. See Miller, 1 : 402.

Copies: FC, LNSW, ML, NL, SLS, SLV, UM. 1152

Lendon, Alfred Austin

Myositis ossificans. ... (With six illustrations.) Reprinted from the Transactions of the First Intercolonial Medical Congress ... Adelaide ... 1887. Adelaide: ... Webb, Vardon, & Pritchard ... 1887.

231 × 147. Pp. 14. 6 litho. pl. P. w. (title rptd).

Copies: EF, KFR, ML, RACP, UA. 1153

———

Clinical lecture on a case of pernicious anaemia cured by bone marrow ... Reprinted from "The Intercolonial Quarterly Journal of Medicine and Surgery", August 1895. Melbourne: Stillwell and Co. ...

204 × 127. Pp. 8 (l.b.). P. w. (cover title).

Copies: NL. 1154

———

Clinical lectures on hydatid disease. ... First series. (Reprinted from "The Australasian Medical Gazette".) Sydney: L. Bruck ... 1896.

185 × 128. Pp. 48 (last 3 blank). P. w. (title rptd).

Author edited *Hydatid Disease*, vol. 2, by J. Davies Thomas.

For A. A. Lendon (1857–1935) MD Lond. & Adel., Hon. Phys. Adel. Hosp., Hon. Surg. Adel. Children's Hosp., see obits, *Med. J. Aust.*, 1935, 2 : 607 and *Proc. Roy. Geog. Soc. (SA) Austsia*, 1936, 36 : 20.

Later publications: *Clinical lectures in hydatid disease of the lungs*, Lond., 1902; *Nodal fever*, Lond., 1905.

Copies: UA. 1155

———

See South Australia—Parliament, No 1985; Thomas, John Davies, No 2186.

Lepper, Sophie

The "Lepper" dietary cure A remedial and curative system, obviating the use of drugs, and nowise weakening the system. By Fräulein Lepper. Late of ... Hannover, Germany, now of ... Kew, Melbourne ... Price—one guinea. Melbourne: Pater & Knapton ... 1889.

214 × 138. Pp. x, 11–36. Woodcut portrait. P. w. (title decorated).

Copies: CC, EF, ML, NL, SLV. 1156

Lesson, René Primèvere

Voyage médical autour du monde, exécuté sur la Corvette du Roi *La Coquille*, commandée par M. L. I. Duperrey, pendant les années 1822, 1823, 1824 et 1825; ou rapport sur l'etat sanitaire de l'equipage ... suivi d'un mémoire sur les races humaines répandues dans l'Océanie, la Malaisie et l'Australie; par R. P. Lesson. ... Paris, Roret, Libraire ... 1829.

217 × 135. Pp. [viii], 244. P. w. (paper label on spine).

Official health report of ship's company, with medical notes on places visited. The ship was at Port Jackson for about two months in 1824. Account of sojourn includes notes on current diseases. Measles and scarlatina were absent; dysentery reigned in summer; chest troubles prevalent. The smallpox epidemic in natives about Sydney in 1789 is discussed. Diseases and degeneration of local aborigines are described and cranial measurements listed.

R. P. Lesson (1794–1849), naturalist, combined this post with that of surgeon in *La Coquille*. See *Biographie Universelle* (Michaud), nouvelle ed., 24 : 330; for other publications: Ferguson, vols 1–4; also Royle, H. G. (1973), 'The state of health in NSW in the 1820's', *Med. J. Aust.*, 1 : 950.

Copies: EF, ML, NL, SLV. 1157

Lewers, Alexander

A plea for rational, if old-fashioned, diet. ... [Text begins.]

206 × 132. Pp. 4. P. w. Repr., *Aust. med. J.*, 1894, ns 16 : 561.

For Alexander Lewers MRCS, LRCP, DPH, who practised at Creswick Vic. and was later Hon. Phys. St Vincent's Hosp., Melb., see *Med. J. Aust.*, 1924, 1 : 379. In 1915 he published *Medicine and meditation*, Melb., Ford & Son.

Copies: EF. 1158

Lewisham Hospital, Sydney

The Little Company of Mary Nursing Sisters, 12 Roslyn Street, off William Street North. The

Nursing Sisters, who have recently come ... from their Central House in Rome ... [Text continues.]

255 × 204. Single leaf, v.b. ND. (1885 or 1886.)

Announces proposed establishment of convent and institution for blind at Petersham.

Copies: Lewisham Hosp. 1159

First annual report for year ending 30th June, 1890. Presented ... 6th August, 1890. [Text continues.]

204 × 127. Pp. 16 (l.b.). NI.

Hospital founded by Nursing Sisters of the Little Company of Mary; opened 9 June 1889.

Copies: Lewisham Hosp. (1890–), ML (1899). 1160

Lhotsky, John

A journey from Sydney to the Australian Alps, undertaken in the months of January, February, and March, 1834. Being an account of the geographical & natural relation of the country traversed, its aborigines, &c. together with some general information respecting the Colony of New South Wales. By Dr. John Lhotsky, Colonist, N. S. Wales, F.R. Bot. S. Bavaria, etc. Sydney: 1835. Sold by J. Innes, Bookseller, Pitt-Street. London:- By commission at R. Ackerman's Repository of Arts, Strand.

214 × 132. Pp. [iv], 3–110, 111–118. Printed at the Australian and Sydney Gazette Offices. Published originally in parts, later collected with above title, prior to completion of the series.

Author travelled through present Aust. Capital Territory—of which he gives the first printed account—and the Monaro District, to the vicinity of Cooma (Kuma). The work, as others below, has no medical content.

Also published: *Illustrations of the present state and future prospects of the Colony of New South Wales*, by an Impartial Observer, Syd., 1835; *Information for the people*, nos 1–3, Hobart Town, [1837].

John Lhotsky (b. 1800) MD Vienna, naturalist and physician, came to NSW in 1833. He travelled widely, probably practised medicine at times, and led a life of want and discontent. In 1836 he moved to Hobart, returning to London in 1838. For biog., see Whitley, G. P., *Aust. Dict. Biog.*, 2 : 114; also Iredale, T. (1924), 'Lhotksy's lament', *Aust. Zoologist*, 3 : 223; MacPherson, J. (1938), 'The turbulent Doctor Lhotsky', *Med. J. Aust.*, 1 : 661.

Copies: DL (pp. 96), ML (pp. 111–118 photo copies). 1161

Liernur, Charles T.

Pneumatic drainage: being some account of the pneumatic system of drainage invented by Captain Liernur. Sydney: Thomas Richards, Govt Printer. 1884.

196 × 145. Pp. [iv] (l.b.), 36. P. w. (title rptd).

About 1880 the Sanitary Reform League, founded in Sydney for improvement of sewage disposal, opposed official scheme of sea disposal of sewage at Bondi and reviewed other measures, including system here described.

Copies: ML, SLV. 1162

Lindeman, Henry John

A few words upon the Wine Bill now before the House, and upon wine matters generally ... [Text begins.]

209 × 132. Pp. 8. ND. Colophon—Gibbs, Shallard and Co. ... Sydney.

For H. J. Lindeman (1811–81) MRCS, founder of the Aust. wine industry, see *Aust. men of mark*, 1889, 2 : 141; *NSW med. Gaz.*, 1871, 1 : 311, and 1874, 4 : 217; Lake, M. (1967), *Vine and scalpel*, Bris.

Copies: ML. 1163

Litchfield, William Frederick

The infants under "The New South Wales Children's Protection Act", with some remarks on infants' asylums. .. [Text begins.]

229 × 165. Pp. 4. Repr., *Austsn med. Gaz.*, 1899.

On the cause and remedy of the high mortality rate in illegitimate infants, with discussion of foundling hospitals and infants' homes.

For W. F. Litchfield (1869–1922) MB Syd., Hon. Phys. Syd. Hosp. for Sick Children, see obit., *Med. J. Aust.*, 1922, 2 : 49; Hipsley, P. L. (1952), *The early history of Roy. Alexandra Hosp. for Children*, Syd. Published: *Diphtheria in practice*, Syd., 1908.

Copies: US. 1164

See also Clubbe, Sir Charles P. B. and Litchfield, W. F.

Little, Robert

Practical observations on the treatment of the epidemic scarlet-fever, recently so prevalent and fatal in New South Wales, by Robert Little, M.D., late Professor of Midwifery and the Diseases of Females and Children, in the Royal Belfast College; Physician to the Belfast Hospital, Lying-in Charity; Dispensary for the Diseases of Females and Children, etc. Sydney: Printed and published by James Tegg, George-street; opposite the Barrack Gate. 1842.

217 × 140. Pp. 36 (l.b.).

The second locally published contribution to clinical medicine. On the first epidemic of scarlet fever reported in Australia, which spread widely and with high mortality. Bland's earlier pamphlet (1841) on the subject also refers. Treatment is exhaustively discussed; prevention is by isolation, free ventilation, and cleanliness.

A preliminary notice of the work (*Colonial Observer*, 29 June 1842) announced price as 1s 6d. Author was then in practice at Hunter St., Sydney.

The unique Dixson Library copy is inscribed: 'From the Author 16th June, 1842.'

Copies: DL. 1165

Little, William

A visit to Topos, and how the science of heredity is practised there ... Ballarat: Berry, Anderson & Co. ... 1897.

183 × 125. Pp. 28. P. w. (title rptd).

A utopian tale of heredity in an imaginary land, by an ex-mayor of Ballarat.

Copies: FC, ML, OL. 1166

Little Company of Mary Nursing Sisters

See Lewisham Hospital.

Liversidge, Archibald

1875. Legislative Assembly. New South Wales. Report to the Sewage and Health Board, upon the Sydney City and Suburban Water Supply. By A. Liversidge, F.C.S., F.G.S., ... Sydney University. ... Sydney: Thomas Richards, Govt Printer. 1875.

342 × 220. Pp. 20.

Chemical analysis of Sydney water supplies, indicating gross contamination.

Copies: EF, ML, NL, SLV. 1167

———

1875. Legislative Assembly. New South Wales. Second Report to the Sewage and Health Board, upon the Sydney City and Suburban Water Supply. ... Sydney: Thomas Richards, Govt Printer. 1875.

346 × 209. Pp. 6.

Water analyses of Sydney sources.

Prof. Archibald Liversidge (1847–1927) FRS, a prolific scientific author, was Prof. Chem. Univ. Syd.

Copies: EF, ML, US. 1168

———

The alkaloid from piturie. ... (Read before the Royal Society of N.S.W., 3 November, 1880.)

209 × 135. Pp. 10. Colophon—Syd.: Thomas Richards, Govt Pr—1880. P. w. (short title).

From *J. & P. Roy. Soc. NSW*, 1880–1, 14 : 123. For piturie, aboriginal stimulant, see papers of Joseph Bancroft.

Copies: EF, LNSW, ML, US. 1169

Loir, Adrien

... Pasteur's vaccine of anthrax in Australia as a preventative against Cumberland disease in sheep, cattle, and horses. By Adrien Loir, Attache a l'Institut Pasteur de Paris. Sydney: C. F. Maxwell (Hayes Brothers) ...

250 × 153. Pp. 10. 3 figs. ND. [?1890.] P. w. (short title, fig.).

Includes history of Pasteur's classical vaccine, its trial at Junee NSW in 1888, and method of use. See also Nos 1481–3.

Copies: FC, ML, NL. 1170

———

La microbiologie en Australie Études d'hygiène & de pathologie comparée poursuivies a l'Institut Pasteur de Sydney par Adrien Loir ... Directeur de l'Institut Pasteur Australien Paris G. Steinheil, Éditeur ... 1892.

242 × 153. Pp. [iv] (ii blank), 96 (4, 8 blank). 12 figs. P. w. (title rptd). Dedicated to Pasteur and others.

Includes: Pasteur's rabbit destruction method (fowl cholera); anthrax vaccination; various diseases of rabbits and cattle; cattle quarantine.

Review (*Austsn med. Gaz.*, 1892, 11 : 391) objects to use of 'l'Institut Pasteur Australien' in title, stating that Loir was allowed to use the Govt laboratory on Rodd Is., Syd. Harbour, built for the Rabbit Commission trials, and to call this a Pasteur Institute is 'entirely devoid of foundation.' This is not to be confused with the short-lived Pasteur Inst. established at Double Bay, Sydney by Dr. E. Rougier in 1898, for supply of calf vaccine.

Adrien Loir (d. 1942) MD Paris, nephew and asst of Pasteur, came to Sydney in 1888 as leader of a mission representing Pasteur in a competition for a prize of £25,000 offered by NSW Govt for a method of exterminating rabbits. Their entry, using fowl cholera, was not accepted as a practical measure. Loir remained in Aust. 1888–93, engaged mainly on anthrax and pleuro-pneumonia vaccination. See his autobiographical *A l'Ombre de Pasteur*, Paris, 1938; also Pasteur, Louis, Nos 1648–9.

Copies: EF, LNSW, ML, NL, OL, SLV. 1171

———

See Bruce, Alexander and Loir, A.

Lombard, Henri Clermond

Traite de climatologie medicale comprenant la meteorologie medicale et l'etude des influences physiologiques, pathologiques, prophylactiques et therapeutiques du climat sur la sante ... Tome I Paris Libraire J. B. Bailliere et Fils ... 1877

4 vols. 217 × 135. Vol. 1, pp. xxiv, 556; vol. 2, pp. [iv], 696; vol. 3, pp. [iv], 772 (l.b.); vol. 4, pp. [iv], 688. Vols 1, 2 : 1877; vol. 3 : 1879; vol. 4 : 1880. Cloth.

Vol. 4 contains section on Aust., Tas. and NZ. Each is dealt with under: geography, climatology, ethnography, demography, and pathology.

Copies: SLV. 1172

Lower Murray District Hospital, Swan Hill, Vic.

See Swan Hill District Hospital.

Lucadou-Wells, Arthur

See Wells, Arthur Lucadou—.

Lucas, Thomas Pennington

The laws of life and alcohol. ... London: William Tweedie & Co. ... 1877.

178 × 122. Pp. xvi, 17–96. Cloth.

Copies: NL, SLV, UQ. 1173

———

My hospital campaign; or reasons against prescribing indiscriminately alcoholic beverages for the sick. ... Melbourne: Mason, Firth & M'Cutcheon ... 1883.

214 × 138. Pp. 20 (l.b.). P. w. (title rptd).

A criticism of excessive use of alcohol at Melb. Hosp. Lucas contested the elective position of Hon. Phys. to the Hosp. with a view to demonstrating the greater success obtainable with treatment without alcohol, but was defeated.

Copies: ML, NL, SLV. 1174

———

Cries from Fiji and sighings from the South Seas. "Crush out the British slave trade." Being a review of the social, political, and religious relations of the Fijians; a consideration of the policy of the English government; the prospects of the white settlers; the labour traffic; and the position and duties of England to the islands of the Pacific. ... Melbourne. Dunn & Collins ...

181 × 117. Pp. 124. Errata slip. ND. [1884.] Cloth.

Denounces Melanesian labour trade, mentioning heavy mortality in native workers.

Copies: DL, EF, FC, ML, NL, SLS, SLT, SLV, SLW, UQ, US, WLC. 1175

———

Life, and how to live: or, how to avoid the doctors. ... Melbourne ...

181 × 117. Pp. 10. ND. Colophon—Donaldson & Hartley ... Emerald Hill. P. w. (title rptd).

Copies: SLV. 1176

———

Do thyself no harm. A lecture to men ... Delivered to Young Men's Christian Association, Melbourne. ...

165 × 102. Pp. 52 (l.b.). ND. (1885.) P. w. (title rptd). Colophon—Mason, Firth and M'Cutcheon ... Melb.

Copies: CC, EF, FC, SLV. 1177

———

Creation and the cross. The harmony of science and revelation. ... Essays and song. Melbourne: Cassell & Company ...

188 × 122. Pp. vi, 7–256. (1886.) Cloth.

Copies: ML, NL, SLV, UQ. 1178

———

The curse and its cure, in two volumes. ... Vol. 1. The ruins of Brisbane, in the year 2000. ... Brisbane, J. H. Reynolds ... 1894.

181 × 120. Vol. 1: pp. 160; vol. 2 : pp. 160 (last advt), with sub-title 'Brisbane rebuilt in

the year 2200.'
An allegorical novel.
Copies: ML, NL, SLV. 1179

———

Social science snobbism, a plea for fair play. . . . To the public of Brisbane. [Text continues.]
220 × 143. Pp. 16. ND. (after 1894.) Colophon—Reynolds, Printer, Brisbane.
Written for a science congress in Brisbane. Author claims it was not allowed to be read because of his attack 'on the unscientific, inhuman ice-bath treatment for typhoid fever.'
T. P. Lucas (1843–1917) LRCP, MRCS, FLS, FES, of Emerald Hill Vic. and later Brisbane, engaged in social and religious work, published in entomology and poetry, and advocated use of paw-paw ferments for cancer and other ailments. See obit., *Proc. Roy. Soc. Qd*, 1918, 30 : 2; Kellow, H. A., *Queensland poets*, Lond., 1930.
Published after 1900: *Domestic medicine*, Bris., 1906 (includes biog. details); *Pawpaw treatment versus German kultur*, Bris., ND.; *The most wonderful tree in the world, the pawpaw tree*, Bris., ND.
Copies: ML. 1180

———

See International Temperance Conference, 1880.

Lumholtz, Carl
Among cannibals An account of four years' travels in Australia and of camp life with the aborigines of Queensland . . . with maps, coloured plates, and 122 illustrations London John Murray . . . 1889.
225 × 157. Pp. xx, 396 (l.b.). 29 pl., text figs., 2 maps. Cloth.
Includes references to food, childbirth, infanticide, ailments and treatment, subincision, medicine men, and population decrease in tribes of the Diamentina and Herbert River districts, Qd.
Author spent four years in Queensland, from Nov. 1880, in zoological and anthropological field work for Univ. Christiania.
Copies: DL, EF, ML, OL, US. 1181

———

The Same. New York, Scribner's Sons, 1889.
Copies: DL, NL, US. 1182

———

The Same. Lond., John Murray; Syd. & Melb., E. A. Petherick; 1890.
Copies: ML, NL. 1183

Lurz, Albin
Ueber die Anwendung der Electricität in der Medicin. Würzburg, C. J. Becker. 1872.
8vo. Pp. 23.
NS. Listed *SGC*, ser. 1.
1184

———

Aphorisms on electricity in medical science. Its worth, indications, and employment; its abuse, and prejudices against its use; points of view. . . . Melbourne: M'Carron, Bird & Co. . . . 1886.
214 × 140. Pp. 22 (l.b.). P. w. (title rptd).
Copies: LNSW, ML. 1185

———

Massage (rubbing treatment). Translated from the Rhenish Westphalian Journal. Melbourne, 1886.
12mo. Pp. 6.
NS. Listed *SGC*, ser. 2.
1186

———

Some remarks on the frequent occurrence of thickenings and callous indurations in chronic rheumatic and traumatic affections of the muscular system. Sydney: L. Bruck, 1886.
12mo. Pp. 8.
NS. Listed *SGC*, ser. 2.
1187

———

On rheumatism and its cure. . . . (Electro-therapeutics, medical gymnastics, and massage.) Melbourne 1886.
214 × 134. Pp. 16 (last—book list). Colophon— M'Carron, Bird and Co. . . . Melb.
'A brief outline of the various . . . rheumatic joint and muscle affections.'
Copies: ML, OL. 1188

———

On combined electric & rubbing treatment (massage) in nervous, rheumatic & joint affections. A practical sketch . . . Cook, Duerre and Co. . . . Melbourne.
178 × 125. Pp. 32. ND. P. w. (title rptd).
Copies: LNSW, ML, SLV. 1189

Indigestion and nervous dyspepsia. Their origin and cure. (Dietetic and hygienic) ... Melbourne: F. C. Cook ... 1897.

214 × 134. Pp. 166. P. w. (amended title).

Albin Lurz MD Würzburg (1872), Staff Surg., German Army, arrived in Melb. in 1884 and practised there for about 20 years as specialist in electrotherapy, medical gymnastics and massage.

Noted as published in works by author, but not seen: *Nervous weakness (neurasthenia) and its successful treatment*, Melb., Robertson; *On paralysis*, Melb., Robertson; *Nervous pain (neuralgia, sciatica, etc.) and its removal*, Melb., Robertson; *Electricity in the service of medicine*, transl. from German; *About joint affections (sprains, strains, etc.)*, Melb., Robertson; *Weltreise-Skizzen*, Dresden, W. Baensch, 1903.

Copies: ML, NL. 1190

Lying-in Hospital of N.S.W.

See Benevolent Society of N.S.W. (note), No 257.

Lyman, H. M., Jones, H. W., Fenger, C., and Belfield, W. T.

Australasian edition. The practical home physician and encyclopedia of medicine: a guide for the household management of disease; giving the history, cause, means of prevention, and symptoms of all diseases of men, women and children, and ... treatment, with ... care of the sick. ... Specially revised and adapted to the colonies of Australia, Tasmania and New Zealand. World Publishing Co. London, Sydney, Melbourne and Christichurch.

236 × 161. Pp. vii-xx, 2–1128 (l.b.), [24], 1129–1142. 37 pl. (16 coloured, 2 with movable superimposed parts), 9 figs. ND. [c. 1888.] Leather.

Copies: BG, KFR, SLV. 1191

M

M., A. C.
See Moon, Alice Caroline.

M., H. D.
How to deal with the refuse of our cities. By H.D.M. T. Dimmock . . . Maitland.
217 × 138. Pp. 16. ND. (1886.) P. w. (title rptd).
Deplores 'barbarian usages' in urban excreta disposal in NSW, and discusses suitable methods.
Copies: ML. 1192

M., J. T.
What to do in cases of accident and everyday complaints. A manual of plain treatment and ready remedies for cases of emergency. By J.T.M. . . . Sydney: James Miller & Co. . . . 1883 . . .
183 × 110. Pp. 33, [15] (advts). Cloth.
Copies: EF, ML, RACP. 1193

———

The Same. 2 ed., 1884.
Copies: ML. 1194

M. B., An
What is homoeopathy? with simple directions for the treatment of common complaints. By an "M.B." Published and sold at the Homoeopathic Pharmacy, Hobart Town, Tasmania.
181 × 125. Pp. (ii), 24, [2] (v.b.).
Copies: CC, SLT. 1195

M. P., An
Compulsory vaccination. Weighed and found wanting. An array of facts and figures *versus* fads and follies. . . . Compiled by an M. P. Tasmania: . . . "Tasmanian News" Office . . . Hobart.
231 × 143. Pp. [iv], 24 (l.b.). ND. (1888.) P. w. (title rptd).
Copies: ML, WLC. 1196

M.R.C.S.E., An
See Beaney, James George, No 212.

Maberly, G. F.
See Electric and Thermopathic Institute, Melb.

MacAdam, John
Testimonials in favour of John MacAdam, Esq. F.R.S.S.A. analytical chemist, and lecturer on theoretical and practical chemistry . . .
204 × 132. Pp. 18 (l.b.). NI. ND. (Items dated 1845–7.)
Copies: ML. 1197

———

Chemistry. Tables, introductory to a course of testing, in qualitative and quantitative analysis. . . . Richard Griffin & Co., London and Glasgow. 1853.
204 × 130. Pp. 24. 2 flg tables.
Copies: ML. 1198

———

A statement submitted to the Council of the Philosophical Institute of Victoria, in reference to a correspondence between Professor McCoy and the Honorary Secretary . . . upon a paper entitled "Museums in Victoria". . . . August, 1857.
204 × 130. Pp. 16. Colophon—Melb. . . . Goodhugh and Hough . . .
Report on a controversy between Prof. Frederick McCoy and MacAdam, Sec. (who signs at end).
Copies: ML, SLV. 1199

———

Report of chemical examination & analyses of waters in the vicinity of Geelong. Scotch College, Melbourne, 28th January, 1857. [Text begins.]
204 × 130. Pp. 12 (l.b.). Colophon—Goodhugh & Hough . . . Melb. P. w.
John MacAdam (1827–65) MD Glas. & Melb., MLA, came to Melb. in 1855. His many appointments included Vic. Govt Analyst, MOH Melb., Lect., Chem. Univ. Melb. Obit.: *Aust. med. J.*, 1865, 10 : 327.
Copies: ML, SLV. 1200

McAlpine, D.

Department of Agriculture, Victoria. Report on a poisonous species of Homeria (Homeria Collina, Vent.—var. Miniata) found at Pascoe Vale, causing death of cattle feeding upon it . . . March, 1893. . . . Robt. S. Brain, Govt Printer, Melbourne.

217 × 134. Pp. 16 (l.b.). 1 flg coloured litho. pl.

Experimental proof of the lethal effect of imported *Homeria*, (Cape tulip).

Copies: SLV, UM. 1201

McCarthy, Charles

On the excessive mortality of infants and its causes. With statistical tables. . . . Read before the Medical Society of Victoria, November 2, 1864, and February 8, 1865. Melbourne: George Robertson . . . 1865.

213 × 135. Pp. 28. 17 tables. P. w. (title rptd).

Infant mortality could be halved by attack on preventable causes—improper diet and clothing, impure air and poor medical care.

Copies: ML, NL, SLV. 1202

———

The Same. 2 ed., 1871. Contains 1 ed., to which is added pp. [29]–32, 4 tables. Read before Med. Assn of Vic., Nov. 11, 1870.

Copies: ML, NL, SLV. 1203

———

Dipsomania or drink-craving Its history, nature, consequences, treatment, and cure . . . Reprinted from the "Melbourne Review" George Robertson Melbourne, Sydney, and Adelaide 1881.

212 × 140. Pp. 16. P. w. (title rptd).

Though Vic. Govt had passed the first Inebriates Act in the world, it had not kept a promise to support an inebriates' institution. State aid is suggested for Northcote Retreat.

Copies: ML, NL. 1204

———

On inebriate retreats: their origin, utility, necessity, and management, showing the result of thirty years' study of the subject, and fifteen years' practical management of the Melbourne Inebriate Retreat, the first in the world having legal compulsory power. By the founder, Charles M'Carthy, M.D. . . . with a short autobiography of the author . . . Melbourne: Stillwell and Co. . . . 1888.

214 × 130. Pp. 72. P. w. (title rptd).

Includes arguments against his projected dismissal from the Retreat, following its assumption by Govt.

Copies: CC, EF, ML. 1205

———

The Royal Commission on Asylums for the Insane and Inebriate: its evidence and report, and the legislation based thereon. . . . The Northcote Retreat is the first in the world having legal power of voluntary and compulsory admittance and detention . . . Melbourne: Stillwell and Co. . . . 1889.

250 × 134. Pp. 32 (l.b.).

Copies: SLV. 1206

———

The Inebriate Retreat Northcote (Copy of letter to the Hon. A McLean, M.L.A., Chief Secretary). . . . April 27, 1891. [Text begins.]

204 × 127. Pp. 12. Colophon—Melb.: Echo Publishing Company . . . North Fitzroy, and . . . Elizabeth Street. 1891.

Protest against closure of Retreat, with outline of events.

For Charles McCarthy (1814–96) MD Melb., LFPS Glas., founder and proprietor of Melb. Inebriate Retreat, see his *On inebriate retreats* . . . (1888); *Austsn med. Gaz.*, 1896, 15 : 119; also items under Melb. Retreat for Cure of Inebriates.

Copies; ML. 1207

———

The Lunacy Bill and inebriate legislation. Melbourne. 1885.

NS. Pp. 4. SLV cat.

———

See Melbourne Retreat for the Cure of Inebriates.

MacCarthy, Charles William

Effects of secular music on mind and morals. . . . read before the first Australasian Catholic Congress . . . Sydney, September, 1900.

220 × 138. Pp. 16. P. w. (title rptd; Matthews & Co. . . . Syd.—added).

For C. W. MacCarthy MD, FRCSI, Hon. Surg. St Vincent's Hosp. Syd., see *Aust. men of mark* (1889), 2 : 205.

Copies: ML. 1208

McConnel, Mrs. Mary

Our Children's Hospital A story of twenty-one years 1876 to 1897 by Mrs. David C. McConnel Published by Thomas Brothers . . . Brisbane.

210 × 135. Pp. 26 (l.b.). 8 pl. On verso of title p.—Bris.: H. J. Diddams & Co., Printers. 1897. Textured p. w. (shortened title).

History of Brisbane Hosp. for Sick Children (opened Feb. 1878) to 1897, by founder and first Pres. See also Fison, D. C. (1970), *History of Royal Children's Hosp., Brisbane*, Bris. Name was changed to Brisbane Children's Hosp. in 1943; to Royal Children's Hosp., 1967.

Copies: OL. 1209

MacCormick, Sir Alexander

See Stuart, Sir T. P. Anderson, and MacCormick, Sir A.

McCrae, Farquhar

Election of medical officers to the Sydney Infirmary and Dispensary.

203 × 130. Pp. xi, 12–24. ND. [1845.] Colophon—Syd.: Printed by W. A. Duncan . . .

Farquhar McCrae (1806–50) MD, candidate for appointment to Syd. Infirmary, presents his testimonials (latest dated 1845) to electors. He became one of two first hon. surgeons to Infirmary.

McCrae, an army surgeon, came to Pt Phillip in 1839, and practised, first in Melbourne and later in Sydney. See Mackay, E. A. (1934), 'Med. men as pastoral pioneers', *Med. J. Aust.*, 2 : 476.

LNSW copy bears McCrae's inscription to James Norton.

Copies: FC, LNSW, ML. 1210

Correspondence between Dr. Farquhar M'Crae and Mr. Surgeon Bland, Sydney. Sydney: . . . Kemp and Fairfax, Lower George Street. 1846.

217 × 130. Pp. 18 (l.b.).

Letters from *Syd. Morning Herald* of March, 1846, republished by McCrae as 'an appeal to the profession' in a dispute arising from Bland's consultation with him on a surgical case. Newspaper publication was resorted to 'in consequence of there being no medical association or publication here . . .' For Bland's reply, see No 338.

Copies: ML, NL, SLV. 1211

McCrea, William

Observations on typhoid fever . . . Melbourne: Samuel Mullen . . . 1879.

198 × 127. Pp. 24 (l.b.).

On cause, pathology, symptoms and treatment; urges use of cold baths in treatment. Review, *Aust. med. J.*, 1879, ns 1 : 295.

For William McCrae (1814–99) MB Lond. & Melb., MRCS, who was in charge of Vic. health administration from 1855 to 1879, see 'Health administration in Vic., 1834–1934', *Health Bulletin*, 1935, 42 : 1180; *Aust. med. J.*, 1879, ns 1 : 343; *Austsn med. Gaz.*, 1899, 18 : 175.

See also items under: Vic.—Cent. Bd of Health, and Vic.—Parliament.

Copies: CC, ML, SLV. 1212

McDonnell, Aeneas John

The statistics and distribution of hydatid disease in the Australian colonies.

218 × 140. Pp. 58 (4, l.b.). 5 maps (2 flg). ND. [1896.] NI. P. w. (cover title).

Collates Aust. statistics (1884–94) and shows disease is increasing. Maps show distribution of 3,940 cases. Anon. author's thesis for MD Syd., 1896.

For A. J. McDonnell (1864–1939) MD, ChM Syd., FRACS, distinguished practitioner of Toowoomba Qd, see obit., *Med. J. Aust.*, 1939, 2 : 816.

Copies: EF. 1213

The Same. 1896. Pp. [ii] (title, v.b.), [iv] (l.b.), [54] (l.b.). 5 maps. Title includes—by Aeneas J. McDonnell . . . Toowoomba: J. E. Stone, Printer . . . 1896. Cloth.

Copies: AMAQ. 1214

McGarvie Smith Institute

See Smith, John McGarvie.

Macgillivray, John

Narrative of the voyage of H.M.S. Rattlesnake . . . during the years 1846–1850. Including discoveries and surveys in New Guinea, the Louisiade Archipelago, etc. To which is added the account of Mr. E. B. Kennedy's Expedition for the exploration of the Cape York Peninsula. By John Macgillivray, F.R.G.S., Naturalist to the Expedition. . . . In two volumes. Vol. 1. London: T. & W. Boone . . . 1852.

2 vols. 216 × 140. Vol. 1 : pp. xii (l.b.), 402, 12 (book advts). plates, chart; vol. 2 : pp. vi (l.b.),

396 (l.b.), 8 (book advts), plates. Cloth.

Facsimile ed., Adel.: Libraries Bd of SA, 1967.

Includes references to foods, infanticide, diseases (including ague), and treatment of Aborigines.

John Macgillivray (1821–67), distinguished naturalist of three scientific expeditions in Aust. and New Guinea waters (1842–55), was elder brother of Paul H. (*infra*). He died in Sydney.

Copies: DL, FC, ML, NL, SLS, SLW, US. 1215

Macgillivray, Paul Howard

Hydatid disease. By P. H. MacGillivray, A. M., Surgeon to the Bendigo Hospital.

204 × 135. Pp. 20 (last—colophon). Colophon—Melb.: Wilson and Mackinnon ... (1866.)

At head of text: 'Hydatid disease, a second series of cases, with statistics of the disease in Victoria, and remarks on the causes of its increased frequency in certain localities. Read before the Medical and Chirurgical Society, April 24th, 1866. ...'

Copies: SLV, UA. 1216

On a case of hydatids in the orbit; with an abstract of cases of hydatid disease treated in the Bendigo Hospital. ... [Text begins.]

209 × 138. Pp. 12 (l.b.). ND. Repr. *Aust. med. J.*

Copies: SLV. 1217

Observations on enteric fever. ... [Text begins.]

209 × 138. Pp. 12. 6 charts. Colophon—Stillwell and Knight ... Repr., *Aust. med. J.*, August 1867.

Observations on 213 Bendigo cases.

Copies: SLV. 1218

Descriptions of some new genera and species of Australian Polyzoa; to which is added a list of species found in Victoria. ... Read before the Royal Society of Victoria, 26th November, 1868. Melbourne: Stillwell & Knight ... 1869.

204 × 130. Pp. 24. P. w. (cover title).

Copies: SLV. 1219

Medical and surgical papers ... Reprinted from the "Australian Medical Journal". Sandhurst: J. W. Pearson & Co. ... 1872.

206 × 132. Pp. [iv] (title, v.b.; contents), 44 papers, each with own pagination.

Papers published 1860–1872.

Copies: SLV. 1220

Inaugural address, delivered to the Bendigo School of Mines Society, June 20, 1881. Sandhurst: G. Young ...

212 × 132. Pp. 8. P. w. (cover title).

Copies: EF, ML, NL, SLS. 1221

(Issued February 21st, 1887.) Royal Society of Victoria. A catalogue of the marine Polyzoa of Victoria. ... Price one shilling.

217 × 138. Pp. 38. Colophon—Mason, Firth & M'Cutcheon ... Melb. P. w. (cover title).

P. H. Macgillivray (1834–95) MA, Hon LLD Aberd., MRCS, FLS, of Sandhurst, one of the foremost Vic. doctors of his time, was an authority on hydatid disease and had wide recognition as a naturalist. See *Austsn med. Gaz.*, 1895, 14 : 349; *Aust. med. J.*, 1895, ns 17 : 325; *Intercol med. J. Austsia*, 1896, 1 : 45; also (for hydatid disease), Graham, H. B. (1953), *Med. J. Aust.*, 1 : 869.

Copies: EF, SLS, SLV, UA. 1222

Macgregor, Sir William

Some notes on disease in British New Guinea. [Text begins.]

242 × 153. Pp. 6 (2 blanks). Repr., *Trans Intercol Med. Cong. Austsia*, 1889 : 46.

See also 'Disease and its treatment', in *Essays on the depopulation of Melanesia*, ed. W. H. Rivers, Cambridge, 1922.

Author's name also appears as MacGregor and McGregor.

Copies: EF, SLS, US. 1223

Handbook of information for intending settlers in British New Guinea. ... Brisbane: James C. Beal, Govt Printer. ... 1892.

220 × 142. Pp. [vi] (3 blanks), 34. Flg map. P. w. (title rptd).

'Health' at pp. 3–4. 'But for fever the country would be a very healthy one for Europeans; and the fever is not nearly so severe as is generally supposed.'

Copies: DL, EF, FC, NL, OL, SLS,

SLT, SLV. 1224

British New Guinea: country and people. By Sir William Macgregor, K.C.M.G., Lieutenant-Governor of British New Guinea. With map and illustrations. London: John Murray . . . 1897.

217 × 143. Pp. [viii], 100. Flg map. Paper boards.

Sir William Macgregor (1846–1919) MD Aberd., DSc, distinguished colonial administrator, after med. service in various tropical colonies (incl. CMO Fiji) became Administrator and later it Governor British NG (1888–98), and Governor Queensland (1909–14). See *Trans Roy. Soc. Trop. Med. & Hyg.*, 1925, 19 : 222; Joyce, R. B., *Sir Wm MacGregor*, Melb., 1971.

Copies: ML, NL, UQ, US. 1225

Mackay, Angus

The semi-tropical agriculturalist and colonists' guide. Plain words upon station, farm, and garden work, house keeping, and the useful pursuits of colonists. With directions for treating wounds, fevers, snake bite . . . Brisbane: Watson & Co. . . . 1875.

217 × 135. Pp. [ii], ii, iv, 224, [6] (advts). Figs. Cloth.

2 ed., 1890. bears title: *The Aust. agriculturalist and colonists' guide.* Sydney: J.W.R. Clarke. 3 ed., 1897, has title: *The Aust. agriculturalist and guide* . . . Melb.: George Robertson.

Includes section on med. help. 2 ed. contains: draining for health, medicinal plants, help in emergencies.

Copies: EF, ML, NL, OL, SLS, SLV, UA, UM, UQ, US. 1226

McKay, William John Stewart

Lawson Tait's perineal operations, and an essay on curettage of the uterus. . . . London: Bailliere, Tindall and Cox . . . 1897. . . .

209 × 135. Pp. x (l.b.), 11–70 (l.b.), 48 (advts). 16 figs. Cloth or paper boards.

The Same. US ed., 1898. Wm Wood & Co., N. Y.

Describes procedures for restoration of ruptured perineum. Author was assistant to Tait, who in preface states that 'writing was to me an intolerable labour.'

Copies: AMAN, AMAV, EF, FF, ML, SLV, UQ, US. 1227

Fifty cases of abdominal section, with two deaths. . . . Reprinted from the "Intercolonial Medical Journal of Australasia", December 20, 1897. Stillwell and Co. . . . Melbourne.

234 × 145. Pp. 20 (l.b.). P. w. (cover title).

W. J. Stewart McKay (1866–1948) MB, ChM Syd., Hon. Surg. Lewisham Hosp. Syd., who was assistant (later biographer) to Lawson Tait of Birmingham, was a prolific writer in many fields. See obit., Skirving, R. Scot (1948), *Med. J. Aust.*, 1 : 353; also Ford, E. (1967), *Med. J. Aust.*, 2 : 927.

Also published: *The history of ancient gynaecology*, Lond., 1901; *The preparation and after-treatment of section cases*, Lond., 1905, and US ed., N. Y., 1905; *Operations upon the uterus, perineum and round ligaments*, Lond., 1909, and US ed., N.Y., 1909; *Lawson Tait. His life and work*, Lond., 1922; *Racehorses in Australia* (with others), Syd., 1922; *Appendicitis*, Syd., 1936; *The evolution of the endurance, speed and staying power of the racehorse*, Lond., [1933]; 2 ed., 1937.

Copies: NL. 1228

Mackellar, Sir Charles Kinnaird

Testimonials in favour of Charles K. Mackellar, Bachelor of Medicine; Master in Surgery. [Text begins.]

252 × 204. Pp. 4 (l.b.). ND. NI.

Copies: RACP. 1229

1883. Legislative Assembly. New South Wales. Quarantine Station, North Head. (Report by Health Officer upon state and condition of, &c.) . . . [Text begins.]

320 × 204. Pp. 14. 5 plans. Colophon—Thomas Richards, Govt Pr—1883.

Recommends stations at Thursday Is. and King George's Sound as part of a federal quarantine service. Signed: Charles K. Mackellar, MD.

Copies: LNSW, ML, NL, SLV. 1230

Federal quarantine. . . . (Read before the Medical Section of the Royal Society of N.S.W., 20 July, 1883.) [Text begins.]

212 × 135. Pp. 14 (l.b.). Colophon—Syd. . . . Govt Pr—1883. P. w. (short title).

Sir Charles Mackellar (1844–1926) MB, ChM Glas., MLC, of Sydney, Pres. NSW Bd Health, Med. Adviser to Govt, was responsible for reforms in the care of neglected and delinquent children in NSW. Obit., *Med. J. Aust.*, 1926, 2 : 196.

Publications after 1900 include: *Parental rights and parental responsibility*, Syd., 1905; *The child, the law, and the state*, Syd., 1907; *The unwanted child*, Syd., 1913; *Evolution of humanitarianism in the treatment of juvenile delinquency*, Syd., 1915.

Copies: NL. 1231

———

See Austsn Sanitary Conference of Sydney; also Clark, Charles Dagnall.

Mackenna, J. William

Mortality of children in Victoria, with means for the prevention and cure of the diseases of children; being a treatise read before the Medical Society of Victoria, March 1, 1858, and enlarged and adapted for general circulation. ... Melbourne: W. Fairfax and Co. ... 1858.

201 × 130. Pp. 24 (last—book notices).

The heavy child mortality of Melbourne is due to prolonged hot dry weather, and cold water baths provide effective treatment for infantile diarrhoea and other serious diseases.

Pamphlet was attacked in *Aust. med. J.*, 1858, 3 : 211, and held by Med. Soc. Vic. to be unduly critical of Melb. doctors.

Copies: AMAV, LNSW, ML, NL, SLV. 2232

———

Mortality of children in Victoria. [Text begins.]

213 × 135. Pp. 16. Colophon—W. Fairfax ... Collins Street East. ND. (1859.)

Extends previous arguments for use of cold baths in fatal summer diseases of infants. Author states that this paper was rejected by *Aust. med. J.*, as insulting to the profession.

Copies: AMAV, NL, SLV. 1233

———

The causes of the diseases of children: with a comparative table of infantile mortality in the Australian Colonies. ... Melbourne: W. Fairfax and Co. ... 1859. ...

198 × 127. Pp. 16. P. w. (cover title).

Copies: NL. 1234

Mackenzie, Eneas

... Mackenzie's Australian emigrant's guide: giving faithful and important advice on the choice of a ship, outfit, preservation of health during the voyage ... with an account of the colony, and the gold diggings ... London: E. Mackenzie, Publisher ...

186 × 122. Pp. 32. ND. [1852.] P. w. (cover title, advts all other sides).

Includes section on health and dietary scale provided by law.

Copies: ML, NL, SLV. 1235

———

The emigrant's guide to Australia. With a memoir of Mrs. Chisholm. London: Clarke, Beeton, & Co. ...

163 × 102. Pp. [ii] (v.b.), vi (2 blanks), 3–188 (l.b.). Frontis. (portrait of Mrs. Chisholm). ND. [?1853.] Paper boards, with title and ship vignette.

Sections on Mrs. Chisholm's rules on board ship including med. comforts and health, surgeon's rules and regs, health on voyage, emigrant's med. chest.

Copies: CC, DL, FC, ML, NL. 1236

MacKenzie, Murdoch

Case of snake bite successfully treated with Calmette's remedy Describing symptoms, treatment, &c. With notes and comments ... Miles & Howell ... Korumburra.

132 × 105. Pp. 8 ND. [?1894.] P. w. (decorated cover title).

Severe snake-bite treated by subcutaneous injections of solution of bleaching powder.

M. MacKenzie FRCS was Dep. Med. Supt of Insane Hosps in Vic., and later practised at Dimboola, Korumburra and St Kilda Vic. In 1900 he was at Westport NZ.

Copies: SLV. 1237

Mackin, Charles Travers

1856 Report on the health and sanitary condition of the town and suburbs of Geelong. ... Geelong ... "Advertiser" Office. 1856.

171 × 110. Pp. 32.

The health of Geelong in earlier and present years, including climate, vital statistics, living conditions, infant mortality.

C. T. Mackin MD Glasgow, MRCS, was Hon. Surg. Geelong Hosp. and GMO Geelong, where he died in 1884. Obit.: *Austsn med. Gaz.*, 1884, 3 : 241.

Copies: ML, NL. 1238

———

A popular treatise on the constitutional origin of nervous disorders with practical hints on treatment—preventive, hygienic, and medical ... Melbourne George Robertson 1875

171 × 110. Pp. 100, P. w. (title rptd).

Copies: EF, ML, SLV, UA. 1239

MacKnight, Charles H. and Madden, Henry

On the true principles of breeding, developed in letters by Chas. H. MacKnight, Esq. and Dr. Henry Madden. Published by the ... Acclimatisation Society of Victoria. Melbourne: Wilson & Mackinnon ... 1865.

198 × 127. Pp. 42.

On advantages of in-breeding with sound stock (C. H. MacKnight); on in-breeding viewed physiologically (H. R. Madden MD).

Copies: LNSW, ML, NL, SLV. 1240

MacLaurin, Sir Henry Normand

1889. New South Wales. Legislative Council. Comparatve view of the mortality of the different colonies from certain diseases ... Address delivered at the Intercolonial Medical Congress ... [Text begins.]

331 × 214. Pp. 26.

Another issue: 1889, NSW Leg. Assembly, Syd., Govt Pr.

Comparative statistics, including tables of deaths from 40 most prevalent diseases in Aust. colonies and NZ.

Copies: LNSW, ML, NL, SLV. 1241

———

Report on sanitary legislation and administration in England. Sydney: Charles Potter, Govt Printer .... 1893.

278 × 220. Pp. [iv] (l.b.), 44. P. w. (title rptd).

Report on 'the various Acts in force in England relating to public health, with a view to the introduction of similar legislation in this Colony.'

Copies: EF, UM. 1242

———

Draft Federation Bill. Speech by Hon. H. N. MacLaurin, M.D., LL.D. ... From the "Parliamentary Debates", 5 August, 1897. [Text begins.]

244 × 147. Pp. 16. Double cols. Colophon—Syd.: William Applegate Gullick, Govt Pr—1897.

Sir Henry Normand MacLaurin (1835–1914) MD Edin., MLC, was Vice Chancr and later Chancr Univ. Syd., Pres. NSW Bd of Health and Med. Adviser to Govt. See *Med. J. Aust.*, 1914, 2 : 241; Mackerras, C. B. (1968), *JRAHS*, 54 : 265.

Copies: ML, NL. 1243

MacLaurin, Charles and Hunt, W. L.

The yachtsman's guide to Sydney Harbour and its neighbourhood. ... Illustrated. Sydney: W. R. Maclardy & Co. ... 1898.

178 × 115. Pp. [6] (advts), 69. 20 pl., 2 flg maps. P. w. (decorated title, cuts of yachts).

For Charles MacLaurin (1872–1925) MB, ChM Ed., FRCSE, of Sydney, Hon. Surg. Roy. Prince Alfred Hosp., see obit., *Med. J. Aust.*, 1925, 1 : 497. Also published: *Post mortem: essays historical and medical*, Lond., 1923; *Mere mortals: medico-historical essays*, Lond., 1925. These were republished with title: *De mortuis: essays historical and medical*, Lond., 1930.

Copies: ML, NL, SLV. 1243a

Maclay, Nicolaus N. Miklucho—, (or Miklouho—)

See Miklucho-Maclay, N. N.

McMurray, Wahab

A case of dermatitis herpetiformis, associated with hyperkeratosis of the palms and soles. Read before the N.S.W. Branch B.M.A. ... Reprinted from the "Australasian Medical Gazette" for September, 1893. L. Bruck ... Sydney. 1893.

229 × 165. Pp. 4 (l.b.). 1 coloured litho. pl.

Wahab McMurray MD QUI & Syd., Hon. Derm. Syd. Hosp., who in 1894 opened a dermatological dispensary for poor patients in Sydney, was a pioneer of radiotherapy in skin diseases and published the first Aust. reports on this subject (*Austsn med. Gaz.*, 1901, 20 : 9). See *Salute to the X-ray pioneers of Aust.*, Syd., 1946, for brief note; also Johnson, A. (1954), *Aust. J. Derm.*, 2 : 149.

Copies: US. 1244

McNeill, John Patrick

A treatise on hydrophobia ... London Henry Renshaw ... 1879.

186 × 120. Pp. viii (l.b.), 9–112 (l.b.). Cloth.

On canine and human infections. Pasteurian treatment was not introduced until 1885.

Copies: ML. 1245

———

A treatise upon the proper management, nursing

and dietary of infancy and childhood, and upon diseases of children, their diagnosis, management and treatment, adapted for the use of mothers or guardians of families. Giving ... full direction ... for the management, feeding and bringing up of a child ... Together with a short description of almost every ... complaint to which children are liable ... and so much of its ... treatment as the mother may safely venture upon ... Sydney: Jas. Miller & Co. ... 1888.

196 × 122. Pp. [viii] (l.b.), iv (l.b.), 232. Cloth.

J. P. McNeill, MD Dubl., LRCSI, practised at Burwood NSW (c. 1888–94).

Copies: AMAV, ML, US. 1246

MacNevin, Thomas E.

Manual of instructions for the guidance of coroners in New South Wales, containing appendices of practical forms and precedents and Acts relating to duties of coroners in New South Wales ... Sydney: Charles Potter, Acting Govt Printer. 1876.

206 × 135. Pp. viii, 46. Cloth.

2 ed., 1884; 3 ed., 1895.

Copies: EF, HDN, ML, SLV. 1247

Madden, Henry

See MacKnight, Charles H. and Madden, Henry.

Madden, Richard Robert

Travels in Turkey, Egypt, Nubia, and Palestine, in 1824, 1825, 1826, and 1827. ... In two volumes. Vol. 1. London: Henry Colburn ... 1829.

217 × 135. Vol. 1 : pp. xvi, 402 (last—errata), engr. coloured frontis. (author in Eastern dress); vol. 2 : pp. xviii, 398.

An account of hazardous journeying, full of incident and medical refs, including a chapter on plague as encountered at Alexandra. Includes practical remarks 'on the epidemic diseases of Egypt and Arabia ... to afford travellers some security from the scourges of the Levant.'

Copies: SLV, SLW, UM, US. 1248

The Same. 2 ed. 1833.

Copies: LNSW. 1249

The infirmities of genius illustrated by referring the anomalies in the literary character to the habits and constitutional peculiarities of men of genius ... In two volumes. ... London Saunders and Ottley ... 1833.

205 × 122. Vol. 1 : pp. [vi], 298; vol. 2 : pp. [iv], 298. Paper boards, linen backstrip with paper label.

Copies: UA. 1250

Phantasmata or illusions and fanaticisms of protean forms productive of great evils. ... In two volumes.—Vol. 1. London: ... T. C. Newby ... 1857

206 × 132. 2 vols. Vol. 1 : pp. xlii, 504, frontis.; vol. 2 : pp. iv, 588. Sub-title: Epidemic mental disorders.

'The madness of the various forms of fanaticism ... have all the distinguishing characteristics of epidemic mental disorders.' A historical survey.

Copies: SLS, SLV, UM. 1251

The memoirs (chiefly autobiographical) from 1798–1886 of Richard Robert Madden, M.D., F.R.C.S., formerly Colonial Secretary of Western Australia; H. M. Commissioner of Inquiry into Slave Trade, West African Settlements. ... Edited by his son, Thomas More Madden, M.D., F.R.C.S.E. London Ward & Downey ... 1891

220 × 135. Pp. [viii] (3 blanks), 328, [4] (book advts). Frontis (engr. portrait). Cloth.

R. R. Madden (1798–1886) MD, FRCS, who was Col Sec. and Acting Governor WA (1847–8), practised in Paris, Naples and Middle East, and thereafter served on anti-slavery administration in W. Indies and Africa. For biog. and extensive bibliog., see *Memoirs*.

Copies: AMAV, DL, EF, ML, NL, SLV, SLW. 1252

The Same. N.Y., Catholic Pub. Co., 1892.

Copies: DL. 1253

Magarey, Sylvanus James

Our climate and infant mortality. [From the Transactions of the Philosophical Society of Adelaide, 1879.] ...

224 × 147. Pp. 10. Title—head of p. 1. ND. (1879.) P. w. (title rptd, abbrev.)

High infant mortality ascribed to the hot, dry climate.

Copies: NL. 1254

The most fatal diseases of infancy and childhood. [Text begins.]

224 × 157. Pp. 22. 2 pl. (charts). ND. NI. [Adel. c. 1880.]

Discusses possible reasons for the infant mortality of SA, which has a higher rate than all other Aust. colonies. After reviewing diseases and other factors, the summer weather of the colony is considered the possible cause.

Copies: UA. 1255

Infant mortality and fatal diseases of infancy & childhood. . . . Adelaide . . . Webb, Vardon, & Pritchard . . . 1880.

250 × 181. Pp. 22, [2] (table, v.b.). P. w. (cover title).

Repeats thesis of previous item.

S. J. Magarey (1850–1901) MD, Melb. & Adel., MLC, was Hon. Phys. Adel. Hosp.

Copies: ML, SLS, SLV, UA. 1256

See International Temperance Convention, 1888.

Maid, Wife, and Mother

Maid, wife, and mother: a book for womankind; containing all the information necessary for the guidance of the sex in pregnancy, labour, maternity, &c., &c. Sydney: Printed for the Publisher. 1883.

215 × 135. Pp. 64. Colophon—Ford & Booth . . . Syd. P. w. (title rptd).

Copies: ML. 1257

Maiden, Joseph Henry

The Technological Museum of New South Wales, Sydney. The useful native plants of Australia. (Including Tasmania.) . . . Sydney: Turner and Henderson. London: Trubner and Co. . . . 1889.

220 × 147. Pp. xii, [ii] (v.b.), 696. Cloth.

Includes chapter on 'Substances reputed medicinal. (Drugs).' Also published: 'Some reputed medicinal plants of New South Wales', *Proc. Linn. Soc. NSW*, 1888 : 355.

J. H. Maiden (1859–1925) FRS, was NSW Govt Botanist and Director, Syd. Botanic Gardens.

Copies: ML, NL, SLT, SLV, SLW, UA, UM, US. 1258

Main, James M.

Palmistry, or, hand-reading explained and illustrated, being an epitome of this revived science from the best authors . . . Melbourne: H. Cordell, Printer . . . 1887.

178 × 120. Pp. 52 (last—colophon). 9 figs. P. w. (title rptd, decorated).

Copies: ML, SLV. 1259

Maitland and Melbourne Hospitals

1844. New South Wales. Maitland and Melbourne Hospitals. Ordered by the Council, to be printed, 4th December, 1844. Message from . . . the Governor, proposing an appropriation of public money in aid of the erection of an Hospital at Maitland; and suggesting the principle on which aid may be given in the erection of Hospitals throughout the Colony. [Text follows.]

311 × 196. Pp. 4 (l.b.). Pale blue paper. From *V&P*, Leg. Council NSW, 1844.

Proposes grant of £1000 for erection of public hospital at Maitland on condition equal sum raised by public subscription; sum of £500 voted for hosp. at Melbourne to be increased to £1000. Correspondence appended.

Copies: LNSW, ML, NL, SLV. 1260

Maitland Hospital, NSW

To His Excellency Major General Sir Richard Bourke, K.C.B., and the Members of the Legislative Council. We, the undersigned, beg leave to . . . call your attention to the extraordinary increase of the Town of Maitland . . . [Petition continues.]

297 × 184. Single leaf, v.b. ND. NI. From *V&P*, Leg. Council NSW, 1835.

Citizens appeal for establishment of hospital.

Copies: LNSW, ML, NL, SLV. 1261

1846. New South Wales. District Hospital of Maitland. Report from the Select Committee on a petition relative to the District Hospital of Maitland. . . . Sydney, Printed by W. W. Davies, at the Govt Printing Office . . . 1846.

316 × 204. Pp. [2]. Blue tinted paper. From *V&P*, Leg. Council NSW, 1846.

On a dispute on the management of Maitland Hosp., causing ill-feeling between Roman Catholic and Protestant sections of the community. Reports public enquiry inadvisable; the only question is whether hospital rules give equal

advantages to both.
Copies: LNSW, ML, NL, SLV. 1262

The annual report of the Committee of Management of the Maitland Hospital, with rules & regulations ... for the year 1858. West Maitland: Printed by George Maxted ... 1859.
206 × 135. Pp. 18 (l.b.).
The report notes a proposal to change the name of the institution to 'The Great Northern Hospital', but this was apparently not acted upon.
Copies: LNSW (1858, 1867), ML. 1263

Mallinson & Co

The Chamberland Pasteur filter described and illustrated. ... Sole agents for Australasia: Mallinson & Co. ... Melbourne. H. W. Mills and Co. ... Melbourne.
212 × 130. Pp. 24. 10 figs. ND.
Copies: DL. 1264

Manning, Frederic Norton

1868. New South Wales. Report on lunatic asylums ... Presented to both Houses of Parliament ... Sydney: Thomas Richards, Govt Printer. 1868. ...
309 × 201. Pp. [ii] (v.b.), iv, 5–216 (l.b.). 5 pl., 17 flg charts.
Information, collected on official visit to Britain, Europe and America, includes accommodation, management, treatment and administration. Manning's reform of the mental health services of NSW was based on this report.
Copies: EF, HDN, LNSW, ML, US. 1265

The Same. 252 × 153. Pp. [ii] (v.b.), vi (l.b.), 7–288 (l.b.). 5 pl., 17 flg plans. Paper boards. 1868.
Copies: EF, HDN, LNSW, ML, SLV. 1266

Address delivered on resigning charge as Medical Superintendent of the Hospitals for the Insane at Gladesville and Callan Park ... Gibbs, Shallard & Co. ... Sydney. ...
217 × 140. Pp. 14. ND. (1879.) P. w. (title rptd).
Copies: EF, HDN, ML, NL. 1267

Ten years at Gladesville. ... (Read ... 5 September, 1879.) [Text begins.]
204 × 127. Pp. 14 (l.b.). Colophon—Syd.: Thomas Richards, Govt Pr—1880. Roy. Soc. NSW paper.
On mental diseases—especially statistics, epilepsy, and general paralysis.
Copies: EF, HDN, ML, US. 1268

The causation and prevention of insanity. ... (read before the Medical Section of the Royal Society of N.S.W., 10 September, 1880.) [Text begins.]
198 × 130. Pp. 18 (l.b.). Colophon—Syd.: Thomas Richards, Govt Pr—1880.
Includes tables showing assigned causes of insanity in 3,077 patients admitted to Gladesville Hosp. for Insane, 1869–1878; and in 13,309 patients to English asylums during 1848.
Copies: HDN, ML, NL. 1269

Is insanity increasing? ... (Read before the ... Royal Society of N.S.W., September, 1881.) [Text begins.]
204 × 127. Pp. 10 (l.b.). Colophon—Syd.: Thomas Richards, Govt Pr—1881.
A statistical study, indicating increase of insanity.
Copies: EF, HDN. 1270

Medical certificates of insanity ... (Read before the Medical Section of the Royal Society of N.S.W., 15 June, 1883.) [Text begins.]
198 × 130. Pp. 12. Colophon—Syd.: Thomas Richards, Govt Pr—1883. P. w. (shortened title).
Another ed., 1891.
Copies: EF, HDN, ML, SLV. 1271

Cases of mental disturbance after injury to the head, with particular reference to loss of memory. ... (Read before the ... Royal Society of N.S.W., 20 June, 1884.) [Text begins.]
204 × 127. Pp. 8. Colophon—Syd.: Thomas Richards, Govt Pr—1884.
Copies: EF, HDN. 1272

A contribution to the study of heredity. ... (Read before the ... Royal Society of N.S.W., 17 July, 1885.) [Text begins.]

204 × 127. Pp. 8. Colophon—Syd.: Thomas Richards, Govt Pr—1886.

An investigation of inherited mental deficiency.

Copies: EF. 1273

Address in psychological medicine, delivered at the Intercolonial Medical Congress in Melbourne on January 11, 1888. ... [Text begins.]

217 × 140. Pp. 30 Repr., *J. Mental Science*, July, 1889. P. w.

Reviews, with statistical data, the incidence and treatment of mental ailments in Australia.

Copies: EF, HDN, ML. 1274

A case of sporadic cretinism, with remarks. ... Reprinted from the "Intercolonial Medical Congress of Australasia Transactions". Melbourne: Stillwell and Co. ... 1889.

214 × 140. Pp. 8 (l.b.). 1 pl. (2 mounted photographs). P. w. (cover title).

Copies: EF, ML. 1275

Insanity in its relation to the law. ... From American Journal of Insanity, January, 1893. Utica, N.Y.

234 × 147. Pp. 12. P. w. (cover title).

F. N. Manning (1839–1903) MD St And., MRCS, was head of NSW Lunacy Dept (1868–98), Med. Adviser to NSW Govt, Pres. NSW Bd Health. See obit., *Austsn med. Gaz.*, 1903, 22 : 317; for his reforms: Parkes, Sir Henry (1892), *Fifty years in the making of Aust. history*, vol. 1, Lond.; for personal account: *Austsn med. Gaz.*, 1898, 17 : 77.

Copies: ML. 1276

Insanity in Australian aborigines, with a brief analysis of thirty-two cases. ... [Text begins.]

214 × 138. Pp. 4. ND. Colophon—Stillwell and Co. ... Melb. Repr., *Trans Intercol Med. Cong. Austsia*, 1889.

Copies: EF, HDN, ML. 1277

See also Dean Case; Gladesville Hosp. for Insane; New Norfolk Hosp. for Insane; Reformatories and reformatory treatment in France; Departmental reps in NSW Parlt Papers.

Marano, Gregori Vincenzo

Respiratory therapeutics. ... Reprinted from the "Australasian Medical Gazette" for September, 1886. L. Bruck ... Sydney. 1886.

181 × 122. Pp. 8.

Copies: NL. 1278

On pneumatic therapeutics by means of the portable apparatus. ... [Text begins.]

212 × 138. Pp. 6. Repr., *Trans Intercol Med. Cong. Austsia*, 1889.

On aero-therapeutics—'the mechanical treatment of certain affections of the respiratory organs by means of alteration in the pressure and composition of the atmospheric air.'

For G. V. Marano (1850–1924) MD, ChD Naples, Cons. Surg. Syd. Benev. Asylum and Consul Gen. for Italy, see *Med. J. Aust.*, 1924, 1 : 474.

Copies: NL. 1279

Marshall, Henry

Abnormal phenomena of the nervous system ... [Quotation] Commenced in London about 1847; concluded in Australia 1883 Adelaide: Carey and Page, Printers ... 1883

209 × 135. Pp. 128 (l.b.). P. w. ('Psychology and evolution ... 1883', on front).

Author, from Angaston SA, announces himself as 'a naturalist and investigator of scientific phenomena.' Two parts: (1) as title (discusses mesmerism, etc.); (2) equatorial development and evolution.

Copies: LNSW, ML, NL, SLS, SLV, UA. 1280

Martin, Sir Charles James

The effect of food on the secretion of bile in man. Read at the Intercolonial Medical Congress, Sydney, 1892.

250 × 153. Pp. [ii] (v.b.), 4, [ii] (v.b.). 5 pl. Colophon—Syd.: Charles Potter, Govt Pr—1893.

Studies on a patient with biliary fistula and complete blockage of common bile duct.

Copies: EF, UM, US. 1281

On the physiological action of the venom of the Australian black snake (Pseudechis porphyriacus). ... (From the Physiological Laboratory of the University of Sydney.) (Read before the Royal Society of N. S. Wales, July 3,

1895) [Text begins.]

201 × 135. Pp. 134 (l.b.). Title at head of p. 2. Short title at p. l. Repr., *J. & P. Roy. Soc. NSW*, 1895–6.

Copies: ML, UM, US. 1282

Snakes, snake poisons and snake bites. ... (Read before the Sydney University Medical Society ... 1895).

244 × 173. Pp. 12. 8 figs. Title at head of p. 2. Repr. from Hermes Med. Supp., *J. Syd. Univ. Med. Soc.*, 4 Dec. 1895.

Copies: UA, UM. 1283

A simple and rapid method of desiccating serum and keeping it sterile during the process. ... [Text begins.]

248 × 155. Pp. 4 (l.b.). Repr., *J. Path. & Bact.*, Jan., 1896. P. w.

Copies: UA. 1284

Explanation of the marked difference in effects produced by the subcutaneous and intravenous injection of the venom of Australian snakes ...

225 × 140. Pp. 8. Read Roy. Soc. NSW, Aug. 1896.

Copies: UA. 1285

A rapid method of separating colloids from crystalloids in solutions containing both. ... (From the Physiological Laboratory of the University of Sydney.) [Text begins.]

240 × 160. Pp. 8. Repr., *J. Physiol.*, 1896, 20 : 364. P. w.

Copies: UA, UM. 1286

Note on a method of separating colloids from crystalloids by filtration. An explanation of the marked difference in the effects produced by subcutaneous and intravenous injection of the venom of Australian snakes. ... Read before the Royal Society of N. S. Wales, August 5, 1896.

225 × 142. Pp. 12 (l.b.). P. w.

Copies: UA. 1287

Australasian Association for the Advancement of Science. Sydney Session, 1898. Section D.—Biology. Presidential address by C. J. Martin, D.Sc., M.B., Acting-Professor of Physiology in the University of Melbourne. ...

212 × 135. Pp. 22 (l.b.). Colophon—Syd.: William Applegate Gullick, Govt Pr—1898. P. w. (cover title).

'The history of the relations between morphology and physiology during the last fifty years.'

For Sir Charles Martin (1866–1955) FRS, who laid the foundations of medical research in Australia and influenced it throughout his life, see *Med. J. Aust.*, 1955, 1 : 809; *Biog. Memoirs of Fellows of Roy. Soc.*, 1956, 2 : 173 (with bibliog.); Bedson, S. P. (1956), *J. Gen. Microbiol.*, 14 : 487.

Copies: US. 1288

See also Dean Case.

Martin, John Wilson

Mind over matter or the influence of will power on disease by Dr. Martin, M.D. ... Sydney: The Commercial Publishing Company ...

178 × 122. Pp. [vi], 78. ND. [?1900.] Cloth.

Another ed., 1903. Includes notice of author's works. (ML.)

Discusses causes and treatment of diseases, stressing importance of exercise of will power for health and treatment.

Author is identified by Univ. Edin. advice that MD thesis on snake-bite (1893), noted in 1903 ed., was presented by John Wilson Martin MD, ChM, b. 1859. He came to Australia in 1888 and practised in turn at Creswick Vic., Urana NSW, Melb. and Syd.

Also published: *The diseases of men and women. A medical handbook for general use*, Syd., R. E. Ambler, 1905.

Copies: EF, ML (2 ed.). 1289

Martin, Lawrence Joseph

In memoriam. Dr. Lawrence Joseph Martin.

117 × 90. Pp. 14, [ii], (colophon, v.b.). Title in black frame. Colophon—Stillwell and Co. ... 1879. Author—J. E. Neild.

L. J. Martin (1826–79) MD, was Hon. Phys. Melb. Hosp. and Melb. Lying-in Hosp. See Forster, F.M.C. (1967) *Progress in obst. and gynaec. in Aust.*, Syd.: 33.

Copies: SLV. 1290

Marvellous Melbourne

"Marvellous Melbourne twenty years hence".

Silting up of Hobson's Bay. Destruction of the port. The plague and fire of Melbourne. ... (Reprinted from the Kew Mercury and Hawthorn Advertiser.) ... Kew: W. Mott and Co. ... 1889.

214 × 140. Pp. 16. P. w. (cover title).

A story of pestilence from insanitary conditions, followed by various disasters. Describes Melb. sanitation as 'more adapted to a community of Yahoos than to a civilised race of human beings.'

Copies: ML. 1291

Maryborough District Hospital, Vic.

Seventh annual report of the Maryborough District Hospital: with the financial statement for the year ending December 31, 1861 ... with the rules and regulations ... Established 1854. Maryborough. ... Evans and Somerton ... 1862.

204 × 127. Pp. 16.

Copies: SLV (7–17; 1862–71). 1292

Maryborough Polynesian Hospital, Qd

See Queensland—Parliament, No 1741.

Mathew, John

Eaglehawk and crow A study of the Australian aborigines including an inquiry into their origin and a survey of Australian languages ... London David Nutt ... Melbourne Melville, Mullen and Slade 1899

234 × 145. Pp. xvi, 288. 5 pl., coloured map. Cloth.

Includes notes on diseases, medicine men, treatment and ritualistic mutilations.

For Rev. John Mathew (1849–1929) MA, DD, Presbyterian minister and anthropologist, see *Aust. Enc.*

Copies: DL, EF, FC, ML, NL, OL, SLV, SLW, UA, UQ, US. 1293

Maughan, James

Adelaide Philosophical Society. Paper read August 15th, 1865 ... "The drainage of Adelaide, considered in its scientific aspects". [Text begins.]

263 × 204. Pp. [4] (l.b.). Colophon—Andrews, Thomas, & Fisher ... Adel.

An appeal for sewerage, especially for abatement of typhoid.

Copies: EF, ML, SLS. 1294

Mault, Alfred

(No. 139.) [Royal Arms] 1886. Parliament of Tasmania. Sanitary conditions of Launceston: report to the Central Board of Health ... Presented to both Houses ...

344 × 214. Pp. [iv], 12 (l.b.). 1 flg chart. Colophon—William Thomas Strutt, Govt Pr, Tas.

Copies: LNSW, NL, SLT, SLV. 1295

———

(No. 136.) [Royal Arms] 1887. Parliament of Tasmania. Outbreak of smallpox at Launceston: Report by Mr. Mault, Engineering Inspector ... Presented to both Houses ...

352 × 204. Pp. [ii] (l.b.), 8 (l.b.). 4 charts. Colophon—William Thomas Strutt, Govt Pr, Tas.

First occurrence of small-pox in Tasmania—33 cases, 11 deaths.

Copies: LNSW, NL, SLT, SLV. 1296

———

Tasmania. Report to the Central Board of Health, by Alfred Mault ... on the sanitary condition of the Municipality of Longford. [Royal Arms] Tasmania: William Thomas Strutt, Govt Printer. 1887.

331 × 204. Pp. 8. 3 flg charts. P. w. (title rptd).

Copies: LNSW, NL, SLT, SLV. 1297

———

Tasmania. Report to the Central Board of Health ... on the drainage and sewerage of the City of Hobart. Tasmania: William Thomas Strutt, Govt. Printer, Hobart. 1886.

331 × 209. Pp. [ii] (v.b.), 22 (l.b.). 1 flg map. P. w. (title rptd).

Copies: NL, SLT. 1297a

———

(No. 20.) 1889. [Royal Arms] Parliament of Tasmania. Disinfection of clothing and bedding: report. Presented to both Houses ...

344 × 214. Pp. 6. Plan of disinfecting station. Colophon—William Thomas Strutt, Govt Pr, Tas.

Copies: NL, SLT. 1297b

———

Tasmania. Report to the Central Board of Health ... on the sanitary condition of the Municipality of Brighton. [Royal Arms] Tasmania: William Thomas Strutt, Govt Printer, Tasmania. 1887.

331 × 204. Pp. 8.

Copies: LNSW, NL, SLT, SLV. 1298

(No. 114.) [Royal Arms] 1887. Parliament of Tasmania. Sanitary condition of Avoca : report to the Central Board of Health . . . Presented to both Houses . . .

339 × 204. Pp. 8. 1 plan.

Copies: LNSW, NL, SLT, SLV. 1299

(No. 34. [Royal Arms] 1890. Parliament of Tasmania. Strahan and Mount Zeehan District: report on sanitary condition. Presented to both Houses . . .

344 × 214. Pp. 10. Colophon—William Thomas Strutt, Govt Pr, Tas.

Copies: LNSW, NL, SLT, SLV. 1300

(No. 36.) [Royal Arms] Parliament of Tasmania. Sanitary condition of part of Glebe Town: Inspector's report. Presented to both Houses . . .

344 × 214. Pp. 6 (l.b.). (1890.) Colophon—William Thomas Strutt, Govt Pr, Tas.

Copies: LNSW, NL, SLT, SLV. 1301

(No. 81) 1891. Parliament of Tasmania. Outbreak of diphtheria at Snug River. Presented to both Houses . . .

344 × 217. Pp. 6 (l.b.). Colophon—William Thomas Strutt, Govt Pr . . .

Considers family outbreak as possibly due to infection from the body of a boy, dead of diphtheria, brought from Hobart Hosp. for burial.

Copies: LNSW, NL, SLT, SLV. 1302

(No. 82.) 1891. Parliament of Tasmania. Diphtheria at Campbell Town. Presented to both Houses . . .

344 × 217. Pp. 6.

Report to Cent. Bd of Health on continuing epidemic of 28 cases with 7 deaths, with consideration of hosp. drainage, cleanliness of housing, spread from animals.

Copies: LNSW, SLT, SLV. 1303

(No. 86 A.) 1891. Parliament of Tasmania. Sanitation of a mining settlement: paper by Engineering Inspector, Central Board of Health. Presented to both Houses . . .

344 × 217. Pp. 6 (2 blanks). Colophon—William Thomas Strutt, Govt Pr . . .

Describes problems of water supply (with gross pollution from sewage and lead), sanitation and living conditions in thickly forested country about Zeehan, where population has grown from 400 to 4000 in 6 months.

Copies: LNSW, NL, SLT, SLV. 1304

(No. 160.) 1891. Parliament of Tasmania. Report on Seventh International Congress of Hygiene and Demography, held in London . . . 1891: and on the latest developments of sanitation and sanitary work in Europe. Presented to both Houses . . .

357 × 212. Pp. vi, 92. 8 pl., 1 fig. Colophon—William Thomas Strutt, Govt Pr, Tas. To Central Board of Health.

Author was official Tas. delegate.

Copies: LNSW, ML, NL, SLT, SLV. 1305

(No. 127.) 1892. Parliament of Tasmania. Metropolitan Drainage Board. Report of Engineer. Presented to both Houses . . .

344 × 204. Pp. 20 (l.b.). 6 flg charts. Colophon—William Thomas Strutt, Govt Pr, Tas.

Includes consideration of various sewage disposal methods for Hobart, including irrigation, chemical precipitation, and discharge into tideways.

Copies: LNSW, NL, SLT, SLV. 1306

Health map of Hobart. Location of diseases notified in 1898—typhoid fever, diphtheria, scarlatina, and deaths of children under one year . . .

370 × 338. ND. (1898.) NI.

Alfred Mault (1829–1902), civil engineer and sanitarian, with experience in Britain and France, was in 1886 appointed Engineering Inspr to newly established Central Bd of Health.

Copies: SLT. 1307

See also Barnard, C. E., and Mault, A.

Maund, J.

See No 2424.

May, J. M.

Notes on some of the charitable institutions of Melbourne. Sydney: Geo. Buckleton & Co. . . .

168 × 112. Pp. 22 (l.b.). ND. (1871.) Paper boards.

Includes: Deaf and Dumb Instn; Asylum for Blind; Prince Alfred Hosp.; Melbourne Hosp., Benev. Asylum.

Copies: ML, NL, UM. 1308

Meares, Edward

Vegetable diet in health and disease. . . . Melbourne: Mason, Firth & M'Cutcheon . . . 1893.

217 × 145. Pp. 16 (l.b.).

Physiological effect of animal food; advantages of vegetable diet; curative properties in disease.

Copies: NL. 1309

Medical and Surgical Review (Australasian)

No. 1, Vol. 1. March 1863. Published monthly. The Medical & Surgical Review. (Australasian) Edited by James Keene, late Surgeon of the West London Hospital. Contents . . . Melbourne: F. F. Bailliere . . .

212 × 135. Pp. 32. P. w. with above title.

Monthly. Vols 1–3; March 1863–Nov. 1865. New Series: vols 1–2; Oct. 1873–April 1875.

Ceased publication Nov. 1865. Recommenced as *Med. and Surg. Review: New Series* in Oct. 1873. See Gandevia, B. (1952), *Med. J. Aust.*, 2 : 184.

Copies: AMAV (complete), ML (v. 1, 1–3), NL (v. 1); SLV (v. 1; ns v. 1–2), UM (v. 1). 1310

Medical and Surgical Sanitarium, Summer Hill, NSW

See Caro, Edgar R.

Medical Association of South Australia

General and by-laws of the Medical Association of South Australia. Approved . . . December 14, 1865. Adelaide: . . . Andrews, Thomas, & Clark . . . 1869.

176 × 110. Pp. 10, [2] (last—colophon).

Founded 1865 for the 'advancement of the scientific and social condition of the medical profession.'

Copies: SLV. 1311

———

The laws and by-laws of the Medical Association of South Australia. Established A.D. 1851. Adelaide: . . . T. Strode . . .

210 × 155. Pp. 12 (two blanks). P. w. (title rptd). (1851.)

Copies: SLS. 1312

Medical Association of Victoria

Founded Jan. 1869; published *Australian Medical Gazette* Jan. 1869–Dec. 1871. Brochure on Assn and *Gazette* was issued. NS.

1313

Medical Bill, New South Wales

The Medical Bill. The following articles are taken from . . . a few of the country papers, and are expressive of the opinions entertained by them on the character and principles of the New Medical Bill now before Parliament . . . [Text continues.]

198 × 135. Pp. 14. (1873.) NI.

Opinions antagonistic to a Bill for regulation of medical practice (i.e. control of unqualified practitioners).

Sir Alfred Stephen's copy in ML, annotated in his hand, has: 'I characterise these comments, one and all, as scandalous: in statement, false—and as to argument ridiculous. All publd. in opposition to a measure which exists in Engld. and every British Colony but this—'

Copies: ML. 1314

———

The proposed Medical Bill. In dealing with this measure, two difficulties are to be met . . . [Text continues.]

239 × 188. Pp. 2. Single leaf. 1873. Colophon —Lee & Rose . . . Syd.

Attacks Bill, extolling certain unregistered practitioners.

Copies: ML. 1315

———

Report of a meeting of the medical profession held at Sydney . . . 2nd June, 1875, to take into consideration the speech recently published by the Dean of the Faculty of Medicine in the Sydney University on the proposed Medical Bill for New South Wales. Sydney: John Sands . . . 1875.

214 × 138. Pp. 22, [2] (resolutions, v.b.).

Meeting protests against a speech derogatory

to the profession, made by Prof. John Smith MLC in opposition to a Bill for the control of unqualified practice, and holds that 'he cannot with propriety continue in the office of Dean.' For Sir Alfred Stephen's agreement with this, see No 2028; for Smith's speech, No 1931.

ML copy, with inserted press cuttings, belonged to Chairman (Geo. Bennett FRCS).

The Bill was defeated, as others, and there was no control of unqualified practice in NSW prior to Med. Practitioners Act 1898 and Amending Act 1900. For the long struggle for this, see McIntosh, A. M. (1951), 'The Aust. Med. Assn', *Med. J. Aust.*, 1 : 533.

Copies: LNSW, ML. 1316

———

New South Wales Parliament. Notes on the Medical Bill, 1892.

247 × 158. Pp. 12 (l.b.). Colophon—Syd.: Charles Potter, Govt Pr—1892. P. w. (cover title).

On evils of unrestricted medical practice in NSW.

ML copy inscribed: 'Drawn up by J. M. Creed, M.L.C. at the request of Sir Geo. R. Dibbs, Prime Minister.'

Copies: ML. 1317

Medical Companion, The

The Medical Companion. Contents: Simple remedies for common ailments. What to do in cases of emergency. Hints to mothers. Health mottoes, etc. (Revised by a medical man.) Price sixpence. Published at the Homoeopathic Pharmacy . . . Launceston . . . "Examiner" and "Tasmanian" Office.

135 × 102. Pp. [iv], 92 (last 10—advts). ND. Cloth.

Copies: CC. 1318

Medical Defence Association, Melbourne

Medical Defence Association. Founded June 12, 1879. Rules and Committee. Melbourne: 1879.

204 × 127. Pp. 4. Colophon—Stillwell and Co. . . . P. w. (cover title).

A later Medical Defence Assn of Vic. was founded in 1895.

Copies: CC, EF, SLV. 1319

Medical Directory for New South Wales, and Queensland

See Australian Medical Association.

Medical Officer in Her Majesty's Service

Western Australia, recommended as a sanatorium, for the restoration to health and usefulness of European soldiers, prostrated by those diseases of India, for which the climate of the hill stations does not afford a remedy, by a Medical Officer in Her Majesty's Service, who has had experience with troops both in Australia and India. Guildford: Printed by E. Andrews, Bookseller . . .

186 × 115. Pp. 8. ND. (1859.) Pref. letter signed H. H. Jones, M.D., Staff Capt., Kurrachee and contrib. to *Bombay Standard* signed 'West Australian.'

Health, climatic and economic advantages. Small-pox, measles, scarlatina, and 'curious enough', venereal disease (except a mild gleet contracted from aborigines) is unknown; syphilis, 'that bane of the British Army', totally absent; dysentery rare; diarrhoea infrequent (and curable by eucalypt gum, 'a remedy known to every settler and native'); and fevers rare 'considering the amount of alcohol drunk.'

Copies: SLW. 1320

Medical Practitioners' Association, Sydney

Founded 1872, by benefit society medical officers for protection of their interests. Publications not seen. For foundation and objects, see *NSW med. Gaz.*, 1872, 2 : 189; *ibid.*, 1873, 3 : 165 (rules). 1321

Medical Record of Australia

The Medical Record of Australia. Edited by Dr. Reeves. Vol. 1. Melbourne: Mason & Firth, Printers . . . 1861.

290 × 215. Pp. ii, 156.

Vols 1–3; May 1861–Dec. 1863. Fortnightly to Sept. 1861, then monthly.

See also *Melb. Med. Record*, which appeared 12 years later (Feb. 1875). This assumed continuity with *Med. Record of Aust.* in its numbering of volumes, commencing with vol. 4, no 1, though further relationship is not evident. See Gandevia, B. (1952), 'A review of Victoria's early med. journals', *Med. J. Aust.*, 2 : 184.

Copies: AMAV (v. 1–3), ML (v. 2, no 7), SLV (v. 1–3). 1322

Medical Register, The—Victoria

The Medical Register, printed and published under the direction of the Medical Board of Victoria, pursuant to . . . "An Act to Amend the

Laws Relating to Legally Qualified Medical Practitioners". 1865. [Royal Arms] Melbourne: . . . John Ferres, Govt Printer; F. F. Bailliere . . .
236 × 148. Pp. 26. Limp cloth.
Lists practitioners, with date of registration, address, and qualifications. Published also in *Vic. Govt Gazette.*
Copies: NL (1863), SLV (1863–). 1323

Medical Society of Queensland
See Queensland Medical Society.

Medical Society of Victoria
Rules of the Medical Society of Victoria. Melbourne: Goodhugh & Hough . . . 1856.
212 × 130. Pp. 8. P. w.
Other editions: 1861, 1864, 1872, 1877, 1880, 1884, 1888, 1898. 1864 ed. includes catalogue of Library.
Society was formed in 1855 by union of Victoria Med. Assn and the Medico-Chirurgical Soc. of Vic.; in 1907 combined with Vic. Branch of BMA. Official organ—*Aust. med. J.* (1856–95). For history, see Graham, H. B. (1952), *Med. J. Aust.*, 2 : 213.
Copies: AMAV (all above), BG (1864–88), CC (1872), DOS (1872–88), EF (1864–88), ML (1864–88), SLV (1856, 1880, 1888). 1324

———

Medical Society of Victoria. Rules for the circulation of books and periodicals. . . . Library kept at T. M. Buzzard's . . . Melbourne. December, 1856.
171 × 107. Single leaf, v.b. NI.
Used as label in books of Library.
Copies: AMAV, BG, EF, KFR. 1325

———

A Bill (recommended by the Medical Society of Victoria) to provide for the registration of duly qualified medical practitioners. [Text begins.]
204 × 132. Pp. 4. ND. (?1870.) Colophon—. . . Goodhugh & Hough . . .
Copies: ML. 1326

———

Medical Society of Victoria. Officers and roll of members. January 1873.
220 × 138. Pp. 4. Colophon—Stillwell and Knight . . . Other editions—1874, 1875.
Copies: AMAV, BG, EF, ML. 1327

———

Medical Society of Victoria. July 4, 1874. Sir, I have the honour . . . to inform you that at a Special Meeting of the Society . . . the Amended Vaccination Bill now before the Legislative Council . . . was the subject of consideration . . . [Text continues.]
255 × 204. Single leaf (v.b.).
Letter to Members of Leg. Council, protesting against appointment of unqualified vaccinators.
Copies: AMAV, BG, EF. 1328

———

Report of the Medical Society of Victoria for the year ending December 1875.
217 × 140. Pp. 10. Colophon—Stillwell and Knight . . . Melb.
Another issue 1878.
Copies: AMAV, BG, CC, DOS, EF, ML, SLV. 1329

———

Report of the Sub-committee of the Medical Society of Victoria on experiments in snake-poisoning. Presented . . . April 5, 1876. [Text begins.]
209 × 135. Pp. 8 (l.b.). Colophon—Stillwell & Knight . . .
Results of animal experiments on Halford's ammonia injection treatment. Reports as ineffective.
Copies: NL, UA. 1330

———

Report on the prevalence of phthisis in Victoria.
214 × 140. Pp. 12. 7 tables. ND. (Committee appointed Oct. 1877). Colophon—Stillwell and Knight . . . Melb.
An attempt to settle a protracted dispute on the trend of tuberculosis in Vic. and the effect of climate on the disease. This inflamed rather than abated local controversy, and met with violent rebuttal by Wm Thomson.
Copies: ML, NL, SLV. 1331

———

Medical Society of Victoria. March 20, 1879. Sir, I have the honour to inform you that the following resolution was unanimously adopted . . . [Text continues.]
252 × 201. Pp. [4] (last 3 blank).
Circular, for despatch abroad, protesting in name of profession 'against being represented in England by Mr. James George Beaney, or in

being, in any way, associated with him.' See *The Medical embassy in England* (No 224), published by Society.
Copies: AMAV, BG, EF. 1332

Medical Society of Victoria. Melbourne ... April 17, 1879. Sir, By the March mail, leaving here for Europe, a circular was forwarded ... containing a copy of a resolution ... repudiating Mr. James George Beaney as a representative of the Medical Profession in this colony. ... [Text continues.]
252 × 201. Pp. [4] (2, 4 blank).
Copies: AMAV, BG, EF. 1333

The Amending Medical Bill. Whereas it is expedient that persons requiring medical aid should be enabled to distinguish qualified practitioners from persons ... [Text continues.]
212 × 135. Pp. 14, [ii] (colophon, v.b.). ND. (1889.) Colophon—Melb.: Stillwell and Co. ...
Proposed amendment to Medical Act of 1865, to control unqualified practice. See *Aust. med. J.*, 1870, 15 : 84 and subsequent discussions in this journal on illegal practice and quackery in Vic. and professional agitation for legislative control. Above draft for proposed amending Bill appeared in *Aust. med. J.*, 1888, ns 10 : 567, and again *ibid.*, 1889, ns 11 : 215, where it is said to have been printed many times over 15 or 20 years.
Copies: AMAV, BG, EF. 1334

Medical Students' Society Review, Adelaide
See Adelaide Medical Students' Society.

Medico Chirurgical Society of Victoria
Medico Chirurgical Society of Victoria. 1854. Melbourne: ... "Herald" Office ... 1854.
204 × 132. Pp. 8. P. w. (title rptd).
Includes rules. Society was formed on 6 June 1854. On 18 July 1855 it combined with Victoria Med. Assn to form Med. Soc. of Vic. See H. B. Graham (1952), *Med. J. Aust.*, 2 : 213; *ibid.*, (1956), 1 : 557.
Copies: NL, SLV. 1335

Medico-Ethical Society of Victoria
For attempts to establish Soc. in Melb., see *Aust. med. J.*, 1868, 13 : 155, 221, 278, 279 (object and rules), and 282. Publications not seen.
1336

Medini, Michael. Case of
Statements and correspondence relative to the case of Michael Medini, who died in the Sydney Infirmary, on the 25th August, 1849. Sydney: Printed by Kemp and Fairfax ... 1850.
217 × 130. Pp. 20.
Correspondence from *Syd. Morning Herald*, published by Charles Nathan, Surg. Syd. Infirmary. Walter Lawrence, Surg. RN., censured by coroner's jury for his conduct of a case, published a statement signed by 20 Sydney doctors disagreeing with verdict and criticising Nathan's evidence. Ensuing correspondence is collected in vindication of Nathan.
For Charles Nathan (1816–72) FRCS, Surg. Syd. Infirm., an Aust. pioneer of anaesthesia, see obit., *NSW med. Gaz.*, 1872, 3 : 43; also Potter, W. L., *Med. J. Aust.*, 1938, 2 : 940; Nathan, C. V. (1968), 'Grim days at the Infirmary', *Med. J. Aust.*, 2 : 688 (outlines Medini case).
Copies: ML. 1337

Mediums and Their Dupes
See Knaggs, Samuel Thomas.

Medlock and Bailey
Medlock & Bailey's patent bisulphite of lime for the preservation of meat, fish, poultry, game, and all other animal substances, in temperate and tropical climates, and on board ship. Melbourne: H. G. De Gruchy & Co. ...
220 × 147. Pp. 16 (l.b.). ND.
Copies: ML. 1338

Meekison, E. R.
1900. Victoria. Department of Mines. Instruction to miners. No. 3. Notes on ventilation in mines. ... Robt. S. Brain, Govt Printer, Melbourne.
265 × 188. Pp. 6 (l.b.). 2 flg plans. P. w. (title rptd).
Copies: EF, SLV. 1339

Melbourne, Royal Commission on Sanitary Condition of
1889. Victoria. Sanitary condition of Melbourne. Progress Report of Royal Commission to Inquire into and Report upon the Sanitary Condition of Melbourne. ... Robt. S. Brain, Govt Printer, Melbourne.
331 × 204. Pp. xliv, 200. 1 coloured flg plan. P. w. (title rptd).
A comprehensive study, basic to future developments. Chairman: H. B. Allen.

Continuation of evidence. 1889. Pp. [ii] (v.b.), 201–388, [ii] (v.b.), 8 plans (6 flg). P. w.

2nd Progress Rep. 1889. Pp. 24, 1 flg plan. On water supply.

3rd Progress Rep. 1889. Pp. xxviii, 88 (l.b.), 2 flg plans. Sewerage, milk, meat, health legislation.

Final Rep. 1890. Pp. 60, 7 plans (5 flg). Noxious trades, abattoirs, refuse disposal, water supplies.

Copies: EF, HDV, LNSW, ML, NL, SLV, SPH, UM, US. 1340

Melbourne Benevolent Asylum

The Fifth Annual Report of the Committee of Management, of the Benevolent Asylum, Melbourne, with the rules of the same . . . for the year 1854. Melbourne: Lucas Brothers, Printers . . . 1855.

204 × 130. Pp. 24.

SLV has first two reports, type-written from ms. originals, with titles : Rep. of Victorian Benevolent Society, 1850, 51.

Founded 1850—to relieve the aged, infirm, disabled, or destitute by care within the Asylum, outdoor relief, or by medical aid through the dispensary. Above title later became Melb. Benev. Asylum. In 1950 (100th an. rep.), name changed to Melb. Home and Hosp. for the Aged. *See also* No 1006.

Copies: ML (1855, 1858–61), SLV (1850–). 1341

Melbourne Convalescent Home for Women

Austsn med. Gaz., 1888, 8 : 81 notes foundation on 20 acre site at Clayton Hill; original site at Oakleigh was sold earlier for £10,000. Publications appeared. NS.

1342

Melbourne Dental Hospital

See Dental and Oral Hospital of Victoria; also Aust. College of Dentistry and Melb. Dental Hosp.

Melbourne Home and Hospital for the Aged

See Melbourne Benevolent Asylum.

Melbourne Homoeopathic Dispensary

See Homoeopathic Dispensary, Melb.

Melbourne Hospital

A meeting of those gentlemen favourable to the establishment of a permanent Hospital in the town, was held at the Royal Hotel; his Worship the Mayor presiding . . . [Text continues.]

293 × 171. Single leaf, v.b. 3 cols. (7 Feb. 1845.) Colophon—Printed by W. Clarke, at the Herald Office . . .

Report of Provisional Committee, notifying completion of arrangements for foundation.

Copy, with ms. corrections, is laid down on verso of leaf bearing earliest entry in first minute book of Melb. Hosp.

Copies: Roy. Melb. Hosp. 1343

The First Annual Report of the Committee of Management of the Melbourne Hospital, with the rules of the same, and a list of subscriptions and donations for the year 1848. Melbourne: William Clarke, Printer, "Morning Herald" Office.

8vo. Pp. 10. Inserted slip. ND. [1849.]

Name later changed to Royal Melb. Hosp.

Copies: ML (1856–60, 1883, 1900), NL (1884), SLV (1848–53, 1856–). 1344

Report of the Select Committee appointed to inquire into alleged abuses in the administration of the Melbourne Hospital. [Text begins.]

212 × 130. Pp. 16 (l.b.). 1865. Colophon—Wilson & Mackinnon, Printers . . . Chairman—Sir James Palmer.

Inquiry into allegations that the hospital was imposed upon by persons able to pay for medical aid.

Copies: SLV. 1345

Pharmacopoeia compiled for use in the Melbourne Hospital Third edition. 1868. Melbourne: Stillwell and Knight . . .

125 × 82. Pp. xvi, 17–78 (l.b.). Cloth.

4 ed., 1878; 5 ed., 1887; 6 ed., 1901.

Copies: AMAV (4, 6 eds), BG (5), EF (4, 5), NL (5), SLV (3), UM (5). 1346

Rules of the Melbourne Hospital. September, 1863. Melbourne: Mason, Firth, & M'Cutcheon . . . 1871.

204 × 132. Pp. 24 (last—colophon).

Other editions— 1863, 1876, 1890.

Copies: EF (1890), ML (1876, 1890), SLV (1863, 1871). 1347

Melbourne Hospital. Report of Sub-Committee

of Enquiry on Trained Nurses. July, 1871.

209 × 135. Pp. 44 (l.b.). Colophon—Mason, Firth, and M'Cutcheon . . . Melbourne.

After correspondence with Syd. Infirm., various Lond. hospitals, and Miss Lucy Osburn, Lady Supt Syd. Infirm. (a Nightingale nominee), it is decided that Matron M'Kie should visit Sydney for one month to obtain instruction from Miss Osburn. Appendix contains correspondence and reports on nursing, espec. from Syd. Infirm.

Copies: NL. 1348

Bye-laws of the Melbourne Hospital. [Text begins.]

204 × 130. Pp. 8. ND. Colophon—Stillwell and Knight . . . Melb.

Other editions: ND, 1876, 1884.

Copies: ML (1876, 1884), SLV (all issues). 1349

Report on the sanitary condition of the Hospital, with appendix.

323 × 204. Duplicated writing on rectos only. Pp. [ii] (v.b.), 12 (report), 30 (appendix). Melbourne Hospital, 21 April 1882, at head p. 1.

Rep. to Hosp. Committee on high mortality from surgical sepsis. 'The lamentably high rate . . . is due beyond doubt to the imperfect adoption on the part of the Hon. Staff of the antiseptic treatment on Mr. Lister's principles. . . . Our misfortunes are due to the single omission throughout the institution of the priceless resource of antiseptic surgery and the Committee looks to the Hon. Staff to have the defect removed immediately.'

Copies: NL. 1350

1886. Victoria. Report of the Select Committee of the Legislative Council on the Melbourne Hospital . . . Ordered . . . to be printed, 7th December, 1886. . . . John Ferres, Govt Printer, Melbourne.

349 × 214. Pp. xvi, 238 (l.b.). 1 pl. (plans).

Principal defects are attributed to overcrowding. Contains much on past and current working of Hospital.

Copies: LNSW, ML, NL, SLV. 1351

See also Maitland and Melbourne Hospitals.

Melbourne Hospital for Sick Children, Melbourne

The Free Hospital for Sick Children, 30 Stephen Street, between Collins Street and Flinders Lane . . . [Committee and Officers] In their first prospectus, issued less than a year since, the Committee expressed a hope that they would soon be enabled to receive in-patients. [Text continues.]

257 × 198. Pp. 4 (l.b.). ND. (Aug. 1870.) NI. Ist an. rep.

In 2 an. rep. (1872) name shows as Melb. Hosp. for Sick Children, becoming Children's Hosp. in 1903, and Royal Children's Hosp. in 1953. For history, see Gardiner, Lyndsay (1970), *Royal Children's Hosp., Melb. A history*, Melb.

Copies: Roy. Children's Hosp. (1870–), SLV (1871–1900 various). 1352

Second Report of the Committee of Management of the Melbourne Hospital for Sick Children. For the period ending December 31st, 1871, with the rules of the institution . . . Melbourne: Clarson, Massina, & Co., General Printers . . . 1872.

205 × 125. Pp. 16.

Copies: Roy. Children's Hosp., Melb. 1353

Pharmacopoeia of the Melbourne Hospital for Sick Children. Melbourne: Stillwell and Co. . . . 1880.

162 × 103. Pp. 40 (l.b.). Cloth.

Another ed., 1899.

Copies: AMAV (1880), EF (1899), ML (1880), RACP (1899). 1354

Childhood in bud and blossom A souvenir book of the Children's Hospital Bazaar Compiled and edited by Joshua Lake [Cut] The Atlas Press Melbourne 1900

286 × 222. Pp. [126]. Frontis., portraits and illustns. Cloth. Also edition-de-luxe, copies numbered.

Includes short illustrated history.

Copies: DOS, EF, FF, ML, SLV. 1355

See also Carmichael, Jennings.

Melbourne Inebriate Retreat
See under Melbourne Retreat for Cure of Inebriates.

Melbourne Institution for Diseases of the Eye and Ear
The Melbourne Institution for Diseases of the Eye and Ear, 101 Spring Street . . . (Removed from Albert Street) Surgeon Oculist and Aurist: A. S. Gray, M.R.C.S. London. Free Dispensary open every Monday, Wednesday and Friday . . . Free ward for in-patients, at present containing three beds, with room for more if required and means are furnished. . . . Melbourne: Fergusson and Moore . . . 1866.

156 × 94. Pp. 8.

An appeal for public assistance. Instsn, founded 1863, was conducted by A. S. Gray. Noted *Aust. med. J.*, 1863, 8 : 279.

Copies: SLV. 1356

First Annual Report of the Committee of Management of the Melbourne Institution for Diseases of the Eye & Ear, for the year ending December 31, 1867, with the rules of the Institution . . . Melbourne: Mason, Firth & Co. . . . 1868.

204 × 127. Pp. 8.

In 1873 Instsn amalgamated with Ophthalmic and Orthopaedic Instsn (founded by T. A. Bowen in 1869), to later become the Vic. Eye and Ear Hosp.

Copies: SLV. 1357

Melbourne Lancet
The Melbourne Lancet or, Every Colonist His Own Doctor. No. 1] [Price 6d. (Or, 6s. per annum, delivered in Town or posted . . . [Quotations] Contents . . . Melbourne: Printed and published by W. J. Wallis No. 1, Church Street, St. James's and sold by all booksellers and newsmen.

168 × 102. Pp. 12. (July 1858.) P. w. (cover title).

No 1 only seen. Advertises 'Neopathic Remedies', purveyed from Richmond by 'Vance and Co., physicians, surgeons, & accoucheurs . . . of 20 years' colonial experience . . .' Opens with 'Doctors' blunders dissected.'

Copies: SLV. 1358

Melbourne Local Board of Health
Town Hall, Melbourne, [Space] 187 . . . In reference to your notice of the [Space] to have the cesspool at [Space] emptied, [Text continues.]

311 × 204. Single leaf, v.b. Pale blue paper. (187–.)

Notice to householder to empty cesspool on property, and fill with earth.

Copies: ML. 1359

City of Melbourne. Local Board of Health. (Order to Amend Cesspools, &c., 31 Vic. No. 310, Sec 37.) [Text begins.]

311 × 204. Single leaf, v.b. Pale blue paper. (187–.)

Order to householder to fill up underground cesspit and substitute watertight receptacle above ground.

Copies: ML. 1360

Melbourne Lying-In Hospital
See Women's Hospital, Melbourne.

Melbourne Medical Association
Founded 1891. See *Aust. med. J.*, 1891, ns 13 : 215 (inaugural meeting), 262 (rules), and 286. Publications not seen.

1361

Melbourne Medical Record
Melbourne Medical Record. Vol. IV.—No. 1. Saturday, February 27, 1875. Price 3d. Annual subscription, 13s. Post Free.

280 × 215. Title from head, pl. 1. Pp. 388 (in vol.).

Vol. 4, no 1—vol. 7, no 5; Feb. 1875–Sep. 1877. Weekly; fortnightly after 1 Oct. 1875. Publisher: R. T. Clarke, Fitzroy.

Vol. numbers are continuous with those of the defunct *Med. Record of Aust.*, though there is little to indicate any connection.

Copies: AMAV (v. 4–7), SLV (v. 4, no 6; v. 6, no 13). 1362

Melbourne Medical Students' Society
Rules of the Melbourne Medical Students' Society. Melbourne: Thos. E. Verga . . . 1880.

183 × 127. Pp. 8 (last 3 blank). P. w. (cover title).

Copies: AMAV. 1363

The Melbourne Medical Students' Society. 1882. Melbourne Printed by Walker, May &

Co. . . . 1882.

217 × 135. Pp. 8. P. w. (cover title).

2 an. rep., with rules.

For history, see *Speculum*, the Soc. journal (No 1, July 1884-present); Gandevia, B. (1948), *The Melb. Med. Students, 1862–1942*, The Soc., Melb.

Copies: UM. 1364

Melbourne Retreat for Cure of Inebriates

Report of the Sub-Committee on the Inebriate Question. Read at a general meeting of subscribers to the proposed retreat, at the Town Hall, Melbourne, 26th April, 1872. . . . Melbourne: Stillwell and Knight . . . 1872.

188 × 120. Pp. 36. Signed: Charles M'Carthy MD, Hon. Sec.

Meeting established the Melbourne Retreat for the Cure of Inebriates at Northcote.

Instsn is also variously referred to as Melb. Inebriate Retreat, Northcote Retreat, and Inebriate Retreat, Northcote.

Copies: LNSW, ML, SLV. 1365

———

The First Annual Report of the . . . Melbourne Retreat for the Cure of Inebriates, with the rules and regulations, the Inebriates Act, and list of subscribers. 1873. Melbourne: Stillwell and Knight . . . 1873.

201 × 127. Pp. 28 (l.b.).

Following 5th an. rep., 1877, publication ceased till 6th rep., 1887.

ML copies belonged to Dr. M'Carthy, and are bound with other papers published by him.

Copies EF (1875), ML (1873–7, 1888), SLV (1873). 1366

———

Report of the Medical Superintendent of the Inebriate Retreat Northcote, from 1st July, 1886, to 31st December, 1887—18 months. [Text begins.]

283 × 143. Pp. 4. Single leaf, v.b., inserted.

On vicissitudes and need for assistance.

Copies: ML. 1367

———

Revised rules & regulations of the Melbourne Retreat for the Cure of Inebriates, Northcote. [Text begins.]

201 × 127. Pp. 4. (1888.) Colophon: Stillwell and Co. . . .

Copies: ML. 1368

———

The Inebriate Retreat Northcote. [Copy of letters to the Hon. A. McLean, M.L.A., Chief Secretary.] [Text begins.]

198 × 130. Pp. 12. Colophon—Melb.: Echo Publishing Company . . . 1891. Signed: Charles M'Carthy.

Copies: ML. 1369

———

See also McCarthy, Charles.

Melbourne Sanitary Protection Association

Founded 1888, on account of prevalence of typhoid and scarlet fever, to provide expert supervision of dwellings for the prevention of contagious diseases and to promote a knowledge of hygiene. Members were entitled to a report on sanitary condition of their premises and to consultation with MO of Assn. (*Aust. med. J.*, 1888, ns 10 : 287). Publications NS.

1370

Melbourne Union Benefit Society

Articles and rules for the regulation of the Melbourne Union Benefit Society instituted in Melbourne, May 8th, 1839. United to relieve not combined to injure. Patron W. Lonsdale, Esq., P. M. Melbourne: Arden and Strode, Printers to the Society, Queen-Street, 1839.

214 × 140. Pp. vi, [7]–24 (l.b.).

The first pamphlet published in Victoria.

For history and reproduction of title, see *Premier Victorian pamphlet*, by J. Gartner, Melb., 1937 (230 copies); also C. A. McCallum, 'Victorian Historical Collection', in *Across the years*, ed. C. Barrett, Melb., Seward, 1948. For account of Society: Graham, H. B. (1956), 'The Hon. David Elliot Wilkie, M.D.', *Med. J. Aust.*, 1 : 557.

NL and SLV copies bear signature of John Pascoe Fawkner.

Copies: NL, SLV. 1371

Melbourne University

See University of Melbourne.

Member of the Medical Profession, A

See Best, John.

Member of the Staff of the Children's Hospital

See Stawell, Sir R. R.

Menzies, Alexander

Letters and journals of the late Alexander Menzies M. B., C. M. Arranged and supplemented by his father. ... Edinburgh: Privately printed 1888.

217 × 140. Pp. [vi], 128. Frontis.—portrait. Cloth.

Biography of young Scottish doctor who, suffering from tuberculosis, came to Aust. in the hope of recovery. He arrived in Melb. in 1887, left for home soon after, and died at sea.

Copies: FC, SLV. 1372

Mercury, The, Hobart

The fluke: What it is. Why it is. How to get rid of it. Dedicated to the Royal Commission on the fluke. ...

209 × 135. Pp. 16 (l.b.). Colophon—Tasmania: ... 'Mercury' Steam Press Office, Hobart Town. Cover title. ND. (1868.)

Three letters on liver fluke in sheep, first published in Hobart *Mercury* (Jan., Feb. 1868).

Copies: ML, NL. 1373

Merewether, Henry Alworth

By sea and land being a trip through Egypt, India, Ceylon, Australia, New Zealand and America all round the world ... London Macmillan and Co. 1874. ...

191 × 127. Pp. xvi, 344, 60 (book advts). Frontis. Cloth.

Small-pox occurred on author's voyage from Colombo to Aust. His account of the passage from WA to NSW is an example of passengers' complaints of the ineptitude of quarantine services, and of the trials of officials with certain influential travellers. Includes account of author's 'hardships' at North Head Quarantine Stn, Syd. (where he was visited by the governors of NSW and Tas.), with criticism of H. G. Alleyne MD, MOH Pt Jackson.

Copies: FC, ML, NL, SLS, SLT, SLV, UA, UQ, US. 1374

Meyer, Felix

British Medical Association. (Victorian Branch) President's address ... December 19, 1894. ... Stillwell and Co. ... Melbourne.

204 × 140. Pp. 14. P. w. (cover title). From *Aust. med. J.*, Jan. 20, 1895.

Reviews recent medical advances.

For Felix Meyer (1858–1937) MD, FRACS, Hon. Surg. Women's Hosp. Melb., see obit., *Med. J. Aust.*, 1937, 2 : 626; for his Jackson Lecture, 'The making of obstetrics' *Med. J. Aust.*, 1933, 1 : 75. He was ed., *The History of Wesley College*, Melb., 1914; author, *Adamson of Wesley*, Melb., 1932.

Copies: LNSW, ML, SLV. 1375

Miklucho-Maclay, or Miklouho-Maclay, Nicolaus N.

Anthropologische Bemerkungen ueber die Papuas der Maclay-Küste in Neu-Guinea ... Overgedrukt uit het "Natuurkundig Tijdschrift". Batavia, Ernst & Co. 1873.

209 × 135. Pp. [ii] (title, v.b.), 26. P. w. (title rptd).

Includes probable first recognition of malarial infection in New Guinea natives.

Copies: EF, LNSW. 1376

———

Meine zweite Excursion nach New-Guinea, (1874) ... [Text begins.]

209 × 135. Pp. 32. 1 flg map. (Tjipanas, Sept. 1874.)

Copies: LNSW. 1377

———

Ueber Brachyocephalität bei den Papuas von Neu-Guinea. ... [Text begins.]

209 × 135. Pp. 4. (l.b.). Bogor, 14 Oct. 1874.

Copies: LNSW. 1378

———

Ethnologische Bemerkungen ueber die Papuas der Maclay-Küste in Neu-Guinea ... Overgedrukt uit het "Natuurkundig Tijdschrift". Batavia, Ernst & Co., 1875.

209 × 135. Pp. 30 (2, last 2 blank). P. w. (title rptd).

Pt 11. Published separately. Pp. 40. ND. NI. (LNSW).

Copies: EF, LNSW, ML. 1379

———

... List of plants in use by the natives of the Maclay-Coast, New Guinea ... With some ... remarks by Baron Ferd. Von Mueller. [Text begins.]

214 × 132. Pp. 14 (l.b.). Repr., *Proc. Linn. Soc. NSW*.

Includes plants for food, stimulants and medicines, and various uses.

Copies: LNSW. 1380

Proposed zoological station for Sydney. ... From the Proceedings of the Linnean Society of New South Wales. Read 26th August, 1878. [Text begins.]

181 × 127. Pp. 10.

See item below; also Syd. Biol. Station.

Copies: LNSW. 1381

... The Committee appointed to consider Baron Miklucho-Maclay's suggestion for the establishment of a zoological station ... [Text continues.]

204 × 130. Pp. [2]. Repr., *Proc. Linn. Soc. NSW*, 30 Sep. 1878.

Approves foundation of Syd. Biol. Station; Wm Macleay provides temporary quarters. Rules.

Station was opened at Watson's Bay about 1881.

Copies: LNSW. 1382

Lettre ouverte a Son Exc. Sir Arthur Gordon ... Sydney, 23 Janv., 1879. Excellence, L'importance du sujet de cette lettre ... [Text continues.]

323 × 204. Single leaf, v.b. Signed: Nicholas de Miklouho-Maclay.

Open letter to British High Commissioner for W. Pacific (Fiji), demanding protection for natives of Maclay Coast NG, by recognition of their land rights and prevention of sale to them of fire-arms and alcohol.

Copies: LNSW. 1383

A short resume of the results of anthropological and anatomical researches in Melanesia and Australia. (March, 1879–January, 1881 ... [Text begins.]

214 × 132. Pp. 6 (l.b.). ND. NI.

Copies: LNSW. 1384

From the Proceedings of the Linnean Society of New South Wales, Vol. VI. Read ... June 29th, 1881. On the practice of ovariotomy by the natives of the Herbert River, Queensland. ... [Text begins.]

214 × 135. Pp. 8 (l.b.).

Unconfirmed hearsay accounts of aboriginal women ovariotomised by native methods. Contains also: 'Remarks about the circumvolutions of the cerebrum of Canis dingo', with 1 litho. pl.; 'Cranial deformation of new-born children at the island of Mabiak, and other islands of Torres Straits ...' (27 July 1881).

Copies: LNSW. 1385

Papers published in Sydney, 1878–84. By N. de Miklouho-Maclay.

214 × 135. Pp. 146 (numbered by hand).

Title to coll. of 23 papers, each with own pagination.

N. N. Miklucho-Maclay (1846–88), Russian scientist and explorer, who made three expeditions to N. Guinea (1870–7), lived in Sydney, active in scientific pursuits, in his later years. For biog., see Thomassen, E. S. (No 2190); Greenup, F. S. (1944), *Who travels alone*, Syd.; Markov, S. (1946), *N.M.M., 1846–1888*, Moscow. Collected works, 4 vols, were published in Moscow, 1950–3.

Copies: LNSW. 1386

Milford, Frederick

A few observations on some cases of cancer of the breast ... Reprinted from the "Intercolonial Medical Congress of Australasia Transactions". Melbourne: Stillwell & Co ... 1889.

220 × 140. Pp. 10. P. w. (cover title).

Copies: ML. 1387

An Australian handbook of obstetric nursing. Designed for the use of midwives and nurses ... with 92 illustrations Sydney Angus & Robertson ... 1896.

168 × 102. Pp. xx (l.b.), [ii] (v.b.), 249 (last—colophon only), 16 (book notices). 92 figs. Cloth.

2 ed., NS. 3 ed., 1911, with title *Aust. midwife's and nurse's handbook*, Melb. (ML.)

The first Aust. manual on the subject. A comprehensive work, with occasional reference to local experience.

For Frederick Milford (1831–1902) MD Heidelberg & Syd., MRCS, of Sydney, see *Austsn med. Gaz.*, 1902, 21 : 430; McIntosh, A. M. (1951), *Med. J. Aust.*, 1 : 533; Miller, D. (1957), 'The med. pioneers of St. Vincent's Hosp.', *BPCMUS*, 13 : 61.

Copies: DOS, EF, ML. 1388

Millar, John

On the supply of water to the town of

Geelong. ... (Reprinted from the Transactions of the Philosophical Institute of Victoria).

204 × 127. Pp. 30 (l.b.). (1857.)

Copies: SLV. 1388a

Miller, John Lindsay

On puerperal fever. ... [Text begins.]

204 × 138. Pp. 22. London, June, 1878—at end of text. Colophon:Dunn and Wright ... Glasgow.

Discusses aetiology and treatment, from Tas. experience.

J. L. Miller MD, FFPS, FRCS Edin., was 'CMO Launceston and one of the Court of Medical Examiners of that Colony.'

Copies: EF. 1389

Miller, William

Health, exercise, and amusement. Athletic sports, and how to train for them. With reminiscences of the world's athletes. By Professor Miller. (Edited by "Andro", of "The Sportsman") ... Melbourne: A. H. Massina & Co. ... 1895.

250 × 156. Pp. 64. 17 figs. Stiff p. w. (with variation of title and 2 cuts).

'Professor' William Miller (1847–1939), exponent of a system of physical training and health culture, was termed the world's finest all-round athlete of his time.

Copies: ML, NL. 1390

Mineral Springs, A sketch of

A sketch of mineral springs and their uses, with references to the properties of the Ballan selters water. Melbourne: Joske and Morton, Proprietors ...

156 × 102. Pp. 36. Colophon—H. Cordell, Printer ... P. w. (title rptd, decorated).

Includes testimonials from Melb. doctors.

Copies: NL. 1391

Ministering Children's Fresh Air League

See Fresh Air League.

Mitchell, Graham

Cumberland disease (the so-called "new disease") in Australian sheep. Reports, letters &c., on the subject. ... Compiled by Graham Mitchell ... Melbourne: Alex. M'Kinley & Co. ... 1877.

217 × 135. Pp. viii (l.b.), 128 (l.b.), xvi (advts). Coloured litho. frontis. 1 map. Stiff p. w. (title rptd) or cloth.

Aust. views on the nature and prevention of anthrax, by numerous contributors. The disease was known in Australia as spleno-enteritis, Cumberland enteritis, 'and more generally ... by the popular name of Cumberland disease—so called from its having made its first appearance ... in the co. Cumberland, N.S.W. It first appeared in 1847 ... near Campbelltown; and since has slowly spread ...'

Graham Mitchell FRCVS, prominent Melb. veterinarian, founder of Austsn Vet. Med. Assn, worked for the organisation of his profession, legislative control of animal diseases, and establishment of a school and hospital.

Copies: EF, ML, NL, SLS, SLV, SLW, UA, UQ. 1392

Mitchell, James

Statement of the case of Jas. Mitchell, Esq., late Surgeon on the Civil Establishment of New South Wales. Printed for private use. Sydney: Printed at the "Herald" Office, Lower George Street.

209 × 127. Pp. 52, cviii (appendix—l.b.). 1 pl. (plan, Civil Hosp., Syd.). ND. (1838.) P. w.

Author's defence against charges of disobedience, which led to his dismissal in 1837.

James Mitchell (1792–1869) LRCSE, Asst Col Surg. in charge of General Hosp. Syd. (1825–37), came to NSW in 1821. He was father of David Scott Mitchell (1836–1907), founder of the Mitchell Library. See McIntosh, A. M. (1956), 'The case of Dr. J. M.', *Med. J. Aust.*, 2 : 161; Smith, C. E. (1966). *Dr. J. M.*, Newcastle, Newcastle Hist. Monograph No 1.

Copies: LNSW, ML, NL, SLV. 1393

Mitchell, James T.

[Laid before the Port Adelaide Board of Health, February 18, 1886.] Dr. Mitchell's report on the drainage of the Port. [Text begins.]

140 × 90. Pp. 8 (l.b.). Title at head of p. 1. Colophon—W. K. Thomas & Co., Register Office.

On recommended replacement of cesspits by pan system.

Copies: SLS. 1394

Moderate Drinking in Relation to Health

Moderate drinking in relation to health. [Text begins.]

206 × 140. Pp. 4. ND. Colophon—McMaster & Savage ... Melb.

Attacks 'the delusion that when used in

moderation stimulants are conducive to health.'
Copies: EF. 1395

Moffitt, Andrew

Papers on blood poisoning, typhoid, typhus, scarlatina, and other zymotic diseases, &c prevalent in N. S. Wales and their treatment ... reprinted from the late N. S. Wales Medical Gazette, and with special notes on Dr. Day's ozone treatment of scarlatina and small pox, and on his own treatment of typhoid ... Sydney: W. E. Smith ... 1878.

212 × 138. Pp. [vi] (ii, v blank), 7–52. 1 fig. Cloth.

Includes, in addition to subjects of title, sections on midwifery difficulties and quinine. Author's treatment of typhoid, for which he claimed success, was with turpentine. Day's treatment of smallpox and scarlet fever consisted of gargles of ozonic ether and the application of ointment containing this to the whole body.

Copies: CC, EF, FC, LNSW, ML, NL, US. 1396

———

No. 11] [October, 1883. Health Society of New South Wales. ... The papers on typhoid of the late A. Moffitt ... Reprinted by permission of his family. ... Sydney ... Turner and Henderson ...

214 × 138. Pp. [ii], 12, [ii] (last—colophon). P. w. (title rptd).

The same. Syd., W. E. Smith. Pp. 14.

Three papers (dated 1873) on the clinical features, treatment and prevention of typhoid.

For Andrew Moffitt (1815–1881) LRCP, MRCS, ex-Surg. RN, of Sydney, see obit., *Austsn med. Gaz.*, 1881, 1 : 32.

Copies: ML, NL. 1397

Mole, Percy

Crown, bar and bridge work. ... Bendigo : J. B. Young, 1893.

NS. Review, *Aust. med. J.*, 1894, ns 16 : 50. 'A well illustrated little brochure' describing methods of repairing the effects of decay in teeth. 1398

Molloy, C. H.

Accidents and emergencies. What to do till the doctor comes. Drawn from the most modern sources and giving the latest methods of treatment. With hints on nursing. Illustrated. Revised by Dr. C. H. Molloy, Resident Medical Officer, Alfred Hospital. Melbourne: A. H. Massina & Co. ...

158 × 102. Pp. 104. Figs. ND. [1888.] P. w. (title rptd, advts other sides).

Copies: SLV. 1399

Moloney, Patrick

The therapeutics of tea drinking ... [Text begins.]

204 × 120. Pp. 8. Repr., *Aust. med. J.*, 1880, ns 2.

Strong tea causes many ills, and 'much of the lunacy in the interior is helped, if not caused' by it. This is ascribed to tannin.

For Patrick Moloney (1843–1904) MB Melb., see obits, *Austsn med. Gaz.*, 1904, 23 : 543, and *Intercol med. J. Austsia*, 1904, 9 : 576; also Hugh McCrae's *My father and my father's friends*, Syd., 1935.

Copies: EF, UM. 1400

———

See also [White, J. H.], (The Shroff.'

Money, Angel

Treatment of diseases in children including the outlines of diagnosis and the chief pathological differences between children and adults. ... London H. K. Lewis ... 1887

181 × 125. Pp. [ii], xiv (l.b.), 560, 16 (book notices). Cloth.

The same, 1887. Philadelphia, Blakiston. 2 ed., 1890. London, H. K. Lewis.

Angel Money (1856–1904) MD Lond., FRCP, Hon. Phys. Syd. Hosp. for Sick Children, and co-editor *Intercol med. J. Austsia*, see obits, *Lancet*, 1904, 2 : 1256 and 1460; *Brit. med. J.*, 1904, 2 : 1196; *Austsn med. Gaz.*, 1904, 23 : 483.

Also published: *The health of children*, Lond., 1888; *The student's text-book of the practice of medicine*, Lond., 1889. NS.

Copies: EF, RACP, UA, UM, US. 1401

Moon, Alice Caroline

No. 11. February, 1881. The Australian Health Society, Melbourne. Preservation of the teeth. [Text begins.]

204 × 140. Pp. 4. Colophon—M'Carron, Bird and Co. ... Melb.

Signed: A.C.M. Writer conducted a physical culture school in Melb., and later engaged in medical journalism in Syd. See *Austsn med. Gaz.*, 1894, 13 : 174.

Copies: CC, EF, ML, NL, SLV. 1402

———

See Bartrop, Mrs. and Moon, Alice C.

Moon, William
See Rutherford, J.

Moore, Joseph Sheridan
See Beer, Frederick.

Moore, William [Surgeon]
Certificates and testimonials of W. Moore, M.D., M. S. Melb. Candidate for the position of Lecturer on Materia Medica, Medical Botany, and Elementary Therapeutics, at the University of Melbourne. ... Melbourne: Stillwell and Co. ...

183 × 125. Pp. 12 (l.b.). ND. (Letters dated 1883–7.)

Copies: AMAV. 1403

———

The treatment of severe and relapsed cases of club-foot. ... Reprinted from the "Australian Medical Journal", April 15, 1894. Melbourne: Stillwell and Co. ... 1894.

217 × 140. Pp. 12. P. w. (cover title).

Copies: AMAV, KFR. 1404

———

Multiple hydatids ... with remarks on hydatids at the root of the neck, simulating thoracic aneurysm. Multiple abdominal hydatids treated by repeated abdominal sections ... Carcinoma of the large intestine-resection, with use of Murphy's button ... Four cases of renal calculus. ... Reprinted from the "Intercolonial Medical Journal of Australasia", June, September and October, 1897. Melbourne: Stillwell and Co. ...

242 × 156. Pp. 24 (last 2 blank). P. w. (cover title).

Copies: AMAV. 1405

———

The operative treatment of varicose veins, with especial reference to a modification of Trendelenburg's operation. "Operation for strangulated inguinal hernia considered in relation to recent advances in surgery". ... Reprinted from the "Intercolonial Medical Journal of Australasia", July and August 1896. Melbourne: Stillwell and Co. ...

247 × 158. Pp. 20. P. w. (cover title).

Copies: AMAV, BG, KFR. 1406

———

Plastic surgery With illustrative cases. ... Melbourne: Stillwell and Co. ... 1899.

247 × 153. Pp. [iv] (l.b.), 116. 5 pl., 6 figs. Cloth or p. w. (title rptd).

Chapters on: incisions, closure, formation and transplanting flaps, Wolfe's and Thiersch grafting, nasal surgery, hypospadias, imperforate anus.

For Wm Moore (1859–1927) MD, MS Melb., Hon. Surg. Melb. Hosp., see obit., *Med. J. Aust.*, 1927, 2 : 857; Graham, H. B. (1954), *Med. J. Aust.*, 1 : 971; Gandevia, B. (1952), "The early history of biliary tract surgery in Aust.', *Roy. Melb. Hosp. Clin. Rep.*, 22 : 19.

Copies: AMAQ, AMAV, BG, CC, DOS, KFR, UM. 1407

Moore, William [Homoeopathist]
(Third edition.) Man! Know thyself; explains by a few facts the origin of contagious sexual diseases; suggested by the perusal of a letter on the prevention of such diseases ... addressed only to those who deem ... self protection from such disorders expedient. ... Sydney: F. Cunninghame and Co. ... 1878. ...

178 × 120. Pp. x (l.b.), [ii] (v.b.), 25, ii. P. w. (short title).

Author, who gives highly original information on sexual complaints, was homoeopathist and proprietor of electric baths. NSW Leg. Council, Sel. Committee on ... Practice of Medicine and Surgery (1887), elicited that he had had no training, and could detect cancer by blood test of his own invention.

Copies: ML. 1408

Morett, R.
Führer für Gesunde and Kranke. Von Dr. R. Morett. Adelaide 1882. Gedruckt von Basedow, Eimer & Co. ... (Office der "Australischen Zeitung".

170 × 106. Pp. 48. Cloth.

Includes advice on healthy living, care and diet in illness, clinical instruction, and list of diseases with numbered remedies.

Copies: SLS. 1409

Morgan, Cosby William
Hydatid disease: remarks on its increasing prevalence in the Australian colonies, with some thoughts as to its causation. ... Reprinted ... from the "N.S.W. Medical Gazette". Sydney: Gibbs, Shallard & Co. ...

212 × 135. Pp. 16 (1874.) P. w. (title rptd).
Copies: ML, SLV. 1410

State medicine in New South Wales, with some remarks on the Medical Acts of the colony ... Read before the Intercolonial Medical Congress ... 1889. Newcastle: ... "Herald" Office ... 1889.

212 × 132. Pp. 12.

Criticises backward condition of NSW health legislation.

C. W. Morgan MD Brux., MRCS, who came to Aust. 1869, practised in many NSW centres, including Sydney (Hon. Surg. Syd. Infirm.), and Newcastle (Hon. Surg. Newcastle Hosp., Port MO, Mayor). See *Aldine Centennial Hist. of NSW*, Syd., 1888; *Aust. men of mark*, Syd., 1889, Champion, B. W. (1952), 'The Newcastle Hosp.', *Newcastle and Hunter R. Hist. Soc. J. & P.*, 6 : 28 and 132.

Copies: ML. 1411

Morris, George Sculthorpe

Convicts and colonies. Thoughts on transportation & colonization, with reference to the islands and mainland of Northern Australia. ... London: Hope and Co. ... 1853.

212 × 140. Pp. iv, [5]–40.

Author, formerly chaplain in VDL, recommends establishment of convict settlements in N. and N. E. Aust. to replace those in the south. He disagrees with the opinion, derived from experience at Melville Is., that the islands of the north coasts would be 'found deadly to Europeans', and states 'this is certainly not the case at Moreton Bay, nor ... in the country between that district and Port Essington.'

Copies: ML, NL. 1412

Morris, Thomas

See Cole, H. S., and Morris, Thomas.

Morrison, Alexander

On lunacy law reform ... George Robertson Melbourne ... 1880.

214 × 147. Pp. 12.

Alexander Morrison (1849–1913) LRCP, LRCSE, was at various times MO Ararat Lun. Asylum, Surg. Alfred Hosp. Melb., and Govt Botanist WA. See *Med. J. Aust.*, 1914, 1 : 112; *J. Nat. Hist. & Sci. Soc. WA*, 1914, 5 : 108; Maiden, J. H. (1921), 'Records of Aust. botanists', *J. & P. Roy. Soc. NSW*, 55 : 164.

Copies: EF. 1413

See also West Australian Settler's Guide and Farmer's Handbook.

Morrison, George Ernest

An Australian in China being the narrative of a quiet journey across China to British Burma ... London: Horace Cox ... 1895.

209 × 138. Pp. xii, 300 (l.b.). Frontis., 26 pl., 2 flg maps, 3 figs. Cloth.

2 ed., 1895; 3 ed., 1902.

For G. E. Morrison (1862–1920) MD, ChM Edin., traveller and 'Times' correspondent in the Far East, see *Med. J. Aust.*, 1920, 1 : 535; Pearl, C., *Morrison of Peking*, Syd., 1967.

Copies: AMAV, BG, EF, FC, ML, NL, RACP, SLS, SLV, SLW, UA, UM, UQ, US, WLC. 1414

Morton, John

A novel view of the causes producing typhoid fever, &c., and plan of treatment. ... Sydney: John Sands, 1875.

NS. 8vo. Pp. vi, 7–14. Review, *NSW med. Gaz.*, 1875, 5 : 274.

Typhoid (and other fevers) are due to self-poisoning, by absorption of gas from the intestines.

1415

Vaccination and its evil consequences Cow-pox and its origin. Small-pox, &c. ... Parramatta: ... C. E. Fuller ... 1875.

217 × 143. Pp. iv, [5]–16. P. w. (title rptd).

John Morton (d. 1887) MB, LRCSE (1850), practised at Potts Point and Tenterfield NSW. In 1884 he offered the NSW Govt a remedy against the venom of black, brown and tiger snakes (*Austsn med. Gaz.*, 1884, 3 : 186).

Copies: FC, LNSW, ML, NL. 1416

Mount Bischoff Provident Hospital, Waratah, Tas.

(No. 5.) [Royal Arms] 1885. Parliament of Tasmania. Mount Bischoff Provident Hospital: Report for 1884. Presented to both Houses of Parliament ...

324 × 206. Pp. 6 (l.b.). Colophon—William Thomas Strutt, Govt Pr, Tas.

4th annual report.

An. reps for 1881–93 appear in Parliamentary

Papers of Tas. (1882–94).
Copies: LNSW, SLT, SLV. 1417

'Mucor'
See Candler, Samuel Curtis.

Mudgee Hospital
See No 1579.

Mueller, Augustus
Psychology as founded on the facts of mesmerism, clairvoyance, and spiritualism. A lecture lately delivered ... at Yackandandah and other places. Melbourne ... W. H. Terry ... 1880.
212 × 140. Pp. 32. P. w. (title rptd).
Copies: ML, SLV. 1418

———

The religious aspect of spiritualism and its relation to the churches. Lecture delivered ... at Yackandandah, etc. ... Published by W. H. Terry ... Melbourne.
212 × 140. Pp. 16. ND. P. w. (cover title).
Copies: EF, SLV. 1419

———

On snake-poison. Its action and its antidote. ... Sydney: L. Bruck, Medical Publisher ... 1893.
247 × 158. Pp. [ii], vi, 86 (l.b.). Frontis.—portrait of author. Cloth.
Snake venom (of any kind) is a specific nerve poison, for which strychnine is the antidote. The drug is recommended in large and repeated injected doses. Review, *Austsn med. Gaz.*, 1893, 12 : 165.
Mueller's treatment caused much controversy in local medical press and was widely adopted, prior to final discredit. See Campbell, C. H. (1968), 'Dr. Mueller's strychnine cure of snake-bite', *Med. J. Aust.*, 2 : 1.
A. Mueller (1828–99) MD, ChD Giessen, who came to Aust. about 1863, practised at Yackandandah Vic. In 1897 he advocated perchloride of mercury by mouth for typhoid fever (*Austsn med. Gaz.*, 1897, 16 : 328.)
Copies: AMAV, BG, DOS, EF, KFR, ML, NL, RACP, SLS, SLV, UA, UM, US. 1420

Mueller, Baron Sir Ferdinand Jakob Heinrich von
... Pitury. To the Editor of the Australian Medical Journal. Sir, Some weeks ago I was asked ... about the origin of Pitury ... a stimulant said to be of marvellous power and known to be in use by the aborigines of Central Australia. [Text continues.]
201 × 132. Single leaf, v.b. (Feb. 15, 1877.) NI.
Identifies preparation as from *Duboisia hopwoodii*—'a new and perhaps important medicinal plant.' As a result of author's advice, Joseph Bancroft studied pharmacological properties of related species *D. myoporoides*, which later proved a source of hyoscine, hyoscyamus, atropine and other alkaloids. See Grimwade R. (1954), 'Duboisia—Australia's own drug plant', *Walkabout*, June; also Bancroft, Joseph.
Copies: ML. 1421

———

Intercolonial Medical Congress, Melbourne, 1889. Address by Baron Ferdinand von Mueller, President of the Section of Pharmacology. [Text begins.]
212 × 138. Pp. 30 Colophon—Stillwell ... Melb.
Reviews Aust. pharmacological contributions.
Sir Ferdinand von Mueller (1825–96), Baron of Würtemberg, MD (Rostock), FRS, illustrious botanist, trained in medicine and pharmacy, was Vic. Govt Botanist. See obit., *Austsn med. Gaz.*, 1896, 15 : 490; Willis, M. (1949), *By their fruits, a life* ..., Syd. Works include over 800 botanical pamphlets and articles. His most complete bibliography is that of Nat. Herbarium, Melb.
Copies: EF. 1422

——— (translator)
Contribution towards the history of the development of the echinococcus, with especial reference to the formation of daughter-cysts. By Vald. Rasmussen ... Copenhagen ... Translation by Ferd. von Mueller, M.D., F.R.S. [Text begins.]
214 × 135. Pp. 18. Repr., *Aust. med. J.*, 1869.
ML copy bears translator's inscription to W. Wools FLS.
Copies: ML. 1423

———

Observations on coccobacteria in the secretions of wounds, and on their transfer to the cornea of rabbits. By Dr. Th. Billroth, Professor of Surgery in Vienna. Translated by Baron Ferd. von Mueller ... [Text begins.]
207 × 130. Pp. 4. ND. Stillwell and Knight, Printers ... Repr., *Aust. med. J.*, Dec. 1876.

'On such vegetable parasites as are recognised as the sources of diseases in man'—Translator's note.
Copies: ML. 1424

Brief excerpts from Professor Carl von Naegeli's recent work on the minutest fungaceous organisms in relation to infectious diseases and sustenance of health ...
207 × 133. Pp. 20. ND. Colophon—Stillwell and Co. ... Repr., *Aust. med. J.*, Nov. 1878.
Copies: ML, NL, SLS, SLV. 1425

Dr. A. Wernich's essay on beri-beri in Japan. A review translated by Baron Ferdinand von Mueller ... [Text begins.]
168 × 143. Pp. 4. Colophon—Stillwell and Co., Printers ... Repr., *Aust. med. J.*, Dec. 1882.
Copies: NL. 1426

Excerpts from Professor Hugo Schulz's treatise on eucalyptus oil. Translated and supplemented by Baron Sir Ferd. von Mueller ... Reprinted from "The Australasian Medical Gazette" for 1883. L. Bruck ... Sydney. 1883.
217 × 135. Pp. 48. P. w. (title rptd).
Chemical, antiseptic and pharmacological actions of eucalyptus oil, with notes on clinical use.
Copies: ML, US. 1427

See also Wilkie, David E. and Mueller, Sir F. von.

Mullen, William Lowell
See Springthorpe, John William and Mullen, W. L.

Mullins, George Lane
Registration of still-births and the protection of infants. ... read before the ... Intercolonial Medical Congress of Australasia, Sydney, September 27, 1892. ...
242 × 153. Pp. 8. Colophon—Syd.: Charles Potter, Govt Pr—1893. P. w. (cover title).
For protection of infant life, author advocates registration of still-births, licencing and inspection of lying-in hospitals and medical supervision of all births in them, proper interment of deceased infants, death certificates for these, and state care of all illegitimate and neglected infants.
Copies: ML. 1428

Register of administrations of anaesthetics for use in hospitals, public institutions and private practice. Sydney: Angus & Robertson.
Qto. Pp. 100. (c. 1892.) Cloth.
NS. Noted in *Austsn med. Gaz.*, 1892, 11 : 365; 'for recording effects of various anaesthetics, local and general.' 1429

Epidemic diseases and their prevention in the eastern suburbs of Sydney. Paper read before the Eastern Suburbs Medical Association ... January 25, 1895. ... J. W. Eedy ... Sydney.
244 × 181. Pp. 8. P. w. (cover title).
Copies: LNSW, SLV. 1430

Notes on hydatid disease in New South Wales. ... (Reprinted from the *Australasian Medical Gazette*, February 15, 1895.) Sydney: J. W. Eedy & Co. ... 1895.
244 × 186. Pp. 4. Frontis. (map). P. w. (cover title).
A statistical study.
Copies: EF, LNSW, SLV, UA, US. 1431

Notes on phthisis in New South Wales and other Australasian colonies. ... read before the Section of Sanitary Science and Hygiene ... (Reprinted from the Australasian Medical Gazette, August 20, 1895.) John Sands ... Sydney.
244 × 186. Pp. 16 (last 2 blank). 1 map, 1 graph. P. w. (title rptd).
Contains comparative statistics.
Copies: EF, LNSW, SLV, UA. 1432

Cancer in New South Wales. ... (Reprinted from *The Australasian Medical Gazette*, January 20, 1896.) John Sands ... Sydney.
245 × 195. Pp. [ii] (title, v.b.), 8. P. w. (title rptd).
A statistical examination.
Copies: EF, LNSW, SLV, UA. 1433

New South Wales as a health resort for British

consumptives. Read . . . at the Annual Meeting of the British Medical Association, held at Carlisle, July, 1896. . . . J. A. Thompson, Printer . . . Sydney.

242 × 172. Pp. [6] (last 2, flg). ND. (1896.) P. w. (title rptd).

Advises British doctors on type of patients likely, or unlikely, to benefit from voyage and sojourn in NSW, and gives form of information which should accompany each patient.

Copies: SLS. 1434

———

A brief history of smallpox and vaccination in New South Wales from the foundation of the colony to the present day. . . . Sydney: Angus & Robertson. London: Young J. Pentland. 1898.

247 × 183. Pp. 16 (l.b.). Double cols. P. w. (cover title).

Extracts reprinted in Cumpston, J.H.L., *Small-pox in Aust., 1788–1908*, 1914 : 175–9.

Copies: EF, ML. 1435

———

Tuberculosis and the public health . . . Read . . . Australian Association for the Advancement of Science, Sydney . . . 1898. Sydney: John Sands . . . 1898.

181 × 117. Pp. 24 (l.b.). P. w. (cover title).

G. L. Mullins (1862–1918) MA, MD TCD & Syd., FSS, Hon. Phys., St Vincent's Hosp. Syd., a leader in St John's Ambulance and Red Cross Soc., had special interests in public health and electro-therapeutics. Obit., *Med. J. Aust.*, 1918, 1 : 294.

Publications after 1900 include: *Camps & camp hygiene* (with W. G. Armstrong), Syd., 1908; *A junior course in first aid*, Syd., 1910; *Medical electricity*, Syd., 1915.

Copies: ML, NL, US. 1436

———

See Springthorpe, John William, and Mullins, G. L.

Murder Made Easy

Murder made easy. [Text begins.]

229 × 165. Single leaf (v.b.). Repr., Editorial, *Austsn med. Gaz.*, 1889, 8 : 277 (with addition). NI.

A criticism of coronial inquiries into deaths not certified by medical practitioners. It is asserted that, 'as a field for . . . exercise of his profession, Australia far surpasses any other country for the average everyday murderer . . . The only essentials wanted here for the successful commission of homicide are determination and self-reliance, the laws of the colonies provide every other requisite . . .'

EF copy bears rubber stamp of L. Bruck, med. publisher, Syd.

Copies: EF. 1437

Murray, James Patrick

Small-pox, chicken-pox, and vaccination: An essay by James P. Murray, L.R.C.S.I., L.K. & Q.C.P.I., late Surgeon to the Immigration Hospital and Western Gaol; late Resident Physician and Surgeon to the Melbourne Hospital; late Resident Surgeon to the Benevolent Asylum; late Resident Surgeon to the Provincial Hospital, Invercargill, New Zealand . . . Melbourne: George Robertson . . . 1869.

212 × 135. Pp. 48 (last—colophon). P. w. (title rptd).

A general account, including section on Vic. small-pox epidemics of 1857–8 and 1868–9.

Author was principal in the slaughter of over 70 kidnapped Solomon Islanders on board his ship *Carl* in 1871—one of the most brutal atrocities of the Pacific blackbirding trade. Though ring-leader in this, Murray later informed on his associates, escaping arrest and serving as Crown witness in the subsequent trials. He was in Manchester in 1879, when he published a letter in *Lancet*, 1: 106. For his clouded earlier years, see Fulton *(infra)*. In 1869 he was ed., *Aust. med. Gaz.*, (1st no) but was dismissed thereafter. (*Aust. med. J.*, 1869, 14 : 94). He was also expelled from Vic. Med. Assn (*Aust. med. Gaz.*, 1869, 1 : 55 and 81). For biog., (in which name is wrongly shown as James Phillip), see Fulton, R. V. (1922), *Med. practice in Otago and Southland*, Dunedin; also Searle, G. S. (1875), *A narrative of the voyage of the brig Carl*, Melb.; *Aust. med. J.*, 1872, 17 : 296 and 343; *NSW med. Gaz.* 1872, 2 : 378; Kreitmeyer's Waxworks Exhib., No 1113.

Copies: EF, ML, SLV. 1438

Muskett, Philip Edward

The health and diet of children in Australia . . . Edwards, Dunlop & Co. Limited Sydney . . . Samuel Mullen Melbourne and London . . .

209 × 168. Pp. [vi], 186 (l.b.). ND. [1889.] Paper boards.

2 ed., [1890]. Pp. [xii], 188. Edwards, Dunlop & Co., Syd.; Melville, Mullen &

Slade, Melb.

Review, *Aust. med. J.*, 1890, ns 12 : 374.

Copies: AMAV, DOS, ML, NL, SLS, SLV, US. 1439

The feeding and management of Australian infants ... Edwards, Dunlop & Co., Limited Sydney, Brisbane and London Melville, Mullen & Slade Melbourne and London ...

212 × 165. Pp. [2] (advts), [iv], 66. ND. (1889.) Stiff p. w. (amended title). [2 ed.]

1 ed., 1888; 2 ed., 1889; 3 ed., 1890; 4 ed., 1896; 5 ed., 1900; 6 ed., 1903; 7 ed., 1906; 8 ed., 1909. Some not seen. Dates from publisher's list.

Includes dietary for breast and hand fed children, recipes. 3 ed. includes 'Mountain air as a remedy.'

Copies: AMAV, CC, EF, KFR, ML, NL, RACP, SLV, SLW, US. 1440

Prescribing and treatment in the diseases of infants and children. ... Edinburgh & London: Young J. Pentland. 1891.

147 × 82. Pp. xii, [ii] (v.b.), 294 (l.b.), [iv] (book notices). Leather.

2 ed., 1892. 3 ed., 1894.

Copies: AMAV, DOS, EF, KFR, ML, MLWA. 1441

An Australian appeal The evil—the cause—the remedy ... Edwards, Dunlop & Co., Limited: Sydney ... Melville, Mullen & Slade: Melbourne ... E. S. Wigg & Son: Adelaide. ...

214 × 135. Pp. 60. 3 pl. ND [1892.] Stiff p. w. (title in red).

High infant mortality is due especially to gastro-enteritis and acute respiratory infections. Author advocates an organisation for reducing this, and suggests mountain stations near all large cities for care of sick infants in summer.

Copies: DL, EF, FC, ML, NL, SLS. 1442

The art of living in Australia (together with three hundred Australian cookery recipes and accessory kitchen information by Mrs. H. Wicken ...) ... Eyre and Spottiswoode ... London ...

181 × 125. Pp. [10] (advts), [ii], xxx (l.b.), 431, [3] (advts). ND. [1894.] Cloth.

Sections on Aust. climate, bathing, ventilation, clothing, diet, exercise, food habits, fish, oysters, wines and cookery.

For comment on the work by an acquaintance of author, see J. R. Tyrrell, *Old books, old friends, old Sydney*, Syd., 1952.

Copies: AMAV, BG, CC, DOS, EF, KFR, ML, NL, OL, SLT, SLV, SLW, UA, UM, UQ, US. 1443

The book of diet (with, also, a collection of savoury, choice, delicious and selected recipes). ... George Robertson & Co., Melbourne ...

227 × 122. Pp. [20] (advts), xvi, [iv], 301, [9] (advts). 3 lines of title in red. ND. [1898.] Stiff p. w. or cloth.

Advocates substitution of fruit, vegetables and salads for part of the heavy Aust. meat diet ('almost a religion'); and cooking training for all girls. Discusses alcohol in health and disease, and properties and actions of various alcoholic drinks.

Copies: EF, ML, NL, SLV, US. 1444

The diet of Australian school children (with, also, health and disease during school life), and technical education. ... George Robertson & Co., Melbourne ...

178 × 127. Pp. [12] (advts), xxviii, 180, [4] (advts). Title partly in red. ND. [1899.] Cloth or p. w.

For P. E. Muskett (1857–1909) LRCP, LRCPE, Surg. Supt of Immigration and Med. Supt Quarantine Stn Syd., and later Hon. Surg. Syd. Hosp., see *Austsn med. Gaz.*, 1909, 28 : 520.

Published also: *The illustrated Aust. medical guide*, 2 vols, Syd., 1903; 2 ed., 1909; *The attainment of health, and the treatment of different diseases by means of diet*, Syd., 1908; 2 ed., 1909.

Copies: AMAV, EF, ML, NL, SLV. 1445

N

Naegeli, Carl von
See Mueller, Sir Ferdinand.

Napier, Alexander Disney Leith
Notes on the treatment of uterine prolapse, with an account of a new modified method of anterior colporrhaphy. Edinburgh: Oliver & Boyd. 1887.
8vo. Pp. 12.
NS. Listed *SGC*, ser. 2.
1446

The thermometer in obstetrics and gynaecology ... (Two lectures delivered at the Midwives' Institute) London H. K. Lewis ... 1890
206 × 130. Pp. 30. 1 chart.
1. Obstetric temperatures, 2. gynaecological temperatures; including treatment of pyrexia and case histories.
Copies: British Museum. 1447

The menopause and its disorders (with chapters on menstruation) ... London The Scientific Press, Limited ... 1897
246 × 147. Pp. xv (l.b.), 307. Plates, figs, tables.
A. D. Leith Napier MD, ChM Aberd., MD Adel., MRCP, qualified 1875, was an experienced gynaecologist with London appointments and ed., *Brit. J. Gynaec.* He became Sen. Res. Surg., Adel. Hosp. about 1896, and later practised in Adelaide.
Copies: Wellcome Inst. Hist. Med. 1448

See also Adelaide Hospital, Nos 16–18.

Narracoorte Hospital, SA
Second Annual Report of the Narracoorte Hospital for the year ended January 12, 1883 ... Also rules and regulations. Narracoorte: J. B. Mather and Co., Printers ... 1883.
204 × 127. Pp. 34.
Copies: SLV (2–8, 1883–9). 1449

Nathan, Charles
See Medini, Michael. Case of

National Bichloride of Gold Institute
A visit to "St. Helen's on the Sea," North Geelong. A delightful home for the treatment of alcoholism. The marvellous cures effected by this institutional and scientific method. ... The National Bichloride of Gold Institute of Australasia Limited. ... Melbourne.
214 × 135. Pp. 14. Woodcut view of Inst. (verso of title).
Institute was founded in 1892 by Rev. Dr. Wolfenden, formerly of Chicago (*Austsn med. Gaz.*, 1892, 11 : 450).
Copies: ML. 1450

Nayler, B. S.
... The battle of science. A lecture, delivered in the Mechanics Institution, Melbourne ... 1869 ... Published by Evans Brothers ... [Text begins.]
201 × 132. Pp. 24 (last 3—book notices).
Accuses clergy of opposing scientific thought. Quotes *Argus* (31 July 1869) stating Melb. Univ. Council had prevented Prof. Halford from giving public lecture on 'Protoplasm', as this was a religious subject.
Copies: SLV. 1451

Naylor, Henry George Horace
How to distinguish and treat diseases of children by G. Horace Naylor ... George Robertson & Co. Melbourne ...
163 × 105. Pp. viii, 126. ND. (1880, in preface from Campbelltown Tas.) Cloth.
A book for parents, including drug list and home dispensing.
H.G.H. Naylor LRCP, LRCSE, Hon. MO to Campbelltown Hosp. at the time of publication, later practised in Hobart and Ballarat (1900).
Copies: RACP. 1452

The Same. 1881. Title amends author's name to

Henry G. H. Naylor.
Copies: CC, ML, WLC. 1453

Neale, Alfred [James]

Facts about the skin. Manchester & London: Deansgate and Ridgefield. 1884.

NS. Listed *SGC*, ser. 1. Pp. 10. Author was at this time Phys. Manchester Hosp. for Skin, Cancer, Scrofula and Chronic Diseases.
1454

———

Eczema. London, Trübner & Co., 1888.

NS. Listed *SGC*, ser. 2. Pp. 40.
1455

———

Scrofula, or King's evil; and what can be done for it. A book for parents. London: Trubner & Co. ND.

NS. Listed *SGC*, ser. 2. 12mo. Pp. 112.
1456

———

Consumption in its modern aspect. Its prevention and cure by climatic and open air treatment. . . . Christchurch . . . Whitcombe and Tombs Limited.

183 × 122. Pp. 74 (l.b.). ND. (?1898.)
Copies: ML, NL. 1457

———

The skin: its disfigurements, diseases and their cure, with notes on baths and bathing. . . . Second edition. . . . Sydney: Turner and Henderson . . . 1899.

178 × 120. Pp. 48. P. w. (title rptd).
Copies: FC. 1458

———

Plague and security . . . [Cut of plague bacilli] Sydney: Turner and Henderson. 1900.

185 × 125. Pp. 36. P. w. (amended title).

A popular account of plague, published at outset of the 1900–1909 epidemic in Australia.
Copies: DL, FC, ML, NL, US. 1459

———

Trichology: a study of baldness & falling hair. . . . Sydney: Turner and Henderson. 1900.

178 × 117. Pp. [6], 7–32 (last—colophon only). 1 fig. P. w. (title rptd).

For A. J. Neale (1857–1937) MD, ChM Edin., an early Sydney specialist in dermatology, see Johnson, A. (1963), "An Aust.—NZ dermatologist of the 19th century", *Aust. J. Derm.*, 7 : 64.

Listed on title: *Common sense about skin diseases*. NS.

Also published: *Toilet and troubles of the skin and hair*, Syd.; *Dyspepsia or indigestion*, Syd., 1903.
Copies: FC, NL, SLT, SLV. 1460

Negus, R. P.

Essay on leeches, a practical hand book by R. P. Negus, leech conservator. Prefaced by Dr. F. Mueller, F.R.S. Melbourne: George Robertson . . . 1868.

178 × 112. Pp. [vi], 24, [4] (l.b.). P. w. (cover title).

The Same, 1868. Pp. [viii] (3 blanks), 24, [6] (advts, 2 blanks). Cloth.

A leech dealer's 'guide to the keeping and preservation of leeches, their application, use, and treatment', including methods of gathering.

Negus and Co. applied for lease of 320 acres of swamp near Dandenong for breeding of leeches; granted 12 acres (*Aust. med. J.*, 1869, 14 : 63). 'Immense quantities' were gathered, particularly from the Murray R., and exported to Europe and US. (*Aust. Med. J.*, 1867, 12 : 29).
Copies: CC, EF, ML, SLV, WLC. 1461

Neild, James Edward

Introductory lecture to the course on forensic medicine, in the Melbourne University. Delivered . . . March 12, 1866. . . .

203 × 133. Pp. 14 (last—colophon only). Melb.: Wilson and Mackinnon, 1866.

Author was 1st Lect. Forensic Med. (1865–1904).
Copies: AMAV, SLV. 1462

———

Valedictory address to the Medical Society of Victoria. By James Edward Neild, MD. President of the Society for the Year 1868 . . . Delivered . . . January 13th, 1869.

212 × 135. Pp. 14. Colophon—Stillwell and Knight . . .
Copies: SLV, UM. 1463

———

Dirt and disease. A lecture, delivered at the Industrial and Technological Museum, Melbourne . . . on 26th July, 1872. [Text begins.]

212 × 135. Pp. 24.

Appeals for improved sanitary conditions in

Melbourne.
Copies: LNSW, ML, SLV. 1464

———

On the advantages of burning the dead. ... (Read before the Royal Society, 8th December, 1873.) [Text begins.]
212 × 135. Pp. 10. Colophon—Stillwell and Knight ... Melb.
Copies: SLV, UM. 1465

———

Address delivered at the annual meeting of the Victorian Branch of the British Medical Association ... Stillwell & Co. ... Melbourne. 1882.
212 × 135. Pp. 12.
Comment on vaccination, quackery, Melb. Hosp., Melb. Med. School, Austin Hosp. for Incurables.
Copies: LNSW, ML, UM. 1466

———

The Medical School of the Melbourne University. An address delivered on the twenty fifth anniversary of the opening of the Medical School ... 1887. ... Melbourne: Stillwell and Co. ...
212 × 135. Pp. 18. (1887.)
The history of School to its 25th year.
Copies: UM. 1467

———

Grand complimentary and special dramatic matinee at the Princess Theatre ... July 26th 1890. Tendered to Dr. James E. Neild by the leading members of the musical & dramatic profession. ... presented by T. A. Alexander, Proprietor of "The Call".
293 × 224. Pp. [4]. Litho. cover title, with portrait and decorations.
For J. E. Neild (1824–1906) MD, medico-legal pathologist, physician, ed. *Aust. med. J.*, and music and dramatic critic, see obits, *Austsn med. Gaz.*, 1906, 25 : 479 and *Intercol med. J. Austsia*, 1906, 11 : 514; also Johnston, Sir Wm (1963), 'Dr. J.E.N. and the early hist. of the St. John Amb. Assoc.', *Med. J. Aust.*, 2 : 563; King, E.S.J. (1951), *Med. J. Aust.*, 2 : 101 (for assn with Univ. Melb).
Copies: ML. 1468

———

See also Bayldon, John; Gilbee, Wm; Martin, Lawrence J.; Sutherland, Alexander, No 2088; Thomas, David John.

———, **'Cleofas'**

A bird in a golden cage. By Cleofas. Christmas, 1867. Melbourne: Charles Muskett, 78 Bourke Street East.
152 × 100. Pp. 80. P. w. (short title). Author identified by inscription in O'Sullivan copy.
A sentimental tale in a theatrical setting.
Copies: DOS, SLV. 1469

———, **and Others**

The Hamlet controversy. Was Hamlet mad? Or, the lucubrations of Messrs. Smith, Brown, Jones, and Robinson. With a preface by the Editor of the "Argus". Melbourne: ... H. T. Dwight, ... 1867.
214 × 140. Pp. 34. P. w. (cover title).
Reprints newspaper discussion by Melbourne citizens: James Smith, J. E. Neild MD, Charles Bright, Sir A. Michie QC, David Blair, and R. H. Horne.
Copies: ML, NL, SLV, UM. 1470

———

The Same. With title: *Was Hamlet mad? Being a series of critiques on the acting of the late W. Montgomery: written in Melbourne in 1867*. Ed. R. H. Horne. Lond., 1871. NS.
1471

Nepean District Hospital, NSW

Rules and regulations of the Penrith Hospital & Benevolent Asylum, with the Annual Report and list of subscribers, &c., for the year 1866. Sydney: ... Edmund Mason ... 1867.
196 × 130. Pp. 12 (l.b.).
Instn was closed and replaced by Nepean Dist Hosp. which, commencing in temporary premises in 1890, opened 1895. Present hosp. opened 1952.
Copies: LNSW (1866, 1867). 1472

[Nesfield, Henry W.]

A chequered career; or fifteen years in Australia and New Zealand. London: Richard Bentley and Son ... 1881. ...
178 × 117. Pp. x, [ii] (v.b.), 370 (l.b.). Cloth.
Describes brief employment as wardsman at Harcourt's private mental hospital at Richmond Vic. (Cremorne Inebriates and Insane Asylum). Anon. Ascribed to Henry W. Nesfield by Miller.
Copies: ML, NL, SLS, UA, UQ, US. 1473

———

The Same. New ed. 1887. Adds 'experience' after 'fifteen years' in title. Pp. viii, [ii] (v.b.), 370 (l.b.), 4 (book advts).

Copies: FC, ML, NL, OL, SLT, SLV, UM, UQ, US. 1474

New Medical Gazette

New Medical Gazette. (Published by authority) Scotch Mary of Bondi having passed her examination . . . [Text continues.]

200 × 128. Pp. 4 (2, 4 blank). ND. [?1876.] NI.

Humourous paragraphs on unqualified practice in NSW, probably propaganda against a Medical Bill. *Bruck's List of Unregistered Practitioners* (1886) shows Scotch Mary then in practice at Blacktown NSW.

Copies: ML. 1475

New Norcia Mission, WA

See Nos 291, 358, 1602.

New Norfolk Hospital for Insane, Tas.

Regulations for the guidance of the officers and attendants of the Lunatic Asylum, New Norfolk. By order of the Commissioners, June, 1856. Tasmania: James Barnard, Govt Printer, Hobart Town. 1856.

220 × 138. Pp. 20 (l.b.). P. w. (title rptd).

Later named New Norfolk Hosp. for Insane, thence Lachlan Park Mental Hosp.

Copies: ML. 1476

———

Evidence taken before Joint Committee on Hospital for Insane, New Norfolk, and returns referred to in Report. [Text begins.]

217 × 140. Pp. 12 (l.b.). (1859.) Colophon—James Barnard, Govt Pr, Tas.

Copies: ML. 1477

———

(No. 11.) [Royal Arms] 1860. Tasmania. Hospital for the Insane, New Norfolk. Annual report of the Commissioners for the year 1859. . . .

332 × 206. Pp. 8 (l.b.), [2] (v.b.). Addendum by Bishop R. W. Willson. Colophon—James Barnard, Govt Pr, Tas.

Hospital was transferred by Imperial Govt to the Colony in 1855, above being 1st Colonial rep. Annual reports from 1859 onwards appear in Parliamentary Papers of Tasmania.

Copies: LNSW, SLT, SLV. 1478

———

(No. 12.) [Royal Arms] 1883. Session 11. Tasmania. Legislative Council. Hospital for the Insane, New Norfolk: Report of Select Committee. . . . Ordered by the Council to be printed, December 18, 1883.

324 × 206. Pp. viii, 54 (l.b.). Colophon—William Thomas Strutt, Govt Pr, Tas.

Inquiry into management.

Copies: LNSW, SLT, SLV. 1479

———

(No. 38.) 1884. Parliament of Tasmania. Hospital for Insane, New Norfolk: Report on: by Doctors Manning, Dick, and Paterson. . . .

323 × 196. Pp. 10 (l.b.). 3 flg maps. Colophon—William Thomas Strutt, Govt Pr, Tas.

Copies: ML, SLT, SLV. 1480

New South Wales—Anthrax Board

1888. Legislative Assembly. New South Wales. Anthrax (Cumberland) disease in sheep and cattle. (Test of efficacy of Pasteur's vaccine of anthrax as a preventive against—Report of experiments at Junee, &c. . . . [Text begins.]

315 × 204. Pp. 6. Colophon—Syd.: Charles Potter, Govt Pr—1888. Signed by members of Anthrax Board.

Copies: LNSW, ML, NL, SLV. 1481

———

The Same. 1889. Queensland. Presented to both Houses. Pp. 6 (l.b.). Govt Pr, Bris.

Copies: LNSW, NL, OL, SLV. 1482

———

1889. New South Wales. Report on experiments demonstrating the efficacy of Pasteur's vaccine of anthrax, as a preventative against anthrax (Cumberland) disease in sheep and cattle. Carried out by representatives of M. Pasteur Paris, under supervision of the members of the Anthrax Board, at Junee during September and October, 1888. Sydney: Charles Potter, Govt Printer, 1889. . . .

242 × 156. Pp. [iv], 38 (l.b.). 5 pl. (inc. portrait of Pasteur). P. w. (title rptd).

Trials with attenuated cultures, performed by Loir and Germont, modelled on those of Pasteur at Pouilly-le-Fort in 1881, had the same dramatic success. Includes: 'The anthrax disease', by E. Stanley; 'The history of the anthrax bacillus', by W. M. Hamlet; 'Anthrax or Cumberland disease', by A. A. Devlin. See also Loir, Adrien.

Copies: EF, LNSW, ML, NL, SLV, US. 1483

New South Wales—Board of Health

1881. Legislative Assembly. New South Wales. Small-pox. (Regulations, &c.) ... [Text begins.]

331 × 204. Pp. 8 (l.b.). Colophon—Syd.: Thomas Richards, Govt Pr. Signed: Alfred Roberts, H. G. Alleyne, for Bd of Health.

Includes organisation, and rules for various groups at risk.

The Board of Health, with statutory executive powers to administer the health legislation, was established by the NSW Govt, faced by a major small-pox epidemic, in 1881. It existed, with an especially proud tradition and reputation of service, to 1973, when it was absorbed by the newly established Health Commission of NSW. For history, see [Cummins, C. J.], NSW, Rep. of Dir Gen. of Pub. Health for 1971, Syd., Govt Pr, 1973 : 5–11.

Copies: LNSW, ML, NL, SLV. 1484

———

Rules for the guidance of surgeons visiting cases of small-pox, or of a doubtful character. [Text begins.]

344 × 217. Single leaf, v.b. (1881.)

Copies: EF, HDN, NL. 1485

———

Regulations for the medical staff. [Text begins.]

344 × 217. Single leaf. Pp. [2]. 1881.

For use in small-pox epidemic. Verso bears: Rules for the guidance of surgeons visiting cases of small-pox, or of a doubtful character.

Copies: EF, HDN, NL. 1486

———

Caution. Small-pox. You are requested to take notice that the house occupied by ... is infected with small-pox. [Text continues.]

344 × 217. Single leaf, v.b. (1881.)

Collection of forms used in small-pox epidemic (1881–2) is held by NSW Health Dept.

Copies: EF, HDN. 1487

———

Sanitary rules for the guidance of householders in the neighbourhoods of houses infected with small-pox. [Text begins.]

344 × 217. Single leaf, v.b. (1881.)

Copies: HDN, NL. 1488

———

Instructions for Disinfecting Corps. [Text begins.]

344 × 217. Single leaf. Pp. 2. (1881.)

For use in small-pox epidemic.

Copies: HDN, NL. 1489

———

Suggestions for the guidance of captains of passenger vessels upon the appearance of small-pox. Board of Health. Sydney ... February, 1882.

344 × 217. Pp. 4 (l.b.).

Copies: HDN. 1490

———

Animal vaccination: being information supplied by the Government of Bombay to that of New South Wales, on the subject of animal lymph and vaccination; and embodying the Bombay Act No. 1 of 1877, for the compulsory vaccination of children in the City of Bombay. Sydney: Thomas Richards, Govt Printer. 1882.

242 × 153. Pp. 16. Woodcut frontis. P. w. (amended title).

Information on manufacture of calf lymph.

For history of vaccination in Aust., see Cumpston, J.H.L. (1914) *The history of small-pox in Aust., 1788–1908*, Melb. : p. 130.

Copies: EF, ML, NL, SLV. 1491

———

1883. Legislative Assembly. New South Wales. Report of the Board of Health upon the late epidemic of small-pox, 1881–1882. ... [Text begins.]

320 × 204. Pp. 30, [ii] (v.b.). 2 flg plans. Colophon—Syd.: Thomas Richards, Govt Pr—1883.

Reports 154 cases, with 40 deaths; also organisation, Coast Hospital, rules for med. and lay staffs.

Board was appointed in June 1881 under the Infectious Diseases Supervision Act 1881, which arose out of this epidemic.

Copies: HDN, LNSW, ML, SLV. 1492

1887. (Second Session.) Legislative Assembly. New South Wales. Report of the Board of Health. (Quarantining of the S. S. "Preussen".) Ordered ... to be printed, 16 March, 1887. [Text begins.]

320 × 204. Pp. 34 (l.b.). Colophon—Syd.: Charles Potter, Govt Pr—1887.

Small-pox on voyage: 114 cases, 14 deaths. Cumpston, J.H.L. (1914), *The history of small-pox in Aust., 1788–1908*, describes as 'the worst case in the history of shipping coming to Australia'.

Copies: HDN, LNSW, ML, NL, SLV. 1493

1887–8. Legislative Assembly. New South Wales. Typhoid fever in Sydney and suburbs. (From 1876 to 1888.) Ordered ... to be printed, 26 June, 1888. [Text begins.]

331 × 212. Pp. 4 (l.b.). Colophon—Syd.: Charles Potter, Govt Pr—1888.

Includes table of deaths and mortality rates 1876–1888, monthly incidence, and hosp. admissions. Reports from 1890 also include information on measles, scarlatina, and diphtheria. Issued annually to 1895 (Syd., 1897).

Copies: HDN, LNSW, ML, NL, SLV. 1494

A map of the City of Sydney. With location of deaths for 1889 from all causes. ...

505 × 380. Single sheet, v.b. (1889.) NI.

3 maps were issued (1889) with location of deaths from: A. (above); B. from diarrhoeal diseases, typhoid, diphtheria, scarlet fever; and C. from phthisis and other lung diseases. B. and C. not seen.

Copies: EF. 1495

Directions for collection and transmission of samples of water for chemical examination. [Text begins.]

320 × 202. Single leaf, v.b. (1889.)

Copies: HDN, ML. 1496

1889. Legislative Assembly. New South Wales. Eureka Patent Sanitary Burning Works, Newcastle. (Report of the Deputy Medical Adviser on.) ...

322 × 204. Pp. 4. Colophon—Syd.: Charles Potter, Govt Pr. 1889.

On excreta disposal at Newcastle. For brochure on method, see No 656.

Copies: HDN, LNSW, ML, NL, SLV. 1497

1889. Legislative Assembly. New South Wales. Board of Health. (Views of, in regard to compulsory vaccination.) Ordered ... to be printed, 7 August, 1889. [Text begins.]

205 × 105. Single leaf, v.b.

Strongly advises compulsory vaccination, which had been adopted 'in the large majority of English-speaking ... colonies, including the whole of the Aust. colonies, except N.S.W.'

Copies: LNSW, ML, SLV. 1498

Board of Health. Rules for disinfection, &c.

312 × 205. Pp. 8. Colophon—Syd.: Charles Potter, Govt Pr ... 1889.

Detailed instructions for local authorities, including special procedures for various diseases.

Copies: HDN. 1499

1890. Legislative Assembly. New South Wales. Bovine tuberculosis in the South Coast district. (Report of the Board of Health on). Ordered ... to be printed, 9 October, 1890. [Text begins.]

330 × 210. Pp. 8. Colophon—Syd.: Charles Potter, Govt Pr—1890.

Copies: EF, LNSW, ML, NL, SLV. 1500

1893. New South Wales. Slaughter-houses throughout the colony. (Their sanitary condition, and inoperativeness of present Acts relating to same.) ... [Text begins.]

331 × 212. Pp. 8. Colophon—Syd.: Charles Potter, Govt Pr—1893.

Bd of Health to Parlt. Review, *Austsn med. Gaz.*, 1893, 12 : 421, states report discloses 'a filthy and horrifying state of affairs' and 'bristles with alarming facts.'

Copies: EF, HDN, LNSW, ML, NL, SLV. 1501

... Board of Health, New South Wales. Manual for the information and guidance of local authorities and of dairymen and milk-vendors registered ... under the "Dairies Supervision Act" ...

263 × 153. Pp. 16 (l.b.). Colophon—Syd.: Charles Potter, Govt Pr—1896.

On hygiene requirements.

Copies: ML. 1502

1897. Legislative Assembly. New South Wales. Board of Health. (Memorandum by the President of the, on prevention of tuberculosis in man and in cattle.)

330 × 210. Pp. 6 (l.b.). Colophon—Syd.: William Applegate Gullick, Govt Pr— 1897.

Copies: LNSW, ML, NL, SLV. 1503

1899. Legislative Assembly. New South Wales. Department of Public Health. (Report of the Board of Health for 1897.) Printed ... 29 March, 1899. [Text begins.]

324 × 305. Pp. 56 (l.b.). Flg plan, 4 figs. Signed: J. Ashburton Thompson.

1st rep. of Bd of Health (created 1881), which administered the health laws, through the Dept of Public Health, to 1973. Includes organisation, administration and functions of Dept. Appendices reprint various publications of Board.

2nd rep. (for 1898) published 1900; no further reports of Dept appeared till 1913.

Copies: HDN, LNSW, ML, NL, SPH, SLV. 1504

1900 New South Wales. The case of A. P. (Report of the Board of Health upon.) [Text begins.]

336 × 212. Pp. 8. 2 mounted microphotographs, 1 fig. Colophon—William Applegate Gullick, Govt Pr—1900.

On the first NSW bubonic plague case in 1900–9 epidemic. Bact. rep. by Frank Tidswell; epidemiology and prevention by J. Ashburton Thompson.

Copies: EF, NL. 1505

See also items under Thompson, John Ashburton.

New South Wales—Department of Agriculture

Flower-farming for perfumes and medicines.

242 × 153. Pp. 26. 2 figs. Colophon—Syd.: Charles Potter, Govt Pr—1883. P. w. (cover title).

Copies: ML. 1506

Department of Agriculture, Sydney ... A fatal case of poisoning by the fruits of a native climbing plant. (Bryonia laciniosa, Linn.) [Royal Arms] Sydney: Charles Potter, Govt Printer ... 1896.

242 × 153. Pp. 4 (l.b.). P. w. (cover title).

Copies: EF. 1507

New South Wales—Department of Public Health

Health Department, New South Wales. Directions for the prevention of hydatid disease; also for the immediate treatment of the apparently drowned, and of snake-bite and sunstroke. Sydney: William Applegate Gullick, Govt Printer. 1897.

215 × 140. Pp. 14 (l.b.). 4 figs. Stiff p. w. (title rptd), cloth backstrip.

Notes each section also issued in poster form.

Copies: EF, KFR, ML. 1508

... Department of Public Health, New South Wales. Suggestions to householders for the prevention of typhoid fever, on domestic isolation and disinfection, and on the law on infectious diseases. ...

250 × 153. Pp. 32. Colophon—Syd.: William Applegate Gullick, Govt Pr—1899.

Copies: NL. 1509

1899. Department of Public Health, New South Wales. Quarterly reports of Local Authorities made under the Public Health Act. [Text begins.]

326 × 209. Pp. 14. Colophon—Syd.: William Applegate Gullick, Govt Pr—1899.

Copies: HDN (1899–1901). 1510

[Royal Arms] By authority. Prevention of plague. Instructions to householders issued by the Department of Public Health. Sydney, 1st March, 1900. Sydney: William Applegate Gullick, Govt Printer. 1900.

209 × 163. Pp. 8. Bluish grey paper.

On rat control and disinfection.

Copies: ML. 1511

New South Wales—Legislative Council

25th August, 1833. The Committee of the

Legislative Council appointed on the 18th June, 1833, to enquire into the mode in which the formation of the tunnel for conducting water to Sydney is carried on, and to report the means by which its progress may be accelerated, and the supply of water rendered more generally useful by leading it to to public fountains, or to private houses . . . [Text proceeds.]

322 × 198. Pp. 6. Blue tinted paper. NI. From *V&P*, 1833.

On the construction of 'Busby's Bore', the tunnel from the site of present Centennial Park to Hyde Park, planned and directed by John Busby to replace the failed supply of the Tank Stream and other sources.

Copies: LNSW, ML, NL, SLV. 1512

Tunnel. Report of the Committee on the Tunnel for Supplying the Town of Sydney with Water. The Committee of the Legislative Council appointed on the 23rd August, 1837, to enquire into, and report upon—[Text continues.]

303 × 181. Pp. 11, [12–14] (tables, l.b.). (13 July 1837.) NI. From *V&P*, 1837.

Copies: LNSW, ML, NL, SLV. 1513

New South Wales. Tunnel. Minutes of evidence taken before the Committee on the Tunnel for Conducting Water into the Town of Sydney. Ordered . . . to be printed, 12th September, 1837. Sydney: Printed by A. Cohen, "Australian" Office . . .

303 × 181. Pp. [iv] (l.b.), 16 (l.b.). Pale blue paper. From *V&P*, 1837.

Account of the scheme and associated circumstances, with evidence of John Busby and Major Barney.

Copies: LNSW, ML, NL, SLV. 1514

Hospital Department. Despatch from . . . Lord Glenelg, to Sir Richard Bourke, K.C.B., directing that no persons but convicts shall be allowed into hospitals maintained for them by the British Government, unless provision for such purpose be made from the Colonial funds. No. 377. Downing Street, 29th September, 1837. [Text begins.]

298 × 209. Pp. 6. Blue tinted paper. NI. From *V&P*, 1838.

Amendment to arrangement by which 'paupers or destitute persons' were admitted gratuitously to convict hospitals, maintenance being a charge on penal funds.

Copies: LNSW, ML, NL, SLV. 1515

New South Wales. Medical Practice Bill. Report from the Committee on the Medical Practice Bill, with minutes of evidence. Ordered . . . to be printed, 2 October, 1838. Sydney: Printed by William Jones . . .

298 × 209. Pp. 42. From *V&P*, 1838.

Recommends appointment of Medical Board; publication of names of all legally qualified practitioners. A Medical Act was passed and Board established in the same year.

Copies: LNSW, ML, NL, SLV. 1516

Report from the Board, appointed on 5th December, 1838, "to inquire into, and report on, the probable causes which have produced, during the present year (1838), a greater degree of sickness on board Immigration Ships chartered by the Government, than in those fitted out under the Bounty System . . ." Immigration Office, 15th January, 1839. [Text begins.]

305 × 184. Pp. 12 (l.b.), [ii] (l.b.). 2 flg charts. NI. From *V&P*, 1839.

Considers migrant selection, clothing and cleanliness, diet, and authority of surgeons-supt.

Copies: LNSW, ML, NL, SLV. 1517

1845. New South Wales. Aborigines. Report from the Select Committee on the condition of the Aborigines, with appendix, . . . evidence, and replies to a circular letter. . . . Sydney: Printed by W. W. Davies, at the Govt Printing Office . . .

331 × 209. Pp. 60 (l.b.). Blue tinted paper.

Copies: LNSW, ML, NL, SLV. 1518

1848. New South Wales. (Vaccine Institution.) . . . Letter from the Health Officer [Arthur Savage], to the . . . Colonial Secretary, 19th Jan. 1848.

312 × 190. Single leaf, v.b. Blue paper.

1st an. rep. announces successful foundation, and distribution of lymph. 'To the best of my knowledge, the true cow-pock is being actively diffused throughout the Colony.' Reports issued

annually.
Copies: LNSW, ML, NL, SLV. 1519

1848. New South Wales. (Military Hospital, Fort Phillip.) Ordered, by the Council, to be printed, 18th April, 1848. [Text begins.]
310 × 190. Pp. 2. Blue tinted paper.
Proposal, through Governor, to transfer Military Hospital at Fort Phillip to the Colony, if expense of building a hospital at the New Military Barracks in South Head Rd, from funds provided for the latter, be approved.
Copies: LNSW, ML, NL, SLV. 1520

1848. New South Wales. Slaughter Houses. Report from the Select Committee on Slaughter Houses, with minutes of evidence. ... Sydney: Printed by W. W. Davies, at the Govt Printing Office ...
310 × 190. Pp. [ii], [2], 46. Blue tinted paper.
Vividly shows the extremely offensive and unhealthy conditions caused by the 78 Sydney butcheries which slaughter in premises within the city. The blood and refuse are carried to the Tank Stream or head of Sydney Cove, where they remain till removed by heavy rains or high spring tides. Recommends removal of slaughter houses 3 miles beyond city limits; establishment of public abattoirs.
Copies: LNSW, ML, NL, SLV. 1521

1849 New South Wales. Aborigines and Protectorate. Report from the Select Committee on the Aborigines and Protectorate, with appendix, ... evidence, and replies to a circular letter. ... Sydney: Printed by W. W. Davies, at the Govt Printing Office ... 1849.
331 × 209. Pp. 40 (l.b.). Blue tinted paper.
Inquiry 'into the state of the Aboriginal Inhabitants of this Colony—more especially in regard to the success or failure of the present Protectorate system at Port Phillip.'
Copies: LNSW, ML, NL, SLV. 1522

1849. New South Wales. Medical Profession Bill. Progress Report from the Select Committee on the Medical Profession Bill, with minutes of evidence. Ordered by the Council, to be printed, 5th October, 1849. Sydney: Printed by W. W. Davies, at the Govt Printing Office ... 1849.
340 × 200. Pp. [iv] (l.b.), 62 (l.b.).
Copies: LNSW, ML, NL, SLV. 1523

1852. New South Wales. Supply of pure water to the City of Sydney. Report from the Board appointed ... to enquire into the best means of affording a supply of pure water to the City of Sydney. With appendix. ... Sydney: Printed by W. W. Davies, at the Govt Printing Office ... 1852.
322 × 190. Pp. [ii] (v.b.), 62 (l.b.), [ii] (v.b.). Pale blue paper.
Copies: LNSW, ML, NL, SLV. 1524

1852. New South Wales. Health Officer. ... Report for the year 1851, from the Health Officer, to the Colonial Secretary, 6th July, 1852.
322 × 190. Pp. [2] (v.b.). NI. Pale blue paper. Signed: Arthur Savage, Health Officer.
Subsequent reports, published 1854–58, appear as HO, Port Jackson.
Copies: LNSW, ML, NL, SLV. 1525

1853. New South Wales. Quarantine Laws. Report from the Select Committee on the Quarantine Laws, with minutes of evidence and appendix. ... Sydney: Printed by W. W. Davies, at the Govt Printing Office ... 1853.
317 × 196. Pp. [iv], 28 (l.b.), 10 (l.b.). Pale blue paper.
Discusses med. views and practice. Quarantine Ground buildings and ship *Harmony*, 'lately fitted as a hospital ship to separate sick and apparently healthy patients', meet requirements.
Copies: LNSW, ML, NL, SLV. 1526

1854. New South Wales. Intemperance. Progress Report from the Select Committee on Intemperance, with minutes of evidence. ... Printed by William Hanson, Govt Printer ... 1854.
315 × 195. Pp. 4, 12, 106 (l.b.). Pale blue paper.
1855. Final report. Pp. [iv], 12 (l.b.).
Inquires 'into the cause of the alarming increase of intemperance in the Colony', and remedies.
Copies: LNSW, ML, NL, SLV. 1527

1854. New South Wales. Destitute Children. Progress Report from the Select Committee on Destitute Children, with minutes of evidence. . . . Sydney: Printed by William Hanson, Govt Printer . . . 1854.

315 × 195. Pp. [iv], 28 (l.b.), 12 (l.b.), [2]. Blue paper.

Copies: LNSW, ML, NL, SLV. 1528

1855. New South Wales. Report from the Commissioners of Inquiry on the Lunatic Asylums of New South Wales, with . . . evidence, appendix . . . Sydney: Printed by William Hanson, Govt Printer . . . 1855.

324 × 202. Pp. 12, 82, 8. Pale blue paper.

On the state of the asylums, the classification and treatment of patients, and their protection and security.

For general appreciation, see Cummins, C. J. (1968), *The administration of lunacy and idiocy in NSW, 1788–1855*, Syd.

Copies: LNSW, ML, NL, SLV. 1529

1854. New South Wales. Lunatic Asylum, Tarban Creek. (Management during the absence of Dr. Campbell.) Ordered by the Council to be printed, 1st December, 1854. [Text begins.]

315 × 195. Pp. 18. Blue paper. NI.

Copies: LNSW, ML, NL, SLV. 1529a

1855. New South Wales. . . . Report from the Select Committee on the Petition of Robert Lakin, with minutes of evidence . . . Sydney: Printed by William Hanson, Govt Printer . . . 1855.

324 × 202. Pp. [iv], 20 (l.b.). Pale blue paper.

Charges against Med. Supt of Tarban Creek Lunatic Asylum, brought by discharged steward of the instn, are dismissed.

Copies: LNSW, ML, NL, SLV. 1529b

1855. New South Wales. Foreign medical practitioners. Ordered by the Council to be printed, 9 August, 1855. [Text begins.]

324 × 202. Pp. 8. NI. Pale blue paper.

Appeals by foreign consuls for legalisation of position of foreign practitioners, and draft of proposed amending Bill.

Copies: LNSW, ML, NL, SLV. 1530

1855. New South Wales. Removal of Resident Surgeon at Port Curtis. Ordered by the Council to be printed, 12 October, 1855. [Text begins.]

324 × 202. Pp. 10. NI. Pale blue paper.

On the dismissal of Wm Greig MRCS, Surgeon to the newly founded Port Curtis settlement, by the Govt Resident, for disobedience. Select Committee later considers dismissal unwarranted.

Copies: LNSW, ML, NL, SLV. 1531

New South Wales—Parliament

The following items are selections from the Parliamentary Papers of New South Wales, as collected in the *Votes and Proceedings of the Legislative Assembly*, 1856/7–1900. See library catalogues for holdings. Detailed listing for LNSW, NL, OL, US, appears in Cope, R. L., *Australian Parliamentary Serials*, Reference Monograph 9, Library of Parliament, Syd., 1973. Individual papers, separately issued, also appear in various collections.

1856. New South Wales. Vaccination. (Report from Medical Adviser to Government.) Ordered by the Legislative Assembly to be printed . . . [Text begins.]

331 × 204. Pp. 4 (l.b.). Blue paper. Signed: R. Greenup.

Annual reports (1856–1900) on number of vaccinations performed.

1532

1859. New South Wales. Health Officer, Moreton Bay. (Report for 1858.) Presented to both Houses . . . Govt Resident, Moreton Bay to . . . Colonial Secretary.

331 × 204. Pp. 2. Blue paper. Colophon—Syd.: Thomas Richards, Govt Pr—1859.

Lists ships inspected, diseases on voyages and causes of deaths.

1533

1859–60. Legislative Assembly. New South Wales. . . . Report from the Select Committee on the Condition of the Working Classes of the Metropolis; . . . with the proceedings . . . evidence and appendix. . . . Sydney: Thomas Richards, Govt Printer . . . 1860.

324 × 195. Pp. 182 (l.b.). Blue paper. Chair-

man: Henry Parkes.

Reviews employment, wages, living conditions, destitute children. Many were in distress through unemployment, with overcrowding and insanitation in poorly built lower class homes. Despite improvidence and depravity in some, the masses were regarded as 'a credit to the country.'

1534

1863. Legislative Assembly. New South Wales. Progress Report from the Select Committee on the Present State and Management of Lunatic Asylums. . . . Sydney: Thomas Richards, Govt Printer. 1863.

322 × 209. Pp. [iv] (l.b.), 14, 110 (l.b.), 40. 3 flg plans.

1535

1865/6. Legislative Assembly. New South Wales. Government Asylums for the Infirm and Destitute. (Report of Board, for 1865.) . . . [Text begins.]

330 × 206. Pp. 4. Colophon—Syd.: Thomas Richards, Govt Pr—1866.

1536

1866. Legislative Assembly. New South Wales. Lunatic Asylums. (Correspondence respecting the internal state and management of.) . . . [Text begins.]

330 × 210. Pp. 12. Colophon—Syd.: Thomas Richards, Govt Pr—1866.

Includes rejected request of Francis Campbell, Med. Supt, for inquiry into newspaper criticism of management of Tarban Creek Lun. Asylum, and his literary effusion criticising Bd of Med. Visitors.

1537

1868. New South Wales. Public Charitable Institutions. (Progress Report of Inspector of Charities, respecting certain.) . . . [Text begins.]

325 × 210. Pp. 22. Colophon—Syd.: Thomas Richards, Govt Pr—1868.

Includes: Syd. Infirmary, Tarban Creek Lunatic Asylum, Deaf and Dumb Instn Syd., Hawkesbury Benev. and Hosp., Penrith Hosp. and Benev. Asylum.

1538

1868. New South Wales. Medical practitioners in the Colonies. (Despatch respecting.) Presented to both Houses of Parliament . . . The Secretary of State for the Colonies to Governor . . . [Text begins.]

300 × 217. Pp. 2 (single leaf). Colophon—Syd.: Thomas Richards, Govt Pr—1868.

Advice on a new Act which allows all persons registered under the Act to practice in any part of the King's dominions. Such persons could be registered, but not re-examined, in the Colonies.

1539

1868–9. Legislative Assembly. New South Wales. Detention in quarantine of the steam-ship "Kaikoura". (Correspondence respecting.) . . . [Text begins.]

331 × 204. Pp. 12. Colophon—Syd.: Thomas Richards, Govt Pr—1869.

Small-pox on voyage from Panama; complaints of passengers and company on detention.

1540

1873. Legislative Assembly. New South Wales. Treatment of criminal lunatics. (Report on.) . . .

325 × 210. Pp. 6. Colophon—Syd.: Thomas Richards, Govt Pr—1873.

E.S.P. Bedford (Pres. Bd of Visitors) emphasises unsatisfactory conditions at Parramatta Asylum.

1541

1873. New South Wales. Public Charities. (Sydney Infirmary.) First report of the Commission appointed to inquire into and report upon the working and management of the public charities of the Colony. . . . Sydney: Thomas Richards, Govt Printer. 1873.

326 × 209. Pp. 104, 262, 34 (l.b.). 6 plans (5 flg).

1st rep. Syd. Infirmary.

2nd and Final rep., 1874. Pp. 168 (l.b.), 342 (l.b.), 92 (l.b.), [2], 110. 1 litho. pl. Orphan schools and benev. asylums. Includes Randwick Asylum, Benev. Asylum, and Instn for Deaf and Dumb and Blind.

1542

1875. Legislative Assembly. New South Wales.

Progress Report of the Sydney City and Suburban Sewage and Health Board . . . to . . . report as to the best means of disposing of the sewage of the City of Sydney and its suburbs, as well as of protecting the health of the inhabitants thereof. . . . Sydney: Thomas Richards, Govt Printer. 1875.

344 × 217. Pp. 10 (l.b.), 28 (l.b.).

Board (Chairman—Prof. M.B. Pell) issued 12 reps. (1875–77).

1st rep. On sewage pollution of water mains.

2nd rep. 1875. Pp. 8, 42. On cesspits.

3rd rep. 1875. Pp. 6. Dry earth excreta disposal.

4th rep. 1875. Pp. 10 (l.b.), 18 (l.b.). Nuisances from Glebe abattoirs.

5th rep. 1875. Pp. 14 (l.b.). Sewage treatment.

6th rep. 1875. Pp. 30, 43–84 (l.b.). Harbour pollution, offensive trades, water supply.

7th rep. 1876. Pp. 20. Crowded dwellings and health.

8th rep. 1876. Pp. 20 (l.b.), 10 (l.b.). Prevalence of scarlet fever (H. G. Alleyne). Urges establishment of infectious diseases hosp.

9th rep. 1876. Pp. 6. Urges action on noxious trades, excreta disposal, water supply. Recommends permanent Bd of Health.

10th rep. 1876. Pp. 12 (l.b.). Recommends piped water to suburbs.

11th rep. 1876. Pp. 10 (l.b.), 112 (l.b.), 3 plans. On crowded areas and dwellings. Board's inspections involved 'great discomfort and risk to health . . . contact with much repulsive moral and physical degradation, and with scenes of filth and wretchedness of which it is impossible to convey any adequate idea by verbal description . . .' A vivid picture of slum conditions of the time. Recommendations: (i) appointment of Health Board, with local boards; (ii) a Building Act; (iii) extended powers for slum clearance; (iv) Govt provision of dwellings for workmen. Appendix: opium and opium smoking.

12th (final) rep. 1877. Pp. 22 (l.b.), 85–154 (l.b.). Recommends ocean disposal of sewage, and again urges establishment of Board of Health.

1543

1875–76. Legislative Assembly. New South Wales. Progress Report from the Select Committee on Employment of Children; . . . with the proceedings . . . ., minutes of evidence, and appendix. . . . Sydney: Thomas Richards, Govt Printer. 1876.

325 × 210. Pp. 52 (l.b.). 1544

1875–6. New South Wales. Legislative Council. Medical Laws Amendment. (Petition from certain members of the medical profession practising in New South Wales.) . . .

326 × 209. Single leaf, v.b.

Petition by 63 practitioners for legislation to control unqualified practice.

1545

1876–7. Legislative Assembly, New South Wales. Public Charities. (Report from Inspector of.) Ordered . . . to be printed, 29 May, 1877. [Text begins.]

330 × 210. Pp. 18 (l.b.).

On condition and management of all Govt asylums for infirm and destitute, and charitable and subsidised institutions (including hospitals). An. reps to 1886.

1546

1876–7. New South Wales. Inspector of the Insane. (Report for 1876.) Presented to Parliament . . . [Text begins.]

304 × 201. Pp. 16 (l.b.). Colophon—Syd.: Charles Potter, Govt Pr—1877.

'On the state and condition of the hospitals and other institutions in this Department.' Signed F. Norton Manning. Changed to 'Reps of Insp. General of the Insane' at 1879 rep. Annual, 1876–1900.

1547

1881. Legislative Assembly. New South Wales. Steamship "Brisbane". (Correspondence) . . .

326 × 214. Pp. 4. Colophon: Syd.: Thomas Richards, Govt Pr—1881.

On reception of vessel with small-pox aboard.

1548

1881. New South Wales. Compulsory vaccination. Opinions of L.H.J. Maclean . . . Henry Normand Maclaurin . . . Carl Frank Fischer . . . Charles K. Mackellar . . . Harman Tarrant . . . George Marshall . . . Arthur Renwick . . . Owen Spencer Evans . . . James C. Cox . . .

George Fortescue . . . John Le Gay Brereton . . . Eben Atherton . . . Andrew Ross . . . P. Sydney Jones . . . Alfred Roberts . . . Presented to Parliament . . . Sydney: Thomas Richards, Govt Printer. 1881.

339 × 217. Pp. 56 (l.b.).

An ineffectual appeal for compulsory vaccination.

1549

1882. Legislative Assembly. New South Wales. Report of the Royal Commission, appointed . . . 1881, to enquire into and report upon the management of the Quarantine Station, North Head, and the Hulk 'Faraway'; together with the minutes of evidence and appendices. . . . Sydney: Thomas Richards, Govt Printer. 1882.

326 × 204. Pp. 14 (l.b.), 118. 1 flg plan. P. w. (title rptd).

During small-pox epidemic of 1881–2, Quarantine Stn, and *Faraway* hulk anchored off shore, acted as isolation hospital. Inquiry arose from charges of mismanagement and neglect. Charges were not sustained in the case of the Station, but conditions on the hulk were 'in every way deplorable.'

For epidemic, see Cumpston, J.H.L. (1914), *The history of small-pox in Aust., 1788–1908*, Melb.: 11; also Gilder, G. A. (1938), 'The "Faraway" and the smallpox outbreak of 1881–1882', *JRAHS*, 24 : 225. The hulk *Faraway* was placed out of commission and sold in 1894 (*Austsn med. Gaz.*, 1894, 13 : 174).

1550

1883. Legislative Assembly. New South Wales. Quarantine Station, North Head. (Report of Health Officer upon state and condition of, etc.) . . . [Text begins.]

331 × 204. Pp. 14. 3 flg maps, 2 charts. Colophon—Syd.: Thomas Richards, Govt Pr—1883. Signed: Charles K. Mackellar MB.

1551

1883. Legislative Assembly. New South Wales. Anthrax (Cumberland Disease.) (Report of Mr. Anthony Willows, M.R.C.V.S.L., on prevalence of anthrax in Lachlan District.) . . . [Text begins.]

328 × 206. Pp. 6. Colophon—Syd.: Thomas Richards, Govt Pr—1883.

Describes epidemic in sheep.

1552

1883. Legislative Assembly. New South Wales. Noxious and Offensive Trades Inquiry Commission. Report of the Royal Commission, appointed on the 20th November, 1882, to inquire into the nature and operations of, and to classify noxious and offensive trades, within the city of Sydney and its suburbs, and to report generally on such trades . . . Sydney: Thomas Richards, Govt Printer. 1883.

326 × 209. Pp. 20, 86 (l.b.), 20 (l.b.). 2 maps. P. w. (title rptd).

Classifies noxious trades; indicates conditions requisite to public health.

1553

1883. Legislative Assembly. New South Wales. Steamship "Gunga". (Quarantining of). . . . Copies of all correspondence, reports . . . and other documents . . .

331 × 204. Pp. iv (l.b.), 52. Colophon—Syd.: Thomas Richards, Govt Pr—1883.

1554

1887. . . . New South Wales. Legislative Council. Report from the Select Committee on Law respecting Practice of Medicine and Surgery . . . Ordered . . . to be printed, 12 July, 1887. Sydney: Charles Potter, Govt Printer. 1887.

331 × 209. Pp. 106 (l.b.). P. w. (title rptd). J. M. Creed, Chairman.

The Same. Pp. 134 (l.b.).

Urges proper regulation of med. practice. 'We find that . . . no law exists for the regulation of the practice of medicine . . . in the colony, and that . . . the public are liable to . . . fraud and imposition which is absolutely appalling from its extent and from the unscrupulous boldness of the many ignorant pretenders who . . . give themselves out as qualified med. practitioners . . .' The evidence displays these vividly.

1555

1887. . . . Legislative Assembly. New South Wales. Report of the Government Asylums Inquiry Board; . . . with minutes of evidence and appendices. . . . Sydney: Charles Potter, Govt Printer. 1887.

331 × 204. Pp. 44, 214, 64, 71–74 (l.b.). 3 flg plans. Stiff p. w. (title rptd).

1556

1887. (Third Session.) New South Wales. Legislative Council. Cockatoo Island. (Reports on sanitary condition of.) . . .

320 × 204. Pp. 12. 1 flg map. Colophon—Syd.: Charles Potter, Govt Pr—1887.

Inquiry arising from occurrence of typhoid and diarrhoeal diseases in crews of ships at Cockatoo Is., Port Jackson, with recommendations on sanitation and water supply.

1557

1887–8. New South Wales. Report [First part] of the Intoxicating Drink Inquiry Commission; together with the epitomes of the evidence. . . . Sydney: Charles Potter, Govt Printer. 1887 . . .

242 × 153. Pp. [iv], 166 (l.b.), 2 flg charts. P. w. (title rptd).

Considers institutional treatment for alcoholism.

1558

1887–8. Legislative Assembly. New South Wales. Quarantine Station at North Head. (Correspondence relating to the removal of.) . . . "Copies of all papers, letters, minutes, &c. in reference to . . ." [Text begins.]

331 × 204. Pp. 2. Colophon—Syd.: Charles Potter, Govt Pr—1888.

1559

1887–8. Legislative Assembly. New South Wales. Deaths under chloroform. (Returns respecting.) Ordered by the Legislative Assembly to be printed, 10 July, 1888. [Text begins.]

323 × 205. Pp. 2.

9 deaths reported for NSW, during 3 years 1885–1887.

1560

1887–8. Legislative Assembly. New South Wales. Rabbit destruction. (Report of Health Board and other papers on proposals to effect destruction of rabbits by means of diseases to be introduced.) . . .

320 × 204. Pp. 18 (l.b.). NI.

Col Sec. seeks advice on possible dangers from introduction of diseases, which formed entries for a £25,000 prize offered by NSW Govt for an effective method of rabbit extermination. The numerous entries included 115 proposing destruction by disease—including small-pox, syphilis, hydrophobia, glanders and tuberculosis. Of these three were considered: fowl cholera (Louis Pasteur); *Sarcoptes cuniculi*—rabbit scab (Prof. Archibald Watson); and Tintinallogy disease, a lethal ailment of unknown aetiology (Drs. Henry A. Ellis and Herbert Butcher). Board recommends non-acceptance of all three. Includes correspondence from entrants, and report from Dr. W. Camac Wilkinson noting drawbacks to these and recommending trials on an island, and establishment of a Govt laboratory.

1561

1889 New South Wales. Royal Commission of Inquiry into Schemes for Extermination of Rabbits in Australasia. Progress report, minutes of proceedings, minutes of evidence, and appendices. . . . Sydney: Charles Potter, Govt Printer. 1890.

331 × 204. Pp. xxxviii (l.b.), [ii] (v.b.), 216. 2 pl., 11 plans. P. w. (title rptd).

Final report. 1889 (Second Session). Pp. [ii], 12.

Following events noted in item above, Commission was appointed in 1889 to report whether introduction of contagious disease in rabbits could be safely achieved, and on methods proposed. Members: H. N. MacLaurin MD, W. Camac Wilkinson MD, and E. Quin (NSW); H. B. Allen MD (Chairman), E. H. Lascelles and A. N. Pearson (Vic.); A. D. Bell (NZ); E. C. Stirling MD and A. S. Paterson MD (SA); J. Bancroft MD (Qd); and T. A. Tabart (Tas.).

Fowl cholera and *Sarcoptes* infestation were investigated by an expert committee of the Commission under W. Camac Wilkinson at its field station on Rodd Is., Pt Jackson, with Dr. O. Katz as bacteriologist; Tintinallogy disease by Joseph Bancroft in the Darling River district where it was said to occur. It was reported that there was no evidence 'that any known disease can be so employed as to exterminate rabbits.' Prize was not awarded.

1562

1890. Legislative Assembly. New South Wales. Deaths under chloroform. (Return of.) ... [Text begins.]

325 × 210. Pp. [2] (l.b.).

Sydney Hosp. (5 deaths), Prince Alfred Hosp. (4); Jan. 1885-May 1890. Details tabulated.

Also: 1891/2. Leg. Assembly. Anaesthetics in metropolitan hospitals. 1891.

1563

1890. Legislative Assembly. New South Wales. Leprosy in the Australasian Colonies. (Report on.) ... [Text begins.]

326 × 204. Pp. 4 (l.b.). Colophon—Syd.: Charles Potter, Govt Pr—1890.

Reports 25 lepers in Australia—all Asian immigrants—and appeals for enactment of a Leper Bill. Leprosy Act, passed the same year, provided for notification, isolation, and establishment of lazarets.

1564

1890. New South Wales. Legislative Council. Report from the Select Committee on the Medical Bill, together with the proceedings ... minutes of evidence, and appendix. ... Sydney: Charles Potter, Govt Printer. 1890.

317 × 214. Pp. 26 (l.b.). Signed: J. M. Creed, Chairman.

1565

1891. Legislative Assembly. New South Wales. Leprosy in New South Wales. (Report on.) Ordered ... to be printed, 26 May, 1891. [Text begins.]

331 × 212. Pp. 12 (l.b.). Colophon—Syd.: George Stephen Chapman, Govt Pr—1891.

An. reps, 1890–1900, include statistics and case records. 1890 rep. records establishment of lazaret at Little Bay; 1898 rep. includes Frank Tidswell on unsuccessful treatment with Carrasquilla serum, prepared by the injection of horse with leprous serum.

1566

1891. (Second Session.) Legislative Assembly. New South Wales. Dairies Supervision Act. (Administration of, during the year 1890.) ...

323 × 204. Pp. 20 (l.b.). Colophon—Syd.: G. S. Chapman, Acting Govt Pr—1891.

On effectiveness of the new Act establishing supervised hygiene of milk supplies, with abstracts of inspections. Annual reports from 1890.

1567

1891. New South Wales. Report on the Department of Charitable Institutions of New South Wales, for the year ended 31 December, 1890, from the Director of Government Asylums and Boarding-out Officer. Sydney: George Stephen Chapman, Acting Govt Printer. 1891.

239 × 153. Pp. iv (ii blank), 60 (l.b.).

Annually, 1890—.

1568

1891–2. New South Wales. Legislative Council. Report from the Select Committee on the Infant's and Children's Protection Bills; ... with the proceedings ... evidence, and appendix. ... Sydney: Charles Potter, Govt Printer. 1892.

331 × 206. Pp. 50 (l.b.).

1569

1891–2. Legislative Assembly. New South Wales. Vessels arriving at and leaving ports in New South Wales. (Returns ... for 1891.) ... [Text begins.]

320 × 204. Pp. 10 (l.b.). Colophon—Syd.: Charles Potter, Govt Pr—1892.

Board of Health on vessels quarantined and especially dealt with at Port Jackson and Newcastle. Annual reports from 1891.

1570

1892. Legislative Assembly. New South Wales. Recent importation of small-pox by the S. S. "Oroya". (Report on.) ... [Text begins.]

321 × 204. Pp. 4. Colophon—Syd.: Charles Potter, Govt Pr—1892.

1571

1892–3. Legislative Assembly. New South Wales. Report of Board appointed to inquire into the prevalence and prevention of lead poisoning at the Broken Hill silver-lead mines to the Honorable the Minister for Mines and Agriculture. ...

Sydney: Charles Potter, Govt Printer. 1893.

331 × 212. Pp. 30 (l.b.), 120. 1 flg map. P. w. (title rptd). Chairman—J. Ashburton Thompson MD.

Evidence on lead hazard; recommendations for prevention.

1572

1894. Legislative Assembly. New South Wales. Diseased Animals and Meat Act. (Report on the administration of, for the year ending 31st March, 1893.) . . . [Text begins.]

331 × 212. Pp. 14 (l.b.). Colophon—Syd.: Charles Potter, Govt Pr—1894.

Appendices: nodular tumours; worm nests in beef; swine diseases; tuberculosis and contagious pneumonia. For later reports, see Reps Dept Pub. Health, 1897, 1898.

1573

1894. (Second Session.) Legislative Assembly. New South Wales. Subsidised Hospitals of New South Wales. (Report on the.) . . . [Text begins.]

336 × 214. Pp. 26 (last—colophon only). Colophon—Syd.: Charles Potter, Govt Pr—1894.

Report by T. P. Anderson Stuart MD, Med. Adviser to Govt, on 102 hospitals receiving Govt subsidy.

1574

1896. New South Wales. Legislative Council. Nuisance from sewer ventilator at Waverley. (Papers respecting.) . . . [Text begins.]

336 × 212. Pp. 8. 1 coloured plan. Colophon—Syd.: Charles Potter, Govt Pr—1896.

Cases of enteric, diphtheria and other ailments are considered due to offensive sewer gas.

1575

1896. Legislative Assembly. New South Wales. Noxious Trades and Cattle Slaughtering Act, 1894. (Report on the working of . . . for the year ended June 30th, 1895.) . . . [Text begins.]

339 × 212. Pp. 2. Colophon—Syd.: Charles Potter, Govt Pr—1896.

1576

1896. Legislative Assembly. New South Wales. Dr. Taylor, Superintendent, Little Bay Lazarette. (Return respecting.) . . . "Copies of all correspondence between Dr. Taylor . . . and Dr. Anderson Stuart, President of the Board of Health in reference to . . . failure to report a case of leprosy".

331 × 204. Pp. 28. 1 chart. Colophon—Syd.: Charles Potter, Govt Pr—1896.

1577

1897. Legislative Assembly. New South Wales. Mining. (Return respecting lead-poisoning in connection with the Broken Hill mines.) . . . [Text begins.]

330 × 210. Pp. 4 (l.b.). Colophon—Syd.: Govt Pr—1897.

Includes 'Regulations . . . lead poisoning.'

1578

1897. Legislative Assembly. New South Wales. Mudgee Hospital. (Report of the Royal Commission appointed to inquire into charges . . . in connection with the treatment of Mary Beattie now deceased.) . . . [Report begins.]

330 × 210. Pp. 32. Colophon—Syd.: William Applegate Gullick, Govt Pr—1897.

Charges not substantiated.

1579

1898. Legislative Assembly. New South Wales. Department of Labour and Industry. Report on the working of the Factories and Shops Act (60 Victoria No. 37) during the year 1897. . . . [Royal Arms] Sydney: William Applegate Gullick, Govt Printer. 1898.

332 × 210. Pp. 40 (l.b.). Blue p. w. (title rptd).

Includes discussion of sanitation, accidents, certificates of fitness, and 'sweating.' Annual reports.

1580

1898. Legislative Assembly. New South Wales. Report of the Royal Commission appointed to . . . report upon the methods of carrying on Government charitable institutions. Part 1.—Institutions dealing with the blind and with the deaf and dumb . . . Sydney: William Applegate Gullick, Govt Printer. 1898. . . .

323 × 209. Pp. iv, 92 (l.b.).

5 reports, same format and imprint, issued 1898–99.

1st rep.—above.

2nd rep. 1898. Pp. xlvii, 100. Benevolent Soc. NSW.

3rd rep. 1899. Pp. xlviii, 36. Subsidised benev. instns.

4th rep. 1899. Pp. cxlii, 114 (l.b.). 2 flg maps. Hospitals. Other subjects include venereal disease treatment and nursing training.

5th rep. 1899. Pp. 30 (l.b.). Recommends legislation for management of hospitals and instns.

1581

———

1899. ... Legislative Assembly. New South Wales. General Fever Hospital for the Metropolitan Districts. (Correspondence respecting establishment of.) ... [Text begins.]

334 × 212. Pp. 6.

Due to local fears of the Diphtheria Branch of Hosp. for Sick Children, an isolated fever hospital is recommended. This is opposed by J. Ashburton Thompson and C.P.B. Clubbe, who consider a centrally placed hospital necessary for acutely ill cases. Letter from the Sec., Hosp. for Sick Children announces closure of Diphtheria Branch, since reduced severity through use of antitoxin now made domiciliary treatment possible.

1582

———

1899. (Third Session.) Legislative Assembly. New South Wales. Interim Report of the Royal Commission to inquire into the prevalence, &c., of tuberculosis and other diseases in stock. ... [Royal Arms] Sydney: William Applegate Gullick, Govt Printer. 1899.

328 × 208. Pp. 8 (l.b.).

2nd Interim Rep., 1899. Pp. [ii], 12. 1 flg map. 1583

N.S.W. Cremation, Funeral and Sanitary Reform Review, The

No. 1. June 26, 1890. Vol. 1. The New South Wales Cremation Funeral and Sanitary Reform Review Circulation, 10,000. Published Monthly by J. R. Bubb, ... Sydney: Gibbs, Shallard, & Co., Printers ... Price One Penny.

217 × 140. Pp. 32. P. w. (cover title).

No 1 includes lecture on cremation by Dr. J. M. Creed and rules of NSW Cremation Soc. See *Austsn med. Gaz.*, 1890, 9 : 119 and 121.

Copies: FC, ML (Nos 1–2), NL. 1584

N.S.W. Home Teaching Society for the Blind

Established 1877. Fifteenth Annual Report of the New South Wales Home Teaching Society for the Blind, and the Ninth Annual Report of the Industrial Home for Blind Women, and Retreat for the Aged Female Blind, for the year ending 31st December, 1892. Moss & Bourcicault, *Australian Courier* Printing Works, Burwood, Sydney.

8vo. Pp. 36. P. w.

Copies: FC. 1585

New South Wales Institution for the Deaf and Dumb and the Blind

Anniversary of the Deaf & Dumb Institution of New South Wales, for the year ending October 1st, 1862. ... Sydney: Joseph Cook & Co. ... 1862.

212 × 135. Pp. 12. P. w. (title rptd).

1st an. rep. Instn, a private project, the Deaf and Dumb School, now becomes a public charity. Up to and including 7th an. rep. (1868), it was named Deaf and Dumb Instn of NSW; in 8th an. rep. (1869), Deaf and Dumb and Blind Instn of NSW; in 10th an. rep. (1871), NSW Instn for the Deaf and Dumb and the Blind.

50th an. rep. (1911) contains illustrated history. See also Peyser, D. (1939), *JRAHS*, 25 : 191.

Copies: EF (1–29, 1862–90), ML (1–, 1862–), OL (35–6, 1896–7). 1586

New South Wales Medical Gazette

The New South Wales Medical Gazette. Published under the auspices of The Association of Medical Officers of the Volunteer Force at Head Quarters, and edited by Three of their Number. Vol. 1—1870–71. Sydney: Gibbs, Shallard, & Co., General Steam Machine Printers ... 1871.

217 × 135. Pp. 378.

Vol. 1, no 1–v. 6, no 2; Oct. 1870–Nov. 1875. Monthly.

See Cumpston, J.H.L. (1939), 'The history of med. journalism in Aust.', *Med. J. Aust.*, 2 : 1.

Copies: See *SSAL*. 1587

New South Wales Medical Union

New South Wales Medical Union (formerly

Sydney Medical Association Defence Fund.) Rules, &c., 1894.

163 × 98. Pp. 16 (l.b.). Title from cover label. Cloth, paper label on front.

Includes 1st an. rep. (1893–4).

Sydney Med. Assn formed 1893, and 'Defence Fund' established (*Austsn med. Gaz.*, 1893, 12 : 170). Object: 'assistance to any member ... involved in any action or prosecution arising out of his practice.'

Copies: ML (1–7, [1893]–1900.) 1588

New South Wales Railways Ambulance Handbook

See Woodward, George P. M.

New South Wales Social Purity Society

The Fourth Annual Report of the New South Wales Social Purity Society. Presented 22nd November, 1886. Sydney: J. L. Holmes and Co. ...

204 × 135. Pp. 16 (l.b.).

Objects: legislative action on protection of young females, establishment of paternity of illegitimate children and their support, civil actions in seductions, and care of fallen juveniles. See also: Olden, Charles.

Copies: ML. 1589

New South Wales Trained Nurses' Association

See Australasian Trained Nurses' Association.

Newbury, James Cosmo

[Issued August 11th, 1885.] Royal Society of Victoria. The examination of waters. ...

214 × 138. Pp. 10 (l.b.). Colophon—Mason, Firth & M'Cutcheon ... Melb. P. w. (cover title).

Discusses chemical analysis from viewpoint of faecal pollution and mentions beginnings of bacteriological examination, and possible purification methods.

Copies: EF. 1590

Newcastle and Northumberland Benevolent Society, NSW

See Newcastle Benevolent Society.

Newcastle Asylum for Imbeciles, NSW

1876–7. New South Wales. Newcastle Asylum for Imbeciles. (Report of Inspector of Insane.) ... [Text begins.]

330 × 210. Pp. [2] (v.b.). NI. Signed: F. Norton Manning.

Copies: LNSW, ML, NL, SLV. 1591

Newcastle Benevolent Society, NSW

Eighth Annual Report of the Newcastle Benevolent Society, New South Wales, for the year ended March 31, 1893 ... Newcastle ... "Herald Office" ... 1893.

204 × 138. Pp. 38. P. w. (title rptd).

Renamed 'Newcastle and Northumberland Benevolent Soc.' prior to 12th an. rep. (1897). Foundation stone of Society's Newcastle Benevolent Asylum and Lying-in Hosp. was laid in 1896.

Copies: ML (1893, 1897, 1900–). 1592

Newcastle Hospital, NSW

Rules and regulations for the management of the Newcastle Hospital. 1861. Newcastle: M'Dicken and Baker, Printers ...

224 × 145. Pp. 8. Plain p. w.

Another ed., 1869. Pp. 12. Printed at the 'Pilot' Office.

Copies: LNSW, ML. 1593

———

Newcastle Hospital. Report. [Text begins.]

286 × 212. Pp. [4] (2, 4 blank). (1872.) Pale blue paper.

An rep. for 1872.

Founded 1817; name changed to Royal Newcastle Hosp. 1949. For history, see Champion, B. W. (1952), 'The Newcastle Hosp. 1815–1891', *Newcastle & Hunter R. Dist Hist. Soc. J. & P.*, 6 (8 parts).

Copies: ML (1872, 1887–99), Roy. Newcastle Hosp. (1887–). 1594

Newcastle Lying-in Hospital

See Newcastle Benevolent Soc.

Newcastle Relief Society

Rules of the Newcastle Relief Society. [Text begins.]

212 × 130. Single leaf, v.b. ND. NI.

Copies: ML. 1595

Newcastle Sanitary Association

Rules and constitution of the Newcastle Sanitary Association. Established 1886. Newcastle, N.S.W. Daily News Printing ... Works ... 1886.

181 × 127. Pp. 8. P. w. (title rptd).

Objects: sanitary reform, removal of the

sources of disease, public and general hygiene, suppression of public nuisances. See *Austsn med. Gaz.*, 1886, 5 : 280 and 310.
Copies: ML. 1596

Newton, A. E.

The better way: an appeal to men on behalf of human culture through a wiser parentage. ... Christchurch, N. Z. : Francis J. Quin, Publisher. A. Wildey, Steam Printer ... 1893.

181 × 120. Pp. 48. Imprint covered by gummed slip bearing: W. E. Gundry, 4 Darlington Road, Sydney, N.S.W. 1894. P. w. (title rptd).

Prenatal regime for parents for betterment of offspring. A mother may by 'exercise and direction of her own mental and psychical forces ... during the development of the embryo ... determine the bent and career of her unborn child.'
Copies: ML. 1597

Nicholas, W. A.

Nicholas' golden cross ... veterinary helping hand book to health. No. 4 containing full & reliable information & advice how to act in case of sickness or accident. ... Published by W. A. Nicholas Fern Mount, New South Wales, Bundanoon.

163 × 115. Pp. [iv], 36, [8]. ND. (c. 1898.) P. w. (title rptd).

Advertises remedies, including No 2 Powder—for cancer, gastric ulcers, cold in head, dropsy, St Vitus dance, leucorrhoea; also Child Birth Powders which shorten duration of labour, prevent pains and check haemorrhage.

Listed for sale: *General helping hand book* ('how to act in over 90 complaints'), pp. 48; *Ladies helping hand book* ('complaints peculiar to women'), pp. 48; *Children's helping hand book*, pp. 48. NS.
Copies: ML. 1598

Nicholson, Sir Charles

Inaugural addresses delivered on the opening of the University of Sydney, on ... October 11, 1852, by the Hon. Sir Charles Nicholson, Speaker of the Legislative Council, Vice-Provost of the University. And the Reverend John Woolley ... Professor of Classics and President of the Professorial Board ... Sydney: Printed by Joseph Cook ...

273 × 209. Pp. [ii] (v.b.), 32. Stiff p. w. (title rptd) or morocco.
Copies: FC, ML, NL, SLV, US. 1599

Inaugural addresses, delivered on the occasion of the opening of the University of Sydney, by the Vice-provost and the Professor of Classics, in 1852; also report of addresses at various commemorations held in subsequent years, and delivered by the Chancellor Sir Charles Nicholson, Bart. ...

275 × 209. Pp. 72 (l.b.). NI. ND. [1878.] P. w. or cloth.

Sir Charles Nicholson (1808–1903) MD Edin., came to Sydney, where he practised, in 1834. He became Speaker of the first NSW Leg. Council, first Chancellor Univ. Syd., and first Pres. Leg. Council of Qd. The gift of his collection of antiquities to Syd. Univ. laid the foundation for the Nicholson Museum. See *Lancet*, 1903, 2 : 1473.
Copies: FC, LNSW, ML, NL, US. 1600

Catalogue of Egyptian and other antiquities. [Egyptian symbols] Collected by Sir Charles Nicholson ... London: ... Reynolds & Co. ... 1858.

204 × 132. Pp. [iv] (ii, iv blank), 64.

Lists 408 items collected during tour of Egypt in 1856–7.
Copies: FC, ML, SLV, US. 1600a

Nightingale, Florence

Sanitary statistics of native colonial schools and hospitals. ... London. 1863.

231 × 127. Pp. 68. Colophon—London: ... George E. Eyre and William Spottiswoode ...

Diseases, racial degeneration, and population decline of native races, are discussed on the basis of statistics and reports from British colonies. Includes Aust. information from various sources.
Copies: ML. 1601

Note on the aboriginal races of Australia. (A paper read at ... National Association for the Promotion of Social Science, held at York, September, 1864.) ... London: 1865.

214 × 140. Pp. 8. Colophon—Emily Faithfull ... Farringdon Street, E. C.

Discusses care and training, based on communication by Bishop Salvado of New Norcia Mission WA.

Copies: FC, ML. 1602

1866. Legislative Assembly. New South Wales. Hospital nurses for Sydney Infirmary. (Correspondence between Colonial Agent General and Miss Florence Nightingale, respecting engagement of.) ... [Text begins.]

330 × 210. Pp. 2. Colophon—Syd.: Thomas Richards, Govt Pr—1866.

Initiation of professional nursing training in Australia. Miss Nightingale expresses interest in a plan to establish a training school for nurses at Syd. Infirmary—'a matter very near her heart'—, and invites interview with Matron, St Thomas's Hosp.

Copies: LNSW, ML, NL, SLV. 1603

Copy correspondence between the Colonial Government, Miss Florence Nightingale and others. With reference to the introduction into the colony of trained nurses for the Sydney Infirmary and Dispensary. Sydney: Joseph Cook & Co., Printers ... 1867.

217 × 135. Pp. 18.

Pamphlet contains correspondence which led to the introduction of modern nursing to Sydney. Through the influence of Miss Nightingale, Miss Lucy Osburn (lady supt) and 5 sisters, trainees of the Nightingale School at St Thomas's Hosp., London, arrived in Sydney in March 1868.

Above transactions are recorded by Sir Henry Parkes in his *Fifty years in the making of Aust. history*, Lond., 1892. See also Watson, J. F. (1911), *The history of the Syd. Hosp.*, Syd. For Lucy Osburn, see Salmon, M. (1911), 'A pioneer of trained nurses', *Austsn Nurses' J.*, 11 : 364; MacDonnell, F. (1970), *Miss Nightingale's young ladies*, Syd.; Bowd, D. G. (1968), *Lucy Osburn*, Syd.

Copies: ML. 1604

See also Nos 380, 1640.

Nightingale Fund

The Nightingale Fund. Hobart Town, July 24th, 1856. Sir, [Text follows.] Thomas D. Chapman, Hon. Sec. [At foot.]

222 × 183. Pp. 4 (last 3 blank). NI.

An appeal for funds for Nightingale nursing school in London. DL copy has inserted page from *Hobart Town Daily Courier* (16 July 1856), which reports public meeting for this purpose.

Copies: DL. 1605

Nixon, Susan. The Case of

See Bruck, Ludwig.

Norman, Herbert Hayes

Arthur Redivivus: or the Arthur system for the prevention of proximate decay of the teeth, revived and extended ... Adelaide June, 1892. Hussey and Gillingham ...

173 × 120. Pp. viii (l.b.), [9]–58, 6 pl. Cloth.

For H. H. Norman (1843–1926) DDS, Adel. dentist, see Chapman, A. (1937) *History of dentistry in SA*, Adel.

Copies: FC, ML, NL, SLS. 1606

North, Franklin H.

Some account of a nursing organization and what it has accomplished in nine years. Being extracts from a paper in the "Century" magazine, New York for November, 1882 ... Printed for private circulation. Sydney: John Woods and Co. ... Sydney.

212 × 132. Pp. 12. (1883.)

On Bellevue School for Nurses, N. Y. Prefatory note (signed WJM, Syd.) expresses disappointment in results of Syd. Infirmary School.

Copies: ML. 1607

North Queensland Medical Society

First annual report of the North Queensland Medical Society ... 17th June, 1890. Townsville: ... Hastings & Jones ...

220 × 135. Pp. 24. P. w. (title rptd).

Includes pres. address by Joseph Ahearne LRCSI, LRCPI. See *Austsn med. Gaz.*, 1890, 9 : 122 for foundation. Meetings were held alternately at Townsville and Charters Towers. *Austsn med. Gaz.*, 1890, 9 : 259 reports lst meeting; *ibid*, 1890, 9 : 319, 2nd meeting, with paper on 'Charters Towers from 1882 to 1890' by G. Browne MD. See also No 28.

Copies: NL. 1608

By-laws of the North Queensland Medical Society, and list of office-bearers for the year 1890–91. Townsville: ... Hastings & Jones ...

168 × 107. Pp. 12. P. w. (title rptd).

Copies: NL. 1609

North Shore Hospital, Sydney

Fourth Annual Report of the North Shore Hospital Committee, 1891. North Sydney ... Sydney: W. A. Pepperday & Co. ... 1892.

209 × 135. Pp. 16.

Name became 'Royal North Shore Hospital of Sydney' at laying of foundation stone for new hospital on the Gore Hill site, June 1902.

Copies: Roy. North Shore Hosp. (4–, 1892–). 1610

Northcote Retreat

See under Melbourne Retreat for the Cure of Inebriates.

Nosological Index—New South Wales

1887. New South Wales. Nosological index or guide to the classification and tabulation of the various causes of death; with instructions to district registrars. [Royal Arms] Sydney: Charles Potter, Govt Printer ... 1887.

209 × 135. Pp. 48 (last 2 blank). P. w. (title rptd). Signed: E. G. Ward, Reg. Gen.

Copies: EF, ML, SPH. 1611

———

The Same. 1892. Pp. 38 (l.b.).

Copies: EF, SPH. 1612

———

The Same. 1898. Pp. [ii] (v.b.), 46.

Copies: EF, ML, SPH. 1613

Nosological Index—Victoria

Registration of the causes of death. A statistical nosology, for the use of those who return the causes of death. Circular to coroners, and a classification of the causes of violent deaths. ... John Ferres, Printer, Melbourne. 1856.

210 × 130. Pp. 80.

Reprint of publication by Reg. Gen. of England.

Copies: SLV. 1614

———

1862–3. Victoria. Nosological index, or guide to the classification and tabulation of the various causes of death; compiled principally for the use of the Registrar-General's Department; with instructions to Deputy Registrars by the Registrar-General of Victoria. ... John Ferres, Govt Printer, Melbourne.

314 × 204. Pp. 28 (2, 4 blank). Blue tinted paper. Preface signed William Henry Archer ... 3rd August, 1863.

Other eds: 2 ed., ND; 4 ed., 1878; 5 ed., 1887; 6 ed., 1892.

Copies: EF (1, 5 eds), ML (1, 2 eds), SLV (4 ed), SPH (6 ed.). 1615

Notes on Homoeopathy

Notes on homoeopathy. ... Hobart Town: ... "Mercury" Steam Press Office. 1871.

198 × 132. Pp. [ii] (v.b.), 152. In 12 numbers, Sep. 1870–Aug. 1871, with running pagination.

NL copy notes Ebenezer Atherton MRCS as editor, and bears inscription from E. A.

Copies: NL, SLT. 1616

Nottage, Charles G.

In search of a climate. By Charles G. Nottage, L.L.B., F.R.G.S. With thirty photographic illustrations ... London Sampson Low, Marston & Company ... 1894.

252 × 161. Pp. xvi (l.b.), 354 (l.b.). Frontis., 29 pl., 1 map. Cloth.

World voyage of an invalid who, after brief calls, reports the climates of Melb. and Syd. as unsuitable for consumptives. 'To send a poor consumptive ... to a country capable of jumbling up winter and summer ... is criminal.'

Copies: ML, NL, SLS, SLV. 1617

Noyes, Alexander Wellesley Finch

Tuberculosis of the skin and cutaneous manifestations occurring in scrofulous subjects. ... Reprinted from the "Intercolonial Medical Journal of Australasia", April 20, 1896. Melbourne: Stillwell and Co. ... 1896.

234 × 147. Pp. 12. P. w. (cover title).

For A.W.F. Noyes (1862–1928) FRCS, Dermatologist to Melb., Alfred and Children's Hosps., Melb., see obit., *Med. J. Aust.*, 1928, 1 : 418. He published *Lectures in dermatology*, Melb., 1918.

Copies: EF, NL. 1618

Nyulasy, F. A.

See Australian Health Society, No 104.

For Francis Armand Nyulasy (1862–1934) MB, ChB Melb., see obit., *Med. J. Aust.*, 1934, 1 : 827; also Egon F. Kunz, *Blood and gold, Hungarians in Australia*, Melb., 1969.

O

[O'Brien, Lucius], 'Lucifer'

Pneumatic high pressure sewerage for cities, towns, and villages. An essay on the sewerage question by "Lucifer" . . . Sydney: Jarrett and Co. . . . 1881.

206 × 132. Pp. 30 (l.b.), [ii] (colophon, v.b.). 1 flg plan. Limp leather.

Note in LNSW copy ascribes to Lucius O'Brien.

Reviews sewage disposal methods and their disadvantages. Disposal by compressed air onto farm-lands is advocated.

Copies: EF, LNSW, ML. 1619

O'Connor, Dr

See West Australian Settler's Guide & Farmer's Handbook.

Odd Fellows, Independent Order of

Laws for the government of the Medical Institute of the Independent Order of Odd Fellows, Manchester Unity, Friendly Society . . . Sydney. Established A.D. 1841. Revised . . . Sydney: F. W. White . . . 1890.

209 × 132. Pp. 16. P. w. (title rptd).

Copies: ML. 1620

Odontological Society of Victoria

Inaugural address read before the Odontological Society of Victoria at the first quarterly meeting, held 5th June, 1884.

213 × 138. Pp. 12. Colophon—Stillwell and Co. . . . Melb.

Includes plea for registration of dentists, and college and hospital for training students.

Copies: SLV. 1621

See also Iliffe, John.

O'Hara, Henry Michael

On some therapeutic uses of iodoform. . . . Read before the Victorian Branch of the British Medical Association, on April 16, 1880.

208 × 133. Pp. 4. Colophon—Stillwell & Co. . . . P. w. (title rptd).

For H. M. O'Hara (1853–1921) FRCSI, Hon. Surg. Alfred Hosp., see obit., *Med. J. Aust.*, 1921, 1 : 512; *Cyclopedia of Victoria*, Melb., 1 : 434.

Copies: SLV. 1622

Old Housekeeper

The Australian housewives' manual: a book for beginners and people with small incomes. By an Old Housekeeper . . . Melbourne: A. H. Massina & Co. . . . 1883.

163 × 102. Pp. [4] (advts), [ii], viii, [9]–116, [2] advts. P. w. (shortened title, decorated; advts all other sides.)

2 ed., 1885.

Includes chapter on infant care.

Copies: FC, ML. 1623

Olden, Charles

Immorality: its fascinating temptations, its awful consequences, and the way to avoid it. A lecture . . . to men only . . . October 8th, 1883 . . . under . . . the New South Wales Social Purity Society . . . Sydney: J. L. Holmes & Co. . . . 1884.

204 × 132. Pp. 36 (l.b.). P. w. (title rptd).

2 ed., 1885. Pp. 36.

See also: NSW Social Purity Society.

Copies: FC, ML, NL. 1624

"The protection of girls and young women and the legislative repression of vice generally". A lecture . . . to men only . . . August 4th, 1885 . . . under the auspices of the Committee of the New South Wales Social Purity Society . . . Sydney: . . . N. S. Wales Social Purity Society. . . . Messrs J. L. Holmes and Co. . . .

206 × 138. Pp. viii, 36. ND. P. w. (title rptd).

Copies: DL, EF, FC, LNSW, ML, NL. 1625

One of the 'Unscientific Mob'

Can disease protect health? The "Age" and vaccination, by One of the "Unscientific Mob", and "The case against compulsory vaccination" by a Physician. (From "The Gentleman's

Magazine"). Melbourne: A. H. Massina & Co., General Printers ... 1890.

214 × 132. Pp. 32. P. w. (title rptd in decorative frame).

Anti-vaccination essays.

Copies: NL. 1626

Ophthalmic and Orthopaedic Institution, Melbourne

See Bowen, Thomas Aubrey.

Ophthalmological Society of Victoria

Founded 1899. *Austsn med. Gaz.*, 1899, 18 : 303 reports 1st meeting. In 1912 merged in Eye, Nose and Throat Sect. of BMA (Vic.) (Williams, D. (1947), *Trans Ophth. Soc. Aust.*, 7 : 5). Publications not seen.

1627

'Opifer'

See Thomson, William

Orange Hospital, NSW

1890. Legislative Assembly. New South Wales. Orange Hospital. (Petition from residents of, as to management.) ... [Petition begins.]

325 × 210. Single leaf, v.b.

Note: bears 1416 signatures.

Copies: LNSW, ML, NL, SLV. 1628

———

1890. Legislative Assembly. New South Wales. Orange Hospital. (Petitions and correspondence for an inquiry into the management of.) Ordered ... to be printed, 15 October, 1890.

325 × 210. Pp. 18. Colophon—Syd.: Charles Potter, Govt Pr—1890.

Copies: LNSW, ML, NL, SLV. 1629

———

1890. Legislative Assembly. New South Wales. Special report from the Select Committee on Management of the Orange Hospital. ... Sydney: Charles Potter, Govt Printer. 1891.

325 × 210. Pp. 4 (l.b.).

Copies: LNSW, ML, NL, SLV. 1630

O'Reilly, Walter W. J.

Testimonials of Walter W. J. O'Reilly, Doctor in Medicine, and Master in Surgery of the Queen's University, Ireland ...

181 × 125. Pp. 8. Colophon—Samuel E. Lees ... Syd. 1874.

Copies: BG, DOS, RACP. 1631

Osborne, Alick

Notes on the present state and prospects of society in New South Wales; with an historical, statistical, and topographical account of Manilla and Singapore. By Alick Osborne, Surgeon Royal Navy. London: ... J. Cross ... also sold by Simpkin and Marshall ... 1833.

161 × 98. Pp. 96, 2 (book notices). Cloth.

Account of voyage to Australia on convict transport *Planter* in 1832, with brief observations, of little medical interest, on sojourn in Sydney.

Copies: FC, ML, NL. 1632

Osburn, Miss Lucy

See Melbourne Hospital, No 1348; Nightingale, Florence.

O'Sullivan, Michael Ulick

The proclivity of civilised woman to uterine displacements: the antidote Also other contributions to gynaecological surgery ... Melbourne: Stillwell and Co. ... 1894.

220 × 140. Pp. 84 (2, 4 blank). 2 pl. Cloth.

Attacks routine treatment of uterine displacements by pessaries and appeals for rational measures and prevention. Section on causes of cancer ranks mental distress as first and most constant, and constipation, tight lacing, excessive use of tea and coffee, and 'cramming' at school as additional serious factors.

For M. U. O'Sullivan (d. 1917) FRCSI, Hon. Surg. Women's Hosp. Melb., Hon. Gynaec. St Vincent's Hosp., see obit.— *Med. J. Aust.*, 1917, 2 : 217; also Macdonald C. (1957), *Med. J. Aust.*, 1 : 25.

Copies: AMAV, BG, CC, DOS, EF, FF, KFR, ML, NL, SLV, RACS, UM. 1633

Otter, Robert Henry

Winters abroad. Some information respecting places visited by the author on account of his health. Intended for the use of invalids. Australia: Melbourne. Tasmania. Sydney. Queensland. The Riverina. Algiers. Egypt. Cape of Good Hope. Davos. [In 2 columns] ... London: John Murray ... 1882. ...

191 × 127. Pp. xii, 236, 32 (book advts). Cloth.

Author visited Australia because of chest trouble in 1872. Includes information on routes, accommodation, weather, etc. 'If precaution be taken to choose the healthiest districts ... a voyage to Australia would be productive of good to many persons with lung complaints.'

Copies: EF, FC, LNSW, ML, NL, SLS, SLV,

SLW, UQ. 1634

Ovens District Hospital, Beechworth, Vic.
The Third Half-yearly Report of the ... Ovens District Hospital with ... the number of in-patients, and classification of diseases, during the half-year ending June 30, 1858. Also the general rules ... Established A.D. 1856. Printed by Abbott and Pepper ... Beechworth 1858.
204 × 127. Pp. 16.
Copies: SLV (1858–1900, various). 1635

P

Packard, John H.
See Vic.—Central Board of Health.

Paget, James
See University of Melbourne, No 2310.

Palmer, Edward
On plants used by the natives of North Queensland, Flinders and Mitchell Rivers, for food, medicine, &c., &c. ... [Read before the Royal Society of N.S.W., 1 August, 1883.] [Text begins.]

212 × 135. Pp. 22 (l.b.). Colophon—Syd.: Thomas Richards, Govt Pr—1884. P. w. (cover title).

Copies: ML, SLV. 1636

Notes on a great visitation of rats in the north and north-western plain country of Queensland, in 1869 and 1870. ... Brisbane: ... Warwick & Sapsford ... 1886.

212 × 135. Pp. 8. From *Proc. Roy. Soc. Qd*, 1885.

For review of plagues of rats and mice in Aust., see Cleland, J. B. (1918), 'Pres. address', *J. & P. Roy. Soc. NSW*, 52 : 123, with occurrences from 1869 to 1917, notes on diseases of mice and associated humans, and control.

Copies: EF, FC, ML, SLV. 1637

Palmer, Sir James Frederick—Editor
See Hunter, John.

Parke, Davis & Co. Catalogue
1892–93 Australasian catalogue of the products of the laboratories of Parke Davis & Co. manufacturing chemists Detroit, Michigan, U.S.A. Revised, November 1, 1892. Australasian Depot: ... N.S.W. ...

173 × 107. Pp. 186 (l.b.). Frontis., 37 pl. P. w. (illust. variation of title).

Copies: ML. 1638

Parker, William R.
The science of life; or, self-preservation, a medical treatise on nervous and physical debility, spermatorrhoea, impotence and sterility, with practical observations on the treatment of diseases of the generative organs ... Sydney: Published by authority of the World's Dispensary Medical Association. Latest edition.

140 × 115. Pp. xvi, 288, 1 pl. ND. (before 1895.)

Advertises practice of World's Dispensary Med. Assn, Sydney (William R. Parker MD, Chief Phys., M. H. Richards MD, Chief Surg.—both unregistered practitioners), and states that author has more than 25, 000 letters testifying to his successes, and has received from National Med. Assoc. 'the most beautiful and expensive gold and jewelled medal ever conferred on anyone, be he prince or potentate.'

Announces issue of *Diseases of the nervous system ..., a treatise of psychological medicine.* Price 10s. NS.

Copies: LNSW. 1639

Parkes, Sir Henry
1883. Legislative Assembly. New South Wales. Hospital construction and management and sanitary subjects. (Papers respecting.) Ordered ... to be printed, 17 January, 1883. [Text begins.]

328 × 206. Pp. 2.

Sir Henry Parkes, visiting London, arranges, through Miss Florence Nightingale, for hospital inspections and public health information. Miss Nightingale sends list of papers forwarded, and notes that there was 'singular dearth of works on hospital management.' See also Nos 1603–4.

Copies: LNSW, ML, NL, SLV. 1640

Parkside Lunatic Asylum, SA
See Adelaide and Parkside Lunatic Asylums.

Parramatta Benevolent Society, NSW
Report of the Parramatta Benevolent Society, for the year ending 31st December 1848 ... Parramatta: Printed by Edmund Mason ... 1849.

213 × 142. Pp. 16 (last 3 blank). Plain p. w.

Founded 1838. See Little, T. D. (1918), 'Parramatta Benev. Soc.', *Parramatta and Dist Hist. Soc. J. & P.*, 1 : 125.

Copies: DL (1848, 1850), ML (1849). 1641

Parramatta District Hospital, NSW

Report of the Parramatta District Hospital, from the 1st of January to the 31st of October, 1865, with a list of subscriptions ... received during the year. Parramatta : Printed by E. Mason ... 1866.

204 × 127. Pp. 16 (last 2 blank).

Hospital, one of the oldest in Australia, originated in the General Hosp. (c. 1790). This was replaced in 1818 by the Colonial Hosp., which in 1848, on cessation of transportation, became Parramatta Dist Hosp., a charitable instn. For history, see Little, T. D. (1918), *Parramatta and Dist Hist. Soc. J. & P.*, 1 : 113; also Brown, K.S.M. (1937), *Med. practice in old Parramatta*, Syd.

Copies: LNSW (1865–7), ML (1854–96 various). 1642

Parramatta Lunatic Asylum, NSW

1876–7. Legislative Assembly. New South Wales. Report from the Select Committee on Lunatic Asylum, Parramatta; ... with the proceedings ... minutes of evidence, and appendix. ... Sydney: Charles Potter, Acting Govt Pr 1877.

330 × 210. Pp. 86 (l.b.).

Copies: LNSW, ML, NL, SLV. 1643

[Parton, James]

Will the coming man drink wine? Reprinted from "The Atlantic Monthly", an American magazine. ... Melbourne: Samuel Mullen ... 1868.

204 × 127. Pp. 16.

Includes medical views on alcohol.

Copies: ML, NL, SLV. 1644

———

The Same. 2 ed. Melb., Samuel Mullen, 1869.

Copies: LNSW, ML, NL, SLV. 1645

———

The Same. Pp. 16. Melb., William Bell ... Independent Order of Rechabites. Mason, Firth and Co., Printers ... 1869.

Copies: ML. 1646

———

Does it pay to smoke? By James Parton, ... to which is added the use and abuse of tobacco: a letter to the "Times". By Sir Benjamin Brodie, Bart. ... Melbourne: Samuel Mullen ... 1869.

206 × 132. Pp. 16.

On the evils of smoking.

Copies: LNSW, ML, NL, SLV. 1647

Pasteur, Louis

A Monsieur [Space for name and address] Paris, le 5 janvier 1888. Sur la destruction des lapins en Australie et dans la Nouvelle-Zélande. [Text begins.]

268 × 218 Colophon: Paris.—Imprimerie Gauthier-Villars et Fils, quai des Grands-Augustins, 55.

Letter, signed 'L. Pasteur, de l'Institut de France et de la Societé royale de Londres', announcing to Agent General (NSW) his intention to send two young savants to compete for the award of £25,000 offered by the NSW Govt for the extermination of rabbits. Includes history of the pest, official notice of award, and observations on fowl cholera as a lethal agent for rabbits. Eng. translation below.

For account of Pasteur mission, see items under Loir, Adrien, and his *A l'Ombre de Pasteur*, Paris, 1938; also N.S.W.—Parliament, Nos 1561–2.

Copies: EF. 1648

———

(Translation.) To [Space for name and address] Paris, January 5, 1888. Upon the destruction of rabbits in Australia and New Zealand. [Text begins.]

268 × 218. Pp. 8.

Translation of Pasteur's letter (above), signed L. Pasteur.

Copies: EF. 1649

Pasteur Anthrax Vaccine Laboratory of Australasia

See Richmond, C. F.

Pasteur Institute of Australia

See Loir, Adrien, No 1171.

Paterson, Alexander

The male generative function in health and disease. ... Second edition. Sydney: L. Bruck, Medical Publisher ... 1887.

206 × 137. Pp. x, 94 (l.b.). Cloth.

A popular treatise on sexual practice and irregularities. The free treatment of the subject, in the manner of a latter day, led to severe professional criticism.

Copies: ML. 1650

Nervous debility. An essay ... Sydney: F. Cunninghame & Co., Steam Machine Printers ... 1889.

220 × 140. Pp. iv, 5–32 (l.b.). P. w. (short title).

Copies: ML. 1651

The male generative function in health and disease ... Marcus & Andrews ... Sydney.

191 × 125. Pp. 8. [c. 1890.]

Advertises work named in title; contains 'Opinions of the press.'

Copies: LNSW. 1652

Physical health of woman. Useful knowledge for maiden, wife, and mother. ... Sydney: Edwards, Dunlop and Co., Limited, Sydney ... 1890.

209 × 135. Pp. vi (l.b.), [ii], 134 (l.b.).

On female sexual physiology and hygiene, including section on contraception.

Alexander Paterson (1844–1920) MD Edin. & Bahia, FRCSE, was born in Brazil, where his father John L. Paterson MD is honoured as a medical pioneer. He was educated in Scotland, returned to Brazil, later practised in Sydney. His advocacy of hypnotism, which he used in obstetrics and minor surgery, brought him into professional conflict. This was intensified by lectures and publications on sexual subjects. He moved to Perth, later to Timaru NZ, where he died. For father, J. L. Paterson MD, see Bacellar, R. C., *Brazil's contribution to tropical medicine*, Rio de Janeiro, 1963.

Also published: *Sobre a ovariotomia e as molestias para allivio ou cura das quaes esta operacão é mais particularmente adaptada*, Bahia, 1868. NS. Listed *SGC*. Also pamphlets on hypnotism. NS.

Copies: LNSW. 1653

Paterson, Alexander Stewart

See New Norfolk Hospital for Insane, No 1480.

Paterson, Hugh

The teeth and their treatment in health and disease popularly explained. By Hugh Paterson, surgeon dentist, Member of the Odontological Society of London. Sydney: Samuel Goold ... 1864.

181 × 112. Pp. xii, 80. Errata slip. Cloth, paper label.

The second dental work published in Australia. (For first, see Jeanneret, Henry.) Advises parents on dental care. See Levine, S. (1967), 'Australia's first two dental works', *Ann. Aust. Coll. Dent. Surgeons*, 1 : 19.

Copies: EF, FC, ML, NL, SLV, US. 1654

Pauper and Invalid Depot, Port Arthur, Tas.

Approved rules and regulations for the Invalid Depot, Tasman's Peninsula. Tasman's Peninsula, July 1868. The following rules and regulations, drawn up by the Comptroller-General of Convicts, having been approved by Governor ... are to be enforced with strict impartiality: [Text follows.]

548 × 339. Single leaf. 3 cols. (1868.) W. Fletcher, Printer ... Hobart Town.

Rules indicate utilisation of prison staff and facilities for care of the aged and infirm.

Copies: DL. 1655

Approved rules and regulations for the Pauper Depot, Tasman's Peninsula. Tasmania: W. Fletcher, Printer ... Hobart Town. 1868.

171 × 98. Pp. 14. Limp vellum wrappers.

Includes medical arrangements, ration scales, and diet lists. Shows 3 ration scales: punishment; for paupers and invalids (industrious and well-conducted); and for paupers and invalids (idle, restless and ill-conducted).

Copies: ML. 1656

Pauper and Invalid Depot, Port Arthur, Tas. [Royal Arms] Regulations made by the Governor in Council for the Pauper and Invalid Depot for Males, Port Arthur.

8vo. Pp. 8 (l.b.). ND. [1876?] P. w. (cover title). Colophon: James Barnard, Govt Pr, Tasmania.

Copies: ML. 1657

Pearson, A. N.

See Australian Health Society, No 104.

Peirce, W.

See Coast Hospital, Sydney.

Penfold, Oliver

From "The Australian Medical Journal", November 15th, 1887. Calf-lymph culture and vaccination. . . . [Text begins.]

217 × 150. Pp. 6. Colophon—Stillwell and Co. . . . Melb.

For Oliver Penfold (1844–1929) MRCS of Sandhurst (Bendigo), see obit., *Med. J. Aust.*, 1929, 2 : 382. In 1881 he prepared calf lymph vaccine, supplying the SA, Tas. and Qd Govts. A musician and composer, he published piano and organ music, songs and choral anthems.

Copies: NL. 1658

Penrith Hospital and Benevolent Asylum, NSW

See Nepean District Hospital.

Péron, Francois Auguste

Voyage de découvertes aux Terres Australes, exécuté par ordre de Sa Majesté l'Empereur et Roi, sur les Corvettes le Géographe, le Naturaliste, et la Geolette le Casuarina, pendant les années 1800, 1801, 1802, 1803 et 1804; . . . rédigé par M. F. Péron, . . . [Arms] A Paris, de l'Imprimerie Impériale. 1807.

300 × 255. 2 vols. Vol. 1 : pp. [iv], xvi, 496, [ii] (errata), frontis.; vol. 2 : pp. xxxii, 472 (l.b.), 3 pl. Vol. 2 published 1816, was completed by Louis Freycinet after Péron's death.

Includes description of the colony at Sydney, where the expedition spent six months. Chapter (vol. 1, pp. 446–84) on the physical strength of aborigines, records dynamometric tests on 12 Tasmanians and 17 Australians, with readings markedly lower than those for similarly tested French (17) and English (14) subjects. The lesser strength of the former is ascribed to poor food and excessive fatigue in obtaining it.

Copies: DL, ML, NL. 1658a

The Same. 2 ed., 1824. 4 vols. 8vo. Paris: Arthus Bertrand.

Copies: DL, ML, NL. 1658b

Perry, Right Reverend Charles

Science and the Bible: a lecture by the Right Rev. Chas. Perry, D. D., Lord Bishop of Melbourne. . . . September 20, 1869. Melbourne: Samuel Mullen . . .

212 × 138. Pp. 24. P. w. (variation of title).

Opposes theories of evolution. See Mozley, Ann (1967), 'Evolution and the climate of opinion in Aust., 1840–76', *Victorian Studies* : 427.

Copies: DL, EF, ML, NL, SLV, SLW, UM. 1659

The Same. 2 ed. Pp. 32 (l.b.). Melb., Samuel Mullen, [1869].

Copies: ML, NL, SLV. 1660

The Same. Pp. 80 (l.b.), [4] (advts). Lond., Soc. Promoting Christian Knowledge, [1869].

Copies: FC. 1661

Perry, Michael

A treatise on nervous debility resulting from diseases of the reproductive organs . . .

158 × 102. Pp. 60. (June 1889.) Colophon—Gibbs, Shallard & Co., Syd. P. w. (title rptd with added: 'Second edition, 50,000.').

Foreword, 'The restoration of sexual health', announces author's Syd. practice.

Michael Perry MRCS was connected with Marsden Remedy Co., run by two Americans for treatment of sexual diseases. See *NSW Leg. Council, Rep. Sel. Com. on . . : Practice of Med. and Surg.*, Syd., 1887, p. 37, for his methods.

Copies: EF. 1662

Perth Hospital

1886. Western Australia. Report of the Select Committee of the Legislative Council appointed to take into consideration the working of the Colonial Hospital. . . . Perth: . . . Richard Pether, Govt Printer. 1886.

317 × 204. Pp. 2.

Recommends that Hospital (Govt institution of 37 beds) be enlarged, with increased nursing efficiency.

Copies: LNSW, SLV, SLW. 1663

1897. Western Australia. Report of the Board of Management of the Perth Public Hospital for the year ended June 30th, 1897. . . . Perth: . . . Richard Pether, Govt Pr. 1897.

323 × 198. Pp. 8.

Annual, 1897—.

Copies: LNSW, SLV, SLW. 1664

1900. Report of the Select Committee of the Legislative Assembly appointed to inquire into the condition of Perth Public Hospital. . .

Perth: ... Richard Pether, Govt Printer. 1900.
305 × 204. Pp. 102.
Copies: LNSW, SLV, SLW. 1665

Peters, Alfred

Massage Its history, its curative uses, and its practical results. ... Melbourne: Pater & Knapton ... 1890.
209 × 138. Pp. 62, [2] (advts). P. w. (title rptd, advts all other sides).
Copies: EF, ML, SLV. 1666

———

The massage cure. Additional facts and testimonials of Alfred Peters, duly qualified masseur ... Being a supplement to his work on "Massage —its history ..." Melb.: Pater & Knapton ... 1892.
180 × 122. Pp. 16. P. w. (title rptd).
Copies: ML. 1667

Peters, Alfred and Aleck

Massage. The system of cure by manipulation, or friction, also known as medical rubbing. As practised for 30 years by the late Mr. J. S. Peters, Newcastle-on-Tyne, England; and, in Australia, by his sons, Messrs. Aleck and Alfred Peters ... Melbourne, Pater & Knapton ... 1890.
210 × 138. Pp. 32.
Copies: SLV. 1668

Petit, A.

Sur l'alcaloide du Pituri par A. Petit ... (Extrait du Journal de pharmacie et de chimie.) Paris Imprimerie Arnous de Rivière ... 1879
214 × 143. Pp. 4. P. w. (cover title).
For pituri, aboriginal stimulant, see Bancroft, J. Author reports analysis of sample sent by Bancroft, and concludes alkaloid is nicotine.
Copies: NL. 1669

Pettigrew, W.

The sanitary condition of Brisbane: read by W. Pettigrew ... at the ... Queensland Philosophical Society, ... 24th December, 1874. [Text begins.]
198 × 105. Pp. 4. Colophon—James C. Beal, Govt Pr ... Bris.
Copies: ML. 1670

Pharmaceutical Society of Victoria

Laws and constitution of the Pharmaceutical Society of Victoria, with a list of members and associates. 1857–8. Melbourne: ... Goodhugh and Hough ... 1857.
195 × 125. Pp. 12 (l.b.).
Other issues: 1872, 1879.
Society founded 1857; incorporated in Pharm. Soc. of Austsia, 1884.
Copies: ML (1857), SLV (1857,–72,–79). 1671

———

Twenty-third Annual Report of the Council of the Pharmaceutical Society of Victoria, 1880, with list of members ... Melbourne: Mason, Firth & M'Cutcheon, Printers ... 1880.
206 × 132. Pp. 12.
Copies: SLV (1878–89). 1672

Pharmaceutical Society of Vic., Quarterly Journal and Trans

Quarterly Journal and Transactions of the Pharmaceutical Society of Victoria. Vol. 1, No. 1. Melbourne, January 1, 1858. Price, 2s. 6d. Contents ... Edited for the Council by J. Bosisto and W. Johnson. Published at the Offices of the Society. ... Melbourne. W. H. Williams, Printer ... Melbourne.
217 × 143. Pp. 32, [4]. P. w. (cover title).
Vols 1–2; 1858–59/61. Publication ceased after vol. 2, no 8.
Copies: See *SSAL*. 1673

Pharmacy Board of New South Wales

Rules and regulations of the Pharmacy Board of New South Wales. Colonial Secretary's Office, Sydney, 28th January, 1891. [Text begins.]
217 × 140. Pp. 4.
Copies: ML, SLV. 1674

Phillip, Arthur (Governor)

See No 2495 (note).

Phillips, James

[No. 137. South Australia. ... Ordered by the House of Assembly to be printed, 10th July, 1872. ... Report of Dr. Phillips on investigation into epidemic diphtheria, at Port Lincoln. [Text begins.]
331 × 204. Pp. 6.
Describes epidemic of 65 cases, with 24 deaths.
James Phillips MRCS (1843) was Hon. Cons. Surg. Adel. Hosp.
Copies: LNSW, NL, SLS, SLV. 1675

Philpots, John Richard

Oysters and all about them. Being a complete history . . . exhaustive on all points of necessary and curious information from the earliest writers to those of the present time . . . John Richardson & Co. . . . London . . . 1890.

186 × 125. 2 vols. Vol. 1 : pp. [ii], [vi], 7–642; vol. 2 : pp. [ii], 643–1370. Cloth. Dedicated to T. H. Huxley.

J. R. Philpots LRCPE, LRCSE, formerly MOH Poole, Dorset, and MOH Swansea Tas., practised at Healesville Vic. in 1911.

Copies: EF, LNSW, SLS, US. 1676

Physician, A

See Guide to Health.

Physician, A

See [Hughes, J. Vaughan].

Pidgeon, Nathaniel

The life, experience, and journal of Nathaniel Pidgeon, City Missionary. Written by himself. Sydney: . . . Smith and Gardiner . . . Printed by R. Barr . . . 1857.

181 × 105. Pp. [iv] (ii, iv blank), 224 (last—errata). Cloth.

Author commenced as missionary with Syd. Wesleyan City Mission, after arrival from Ireland in 1841. Records work among poorer classes of Sydney to 1857, with incidental information on living conditions.

Copies: EF, ML, NL, SLV, UQ, WLC. 1677

———

The life, experience, & journal of Nathaniel Pidgeon, who has been upwards of twenty years, an open-air preacher and City Missionary, in the City of Sydney: being a continuation of the work up to January 1st, 1864, with a splendid portrait, engraved by W. G. Mason, Esq. . . . Written and published by himself. Sydney: Mason and O'Connor . . . 1864.

201 × 127. Pp. [vi] (3 blanks), 224 (last—errata), 104. Woodcut portrait frontis. Cloth.

Part 1 consists of earlier work with amended preface. Part 11 (with own pagination) added.

ML copy has inserted note of author—'d. Milson's Point 17 Feb. 1879, aged 77. He was 37 years a City Missionary.'

Copies: EF, FC, ML, NL, SLT, SLV, UQ, US. 1678

Placebo Aspen

Experiences of a medical man in New Zealand or our hospital at Sopemdown By Placebo Aspen, M.D. Melbourne & Sydney George Robertson 1883

212 × 135. Pp. 24. P. w. (title rptd).

Experiences in a fictional NZ hospital, based on actual events in various places and institutions. These call for 'broad and liberal reform in hospital management.'

Copies: ML, NL. 1679

Pleasant Creek Hospital, Vic.

See Stawell Hospital.

Pocket Guide to Water-Cure

A pocket guide to water-cure for the million. Pro bono publico. . . . Sydney: Printed by G. R. Addison . . .

181 × 110. Pp. 24. ND. P. w. (title rptd, poem on verso of back wrapper).

Copies: ML. 1680

Pocock, *Zachary* Pearce

Transportation and convict discipline considered in a letter to the Right Honourable Earl Grey . . . Showing the evils attendant upon the system pursued in Van Diemen's Land, and the remedy for those evils . . . London: Simmonds and Co. . . . Bucklersbury. . . .

201 × 130. Pp. 30 (l.b.). ND. (1847.) P.w. (cover title). Colophon: George Pierce, Printer, 310, Strand.

Z. P. Pocock LSA (1840), MRCS, colonist of 45 years standing, died at Summer Hill NSW 1895, aged 79 (*Austsn med. Gaz.*, 1895, 14 : 508). He served as Supt of Public Works VDL. Also published: *Emigration and colonisation in a letter to . . . Earl Grey*, Lond., (1847).

Copies: DL, ML, NL. 1681

Port Fairy Hospital, Vic.

Belfast Hospital and Benevolent Asylum. Established 1850. . . . [List of office bearers.] Belfast: . . . Smith & Osborne, "Gazette" Office.

204 × 130. Pp. 12. [1868.]

18th an. rep., for 1867, with rules and regulations.

After 36th an. rep. (1885–6), instn was known as Hosp. and Benev. Asylum, Port Fairy.

Copies: SLV (1867–72); 1885–90). 1682

Port Macquarie Asylum for Infirm and Destitute, NSW

1867. Legislative Assembly. New South Wales.

Port Macquarie Asylum for Infirm and Destitute. (Report of inspection of.) The Secretary of the Government Asylums Board to Princ. Under Secretary. [Text begins.]

326 × 205. Pp. 4 (l.b.).

On newly established institution.

Copies: LNSW, ML, NL, SLV. 1683

Port Phillip Medical Association

Rules and regulations of the Port Phillip Medical Association. March 5th, 1850. Melbourne: John Ferres, Printer, M. M. Herald Office.

173 × 110. Pp. 8.

The first Aust. medical society. Founded 1846; disbanded 1851. For history, see Graham, H. B. (1952), *Med. J. Aust.*, 2 : 213. AMAV has minute book of Assn.

Copies: AMAV, SLV. 1684

Port Phillip Medical Association. This book belongs to the Port Phillip Medical Association. [Space] days are allowed for reading it. If kept beyond the prescribed time, a fine of one penny per day will be charged for each day so kept. [Text continues.]

95 × 71. Single leaf, v.b. ND. NI.

Book label, signed (by hand: Edw. Barker) Secretary.

Copies: AMAV, BG, EF. 1685

[Potter, Robert]

The germ growers. An Australian story of adventure and mystery. By Robert Easterley and John Wilbraham. ... Melbourne: Melville, Mullen, & Slade. London: Hutchinson & Co. 1892. ...

181 × 125. Pp. vi, 274. Cloth.

A tale of evil supernatural beings and their secret base in the Kimberleys. They used aircraft and other unbelievable methods, and cultured organisms to spread pestilences.

Author identified as Robert Potter, Canon of St Paul's, Melb. (Miller).

Copies: EF, ML, NL, OL, SLT, SLV, UQ. 1686

Poulton, Robert Joseph

The reproductive organs. Snares & pitfalls of youth: a treatise on the derangements and diseases incident to the organs of generation. Their symptoms, consequences and cure. ... Third edition. Printed and published by the Author ... Melbourne.

135 × 102. Pp. 32 (l.b.). ND. [?1880.]

Includes advt for treatment by pharmacist, and anti-vaccination section.

Copies: SLV. 1687

Pound, Charles Joseph

Tick fever. Observations on ticks and tick fever at the Indooroopilly Experiment Station and at St. Helena. ... [Text begins.]

247 × 163. Pp. 6. 2 pl. Colophon—Edmund Gregory, Govt Pr ... Bris. Repr., *Qd Agric. J.*, 1890.

Copies: ML. 1688

The discovery of chicken cholera in Queensland. Part 1. ... Read before the Royal Society of Queensland, August 10, 1895.

220 × 134. Pp. 6 (l.b.). P. w. (cover title).

Announces discovery of fowl cholera (avian pasteurellosis) for first time in Australia.

Copies: ML. 1689

Department of Agriculture, Sydney. Miscellaneous publication, No. 174. The destruction of rabbits by means of the microbes of chicken-cholera. Sydney: William Applegate Gullick, Govt Printer. 1897.

244 × 153. Pp. 38. Repr., *Agric. Gaz. NSW*, Aug. 1897. P. w.

Report occurrence of fowl cholera in Brisbane. This had been recommended as rabbit extermination measure by Pasteur (No 1648), when it appeared that a new disease could consequently be introduced. In view of its local discovery, author urges further trials.

Copies: ML. 1690

1897. Queensland. Reports relating to the microbes of chicken cholera. (By C. J. Pound ... Government Bacteriologist.) Presented to both Houses ... [Text begins.]

326 × 204. Pp. 22. 2 pl. Colophon—Edmund Gregory, Govt Pr, Bris. Addressed to Minister for Lands. Four reports (1895–7).

Copies: LNSW, ML, NL, SLV. 1691

The stockowners' indebtedness to the microscope. ... Presidential Address ... of the Royal Society of Queensland. 31st January, 1898.

217 × 140. Pp. 30 (l.b.).

Discusses anthrax, tetanus, actinomycosis and tuberculosis. Repr., *Proc. Roy. Soc. Qd*, 1898, 13 : vi.

Copies: ML. 1692

———

Preventive inoculation for tick fever. ... [Text begins.]

250 × 156. Pp. 4 (l.b.). ND. Colophon—Edmund Gregory, Govt Pr ... Bris.

Copies: ML. 1693

———

Tick fever. Technique of the method of preventive inoculation. ... [Text begins.]

247 × 153. Pp. 8. 1 pl. Repr., *Qd Agric, J.*, 1899.

C. J. Pound FRMS, bacteriologist, Pres. Roy. Soc. Qd, was Director of Stock Inst. and Govt Bacteriologist, Brisbane.

Copies: EF. 1694

Powell, R. D. and Mahomed, W.

Terms used in a technical sense necessary for describing sounds met with in chest diseases ... Selected by Drs. R. D. Powell and W. Mahomed from the terminology of auscultation compiled by a committee appointed by the International Medical Congress held in London in 1881.

217 × 138. Pp. 4. ND. Colophon—W. E. Smith ... Syd. P. w. (cover title).

In columns—terms, definition, synonyms, significance.

Copies: EF. 1695

Practical Home Physician and Encyclopaedia of Medicine

See Lyman, Henry M. and Others.

Pratt, Eustace Henry Lever

On the treatment and permanent cure of stricture of the urethra, with notes of fifty cases cured by the author. ... Sydney: C. T. Sandon, Publisher ... 1875.

181 × 122. Pp. 16. P. w. (title rptd).

New treatment consists of instrumental introduction of iodoform in glycerine, on both sides of stricture.

Noted to be shortly published: *On stricture and diseases of bladder and prostate*. NS.

Copies: ML. 1696

———

Notes on tumours and cancers: with remarks on a new and painless method of treating them. ... Second edition. Sydney: S. T. Leigh and Co. ... 1875.

179 × 122. Pp. 12. P. w. (title rptd).

Recommends trial of local injections of iodoform for treatment of epithelioma.

For E.H.L. Pratt (1841–99) MD St And., MRCS, see Kennedy, R. T. (1946), *Med. J. Aust.*, 2 : 699.

Copies: LNSW, ML, WLC. 1697

Pressey, George Shaddack

Teeth in Australia ... 1883: A. Asher ... Melbourne, Richmond and Kew ...

275 × 214. Pp. 48. P. w. (amended title).

Tooth structure, teething, caries, stopping and extracting, diseases, nitrous oxide *versus* chloroform, artificial teeth.

Author, of Hawthorn Vic., was Hon. Sec. Dental Soc. Vic.

Copies: ML, SLV. 1698

Price, W. R.

Curative mesmerism. In submitting a few extracts from recent unsolicited London testimonials Mr. W. R. Price begs to announce that he receives patients for treatment at 159 Collins Street East, Melbourne ... [Text continues.]

191 × 122. Pp. 4. Mauve paper. (1887.) NI.

Testimonials refer to author's cure of consumption and other ailments.

Copies: ML. 1699

———

Mesmerism: its use and abuse. ... (From the "Proceedings of the Athenaeum Society".)

214 × 140. Pp. 12 (l.b.). 'Read July 13, 1887.' P. w. (cover title).

Copies: LNSW, ML. 1700

Prince Alfred Hospital, Melbourne

See Alfred Hospital.

Prince Alfred Hospital, Sydney

Prince Alfred Hospital. For the relief of the sick, the maimed, and the convalescing from all parts of the Colony. The following resolutions were passed ... at the Public Meeting of Colonists held in Sydney, on the 20th March, 1868: [Text continues.]

300 × 210. Single leaf, v.b. NI.

An appeal for funds, 'left at every house in the

Colony.' Resolved: a hospital, named 'Prince Alfred Hosp.', memorial to Duke of Edinburgh, should be erected on site of Syd. Infirmary.
Copies: RACP. 1701

Report of the Organization Committee. Appointed on the 19th August, 1873. To consider and report upon the organization of the Hospital . . . [Text begins.]
201 × 132. Pp. 32. Colophon—J. Reading and Co. . . . Syd.
Copies: ML. 1702

Prince Alfred Hospital, Sydney. Description of the proposed building. Mansfield Bros., architects. December, 1874. Sydney: Thomas Richards, Govt Printer. 1874.
278 × 210. Pp. 18. 8 plans, including 1 double leaf, and 4 flg.
Contains notes on foundation of hospital, organization and administration, duties of medical and nursing staffs, accommodation and costs.
Copies: LNSW. 1703

To the Honorable the Colonial Secretary. The petition of the [Space for name] 1.—That your petitioners understand that the Government have been asked to place a large sum of money . . . towards the erection of the Prince Alfred Hospital. [Text continues.]
212 × 125. Single leaf. ND. NI.
Petitions for inclusion of homoeopathic treatment.
Copies: ML. 1704

Leading features of the origin and progress of the Prince Alfred Hospital . . . April, 1881. [Text begins.]
250 × 178. Pp. [4] (2, 4 blank). NI. Signed Alfred Roberts, Edward Knox, Hon. Secs.
Copies: ML. 1705

1881. New South Wales. Legislative Council. Report from the Select Committee of the Royal Prince Alfred Hospital; together with the proceedings . . . and . . . evidence. . . . Sydney: Thomas Richards, Govt Printer, 1881.
326 × 212. Pp. 8, 24.
On the state of the Hospital (opened following year), and provision for contagious diseases.
Copies: LNSW, ML, NL, SLV. 1706

Rules. General Rules. [Text begins.]
204 × 127. Pp. 24 (l.b.). (?1882.) Colophon—Gibbs, Shallard, and Co. . . . Syd.
Another ed., 1883. (ML.)
Copies: ML. 1707

By-laws made in pursuance of the provisions of "The Prince Alfred Hospital Act" and "The Prince Alfred Memorial Hospital Site Dedication Act". [Text begins.]
204 × 127. Pp. 16. ND. Colophon—Syd.: Gibbs, Shallard, & Co.
Other editions: ND; 1889.
Copies: ML. 1708

Prince Alfred Hospital. Report of the first Board of Directors to the annual subscribers, October 22, 1883.
204 × 132. Pp. 20. Colophon—Syd.: Gibbs, Shallard and Co. . . . P. w. (cover title).
1st annual report.
Hospital opened 1882; title became 'Royal Prince Alfred Hosp.' 1904. For history: Epps, Wm (1918), *The story of an Aust. hospital*, Syd.; Schlink, Sir H. (1956), 'Alfred Roberts and the foundation of the RPAH', *BPCMUS*, 12 : 69.
Copies: EF (1883, 1895), ML (1883–), Roy. Prince Alfred Hosp. (1883–). 1709

Prince Alfred Hospital, Sydney. Rules. Honorary medical staff, ministers of religion, resident medical officers, various medical officers, hospital students, dispensers. Sydney: F. Cunninghame & Co. . . .
217 × 140. Pp. 24 (last 2 blank). ND. P. w. (title rptd).
Copies: ML. 1710

Resolutions affecting the appointment of the medical staff of the Prince Alfred Hospital. [Text begins.]
344 × 217. Single leaf, v.b. (1889.)
Copies: EF. 1711

Prince Alfred Hospital. Conditions under which patients are admitted. [Text begins.]

204 × 132. Single leaf. Pink tinted paper. (1891.)

Copies: ML. 1712

Directions to mothers respecting the feeding of infants and children. [Text begins.]

204 × 130. Pp. 4. Colophon: 'Christian Work' Print . . . Syd. ND. (c. 1898.)

Copies: EF, ML. 1713

Prince Alfred Hospital Pharmacopoeia [Text begins.]

120 × 85. Pp. 62 (l.b.). (1898.) Cloth. Includes case-taking card for students.

Copies: RACP. 1714

Prince Henry's Hospital, Melbourne

See Homoeopathic Hospital, Melbourne.

Pringle, George Hogarth

Communications to the Australian Medical Journal. By Dr. G. Hogarth Pringle, F.R.C.S.E. Parramatta, N.S.W. Melbourne: Stillwell and Knight, Printers . . . 1871.

214 × 107. Pp. 20.

Seven papers (1868–70), including early accounts of Listerian surgery: 'Three cases of extensive burn and scald treated with carbolic acid'; 'Surgical cases illustrating the advantages of the use of carbolic acid in compound fractures.' ML copy bears author's inscription.

Copies: ML. 1715

Papers on surgery, &c., reprinted from the New South Wales Medical Gazette, by G. Hogarth Pringle, F.R.C.S.E. Parramatta. Sydney: Gibbs, Shallard & Co. . . .

214 × 140. Pp. [ii] (title, v.b.), 34 (l.b.). 1 litho. pl. ND. P. w. (title rptd).

Papers, dated 1870–1. ML copy has author's inscription.

G. H. Pringle FRCSE, a local pioneer of Listerian surgery, settled at Parramatta in 1860. He was friend and associate of Lister, and Brown states that 'there is little doubt that he had been using carbolic acid as a dressing several months before Lister announced his new theory of wound infection to the world.' He died at sea in 1872. See Brown, K. M. (1937), *Med. practice in old Parramatta*, Syd.; *NSW med. Gaz.*, 1872, 2 : 372; O'Sullivan, D. M. (1967), *Med. J. Aust.*, 2 : 896.

Copies: ML. 1716

Proctor, T. R.

A treatise on the optical diseases of the eye and their results. The use of spectacles and the mode of manufacture. Anatomy and physiology of the eye by T. R. Proctor, oculist, optician, and scientific ophthalmologist . . . 388 Albert Street, East Melbourne. [Text follows.]

209 × 147. Pp. 20. 20 figs. ND. P. w. (cover title).

Also published: *Optical diseases of the eye*, Christchurch, ND.

Copies: ML. 1717

Pugh, William Russ

A letter to the medical profession of Van Diemen's Land: accompanied by the particulars of an operation for strangulated congenital hernia, &c. &c. By W. R. Pugh M.D. "Oh! if there be justice in Heaven, and we are assured there is, a day must come of ample retribution!" Foscari. Launceston, V.D.L. : . . . "Launceston Examiner" Office . . . 1845.

209 × 127. Pp. 70 (2, l.b.). P. w. (title rptd, slightly shortened).

This earliest separate Aust. publication on a surgical subject discusses the fatal case of a patient operated upon by author for strangulated inguinal hernia in 1841. This was criticised by a local faction, which was joined by Dr. Haygarth on his arrival in VDL some months after the event. As the result of information laid by him, Pugh was charged in police court with 'gross negligence, ignorance and rashness.' The case was dismissed, Pugh sued Haygarth and was awarded £250 damages, and Haygarth, unable to pay, was imprisoned for 12 months.

W. R. Pugh, first to use surgical anaesthesia in Australia (7 June 1847), was Supt St John's Hosp., Launceston. For above pamphlet, see Craig, C. (1941), *Med. J. Aust.*, 2 : 266; for anaesthesia, Dunlop, N. J. (1927), *Med. J. Aust.*, 1 : 144; Potter, W. L. (1938), *Med. J. Aust.*, 2 : 940; Crowther, W.E.L.H. (1947), *Med. J. Aust.*, 2 : 561.

Copies: CC, FC, ML, NL, SLV. 1718

See also St John's Hospital, Launceston.

Pupil of the Late Prof. John Woolley

See [Banks, Samuel Hawker].

Pythagorean, A

See Campbell, Francis.

Q

Quaife, Barzillai

The intellectual sciences; outline lectures delivered chiefly at the Australian College, Sydney, in the years 1850, 1851 ... Vol. 1 Mental philosophy or psychology, and metaphysical science ... Sydney: Gibbs, Shallard and Co. ... Melbourne: Robertson, Elizabeth Street. ...

186 × 117. 2 vols. Vol. 1 : pp. x, 238, [2] (colophon, v.b.); vol. 2 : pp. viii, [ii] (v.b.), 352. (1872.) Cloth.

Vol. 2 : Moral philosophy and logic. Shows Melb. publisher as William Robertson.

Copies: EF, ML, NL, SLT, SLV, US. 1719

Quaife, Frederic Harrison

Notes on the sanitary condition of the Eastern Suburbs, etc. ... (Read before the Sanitary Section of the Royal Society of N.S.W., 19 October, 1886.) [Text follows.]

217 × 143. Pp. 4. Colophon—Syd.: Charles Potter, Govt Pr—1887. P. w. (title rptd).

F. H. Quaife, MD, ChM Glas., who practised at Woollahra, was Hon. Phys. Syd. Infirm. (1871–8) and Hon. Cons. Phys. (1879–1911).

Copies: HDN, SLW. 1720

Quarterly Clinical Reports

See Reid, David Boswell.

Queen Victoria Homes for Consumptives Fund

Second Annual Report The Queen Victoria Homes for Consumptives Fund for the year ending 31st August, 1899. Marchant & Co. ... Sydney. 1899.

220 × 140. Pp. 16. P. w. (cover title).

Includes 1st an. rep. of Queen Vic. Home for Consumptives, Thirlmere. For notes on Homes, see Purser, C. (1899), *Austsn med. Gaz.*, 18 : 554; O'Neill, W. H. (1900), *ibid.*, 19 : 39.

Copies: ML (1898–). 1721

Souvenir book. Published in connection with the grand fair and press bazaar In aid of the Queen Victoria Homes for Consumptives Edited by His Excellency Lord Beauchamp Governor of N.S.W. Sydney, 1899.

295 × 191. Pp. [12] (l.b.). 65 pl. Cloth.

Copies: ML. 1722

Queen Victoria Hospital, Melbourne

Queen Victoria Hospital. Statement of receipts and expenditure from 11 December, 1896 to 30th June, 1897. [Text begins.]

193 × 132. Single leaf, verso—colophon only. Jas Arbuckle & Co., Print ...

1st an. rep. 2nd an. rep. shows title as Queen Vic. Hosp. for Women and Children. For history—Swinburne, G. H., *Queen Vic. Memorial Hosp.: A history of the first fifty years*, Melb., 1951.

Copies: SLV (1896/7–1899/1900). 1723

Queen's Asylum for Destitute Children, Hobart

Rules and regulations of the Queen's Asylum for Destitute Children. [Arms] Tasmania: James Barnard, Govt Printer, Hobart Town. 1862.

231 × 147. Pp. [iv], 26 (l.b.). P. w. (title rptd).

Another ed., 1866. Pp. 32 (l.b.).

Copies: ML (1862, 1866). 1724

[Royal Arms] 1867. Tasmania. Queen's Asylum. Report of the Royal Commission, with the evidence ... printed, 10 September 1867.

198 × 140. Pp. xiv, 92 (l.b.). Colophon—James Barnard, Govt Printer ...

Copies: SLT, SLV. 1725

Queensland—Parliament

The following items are selections from the *Votes and Proceedings of the Legislative Assembly of Queensland*, 1860–1900. See library catalogues for holdings. Detailed listing for LNSW, NL, OL, US, appears in Cope, R. L. *Australian Parliamentary Serials*, Reference Monograph 9, Library of Parliament, Syd., 1973. Separately issued papers of the series occur in various collections.

1868. Queensland. Legislative Assembly. Report on water supply to the various municipalities, by Joseph Brady, Esquire. ... [Text begins.]

326 × 204. Pp. 6 (l.b.). Blue paper. Colophon —James C. Beal, Govt Pr, Bris.

On the supplies of Ipswich, Rockhampton, Bowen, Gladstone, Maryborough, Toowoomba, Dalby and Mackay, mainly limited and poor quality, with methods for provision of a suitable supply to each.

1726

1871. Queensland. The dry earth system (Despatch respecting) ... The Secretary of State for the Colonies to the Officer administering the Government of Queensland. [Text begins.]

326 × 204. Pp. 14. Colophon—James C. Beal, Govt Pr, Bris.

Report by Dr. Buchanan, of Med. Dept of Privy Council, on a method of excreta disposal by adding earth, with removal for agricultural use. Recommends as a cheap alternative to water carriage.

1726a

1876. Queensland. Report of the Board appointed to enquire into the causes of disease affecting live stock and plants. Brisbane: ... James C. Beal, Govt Printer ... 1876.

229 × 147. Pp. 42 (l.b.). 4 litho. pl. Stiff p. w. (cover title). Signed: A. C. Gregory, Chairman.

Includes information on pleuropneumonia, worm diseases of sheep, fluke, hydatids, and poisonous plants. Annual reports, 1876–82.

1727

1877. Queensland. Progress Report of the Central Board of Health. Presented to both Houses ... To the ... Colonial Secretary. [Text begins.]

320 × 204. Pp. 4. Colophon—James C. Beal, Govt Pr ...

Central Bd of Health was established in 1865 and functioned till a Commissioner of Public Health was appointed under Public Health Act of 1900. Reports: 1865, 1877, 1880.

1728

1878. Queensland. Report with ... evidence taken before the Board appointed to inquire into the causes of the prevalence of typhoid fever at Toowoomba, and the best means ... for the suppression of the same. ... Presented to both Houses. Brisbane: ... James C. Beal, Govt Printer, Brisbane.

326 × 204. Pp. 16 (l.b.).

Cause held to be cess-pits in close proximity to wells, and general insanitation.

1729

1878. Queensland. Lunatic Reception House, Brisbane. (Report from the Medical Officer on the management of the) Presented to both Houses.

326 × 204. Pp. 2. Colophon— ... James C. Beal, Govt Pr ... Bris. Signed: W. Hobbs.

1730

1878. Queensland. Legislative Council. Report of Board on Dr. Seaton's minute, re quarantine and medical inspection ...

331 × 204. Pp. 6. Colophon— ... James C. Beal, Govt Pr ... Bris.

Includes opinion of Central Bd of Health that quarantine of vessels was essential, together with medical inspection of ships.

1731

1878. Queensland. Quarantine matters. (Report from the Health Officer.) Presented to both Houses ... [Text begins.]

331 × 204. Pp. 4.

Supports quarantine of vessels, as opposed to inspection and isolation of patients only, as in Britain, stressing that undeveloped services render the latter impossible here. Signed: Henry Challinor.

1732

Report ... of Board appointed to ascertain ... the cause of excessive mortality among the South Sea Islanders on the sugar plantations ... Maryborough.

330 × 204. Pp. 14. (1881.) Colophon—James C. Beal, Govt Pr, Bris. Signed: John Thomson MB, C. J. Hill-Wray.

Severe indictment of native labour conditions

throughout Maryborough district. All plantation hospitals are inadequate and insanitary, with total lack of med. care and med. certification of deaths. Concludes mortality due to poor diet, insanitation, overwork, medical neglect. Recommends full-time Govt doctor, large native hosp. at Maryborough.

1733

1881. Queensland. Cinchona. (Despatch respecting the cultivation of) Presented to both Houses ... [Text begins.]

320 × 204. Pp. 6 (l.b.). Colophon—James C. Beal, Govt Pr, Bris.

Information by Director of Gardens and Plantations, Jamaica.

1734

1884. Queensland. The temporary closure of the Hospital for Pacific Islanders at Mackay. (Correspondence respecting.) Presented to both Houses. [Text begins.]

326 × 204. Pp. 28 (l.b.). Colophon— ... Edmund Gregory, Acting Govt Pr ... Bris.

1735

1884. Queensland. The prevalence of typhoid fever in Brisbane and suburbs. (Report of Committee of Central Board of Health upon) Presented to both Houses ... [Text begins.]

323 × 204. Pp. 2. Colophon— ... Edmund Gregory, Govt Pr, Bris. Signed: K. Cannon MRCS, John Thomson MB, Charles F. Marks MD.

1736

1885. Queensland. Water Supply. Presented to both Houses ... [Text begins.]

320 × 204. Pp. 4 (l.b.). Colophon—James C. Beal, Govt Pr, Bris. Signed: J. B. Henderson, M.I.C.E.

Summarized information for Bd of Health on nature and efficiency of water supplies of Brisbane and 14 other centres.

1737

1885. Queensland. Charters Towers Water Supply. Presented to both Houses ... [Text begins.]

320 × 204. Pp. 6 (l.b.). Colophon—Edmund Gregory, Acting Govt Pr, Bris. Signed J. B. Henderson and W. M. Mackinnon.

1738

1885. Queensland. The employment of coloured labour in connection with the sugar industry. Presented to both Houses ... [Text begins.]

320 × 204. Pp. 4 (l.b.). Colophon—James C. Beal, Govt Pr, Bris. To Col Sec. per M. Hume Black MLA.

White labour is entirely unfitted, physically and economically, for heavy work of the sugar industry, leads to premature decay and physical wreck, and may ruin the industry. Urges that Pacific or Indian labourers be employed.

1739

Queensland. 1886. "Dorunda" Inquiry. Report, with ... evidence ... before the Board appointed to inquire into the alleged cases of cholera among the passengers on ... S. S. "Dorunda" ... between London and Brisbane (October, November, and December, 1885) ... Presented to both Houses ... Brisbane ... James C. Beal, Govt Printer ... 1886.

331 × 204. Pp. 54. 2 flg charts. Chairman : J. Bancroft, MD.

Asiatic cholera, contracted at Batavia, resulted in 17 deaths (6 in quarantine at Peel Is.). Recommends quarantine stations at Thursday Is., Cooktown and Townsville.

1740

1887. Queensland. The Pacific Islanders' Hospitals. (Report upon financial condition of) Presented to both Houses ... [Text begins.]

326 × 204. Pp. 8. Colophon—James C. Beal, Govt Pr, Bris.

Hospitals for the care of Pacific Islands labourers—here termed the 'Maryborough Polynesian Hospital', etc.—were maintained in sugar-growing districts at Maryborough, Mackay, Ingham and Johnstone. Statistical information includes number in district, staffing, average daily admissions.

1741

1890. Queensland. Epidemic influenza in Queensland. (Replies received from surgeons of hospitals and Government medical officers to questions forwarded ... by the Local Government Board, Whitehall ...) Presented to both Houses ...

323 × 206. Pp. 2. Colophon—... James C. Beal, Govt Pr. ...

Brief notes on incidence, time of first infection, place of origin, spread, clinical features.

1742

1891. Queensland. Shops, Factories, and Workshops—Royal Commission of Inquiry. Report with ... evidence taken before the Royal Commission appointed to inquire into ... the conditions under which work is done in the shops, factories, and workshops in the Colony; ... with proceedings ... and appendices. Presented to both Houses ... Brisbane: ... James C. Beal, Govt Printer ... 1891.

320 × 204. Pp. xlvi, 356 (l.b.).

Discloses conditions of juvenile and sweated labour, and gross insanitation. Recommendations include: restrictions on juvenile employment, improved sanitation, ventilation, fire and machinery protection, establishment of technical education.

1743

1892. Queensland. Imperial and Colonial Acts relating to the recruiting, etc., of Pacific Island labourers, and regulations made thereunder; together with instructions for the guidance of government agents appointed to accompany vessels licensed to carry Pacific Islanders. Brisbane: ... James C. Beal, Govt Printer. 1892.

217 × 140. Pp. 72, [ii] (inserted leaf, v.b.). P. w. (title rptd).

Includes provisions for medical treatment, establishment of native hospitals in certain districts, and rations.

1744

1897. Queensland. Report upon the working of "The Factories and Shops Act, 1896", from 1st May to 1st November 1897. Presented to both Houses ... [Text begins.]

323 × 204. Pp. 4. Colophon—Edmund Gregory, Govt Pr, Bris.

Includes reports by first inspectors appointed.

1745

1897. Queensland. Regulations dealing with cholera, yellow fever, and plague at ports in the United Kingdom. Presented to both Houses ... Secretary of State for the Colonies to the Governor of Queensland. [Text begins.]

326 × 204. Pp. 4 (l.b.). Colophon—Edmund Gregory, Govt Pr, Bris.

1746

1899. Queensland. Legislative Assembly. Health Officer, Thursday Island. ... Return to an order ...

340 × 204. Pp. [4] (2 blanks). Colophon—Edmund Gregory, Govt Pr, Bris.

Relates to objections by residents to relief of Dr. Tilson, HO, while on leave, by Dr. Salter.

1747

1900. Queensland. Publications of Berlin Imperial Health Office dealing with bubonic plague. Presented to both Houses ...

320 × 204. Pp. 18 (l.b.). Colophon—Edmund Gregory, Govt Pr ... Bris.

Transactions of official conference of German scientists on plague—bacteriology, pathology, epidemiology and prevention, including inoculation.

1748

1900. Queensland. Venice International Sanitary Conference and Convention regarding Bubonic Plague. (Correspondence respecting.) Presented to both Houses ... [Text begins.]

326 × 204. Pp. 26 (l.b.). Colophon—... Edmund Gregory, Govt Pr ... Bris.

Further despatch respecting ... Pp. 2 (l.b.). 1900.

1749

Queensland Association for the Prevention of Consumption

Queensland Association for the Prevention of Consumption. Annual Report, 1900. Alex. Muir & Co. ... Brisbane & Rockhampton. 1901.

212 × 140. Pp. 12 (l.b.). P. w. (title rptd).

Society founded 1899. Issued prior to this report, and reprinted here: *How to prevent the spread of consumption; Regulation for the disinfection*

of premises following a death from consumption. Originals NS.
Copies: ML. 1750

Queensland Medical Society

Queensland Medical Society. Office-Bearers: Kearsey Cannan, President, Hugh Bell, Treasurer. Joseph Bancroft, Secretary . . . [Text follows.]

204 × 127. Single leaf. Pp. [2]. Bris.: A. Cleghorn . . . (1871.) Rules.

For history from foundation in 1870 to 1900, see Hardie, Sir David (1900), *Austsn med. Gaz.*, 19 : 1.
Copies: AMAQ. 1751

———

By-laws of the Medical Society of Queensland. Brisbane.

214 × 107. Pp. 12 (l.b.). (1882.)
Copies: AMAQ. 1752

Queensland Medico-Ethical Association

Brochure, 1893, recommends health legislation to parliamentary candidates. (NS.) Includes establishment of health dept, federal quarantine, infectious disease notification, establishment of public abattoirs and inebriate asylums. (*Austsn med. Gaz.*, 1893, 12 : 166.)

Assn founded Brisbane, 1890 (*Austsn med. Gaz.*, 1890, 10 : 53).
1753

Quong Tart

See Tart, Quong

R

R., H. K.

See Rusden, Henry Keylock.

Radam's Microbe Killer

History and discovery of the greatest medicine, in the world. Wm. Radam's microbe killer. Germ, bacteria & fungus destroyer. [Emblem] Registered March 14th, 1890 . . . Cures disease, by removing the cause—microbes. Headquarters . . . Sydney.

209 × 138. Pp. 32. P. w. (cover title).

A cure for all diseases, composed of 'pure water charged with gases', discovery of a Texan nurseryman.

Copies: ML. 1754

Ralph, Thomas Shearman

Elementary botany, (Australian edition,) for the use of beginners . . . Melbourne: Bailliere . . . 1862.

171 × 107. Pp. viii, 72, [16]. 24 pl. Inserted slip (notice of classes in botany). Cloth.

Adapted from earlier English ed.

Copies: FC, ML, NL, SLV, WLC. 1755

———

Observations and experiments with the microscope on the effects of prussic acid on the animal economy. . . . (Read before the Medical Society of Victoria, December 6, 1865.) [Text begins.]

212 × 130. Pp. 12. Colophon—Wilson and Mackinnon . . . Melb.

Copies: AMAV, NL, SLV. 1756

———

On the parasitic origin of pleuro-pneumonia in cattle. [Text begins.]

255 × 163. Pp. 4 (l.b.). ND. NI. Signed at foot, with ms. addition: 'Kew, Melbourne. 20 Jan. 65.'

Copies: NL. 1757

———

Observations and experiments with the microscope on the effects of various chemical agents on the blood. . . . [Text begins.]

204 × 122. Pp. 10. 1 pl. ND. (1866.) Colophon —Wilson and MacKinnon . . . Collins Street East.

Copies: EF, SLV. 1758

———

Micro-chemical observations on the blood in health and in typhoid fever. Read before the Victorian Branch of the British Medical Association . . . Reprinted from the "Australasian Medical Gazette" for July, 1885. L. Bruck . . . Sydney. 1885.

212 × 135. Pp. 12. 1 pl. P. w. (title rptd).

For T. S. Ralph (1812–91) MRCS, founder of Microscopical Soc. of Vic., see obit., *Austsn med. Gaz.*, 1892, 11 : 117.

Copies: EF, SLV. 1759

Randwick Asylum

See Society for Relief of Destitute Children, Sydney.

Rasmussen, Hans P.

The natural doctor or the mysteries of nature explained. Being a description . . . of the human body, together with its principal diseases and nature's remedies for their cure. By H. P. Rasmussen, F.H.S., herbal specialist in blood and nervous diseases. Professor of medical botany . . . Sydney. 1890.

181 × 120. Pp. viii, [iv], 328. Frontis. (portrait), 18 figs. Colophon—Marcus & Andrew . . . Syd. Cloth or p. w.

Includes: general ailments, herbal mat. med., midwifery, health preservation, marriage, venereal dis., nervous debility. Among diagnostic services available: 'Patients may forward a few drops of their urine, dried on a small piece of glass, and Herr Rasmussen will examine it under his powerful microscope, which will . . . reveal any seminal losses, or whether (he) suffers from Bright's disease, or any other organic complaint.'

Author came from Denmark in 1879 and practised at Paddington and later Sydney. His Alfaline remedies were still being advertised, in his name, in 1958.

Copies: EF, WLC. 1760

———

The Same, 1890. Pp. viii, [iv] (3 blanks), 216. Frontis., 1 pl.
Copies: RACP. 1761

———

The Same, 1897. 10th ed. Pp. 165, [3]. P. w. (title rptd, dated).
Copies: ML. 1762

———

The Alfaline natural doctor by Herr Hans P. Rassmussen, the Danish herbalist, discoverer and proprietor of the celebrated registered Alfaline remedies. [Reproduction of label, with portrait, laurels, medals] . . . Cured over 100,000 sufferers. . . .

117 × 72. Pp. 112. Portrait, 6 figs. (1891.) Colophon—Marcus & Andrew . . . Syd. Title on verso of front cover. Cloth (portrait, 'The revised and condensed Natural Doctor . . .' on front).

Author's name is spelled 'Rassmussen' throughout, with exception of inscription (Rasmussen) on fig. of medal, dated 1887.
Copies: EF. 1763

———

The Alfaline medical guide to health or the natural doctor. The mysteries of the human body explained. [Portrait of author] Outlines of the principal diseases and how to cure them. . . . Herr Rasmussen . . . Sydney. . . .

147 × 100. Pp. 98. Figs. Paper boards (title rptd). ND. (Includes calendar for 1895/6.)
Copies: NL. 1764

———

Denmark female restorer pills . . . Best anti-barrenness pills in the world. This world-famed remedy for female complaints is unequalled for its wonderful virtues, in the treatment of all complaints peculiar to females. . . . 10,000 cures last year. A guaranteed cure for closing, falling, displacements, the whites . . . and prevents barrenness or sterility. . . . Herr Rasmussen, specialist . . . Paddington, Sydney. [Text follows.]

191 × 135. Single leaf, v.b. ND. NI.
Copies: E. M. Christie coll., Melb. 1765

Rasmussen, Vald.
See Mueller, Sir Ferdinand.

Rattray, Alexander
Notes on the physical geography, climate and capabilities of Somerset, and the Cape York Peninsula, Australia. . . . (Read before the Royal Geographical Society of London . . . 22nd June, 1868.) London: . . . W. Clowes and Sons . . .

214 × 132. Pp. 42. 2 maps. P. w. (cover title).

Author (MD Edin., RN) reports that though 'no malaria or other morbific influences beyond those of the climate exist' the area, like all tropical places, is unsuitable for prolonged white residence.
Copies: ML, NL, SLS. 1766

Ray, James
A voice from the inquest room; being the subject of a letter addressed to the medical gentlemen of Van Diemen's Land, and the public. By James Ray, Surgeon, &c. Hobart Town: Printed by James Burnet . . . 1849.

204 × 128. Pp. 12 (last 2 blank).

Defence of North West Bay doctor, 'stigmatized' by the evidence of Dr. Richard Bright, of Hobart, at inquest on a woman, his patient, who had died of protracted sepsis following suspected abortion.

See also: Bright, Richard.
Copies: SLT. 1767

Raymond, E. N.
Physical culture for women. The Sandow system. . . . [Cut—Venus de Milo] . . . The Sydney School of Physical Culture . . . Moore Street. . . .

186 × 125. Pp. 8. ND. Colophon—Commercial Publishing Co. of Sydney, Ltd. . . . P. w. (cover title).
Copies: ML. 1768

Raymond, Walter
A few brief remarks on the preliminary arrangements for collecting and the conducting of poor emigrants. With suggestions to guard against many of those fatal disasters that have occurred, particularly to emigrant, troop, and convict ships. . . . London: . . . W. S. Johnson . . .

209 × 127. Pp. 20 (l.b.). ND. [1849.]

A master mariner indicates the miserable conditions under which emigrants are transported, with heavy risk from disease and accident, and suggests preventive measures. ML copy has date, March 1849, at end in contemporary hand.

Copies: ML, NL. 1769

Redfern, William

See No 2070n.

Reeves, Charles Evans

An address on homoeopathy. London: Simpkin, Marshall and Co. 1853.

NS. Pp. 24. 1770

———

Diseases of the stomach. By Evans Reeves, B.A., M.D. [Quotation] London: S. Highley, and Son . . .

178 × 102. Pp. [viii] (l.b.), 195. 1 leaf removed after p. [viii]. ND. [1854.]

Copies: Roy. Coll. Phys. Lond. 1771

———

Diseases of the stomach and duodenum. . . . London: Simpkin, Marshall and Co. . . . 1856.

198 × 125. Pp. xvi (last—book notice), 354, [ii] (colophon, v.b.). Cloth.

Copies: AMAV, KFR, SLV. 1772

———

Diseases of the spinal cord and its membranes, and the various forms of paralysis arising therefrom,—chorea and tetanus. . . . London: Simpkin, Marshall and Co. . . . 1858.

198 × 125. Pp. xvi (last—list of author's books), 406 (last—colophon only). Cloth.

Chapters on spinal meningitis, myelitis, softening, apoplexy and atrophy of cord, tumours, chorea and tetanus.

Copies bear author's written inscriptions, with 'and 159 Collins St. East, Melb.' after London address in introduction.

Copies: AMAV, CC, EF, SLV. 1773

———

Acute cerebral meningitis, or hydrocephalus. . . . (From the Glasgow Medical Journal, Part XXI., April, 1858.) Glasgow: . . . William Mackenzie . . . 1858.

212 × 135. Pp. 60.

Causes, morbid pathology, course, diagnosis, prognosis, treatment.

Copies: EF, SLV. 1774

———

On a new method of treating swelled testicle, and on the employment of resine as a substitute for copaiba and cubebs. London: Simpkin, Marshall and Co.

NS. (c. 1858.)

1775

———

The Queen v. Beaney. Extraordinary charge of murder against a medical man, in consequence of a diseased womb being ruptured after death. With medical notes and observations . . . [Quotation] Melbourne: W. B. Stephens . . . 1866.

224 × 138. Pp. xii (l.b.), 244. Inserted yellow leaf of book notices, v.b. Cloth.

Report of the two trials of J. G. Beaney for the murder of Mary Lewis by procuring abortion, with comment by author, who prepared med. evidence for defence. Death was held due, by Crown witnesses, to rupture of uterus. In first trial jury disagreed; in the second, a verdict of 'Not guilty' was given. Bitter attacks are made upon med. witnesses for prosecution.

For further accounts: *Dr. Beaney's vindication* (No 193); *Aust. med. J.*, 1866, 11 : 240.

Copies: AMAV, BG, CC, DOS, EF, KFR, LNSW, ML, NL, SLT, SLV, UA, UQ, WLC. 1776

———

Softening of the stomach in children in Australia, with some observations on the disease in adults. . . . Melbourne: George Robertson . . . 1867.

212 × 135. Pp. [ii] (v.b.), 66. Cloth.

On gastroenteritis. In book list in author's *Consumption in Australia*, 1874, title is included as *Softening of the stomach in children in Australia, usually called dysentery*. 'Softening of the mucous membrane of the stomach' was accepted as a diagnosis in nosological indices of the time.

Copies: CC, LNSW, NL, SLV, UA, UM. 1777

———

On the cure of stricture by a new mode of dilation. And on the injection of the preparations of mercury under the skin in syphilis. . . . Melbourne: Clarson, Massina, and Co. . . . 1870.

217 × 135. Pp. 52 (l.b.). Cloth.

Gradual dilation with bulbed wires, tubes and rods.

Copies: ML, RACS, SLV, UM. 1778

———

The Same. 2 ed., 1872, with title: *On the cure of stricture by a simple mode of dilatation. And on the beneficial effects of the introduction of mercury* . . . Pp. xii (2 blanks), [3]–52 (l.b.).

Copies: AMAV, CC, EF. 1779

———

Heart diseases in Australia, with observations on aneurism of the aorta. . . . Published by the Author, and sold by J. Brooks . . . Melbourne. 1873.

220 × 138. Pp. xvi, 188. Cloth.

Contains 'the results of . . . examination of between five and six hundred cases of diseases of the heart', with tables from records of the Instn for Diseases of the Chest (established 7 years before). See Bauer, G. E. (1970), 'Four chapters in the history of Aust. cardiology', *Postgrad. med. J.*, 46 : 229.

Copies: AMAV, DOS, EF, KFR, LNSW, ML, NL, RACP, SLV, SLW, UA, UM, US. 1780

———

Consumption in Australia. . . . Published by the Author, and sold by J. Brooks . . . Melbourne. 1874.

217 × 135. Pp. [ii], viii, 154. Cloth.

Based on review of several thousand cases at Melb. Hosp. Warns against sending consumptive patients to Australia with the idea they can earn enough to keep themselves, and yet get well. Also discusses hydatids and cancer of lung.

Book notice includes *Diseases of Australia* as 'in the press.' NS.

Copies: AMAN, AMAV, BG, CC, DOS, EF, KFR, ML, NL, RACS, SLV, UM. 1781

———

On the cure of fluke in sheep with observations on fluke in man . . . 1878. . . . V. S. Azzoppardi & Hildreth . . . Melbourne.

201 × 130. Pp. 38 (last—author's book advt). 19 figs. Cloth.

C. E. Reeves (?1828–1880) MD published in London to 1858. He came to Melbourne soon after, following conviction in Dublin for defrauding the College of Physicians by obtaining diploma (LKQCPI) on another's behalf. (*Med. Times & Gaz.*, 1859, 39 : 89 and 176.) He was ed. and proprietor of *Med. Record of Aust.*, which ceased publication owing to his ill-health, and practised in Melb. till his death. See Gandevia, B. (1952), 'A review of Vic.'s early med. journals', *Med. J. Aust.*, 2 : 184; Bauer, G. E., *Postgrad. med. J.*, 1970, 46 : 229.

Copies: AMAV, EF, ML, NL, UA, UM. 1782

———

See *Medical Record of Australia, The.*

Reformatories and Reformatory Treatment in France

Reformatories and reformatory treatment in France. Translated from the French, by direction of the Government. [Royal Arms] . . . Sydney: Thomas Richards, Govt Printer. 1868.

222 × 135. Pp. [iv] (2 blanks), 126 (l.b.). Engraved frontis. Cloth.

Pamphlet collected by F. Norton Manning on tour of inspection of mental care institutions abroad.

Copies: EF, FC, HDN, ML, NL, SLV. 1783

Reid, David Boswell

Quarterly Clinical Reports. By David Boswell Reid, Junr., Surgeon to the Geelong Hospital, late House Surgeon to University College Hospital and Demonstrator of Anatomy to the University College, London. No. 1. January, 1861. Geelong: Heath and Cordell . . . 1861.

217 × 135. Pp. 30 (l.b.). 3 litho. pl. P. w. (title rptd; notice of anat. and surg. demonstrations at Geelong Hosp. inside back wrapper).

Record of cases treated at Geelong Hosp. Review, *Aust. med. J.*, 1861, 6 : 42 and 48. No 1 only seen.

Copies: LNSW, ML, SLV. 1784

———

Memo. on the case of Mrs. Barnett, by D. B. Reid, Surgeon to the Geelong Hospital . . . [Text begins.]

175 × 120. Pp. 12. ND. (1868.) Colophon—Henry Franks . . . Geelong.

Author, exonerated at enquiry, justifies his procedure. See also Geelong Infirm. and Benev. Asylum.

D. B. Reid (1834–1913) MRCS, became Res. Surg. Geelong Infirm. after arrival from London in 1859, and was associated with this till 1893. About 1896 he returned to London.

Copies: SLV. 1785

Reid, George Marr

Treatment of acute phthisis, by continuous and

persistent reduction of body temperature; lowering the vitality, and consequent virulence of the tubercle bacillus. ... [Text begins.]

204 × 132. Pp. 6. Colophon—Melb.: Stillwell and Co. P. w. Repr., *Aust. med. J.*, 20 Feb. 1895.

Advocates trial of treatment based on theory that continued lowering of the raised body temperature will diminish activity and virulence of organisms. Anti-pyretics and cooling applications are suggested, together with creosote as bactericide.

G. M. Reid MB, ChM Aberd. (1886), who came to Vic. for health reasons, practised at Kew (1892), Cobden (1896), and Heathcote Vic. (1911–).

Copies: EF. 1786

Reid, John

Drumine—A new Australian local anaesthetic. Discovered and described by John Reid ... L. Bruck ... Sydney. 1887.

234 × 173. Pp. 4. Repr., *Austsn med. Gaz.*, 1886.

Reports pharmacological experiments on 'drumine', an extract of *Euphorbia drummondi*, later marketed as a local anaesthetic. See *Austsn med. Gaz.*, 1886–1889, vols 6–8.

John Reid MA, MD ChM Aberd., was in practice at St Germein SA in 1886. He moved to Melb. in 1887, and in 1892 was MO, Yarra Bend Asylum.

Copies: US. 1787

———

Reprinted from the Australasian Medical Gazette. Burns and scalds. ... [Text begins.]

196 × 122. Pp. 8. ND. [1887.]

Copies: SLV. 1788

———

Croup and diphtheria. ... Reprinted from "The Australasian Medical Gazette" for December 1887. L. Bruck ... Sydney. 1887.

201 × 130. Pp. 16.

'I hold diphtheria and croup to bear the same pathological relationship as do scarlet fever and measles in their skin action, and that croup is not confined to the larynx, but affects the follicles of the thyroid gland.'

Copies: EF, LNSW, NL, WLC. 1789

Reid, Thomas

Two voyages to New South Wales and Van Diemen's Land, with a description of the present condition of that interesting colony: including facts and observations relative to the state and management of convicts of both sexes. Also reflections on seduction and its general consequences. ... London: ... Longman, Hurst, Rees, Orme, and Brown ... 1822.

224 × 135. Pp. xxiv (l.b.), 392 (last—errata). Paper boards.

Author (MRCS, RN) describes two voyages as surg. supt of convict transports *Neptune* (1817–18) and *Morley* (1820), including account of duties and measures for convict reform. Dedicated to Mrs. Elizabeth Fry, who influenced his acceptance of duty on latter vessel, in charge of female prisoners whose depravity made this 'extremely repulsive.'

Copies: DL, FC, ML, NL, SLS, SLT, SLV. 1790

Reissmann, Charles Henry—Editor

See Cayley, C. H.

Rendle, Richard

Notes on scarlet fever, also called scarlatina. Brisbane. 1892.

NS. Listed in *Cat. of additions to Parlt. Library of Qd*, 1892. 1791

———

Notes on the teeth. Why they decay; how to preserve them; how to restore them; how to replace them. Brisbane, 1892.

NS. Listed in *Cat. of additions to Parlt. Library of Qd*, 1892.

1792

———

Notes on snake bite, what to do, including the use of strychnia, (Dr. Mueller's antidote). Arranged by Richard Rendle, surgeon and apothecary, Brisbane. March, 1892. ...

105 × 66. Pp. 34 (last—colophon). 15–34 on yellow paper. Errata leaf. Paper boards (cover title on label).

Includes: treatment (ligation, incision), Mueller's strychnine treatment, information on Queensland snakes.

Richard Rendle FRCS, Surg. Lady Bowen Hosp. and Hosp. for Sick Children Bris., formerly Surg. Seamen's Hosp. Lond., and 'teacher of practical surgery', Guy's Hosp., was in practice in Brisbane to 1896, in Normanton Qd in 1900.

Copies: ML. 1793

Renwick, Sir Arthur

1882. New South Wales. State Children's Relief

Department. Report of the President, the Hon. Arthur Renwick, M.D., M.P., for the year ended 5 April, 1882. Presented to Parliament . . . Sydney: Thomas Richards, Govt Printer. 1882.

320 × 209. Pp. 20.

Sir Arthur Renwick (1837–1908) MD Edin., FRCSE, MLA, Hon. Phys. Syd. Hosp., was Vice Chancr, Dean of Med. and one of founders of Med. School Univ. Syd. He founded and was first Pres. of State Children's Relief Dept, and Pres. of original committee on the old age pension scheme and influenced its introduction. Obit.: *Austsn med. Gaz.*, 1908, 27 : 688.

Copies: ML. 1794

———

See Charity Organization Society of Melbourne.

Report of a Meeting of the Medical Profession at Sydney

See Medical Bill, NSW, No 1316.

Restoring the Apparently Drowned

Directions for restoring the apparently drowned. (Vide Government Gazette, 25th November, 1864) [Text begins.]

217 × 134. Pp. 8. 4 woodcut figs. Colophon—Syd.: Thomas Richards, Govt Pr . . . 1885. P. w. (short title).

Reprints instructions of Royal National Life-boat Instn Lond., 1864.

Copies: EF, UM. 1795

Retreat for the Aged Female Blind, Sydney

See N.S.W. Home Teaching Society for the Blind, etc.

Review, The

See Adelaide Medical Students' Society.

Richards, William N.

[Cut of premises] Dr. Richards on lost manhood: its causes and cure by medicine and electricity. Sydney: Gibbs, Shallard & Co. . . .

173 × 125. Pp. viii, 152. ND. [c. 1886.] Cloth.

On sexual impotence.

Copies: NL. 1796

Richardson, Walter Lindesay

Seven years' experience of diphtheria. By W. Lindesay Richardson, M.D., one of the physicians to the Ballarat District Hospital.

209 × 135. Pp. 8 (l.b.). ND. Colophon—Wilson and Mackinnon . . . [Melb.].

Copies: ML. 1797

———

Why I do not practise homoeopathy: being a letter to Mr. W. H. Barnard, in reply to a lecture recently delivered by him on that subject . . . Ballarat: Sold by Holmes . . . ; Vale . . . and all booksellers. Lewis & McKee, Printers . . .

171 × 102. Pp. 20. ND. [186–.]

W. L. Richardson (1826–79) MD Edin. & Melb., commenced practice at Ballarat in 1850s and was Hon. Phys. Ballarat Hosp. Successful in mining investment, he retired in his early 40s, lost his fotune, and in increasing ill-health, practised in turn at E. Melb., Queenscliff and other places. He became mentally ill and died at Koroit Vic. His daughter, Ethel Henrietta, Mrs. J. G. Robertson (1870–1946), the distinguished novelist, assumed the name of Henry Handel Richardson. Craig *(infra)*, referring to her trilogy *The fortunes of Richard Mahony*, states that without doubt the tragedy of Mahony is the tragedy of her father, and that her experiences 'must have burned into her very soul.' See obit., *Aust. med. J.*, 1879, ns 1 : 407; Craig, C. (1958), *Med. J. Aust.*, 2 : 1.

Copies: SLV. 1798

Richmond, C. F.

Anthrax and its treatment. . . . (Reprinted from the "Sydney Wool and Stock Journal".) . . . S. T. Leigh, & Co., Printers . . . Sydney. 1899.

181 × 120. Pp. 16. P. w. (cover title).

Discovery and tests of Pasteur's anthrax vaccine, including Aust. trials at Junee in 1888; spread and treatment of anthrax; advts of Pasteur Anthrax Vaccine Laboratory Ltd., Syd.

Copies: ML. 1799

[Riely, John]

Startling disclosures in connection with Tamworth water supply. Revelations of circumstances hitherto unduly suppressed, or kept carefully in the background, by those interested on behalf of departmental and legislative misfearants. An appeal to citizens, and a direct challenge to the Works Department to justify their action in this matter as other than maleficent.

178 × 127. Pp. 8. Colophon—Tamworth: Geo. Brunsdon, Printer . . . 1895. Author's name shown at p. 7 as John Riely, Moonbi.

Copies: ML. 1800

Ritchie, Daniel

The voice of our exiles or stray leaves from a convict ship. Edited by Daniel Ritchie, Esq. Surgeon, R. N. Edinburgh: John Menzies; London: W. S. Orr & Co. 1854.

158 × 107. Pp. [iv] (l.b.), ii, ii, 278. Cloth.

In 1852 author was Surg.-Supt of *Pestonjee Bomanjee*, with 292 convicts for VDL. A ship's journal, to which convicts contributed, forms the main part of the book.

Copies: FC, ML, NL, OL, SLT, SLV. 1801

Roberts, Sir Alfred

On pauperism in New South Wales ... Letts, Son & Co. (Limited), London.

217 × 138. Pp. 14. ND. [1870.] P. w. (title rptd, ornamented).

Copies: ML, NL. 1802

———

Paper on hospital accommodation ... Sydney: Thomas Richards, Govt Printer. 1874.

212 × 143. Pp. 16. Flg pl. (facsimile of letter in author's hand). Stiff p. w. (title rptd). Read at Roy. Soc. NSW, July 1874.

Another issue—P. w.; without letter.

Hospital services and needs of Sydney, induced by proposals for removal of Syd. Infirm. and foundation of Prince Alfred Hosp.

Sir Alfred Roberts (1823–1898) MRCS, Hon. Surg. Syd. Infirm., was a leader in hospital and public health organization in NSW. See obit., *Austsn med. Gaz.*, 1899, 18 : 38; Skirving, R. S. (1926), *Med. J. Aust.*, 1 : 290; Schlink, Sir H. (1956), 'A. R. and the foundation of the Royal Prince Alfred Hosp.', *BPCMUS*, 12, 3 : 69.

Copies: FC, LNSW, ML, NL. 1803

———

"May I tell you how I should like to be mourned! This will explain what I think is beautiful in such sorrow. [Text continues.]

175 × 112. Pp. [4] (last 3 blank). (1898.)

Message to his friends, prepared and signed by hand at foot, and distributed after his death.

Copies: EF. 1804

[Roberts, Charles Frederick]

Iniquities of lunacycraft and hocus-pocus of three learned judges in the first law case of the kind on this side of the world. By a great victim to them. ... Melbourne. Printed and published for the public good, by Charles F. Roberts ... Fitzroy. 1883.

201 × 135. Pp. 96. Plain p. w.

Curiously printed for author on a press of his own making, since 'no printer, for reasons which will be obvious, would print it ...' Attacks Dr. Hadden of Fitzroy Vic., and others, following author's commitment to Yarra Bend Mental Asylum, and receipt of Supreme Court judgement of a farthing damages for wrongful certification. Followed by *Worse than murder* (NS) and other publications, including *A courtship: a cat and a carrot or the marriage question solved at last*, Fitzroy (NS).

Copies: EF, ML, NL, SLV. 1805

———

Roberts' Occasional. In the sacred names of justice and humanity. No. 1. Melbourne, May 6, 1885. Gratis. [Text begins.]

217 × 138. Pp. 4.

Mainly devoted to personal attacks on those believed to have wronged him, including those associated with his commitment to mental asylum.

Copies: SLV (1–9, 1885–6). 1806

———

Jokers! [on woodcut fig. of coffin] Grave, ghastly and great. "Cast the full light of publicity on this dark villainy and it will wither, and your fellow citizens will be safe", says Charles Reade. The dark villainy he means, is the atrocious wickedness of ensnaring sane persons into madhouses ... [Text continues.]

224 × 140. Pp. [4]. Colophon—C. F. Roberts ... Fitzroy: Melb. April 1888.

Continues scurrilous campaign, mentioning many Melb. doctors.

Copies: SLV. 1807

Robertson, Alexander Milne

For the information of gentlemen of the medical and other scientific professions. Report ... upon certain peculiar habits and customs of the aborigines of Western Australia. ... Perth ... Richard Pether, Govt Printer. 1879.

209 × 105. Pp. 8.

Another issue omits 'For the information ... professions' from title.

Includes accounts of circumcision, subincision, scarring, performation of nasal septum, and physical measurements. Signed: A. Milne Robertson, Surgeon, Convict Establishment, WA.

Copies: FC, ML, NL. 1808

Robertson, Alexander P. L.

Medical reform: an inquiry into the relation existing between the public and the profession. . . . Melbourne: Wm. Fairfax and Co. . . . 1858.

209 × 132. Pp. 16 (l.b.). P. w. (cover title).

Author inquires into public and parliamentary indifference to medical legislation, and concludes that this can only be rectified by general education.

A.P.L. Robertson (d. 1878) MD Edin. was in turn Health Officer Port Phillip Heads, Supt Ararat Lun. Asylum, and first Supt Kew Lun. Asylum. Obit.: *Aust. med. J.*, 1878, 23 : 82.

Copies: ML, SLV. 1809

Robertson, George

Catalogue of standard works on medicine, surgery, pathology, anatomy, &c. British, American, & Colonial on sale by George Robertson Melbourne . . . Sydney . . . Adelaide . . .

204 × 127. Pp. 16. (1877.)

Copies: SLV. 1810

Robertson, James [Melbourne]

The University of Melbourne. Inaugural lecture to the course on the theory and practice of medicine. Delivered at the University Medical School, March 6th, 1865 . . . [Text begins.]

204 × 127. Pp. 16. Colophon—Melb.: Wilson & Mackinnon . . . Repr., *Aust. med. J.*, 1865, 10 : 97.

First lecture on clinical medicine, Univ. Melb. James Robertson (1822–93) MD Aberd., Hon. Phys. Melb. Hosp., was Lect. in Med. Melb. Univ. The so-called 'colonial fever' was identified by him as typhoid. Obit., *Aust. med. J.*, 1893, ns 15 : 85.

Copies: UM. 1811

———

Intercolonial Medical Congress of Australasia, Third Session, Sydney, 1892. Section of Medicine. President's Address . . . Reprinted from the "Australian Medical Journal", October 15, 1892. Melbourne: Stillwell and Co., Printers . . . 1892.

217 × 138. Pp. 20. P. w.

Univ. Melb. has author's copy, with galley and page proofs.

Copies: UM. 1812

Robertson, James [Sydney]

To the subscribers to the free hospital proposed to be erected in Sydney under the special care of the Sisters of Charity. [Text begins.]

214 × 138. Pp. 8 (l.b.). (1856.) Plain p. w.

Application for post of Surg., St Vincent's Hosp. Syd., by James Robertson MD St And., MB Lond., FRCS—who received appointment.

James Robertson founded Aust. Med. Assn, and was its first Sec., in 1859. He retired from practice the same year, suffering from tuberculosis, and died at Woodside near Parramatta in 1862, aged 40. See Miller, D. (1957), 'The med. pioneers of St Vincent's Hosp.', *BPCMUS*, 13 : 61; McIntosh, A. M. (1951), "The Aust. Med. Assn', *Med. J. Aust.*, 1 : 533.

Copies: ML. 1813

Rochlitz, Koloman

An essay on sea-sickness, explaining its real nature, and giving practical advice for its prevention and treatment. By Colomanus De Rochlitz, M.D. and Ch.D (Vienna). . . . London: Longmans, Green, Reader & Dyer. 1872.

8vo. Pp. 30.

Sea-sickness is caused by inactivity, aggravated by claustrophobia, and relief is by amendment of these. Refers to personal suffering on voyage to Australia, Port Phillip trips, Manly ferry crossings, and journeys by Cobb and Co's coach in NSW.

Koloman Rochlitz (b. 1825) graduated Vienna 1858–9; was in Aust. 1860–9. After practice in Melb. and Syd. he returned to Europe. For biog., see Kunz, Egon F., *Blood and gold, Hungarians in Aust.*, Melb., 1969.

Copies: British Museum, NL (photo.). 1814

Roebuck, Henry

Homoeopathy and the late Mrs. Tuckfield. Dr. Day's assertions; are they true or false? Geelong: Printed by Heath and Cordell . . . 1860.

175 × 110. Pp. 8. Signed by author at end.

'To the Public of Geelong', by homoeopath who had treated a woman in the early stage of a fatal illness later diagnosed as typhus, replying to the 'impudent abuse' of Dr. [John] Day, who attended her in the later phase.

Copies: WLC. 1815

Rolleston, C.

See No 2124.

Rooke, Charles

The handy pocket-guide to health & health-restoring places ... Published ... 1884, by C. Rooke, M.D., Scarborough. ...

138 × 100. Pp. [iv], 86, [ii] (advts). 27 figs. Paper boards.

Australia as health resort, pp. 75–7. The sea voyage is recommended for early phthisis, and climatic disadvantages indicated.

Copies: EF. 1816

Rose, James Marmaduke

For private circulation only. Testimonials of J. Marmaduke Rose, M. B., C. M., panopathist, consulting physician and surgeon. ... Melbourne. ...

217 × 140. Pp. x (l.b.), 88. ND. (c. 1891.) P. w. (title rptd, adds Sands & McDougall ... Melb.)

Preface notes author as founder of new system of treatment he names 'panopathy', which cures more effectively and rapidly than the defective 'old system.'

For J. M. Rose MB, ChM Edin., see Leavitt, T.W.H., *Jubilee history of Vic. and Melb.*, vol. 1 : 79.

Copies: CC, NL. 1817

Ross, Andrew

Jottings on vitality; or the physical basis of life. Reprinted from the "N.S.W. Medical Gazette". ... Sydney: Gibbs, Shallard, and Co. ... 1872.

193 × 127. Pp. 32 (l.b.). P. w. (title rptd).

Copies: LNSW, ML. 1818

———

The power of mind over matter: or, thoughts suggested on reading Nichols' confession of the Parramatta River murders. ... Sydney; Gibbs, Shallard, & Co. ... 1872

217 × 138. Pp. 24 (l.b.). P. w. (title rptd).

Copies: EF, FC, LNSW, ML, NL. 1819

———

Typhoid fever; its pathology and treatment, based on rational physiological principles, coupled with a cursory glance at diphtheria, Cumberland disease, and pleuro-pneumonia. Also, a few practical hints on the preservation of health in tropical countries. ... Sydney: Gibbs Shallard, & Co. ... 1873.

217 × 140. Pp. v, [6]–60. 4 figs. P. w. (title rptd).

Copies: EF, LNSW, RACP, SLV. 1820

———

Public health. (Read before the Intercolonial Medical Congress meeting, 28 September, 1892.) Sydney: W. A. Gullick, Govt Printer. 1900.

8vo. Pp. 8.

NS. Listed *SGC*, ser. 2. Noted only in Congress *Transactions*.

Andrew Ross (1829–1910) MD, ChM Glas., came from Scotland in 1857 and practised at Molong NSW, where he served as mayor, magistrate, and MLA. Obit.: *Austsn med. Gaz.*, 1910, 29 : 105.

Also published: *Guiding principles in the production of wool and mutton*, Syd., 1878; *Philosophy of mind and matter*, Syd., 1881; *On the influence of Aust. pastures on the growth of wool*, Syd., 1883; *The climate of Aust. ... in relation of health*, Syd., 1904 (reprints *NSW med. Gaz.* series, from 1871, 1 : 131.)

1821

Ross, Robert

Rev. Robert Ross (1792–1862) MD Edin., pastor of Congregational Church, Syd. and Director of Syd. Infirm. (1846–60), was a former med. missionary in Tartary, where he received royal commendation for work in a cholera epidemic. For devotional works, see Ferguson.

1822

Rossiter, Frederick M.

The practical guide to health A popular treatise on anatomy, physiology, and hygiene, with a scientific description of diseases, their causes and treatment. Designed for nurses and for home use ... Signs Publishing Company Limited, Melbourne ...

214 × 145. Pp. [ii] (v.b.), 636 (last, advt). 12 col. pl., 70 figs. ND. (EF copy bears inscription dated 1900.)

Reprint of US publication.

Terminal advt— Sydney Sanitarium, Wahroonga NSW.

Copies: EF. 1822a

Roth, Henry Ling

The aborigines of Tasmania by H. Ling Roth assisted by Marion E. Butler; with a chapter on the osteology, by J. G. Garson, M.D. ... and a preface by Edward B. Tylor ... London Kegan Paul, Trench, Trübner & Co. ... 1890.

222 × 130. Pp. xxviii (l.b.), 224, cx (appendices and index). 21 pl., 10 figs. Cloth. 200 copies, initialled by author.

2 ed., 1899. F. King & Sons, Halifax (England). 225 copies. Another ed., [?1968], Hobart, Fuller's Bookshop.

Many references of medical interest. For author, see Aust. Enc.

Copies: ML, NL, OL, SLT, SLV, UA, US, WLC. 1823

Roth, Reuter Emerich

Sitting in school as a cause of deformity ... [Text begins.]

209 × 140. Pp. 4. Repr., *Austsn med. Gaz.*, Nov. 1885.

R. E. Roth (1859–1924) MRCS, Med. Adviser NSW Educ. Dept, Hon. MO Prince Alfred Hosp., was an exponent of phys. culture and physiotherapy. Obit.: *Brit. med. J.*, 1924, 2: 1083.

Copies: NL. 1824

Roth, Walter Edmund

The elements of school hygiene: for the use of teachers in schools With a bibliography. London: Bailliere. 1886.

8vo. Pp. [4], 88. Cloth.

NS. Listed in Dawson (Lond.) cat., 206/1970. 1825

———

Theatre hygiene: a scheme for the study of a somewhat neglected department of the Public Health. ... London: Bailliere, Tindall and Cox ...

217 × 142. Pp. viii (3 blanks), 54 (l.b.). P. w. (title rptd). ND. Preface dated 1888, from College St, Syd.

Considerations of health, comfort, safety, including ventilation, sanitation, lighting, fire protection, seating and construction Lists features of Sydney theatres.

Copies: UA. 1826

———

Ethnological studies among the North-West-Central Queensland aborigines. ... With 438 illustrations. Brisbane: ... Edmund Gregory, Govt Printer ... London: Queensland Agent-General's Office ... 1897.

250 × 155. Pp. xvi, 200, 24 pl. (4 coloured). Inserted slip: 'This work is intended for scientific purposes only.' Cloth.

Notes collected while surgeon to Boulia, Cloncurry and Normanton Hosps (1894–7). Includes accounts of pituri *(Duboisia)*; ear, nose piercing and tooth avulsion; the death bone and other lethal magic; med. treatment. Chapter 'Ethno-pornography', noted as 'not suitable for perusal by the general lay reader', describes initiation rites, including circumcision and subincision; pregnancy and parturition.

For W. E. Roth (1861–1933) MRCS, LRCP, see *Aust. Enc.*

Copies: EF, KFR, ML, NL, OL, SLS, SLT, SLV, UA, UQ, US, WLC. 1827

Royal Adelaide Hospital

See Adelaide Hospital.

Royal Alexandra Hospital for Children, Sydney

See Sydney Hospital for Sick Children.

Royal Blind Society of New South Wales

See Industrial Blind Institution, Sydney.

Royal Children's Hospital, Brisbane

See McConnel, Mrs. Mary.

Royal Children's Hospital, Melbourne

See Melbourne Hospital for Sick Children.

Royal Hobart Hospital

See Hobart General Hospital.

Royal Industrial School for the Blind, North Adelaide

See Industrial School for the Blind.

Royal Melbourne Hospital

See Melbourne Hospital.

Royal Newcastle Hospital

See Newcastle Hospital.

Royal North Shore Hospital of Sydney

See North Shore Hospital.

Royal Polytechnic Institute and Museum, Melbourne

Catalogue of the Royal Polytechnic Institute and Museum of Natural History & Science, Bourke Street East ... Melbourne and Sydney: Printed by Clarson, Shallard, & Co.

204 × 132. Pp. iv, 5–32 (last 2 blank). ND. (c. 1862.) Cover title.

Lists items on display, mainly 'an introduction to anatomy', with 'natural' anatomical and embryological specimens.

Institute, conducted by Dr. L. L. Smith as a commercial project, opened in Dec. 1861. Lectures were given in various subjects, those on anatomy and physiology by proprietor. See Robertson, E. G. (1956), 'Melbourne's public anatomical and anthropological museums', *Med. J. Aust.*, 1 : 164.

Copies: SLV. 1828

Royal Prince Alfred Hospital, Sydney

See Prince Alfred Hospital.

Royal Society of Tasmania, Medical Section

Medical Section of Royal Society of Tasmania. Hobart: Printed at "The Mercury" Office ... 1897.

165 × 107. Pp. 4. P. w. (cover title.)

Rules and regulations.

Copies: NL. 1829

Royal Victorian Eye and Ear Hospital

See Victorian Eye and Ear Hospital.

Royal Women's Hospital, Melbourne

See Women's Hospital, Melbourne.

Rudall, James Thomas

With the Author's compliments ... Colour-blindness and other defects of sight in some of their medico-legal aspects ... George Robertson and Company Melbourne ... 1887

204 × 127. Pp. 20. P. w. (title rptd).

Demands exclusion of visually defective officials from pertinent posts in railways and at sea.

Copies: CC, EF, SLV, UA. 1830

———

Responsibility of government in regard to sight-testing for land and sea service. ... Read at the Intercolonial Medical Congress, Adelaide, 1887. Adelaide: ... Vardon and Pritchard ... 1888.

231 × 145. Pp. 10. P. w. (title rptd).

J. T. Rudall (1828–1907) FRCS, Hon. Surg. Melb. and Alfred Hosps, 'was the first, or one of the first, in Aust. to operate to relieve oesophageal obstruction, to use the ophthalmoscope, to perform tracheotomy for diphtheria, to employ microscopy in clinical diagnosis, and ultimately to confine his practice to opthalmology.' See Gandevia, B. (1954), 'J.T.R., his life and journal', *Med. J. Aust.*, 2: 989; Williams, D. (1947), *Trans Ophth. Soc. Aust.*, 7 : 5.

Copies: SLS, SLV. 1831

———

... On the surgical use of perchloride of mercury as an antiseptic. By James T. Rudall, F.R.C.S. Surgeon to the Alfred Hospital, &c. [Text begins.]

214 × 144. Pp. 4. Colophon—Stillwell and Co. ... Melb. Repr., *Aust. med. J.*, 15 June, 1887.

Trials of corrosive sublimate, 'the most powerful antiseptic known', performed 'in the hope of avoiding the dangers and inconveniences of carbolic acid.'

Copies: UA. 1832

——— (translator)

The pathology and therapeutics of mental disease. By J. L. C. Schroeder van der Kolk, Professor of Physiology in the University of Utrecht. Translated from the German by James T. Ruddall ... Melbourne: Samuel Mullen ... 1869.

222 × 140. Pp. xii, 158. Cloth.

Physiological anatomy of the brain, pathology and therapeutics of insanity. Translator's ms. revised by F. von Mueller FRS. Review, *Aust. med. J.*, 1870, 15 : 312.

Copies: HDN, KFR, ML, NL, SLV, UA, US. 1833

——— **and Jamieson, James**

No. 9. November, 1879. The Australian Health Society, Melbourne. Summer diseases. 1. Ophthalmia. By J. T. Rudall, F.R.C.S. 11. Sunstroke. By James Jamieson, M.D. M'Carron Bird and Co. ... 1879.

206 × 135. Pp. 8. P. w. (cover title).

2 ed., 1881. Reprinted 1883, 1887. 4 ed., ND.

Copies: EF, ML, NL, SLS, SLV. 1834

Ruddock, E. Harris

The homoeopathic vade mecum of modern medicine and surgery ... Seventh edition. Thirty-eighth thousand. Melbourne: B. Poulton & Sons, Homoeopathic Chemists ... London: The Homoeopathic Publishing Company ... 1877.

196 × 135. Pp. xxiv, 25–920, 8 (advts). Title p. tipped in. Colophon—London: R. K. Burt and Co., Printers ... Cloth.

A number of works of E. H. Ruddock MD, by the Homoeopathic Pub. Co., Lond., were

issued in Australia by homoeopathic chemists. These are English editions, with title replaced by tipped-in leaf bearing Aust. imprint above the usual London one. The author's approach is not purely homoeopathic; he adds homoeopathic methods to the standard practice of the day.
Copies: EF. 1835

Essentials of diet; or, hints on food, in health and disease. By the late E. Harris Ruddock, M.D. ... Corrected and revised by E. B. Shuldham, M.D. ... Melbourne: Martin & Co., Melbourne Homoeopathic Pharmacy ... London: The Homoeopathic Publishing Company ... 1877.
163 × 105. Pp. viii, 252, [20] (advts). Cloth.
Copies: RACP. 1836

The Same. 2 ed., 1879. Syd., F. N. Collins ...
Copies: AMAV, EF. 1837

The diseases of infants and children, and their homoeopathic and general treatment. ... Third edition, revised and enlarged, by George Lade, M.D. ... Adelaide: G. N. & W. H. Birks, Homoeopathic Chemists ... London: The Homoeopathic Publishing Company ... 1880.
178 × 122. Pp. viii, 9–240 (last—advts). Title p. tipped in. Cloth.
Copies: SLV. 1838

The Same. 3 ed., 1880. Syd., F. N. Collins ...
Copies: EF. 1839

The Same. 6 ed., ND. Melb., Martin & Pleasance ...
Copies: EF. 1840

The lady's manual of homoeopathic treatment in the various derangements incident to her sex. ... Seventh edition. Thirty-sixth thousand. ... Melbourne: Martin and Co., Melbourne Homoeopathic Pharmacy ... The Homoeopathic Publishing Company ... 1881.
178 × 120. Pp. viii, 9–280 (267–280 advts). Title p. tipped in. 2 figs. Cloth.
Copies: EF. 1841

The Same. 3 ed., 1869. Melb., Gould & Martin.
Copies: WLC. 1842

The Same. 6 ed., 1876. Adel., E. S. Wigg ...
Copies: UA. 1843

The Same. 9 ed., 1886. Melb., Martin & Pleasance ...
Copies: EF, SLV. 1844

The Same. 9 ed., ND. Melb., Martin & Pleasance ...
Copies: EF. 1845

Rusden, Henry Keylock

The treatment of criminals in relation to science; or, suggestions for the prevention of cruelty to honest men and women. ... read before the Royal Society of Victoria ... 11th November, 1872. ... Melbourne: George Robertson ... 1872. ...
202 × 130. Pp. 24.
Another ed., 1872, with shortened title.
Convicted criminals should be used 'as subjects for physiological, medical and surgical experiment', graded according to the type of criminal, the worst being utilised for trials 'involving so much risk or certainty of death, as would ... reduce their numbers.'
Copies: ML, SLV. 1846

Selection: natural and artificial. A lecture ... in the Wangaratta Athenaeum ... October 26th, 1874. Beechworth: Richard Warren, Printer, the Ovens and Murray Advertiser General Printing Offices ... 1874.
204 × 132. Pp. 16.
ML copy has author's notes and corrections.
Copies: ML, SLV. 1847

Essay on suicide. By H.K.R. Read before the Eclectic Association of Melbourne. Melbourne: ... Robert Bell ...
209 × 138. Pp. 8. ND. [1875.]
Copies: ML, NL, SLV. 1848

Mr. Bradlaugh's conviction for free printing on

the population question. A lay sermon ... Read to the Sunday Free Discussion Society ... August, 1877. Trades Hall, Melbourne. [Text begins.]

183 × 125. Pp. 16. Colophon—E. Purton & Co. ... Melb.

Advocates contraception and protests against prosecution of Bradlaugh and Besant for publication of Knowlton's *Fruits of philosophy*. For latter, see Knowlton, Charles.

Copies: ML, NL, SLV. 1849

The value of human life. ... Melbourne. J. Wing ... Collingwood, 1884.

178 × 122. Pp. 18.

Fictitious value is placed on life in infanticide, suicide, capital punishment, and maintenance of incurable insane; disregard for life in inadequate prevention of disease and child mortality. Social improvement would result from birth control and removal of criminal and insane persons.

Copies: ML. 1850

Cremation: a sanitary necessity. A paper read to the Australasian Association for the Advancement of Science. (Revised and enlarged.) ... Melbourne: J. Wing ... Collingwood. 1890. ...

183 × 122. Pp. 24, [ii] (v.b.). 1 pl. P. w. (cover title).

Includes objects of Vic. Cremation Assn.

H. K. Rusden (b. 1826), writer of many pamphlets, was Sec. Roy. Soc. Vic. and Vic. Cremation Assn.

Copies: ML (incomplete). 1851

Russell, Henry Chamberlain

Climate of New South Wales: descriptive, historical, and tabular. ... Sydney: Charles Potter, Acting Govt Printer. 1877.

231 × 156. Pp. [ii], viii, 190 (l.b.), [ii] (v.b.), 66 (last—colophon). 6 charts. Paper boards (title rptd), cloth backstrip.

Information of medical interest included.

Copies: EF, FC, ML, SLS, SLT, SLV, US. 1852

Russell, Robert Hamilton

The early diagnosis of hip-joint disease. By R. Hamilton Russell, F.R.C.S. Eng., of Melbourne, Victoria. Hon. Surgeon to the Melbourne Hospital for Sick Children. (Read ... Medical Society of Victoria.) [Text begins.]

229 × 140. Pp. 12 (l.b.). Repr., *Intercol med. J. Austsia*, 1897, 2 : 582.

For R. Hamilton Russell (1860–1933) FRCS, FRACS, Hon. Surg. Children's and Alfred Hosps Melb., distinguished and highly original surgeon who gained wide recognition for his work on congenital inguinal hernia, see *Med. J. Aust.*, 1933, 1 : 752; *Aust. NZ J. Surg.*, 1933, 3 : 110. See also, author's *Papers and addresses in surgery*, Melb., 1923.

Copies: US. 1853

Rutherford, J.

William Moon, ... and his work for the blind ... London Hodder and Stoughton ... 1898

200 × 132. Pp. viii, 280. 13 pl. Cloth.

William Moon LLD, of Brighton, England, himself blind, introduced his 'Moon System' of reading for the blind by embossed type in 1845–7, and achieved its wide use through home teaching societies and free-lending libraries. Chap. XI (pp. 111–5) notes the origin of this work in Australia, which is earlier mentioned in Moon's *Light for the blind*, Lond., 1873, p. 65; 3 ed., 1877.

Copies: LNSW, ML. 1853a

Ryan, Charles Snodgrass

Under the Red Crescent : adventures of an English surgeon with the Turkish Army at Plevna and Erzeroum, 1877–1878. Related by Charles S. Ryan, M. B., C. M. Edin., in association with his friend John Sandes, B.A. Oxon. With portrait and maps. London: John Murray ... 1897.

204 × 135. Pp. xx (l.b.), 436 (l.b.). Portrait, 2 maps. Cloth.

Sir Charles Ryan (1853–1926) MB, ChM. Edin., recently graduated, enlisted as surgeon in Turkish Army (1877–8). His hazardous service in the Russo-Turkish War is vividly described. He later served as Hon. Surg. Melb. and Children's Hosps and with AIF in World War 1 (KBE, CB, CMG). See *Med. J. Aust.*, 1926, 2 : 746; Casey, M. (his daughter) (1959), *Med. J. Aust.*, 2 : 390 and *An Australian story*, Lond., 1962.

Copies: AMAV, LNSW, NL, SLS, SLV, SLW, UQ. 1854

Ryan, James Patrick

No. 13] [July 1881. The Australian Health Society, Melbourne. Small-pox & vaccination.

By James P. Ryan (Chevalier of the Legion of Honour). [Text begins.]

217 × 140. Pp. 4. Colophon—Mason, Firth & M'Cutcheon . . . Melb.

Other issues: 1897; ND.

J. P. Ryan (1840–1918) MD, LRCSI practised in Panama, Peru and Chile (1865–70), and was surgeon in French Army in Franco-Prussian War. In 1873 he came to Melb., and was Hon. Surg. Vic. Eye and Ear Hosp. See *Med. J. Aust.*, 1918, 1 : 401; Williams, D. (1947), *Trans Ophth. Soc. Aust.*, 7 : 5.

Copies: EF, LNSW, ML, NL, SLS, SLV. 1855

S

Sadleir, Richard

A shot at the Medical Bill. The supporters of the Bill profess it is for the protection of the public, but . . . we must come to a contrary conclusion. . . . [Text continues.]

247 × 215. Single leaf (v.b.). Double cols. ND. [1876.] NI. Signed at foot: Richard Sadleir, R. N.

Attacks Bill for the regulation of medical practice.

Copies: ML. 1856

What is the Medical Bill? [Text begins.]

215 × 120. Single leaf (v.b.). ND. (probably 1876.)

Criticism of Medical Bill. Signed at foot.

Copies: ML. 1857

St John Ambulance Association, NSW

St. John Ambulance Association. New South Wales Centre. General rules and regulations of the Centre, together with instructions for the branches in New South Wales. 1890. Sydney: W. M. MacLardy . . . 1890.

196 × 132. Pp. 16. (l.b.).

Includes courses in first aid, home nursing and hygiene.

Copies: ML. 1858

First aid to the injured. St. John Ambulance Association, New South Wales Centre. Established 1890. Annual Report, April 29th, 1892. Sydney: F. Cunninghame & Co. . . . 1892.

212 × 132. Pp. 8 (l.b.). P. w. (cover title).

2 an. rep. (1891/2). 1 an. rep. (presented 28 Apl. 1891) was not printed.

Copies: ML (1891–1900). 1859

St John Ambulance Association, Vic.

Sir William Johnston (1963), "Dr. James Edward Neild and the early hist. of the St. John Amb. Assn in Aust.", *Med. J. Aust.*, 2 : 564, notes that early records of Assn in Vic. are in the possession of Secretary, Vic. District. 1859a

St John's Hospital, Launceston, Tas.

St. John's Hospital, Launceston. 1846. Launceston: Henry Dowling, Printer and Stationer . . .

324 × 194. Pp. 4(last—title and imprint as endorsement).

Letter to subscribers from Dr W. Russ Pugh, founder of Hospital.

Copies: Archives Office of Tas. (CSO 8/166/2097). 1860

St. John's Hospital, Launceston. Report, 1851. . . . Launceston: Henry Dowling, Printer and Stationer . . .

198 × 127. Pp. 8. P. w. (short title).

Opened Sep. 1845. For early history and association with introduction of anaesthesia, see refs under Pugh, William Russ.

Copies: ML. 1861

St Kilda Local Board of Health, Vic.

Town Hall, St. Kilda . . . Council of the Borough . . . with the view of obviating the unpleasantness arising from the present system of cleaning closet pans . . . [Text continues.]

204 × 127. Pp. [4] (1, 4 blank). ND. (1885.)

Circular to rate-payers on improved sanitation.

Copies: AMAV. 1862

St Luke's Clerical Sanatorium, NSW

St. Luke's Clerical Sanatorium. Prospectus of a clerical sanatorium, to be erected on Douglas' Hill, Kurrajong, in the neighbourhood of Richmond . . . [Text begins.]

206 × 132. Pp. 2. Single leaf. ND. Colophon—Sherriff & Downing . . . Syd.

Proposed NSW institution for health and relaxation of Presbyterian clergy.

Copies: ML. 1863

St Mary's Hospital, Hobart

Prospectus of a self-supporting dispensary and hospital, to be opened the first day of January, 1841.

231 × 172. Pp. [4] (last 2 blank). ND. NI.

[Hobart, Dec. 1840.]
Copies: Archives Office of Tas. (CSO 8/166/2097). 1864

St. Mary's Hospital, Patron, His Excellency Sir J. E. Eardley-Wilmot, Baronet, Lieutenant-Governor. Vice Patrons . . .

8vo. Pp. 4 (l.b.). ND. NI.

Opened 1 Jan. 1841 'as a self supporting Hospital, for the benefit of the labouring classes of Society, to afford at a small cost, medical attendance to the poor, and to enable the rich to aid the destitute sick.'

Copies: Archives Office of Tas. (CSO 8/166/2097). 1865

Report St. Mary's Hospital. 1856.

204 × 133. Pp. 16 (l.b.). 1 flg list. Colophon— . . . Pratt & Son . . . Hobart Town. P. w. (cover title).

Earlier report published July 1846. NS.

Appends letter (18 Nov. 1853) from E.S.P. Bedford to Royal College of Surgeons announcing a projected 'preparatory medical school' at the hospital and requesting recognition for course. Further appendix discusses student training.

See Crowther, W.E.L.H. (1944), 'Dr. Bedford and his Hosp. and Med. School of St. Mary's V.D.L.', *Med. J. Aust.*, 2 : 25.

Copies: FC, ML, SLT. 1866

See also Bedford, Edward Samuel Picard.

St Vincent's Hospital, Melbourne

St. Vincent's Hospital, Melbourne. Under the care of the Sisters of Charity. The opening ceremony, 6th November, 1893, by Lady Clarke. His Grace the Archbishop will preside. Melbourne: Sands & McDougall Limited . . . 1893.

208 × 130. Pp. 12. P. w. (variation of title).

Copies: SLV. 1867

The First Report of St. Vincent's Hospital, Melbourne. Under the care of the Sisters of Charity. Founded from Sydney, 1893. List of subscriptions and donations, etc., from 1st May, 1893, to 31st December, 1894.

214 × 138. Pp. 28.

Includes report on opening ceremony, 6 Nov. 1893.

Copies: ML (1862–9, 1894–), SLV (1893/4, 1895–). 1868

St Vincent's Hospital, Sydney

St. Vincent's Hospital, Sydney. Under the care of the Sisters of Charity. Surgeon: James Robertson, M.D., F.R.C.S. . . . Treasurer: The Hon. J. H. Plunket . . . Secretary: Francis MacNab, Esq. . . .

204 × 130., Pp. 8. Colophon: Printed by F. Cunninghame . . . P. w. (with 'St. Vincent's Hospital, Sydney. Under the care of the Sisters of Charity. 1857.').

Preliminary statement, dated Dec. 1857, on establishment of Hospital at 'Tarmons', Potts Point. It opened in its present situation in 1870. See also No 1813.

Copies: ML, SLV. 1869

The Same. [1858.] Pp. 16. Colophon: Joseph Cook & Co., Printers . . . P. w. (with 'St. Vincent's Hospital. Sydney. Under the care of the Sisters of Charity. 1858.' on front and v. of back wrapper).

Preface dated April 10th, 1858. Second progress report.

Copies: EF, ML. 1870

The First Annual Report of St. Vincent's Hospital, Sydney. Under the care of the Sisters of Charity. Surgeon: James Robertson, M.D., F.R.C.S. . . .

206 × 132. Pp. 24 (last 3 blank). Colophon: Joseph Cook & Co. . . . Syd.

Report for 25 Aug. 1857–31 Dec. 1858. Surgeon's Report states that consumption is the most frequent disease of in-patients, followed by chronic lead poisoning from lead water pipes.

For review of first 12 years, see Oliver, T. J. (1871), *NSW med. Gaz.*, 1 : 107; for early history, *Fifty years. St. Vincent's Hosp.*, Syd., 1907; also Miller, D., *Earlier days, the story of St. Vincent's Hosp.*, Syd., 1969.

Copies: EF (1857/8–1862), ML (1857/8–), St Vincent's Hosp. (1857/8–), SLV (1859). 1871

Salisbury, A.

The book of the nineteenth century, containing instructions for the safe & certain cure of every form of pain & disease known to mankind, without the aid of any medicine whatever . . .

Sydney: J. J. Cousins, Printer, Surry Hills. 1892.
173 × 117. Pp. 36 (l.b.), [4] (l.b.). P. w. (cover title).
Hydrotherapy. 'The doom of medicines and vile and noxious drugs has been written in one magic word—Water!' Title shows unidentified author as MD, FRCS.
Copies: ML. 1872

Sanderson, Archibald
Points for the electors. Dedicated to the electors of East Perth . . . Killing no murder by "Sandy" (Mr. Archibald Sanderson). (Reprinted from the Perth "Morning Herald" of February 3, 1897 . . .)
217 × 145. Pp. 12.
'A damning indictment' of WA Government for the 'appalling insanitary condition and loss of life in WA'—especially from typhoid.
Copies: NL. 1873

Sando, William Robert
The evil effects of alcohol on the human system as shown by phrenology, physiology, and toxicology . . . Adelaide: Frearson Bros., Booksellers, &c. . . . T. Smith, Printer . . . Fitzroy, Melbourne.
154 × 98. Pp. 64 (l.b.). ND. [1871.] P. w. (title rptd).
Copies: SLS. 1874

Sanitary Reform League, NSW
See Liernur, Charles T.

Saunders, John
Comparative tables of sickness in friendly societies. "Compiled from the Government Statistics for Victoria for 1874 . . ." [Table begins.]
173 × 112. Single leaf, v.b. ND. NI.
Compares duration of sickness, by ages, in various societies and shows lower figures for temperance groups.
Copies: ML. 1875

Sawtell, Charles
The children's eyes. Defective vision and how to deal with it, by Charles Sawtell. From the South Australian Register. July 16, 1892 [Text begins.]
265 × 210. Pp. 4 (l.b.). Triple cols. Title at head of p.1. Colophon—W. K. Thomas & Co., Printers . . . Adel.
Copies: SLS. 1876

'Scalpel'
See Blair, John.

Scherzer, Karl, and Eduard Schwarz
Printed for private circulation only. On measurements as a diagnostic means for distinguishing the human race. A systematic plan established and investigated by the undersigned, for the purpose of taking measurements on individuals of different races during the voyage of H.I.R.M's Frigate "Novara" round the world. [Text begins.]
263 × 204. Pp. 26. Colophon—W. Hanson, Govt Pr, Syd. . . . 1858.
Signed by K. Scherzer PhD and E. Schwarz MD, of the Austrian Expedition of Circumnavigation, on board frigate *Novara*, Port Jackson, November, 1858.
Copies: ML, SLV. 1877

Schmidlon, F.
Electro-medical instruments and their management. By F. Schmidlon, 44, Elizabeth Street, Sydney. . . . Bristol: John Wright & Co. . . .
236 × 156. Pp. [iv], 46, [ii] (colophon, v.b.). ND. [?1892.] P. w. (shortened title).
Copies: ML. 1878

Schmiedeberg, Oswald
See Dixson, Thomas—Translator.

Schomburgk, Richard Moritz
On the urari: the deadly arrow-poison of the Indian tribes in British Guiana. Read before the Philosophical Society, on April 10th, 1866. [Text begins.]
204 × 127. Pp. 29–42. In 'Papers read before the Phil. Soc. and the Chamber of Manufactures', Adel., Govt Pr, 1873.
Also summary, pp. [2]. Colophon—Andrews, Thomas & Clark . . . Adel. (SLS, SLV.)
Copies: EF, FC, ML, NL, SLS, SLV, SLW, UQ. 1879

Papers read before the Philosophical Society and the Chamber of Manufactures. . . . Adelaide: W. C. Cox, Govt Printer . . . 1873.
204 × 127. Pp. [vi] (3 blank), 120. Stiff p. w. (title rptd).
Contents include: On the urari: the deadly arrow-poison of the Indian tribes in British

Guiana; Poisonous plants; Capabilities of the various districts in the colony (suggests cinchona culture at Darwin); Uses and properties of pl.nts (describes many of med. interest).

Copies: EF, FC, LNSW, ML, NL, SLS, SLV, SLW, UQ. 1880

———

On the urari: the deadly arrow-poison of the Macusis, an Indian tribe in British Guiana. ... Adelaide: E. Spiller, Acting Govt Printer ... 1879.

242 × 183. Pp. 20 (last 2 blank). Stiff p. w. (title rptd).

An account of urari (curare), from personal experiences in S. America. Includes notes on native manufacture, use, action, results of animal experiments, and curare treatment of tetanus.

For R. M. von Schomburgk (1811–91) DPh, Director of Adel. Botanical Gardens, see *Aust. Enc.;* Maiden, J. H. (1907), 'Records of Aust. botanists', *Rep. Aust. Assn Adv. Sci.*, : 176.

Copies: ML, SLS, SLV, UA, US. 1881

Schrader, Christian Urich Detlef

Popular medical guide imparting instruction in the knowledge & rational treatment of diseases ... Sydney: Printed by the Direct Supply Company ... 1887.

161 × 102. Pp. [viii], 128. Cloth.

Diagnosis and treatment 'of the diseases which most often perplex the dwellers in the bush.'

C.U.D. Schrader (1819–92) MD Kiel, came to Aust. from Prussia in 1855 and practised at Walcha NSW.

Copies: ML. 1882

Schroeder van der Kolk, J.L.C.

See Rudall, James Thomas—Translator

Schwarzbach, Bruno Beheim

The eye and its care. Some advice ... [Quotation] Sydney: Turner and Henderson ... 1878.

222 × 140. Pp. [iv], iv-v, 6–41. 3 figs. P. w. (amended title).

Sections on: shortsight and longsight, squint, shortsight in school children, sandy blight, an eye infirmary is a necessity in a large city, appendix on ear diseases.

Copies: ML, NL, SLV. 1883

———

Weak eyes; lecture ... delivered at Sydney Protestant Hall ... Publishers—George Robertson & Co. Sydney ... 1885.

201 × 140. Pp. [vi], 7–32. P. w. (title rptd).

For B. B. Schwarzbach MD Wurzburg, LFPS Glas., who opened a 'free dispensary for the poor suffering from diseases of the eye, ear and throat' in King St, Sydney, in 1894, see Williams, D. (1947), *Trans. Ophth. Soc. Aust.*, 7 : 5; also *Austsn med. Gaz.*, 1894, 13 : 216.

Copies: LNSW, ML, NL. 1884

———

Report on operations on the eye and ear. ... [Text begins.]

255 × 206. Pp. 4 (2, l.b.). Repr., *Austsn med. Gaz.*, Oct. 1890.

On operations performed by author in previous 18 months.

Copies: ML, NL, SLV. 1885

Scoresby-Jackson, R. E.

See Jackson, R. E. Scoresby—.

Scott, Robert

A review of hydatid disease in Australasia during the decennial period 1888–1897. By Robert Scott, M.D., Ch.M., Hon. Surgeon Ballarat Hospital.

217 × 140. Pp. 34. Colophon—J. Anderson & Co., Printers ... Ballarat. P. w. (cover title).

Parasite, distribution, statistics, treatment, case histories.

Robert Scott MD Glas. & Melb., commenced practice at Ballarat 1886; died at Scotsburn 1940. For his gall-bladder surgery, see Gandevia, B. (1952), *Roy. Melb. Hosp. Clin. Rep.*, 22 : 19.

Copies: EF. 1886

Searle, G. S.

Mount & Morris exonerated A narrative of the voyage of the brig "Carl" in 1871, with comments upon the trial which followed the massacre on board that vessel. Compiled from documents published and unpublished ... Melbourne : Evans Brothers, Printers ... 1875.

196 × 127. Pp. 40. Cover title.

'The true story of the "Carl" massacre in 1871.' See Murray, James Patrick.

Copies: DL, FC, LNSW, ML, SLV. 1887

Second Midnight Cry, The

The second midnight cry; a divinely authorized

alarm and warning in connection with the Adelaide water supply, revealing the positive danger now threatening the welfare of these colonies, by the reason of the long-continued anti-Christian rejection of divine spiritual evidence ... Adelaide: Frearson & Brother, Printers ... 1896.

183 × 122. Pp. 12. P. w. (title rptd).

Adelaide water supply appears only in title. It was evidently of such repute as to serve as indication of divine wrath against the wickedness of the city.

Copies: ML. 1888

Secrets of Clairvoyance, The

The secrets of clairvoyance!! and how to become an operator. Mesmerism and psychology, and how to become a mesmeriser and psychologist. Being a complete embodiment of all the curious facts connected with the above strange sciences, with instructions how to become a medium. Sydney: The Research Publishing Company. E. T. Radcliffe, Printer. ... Sydney.

183 × 120. Pp. 72. ND. P. w. (title (abbrev.) rptd, advts all other sides).

Copies: BG. 1889

Selby, Richard Thomas

Truth: illustrations of the evils caused by tobacco, alcohol, under-surface evils, celibacy, &c., with advice by Richard Thomas Selby, Professor of Medical Herbs, who heals all diseases with herbal preparations only. ... Surry Hills, Sydney. ...

153 × 107. Pp. 48 (l.b.). ND. [c. 1883.] P. w. (title rptd, decorated, with added: Syd.: Thomas Renn, Austral Steam Printing Works ...).

Copies: FC. 1890

———

... What every bachelor should read. Social physiology by Professor R. T. Selby "... I condemn the use of all minerals as medicines, but mercury is the leading and notorious offender". N. Swainson. ...

153 × 105. Pp. [ii] (v.b.), ii, 96. ND. P. w. (title rptd).

A treatise on sexual troubles, advertising the practice of a Redfern NSW herbalist.

Also published: *Treatise on nervous disorders, celibacy, marriage; Nature's design.* NS.

Copies: ML. 1891

Self-supporting Infirmary for Diseases of Throat, Chest, Eye and Ear, Melb.

See Wilkins, John.

'Seneca'

See District Trained Nursing Society of SA.

'Senex'

See No 2130.

Serjeant, Mrs. G.

Proceedings of the Second Australian Conference on Charity ... Melbourne ... 1891. Mrs. Serjeant read a paper on—The Consumptive Sanatorium at Echuca. [Text begins.]

217 × 143. Pp. 8 (2 blanks). NI.

Instn, described as the only one in Aust. for the care of friendless consumptives, was founded by George Serjeant MRCS and his wife. Dr. Serjeant came to Aust. in 1888 as a tuberculosis sufferer and died in 1890, aged 33. Referred to also in *Henry Varley's life story*, by H. Varley, Lond., ND : 149.

Appended discussion on 'deportation of consumptives' to Aust.

Copies: SLV. 1892

Service, John

The life and recollections of Doctor Duguid of Kilwinning. Written by himself, and now first printed from the recovered manuscript. ... Edinburgh: Young J. Pentland. Sydney: Angus & Robertson ... 1887.

191 × 127. Pp. xiv (l.b.), [ii] (v.b.), 288 (l.b.). Errata slip. Cloth.

2 ed., 1888, Edin.: Young J. Pentland. 3 ed., ND.

A story, in Scottish dialect, purporting to be the memoirs of an 18th century doctor, discovered by author in the village of his birth.

Copies: AMAV, BG, CC, EF, LNSW, ML, OL, SLV, UQ, US. 1893

———

On the natural and artificial feeding and care of infants. ... Edinburgh and London: Young J. Pentland. Sydney and Brisbane: Edwards, Dunlop ... 1890

186 × 122. Pp. x, [ii] (v.b.), 68 (l.b.), [4] (book notices, l.b.). Cloth.

Breast feeding, care of nursing mothers, after-weaning diet, artificial feeding, treatment of diarrhoea.

Also published: *Thir notandums, being the*

literary recreations of Laird Canticarl of Mongrymen, Syd., 1890; *The smugglers of Marsden Rock*, NS; *The memorables of Robin Cummell*, Paisley, 1913.

John Service (1851–1916) LRCPE, LRCSE settled in Sydney in 1884 and in 1885 was Supt of quarantine ship *Faraway*, Syd. He practised at Newtown, Syd. (1885–92) and later moved from place to place in NSW. For obit., see *Daily Telegraph*, Syd., 1 April 1916. ML has typed mss of three of his novels, presented by him.

Copies: EF, US. 1894

Seventy Years of Life in the Victorian Era

See [Hughes, J. Vaughan—].

Shanasy, W. Theo.

Australia's teeth and how to save them. By W. Theo. Shanasy, ... Hussey & Gillingham, Printers ... Adelaide. 1900.

206 × 162. Pp. 8.

Copies: SLS. 1895

Sharp, Albert

With later reports. Copy. The prevention and cure of sea-sickness. To owners and agents of passenger vessels. [Circular letter begins.]

212 × 135. Pp. [4]. ND. Aust. testimonials dated 1898.

'Seajoi', a secret preventive and remedy.

Copies: ML. 1896

Sharp, W. Hey

The water of Sydney Harbour. ... [Read before the Royal Society of N.S.W., 4 August, 1879.] Introductory.—There are not wanting in ... Sydney ... forcible reminders that the citizens have not yet successfully solved the pressing ... problem of keeping their surroundings pure and wholesome. [Text continues.]

214 × 132. Pp. 6 (l.b.). P. w. (title rptd). Colophon—Syd.: Thomas Richards, Govt Pr—1880.

Analyses of free and albuminoid ammonia, as tests of pollution. Author was Warden of St Paul's College.

Copies: ML. 1897

Shaw, John

A tramp to the diggings: being notes of a ramble in Australia and New Zealand in 1852. ... London: Richard Bentley ... 1852.

186 × 125. Pp. vi, 318. Cloth.

John Shaw MD arrived in Sydney from NZ in 1851 and visited Sofala and Turon diggings, and Wollongong. General information, with descriptions of Syd. and country visited.

Copies: ML, SLS, SLV, SLW, UA, UQ, US. 1898

———

A gallop to the Antipodes, returning overland through India. ... London: J. F. Hope ... 1858.

183 × 117. Pp. iv, 392, 16 (book list). Cloth.

Account of voyage from Plymouth to Aust. on emigrant ship *Undaunted* in 1857, with descriptions of Melb., Syd. and NZ.

Copies: DL, EF, FC, ML, NL, SLT, SLV, UA. 1899

Sheffield, Vaccination, and False Prophets

Sheffield, vaccination, and false prophets. [Text begins.]

217 × 144. Single leaf, v.b. ND. [c. 1889.] Hobart: Calder, Bowden, & Co.

Anti-vaccination leaflet.

Copies: EF, NL. 1900

Shelton, Charles M.

See Vitadatio.

Sheridan, John J.

Phrenology A few words on the subject by John J. Sheridan, M.T.P.S., inventor of the crianocentiometer, &c. Perfecter of the water test system. ... Hobart: Published by the Tasmanian Phrenological Society. ... Printed at the "Tasmanian News" Office, Hobart. 1890.

190 × 140. Pp. 16, [2] (v.b.). P. w. (cover title).

Author noted as inventor of an instrument for measuring the head.

Includes notice of Tas. Phrenological Soc. inviting gifts of human and monkey skeletons and skulls.

Copies: CC, EF, SLT. 1901

Sherwin, William

On the primum mobile of the blood in the lungs at birth: its complete vitalization or animalization; and its subsequent circulation. By William Sherwin, M.R.C.S. of London. Sydney: Printed by James Reading, King Street. 1844.

214 × 127. Pp. 8.

The first medical publication by a native-born Australian. Explains changes in foetal circulation at birth.

Copies: ML. 1902

———

Physiology and pharmacodynamics. By William Sherwin, F.R.C.S.E. & M.D. Delivered at the School of Arts, Sydney, on ... the 8th of January, 1863. Sydney: Printed by Hanson and Bennett ... 1863.

209 × 130. Pp. 26. Colophon—W. Davey & Son, Printers, 8 Gilbert-street, Oxford-street.

In support of homoeopathy. Author believes in 'the general correctness of the doctrine' and correctly forecasts resultant criticism.

Copies: LNSW, ML, RACP. 1903

———

Evidence of the benefits of homoeopathy, and statistics of its success ... Delivered at the School of Arts, Sydney, on ... the 24th January, 1863. Sydney: Printed by Hanson and Bennett ... 1863.

212 × 145. Pp. 26 (l.b.). P. w. (title rptd).

William Sherwin (1804–1874) MD, FRCS, b. Parramatta, was apprenticed to Wm Bland in 1817 and completed his studies in London—the first Australian youth to do so. He served as asst surg. to Melville Is. settlement (N. Aust.); established the first fully private practice in Parramatta in 1829; moved to Sydney in 1840. In 1862 he qualified FRCS, and on return practised homoeopathy.

See *NSW med. Gaz.*, 1874, 4 : 212; also Brown, K. M. (1937), *Med. practice in old Parramatta*, Syd.; McIntosh, A. M. (1954), 'The life and times of William Bland', *BPCMUS*, 10 : 109.

Copies: LNSW, ML. 1904

———

See Bennett, George; Gibson, A.; and Sherwin, William.

Shirley, John

International catalogue of scientific literature. Queensland Volume. By John Shirley, B.Sc. (Lond.), ... Brisbane: ... Edmund Gregory, Govt Printer. 1899.

220 × 140. Pp. iv, vi, ii (errata, v.b.), 154. P. w. (title rptd).

Lists Queensland publications to June 1898; prepared for Roy. Soc. Qd. Includes some med. authors. *Proc. Trans Roy. Geog. Soc. Austsia*, 1899, 14 : 13 (also as pamphlet), states that not more than half the literature is included.

Copies: EF, LNSW, ML, NL, SLV, UA, UM, UQ, US. 1905

———

A fish-poison of the aborigines ... (Read before the Royal Society of Queensland, October 5, 1895.) [Text begins.]

218 × 145. Pp. 2.

On the use of *Stephania hernandiaefolia*.

Copies: EF, SLV. 1905a

Shirres, George

See Gresswell, Dan Astley, No 777.

Shoobridge, Margaret

Something about our bodies, and what to do when we are ill. ... Tasmania: Published by J. Walch and Sons, Hobart; Walch Bros. and Birchall, Launceston. Printed at "The Mercury" Office ... Hobart. 1889.

180 × 122. Pp. 52 (l.b.). P. w. (title rptd).

Lectures by Matron, Cottage Hosp. and Convalescent Home, New Norfolk.

Copies: SLT. 1906

Shroff, The

See [White, J. H.].

Sidders, T. A.

Burnett refuted! Total abstinence, anti-scriptural, anti-social, and opposed to the common sense of mankind, in all ages and countries. ... Geelong: Wise & Downie ... 1868.

173 × 107. Pp. 32. P. w. (title rptd).

On the value of alcoholic drinks, which increase health and longevity, protect from infectious diseases, etc. 'Shall there be no more cakes and ale, because Bannister takes raw carrots and turnips, and Jenkins sings to the praise and glory of the poisonous Yan Yean, or the filthy liquid of the Barwon ...?'

Copies: ML. 1907

Silverton Hospital, NSW

Rules and regulations for the management of the Silverton Hospital. Adel. : W. K. Thomas & Co., Printers ... 1890.

211 × 132. Pp. 8.

Copies: SLS. 1908

Simon, Sir John

See Greenup, Richard.

Simple Household Recipes

Simple household recipes, collected from most reliable sources. No home should be without this book. ... Ballarat: Printed by A. A. Herberts, "Sport" Office ... 1894.

186 × 125. Pp. 48 (last 2 blank).

Remedies for all complaints; e.g., 'Cancers ... In ten cases of cancer this simple remedy has failed in none. Red clover tops are to be used in the manner of tea. ...'

Copies: BG. 1909

The Same. Ballarat: W. B. Macdonald, Printer ... 1899.

Copies: DOS. 1910

Simpson, Stephen

A practical view of homoeopathy, being an address to British practitioners on the general applicability and superior efficacy of the homoeopathic method in the treatment of disease. With cases. London: J. B. Bailliere, 1836.

8vo. Pp. xviii, 352.

NS. Listed *SGC*. One of the earliest English books on homoeopathy.

Stephen Simpson (c. 1800–69) MD, MLC, a pioneer of Moreton Bay District, where he practised and held various official posts, qualified in Britain and later studied homoeopathy under Hahnemann. His migration to Australia in 1840 is ascribed to antagonism aroused by this publication. For biog., see Stevens, E. V. (1953), 'Stephen Simpson', *J. Hist. Soc. Qd*, ns 5 : 794; Jackson, E. S. (1922), 'Historical notes from ... the Brisbane Hosp.', *Med. J. Aust.*, 1, 685; Russell, H. S., *The genesis of Queensland*, Syd., 1888 : 211.

1911

Aborigines (Australian Colonies). Return to an address of the Honourable The House of Commons, dated 5 August, 1844:— for, copies or extracts from despatches of the Governors of the Australian Colonies, with the reports of the Protectors of Aborigines, and any other correspondence to illustrate the condition of the aboriginal population of the said Colonies ... Ordered, by the House of Commons, to be printed, 9 August 1844. [627.]

333 × 213. Pp. viii, 438 (l.b.). 6 maps.

See 'Aborigines, Aust. Colonies. (No 3). Journal of an excursion to the Bunya Country, situated to the north of Moreton Bay', pp. 299–303, signed (at end): S. Simpson, Commr Crown Lands.

See also 'Rep. of the present state of the aborigines in the District of Moreton Bay', 1844, *HRA*, ser. 1, 23 : 485 (similarly signed).

Copies: DL, ML, NL, OL. 1912

Singleton, John

Lecture delivered ... Melbourne, July 29, 1853 ... "The effects of intoxicating drinks upon the community considered in their moral and physical relations". Melbourne Printed by B. Lucas ... 1853.

196 × 127. Pp. 16 (l.b.).

Copies: LNSW, NL. 1913

Alcohol as a medicine. ... read at ... Medical Society of Victoria. Copied from the *Australian Medical Journal* of November, 1874. ... [Text begins.]

183 × 122. Pp. 8. Colophon—Mason, Firth & M'Cutcheon ... Melb.

Attack on medicinal use of alcohol, circulated by author 'with a lithograph letter.' Review, *NSW med. Gaz.*, 1875, 5 : 273. Also as appendix to *Narrative of ... eventful life*.

Copies: LNSW, ML, NL, SLV. 1914

Phthisis in Victoria. ... read ... Medical Society of Victoria, 6th September, 1876. (Extracted from the Australian Medical Journal.) [Text begins.]

215 × 138. Pp. 8 (l.b.). Colophon—Stillwell and Knight ...

Denies W. Thomson's statement that local climate fails to modify or prevent tuberculosis.

Also appears as appendix to *Narrative of ... eventful life*.

Copies: CC, FC, SLV. 1915

From the Australian Medical Journal, March, 1878. On fever and the mode of treatment adopted at the Free Medical Mission Dispensary, Wellington Street, Collingwood: being a paper read before the Medical Society, Melbourne ... Melbourne: Mason, Firth & M'Cutcheon ... 1878.

198 × 127. Pp. 6. Cover title (decorated border).

Copies: NL. 1916

Narrative of incidents in the eventful life of a physician . . . Melbourne: M. L. Hutchinson . . . 1891.

209 × 132. Pp. xxiv, 414, [ii] (colophon, v.b.). Frontis. (photo. portrait of author, laid down, with facsimile signature), 28 pl. Cloth.

Author's life, especially describing his med. and social welfare work in Vic. from 1851 to 1891. Appendix: selected papers. The book was drawn on freely by author's great-grand-daughter, Dr. Mary Kent Hughes, for her Singleton biog., *Pioneer doctor*.

John Singleton (1808–91) MD Glas. & Melb., founded Collingwood Free Med. Mission Dispensary in 1869, was later one of the founders of the Children's Hosp., and established numerous other early Melb. charities. For biog., see author's *Narrative* . . .; Hughes, Mary K. (1950), *Pioneer doctor*, Melb.

Copies: AMAV, BG, CC, DOS, EF, FC, KFR, ML, NL, RACS, SLS, SLT, SLV, UA, UM, UQ, US. 1917

The Same. Melb. : Thompson & McCutchan, General Printers . . . Richmond. M. L. Hutchinson . . . 1891. Photo. frontis. replaced by woodcut port.; lacks imprint on v. of title. Paper boards.

Copies: CC, EF, FF. 1918

See also Collingwood Free Med. Mission Dispensary; International Temperance Convention, 1888.

Singleton and Patrick's Plains Benevolent Society, NSW

Rules and regulations for the management of the Singleton and Patrick's Plains Benevolent Society. Approved and adopted, August 30, 1861. Maitland: Tucker, Cracknell, and Falls, Printers. 1861.

185 × 108. Pp. 12.

Copies: LNSW. 1919

Sisca, Natale

Chronic indigestion, biliousness, and management of children . . . Ballarat: J. Anderson & Co. . . . 1889.

178 × 115. Pp. 54 (l.b.). P. w. (title rptd).

Copies: LNSW. 1920

Miners' disease: what it is, its causes, and treatment. . . . Ballarat: J. Anderson & Co. . . . 1890.

209 × 138. Pp. 36. 1 flg woodcut plate.

Published to bring the problem of silicosis to legislators and the public.

Copies: NL, SLV. 1921

Management of children in health and disease . . . George Robertson & Co., Melbourne, Sydney and Adelaide.

175 × 117. Pp. (x), 198. P. w. (title rptd).

Advice to mothers. Parts on management of pregnancy, of healthy children, of sick children. Preface addressed: Hawksburn, 1892.

Natale Sisca MD Naples (1885) practised at Mt Egerton Vic., later at Hawksburn and Melb., and was in NSW in 1904.

Copies: NL, SLV. 1922

Skirving, Robert Scot

Testimonials in favour of R. Scot Skirving M.B., C. M., Edin. (with honours) . . . [Appointments follow.]

214 × 140. Pp. 12. (1883.) P. w. (cover title). Colophon—A. W. Beard . . . Syd.

R. Scot Skirving (1859–1956) MB Edin., FRACP, FRACS, FRCS, trained for the merchant service and left the sea to study medicine in Edinburgh. In 1883 he came to Sydney, became a leading practitioner, and remained to the age of 97 a vivid and instructive link with earlier days. For biog., see obit., *Med. J. Aust.*, 1956, 2 : 734 (with bibliog.); Greenaway, T. (1964), *BPCMUS*, 20 : 281.

Later publications: *Our Army in S. Africa*, Syd., 1901; a novel *Love and longitude*, Syd., 1901; and *Wire splicing for yachtsmen*, 1,2,3 eds., Glasgow; Aust. ed., Syd., 1931.

Copies: EF. 1923

Smith, Abbotts

On ventilation. . . . Melbourne: Walker, May and Co. . . . 1875.

217 × 130. Pp. 8. 1 fig.

Copies: ML. 1924

Smith, Alfred Mica

1892. Victoria. Department of Mines. Special reports . . . Report on the foul air in the Allendale mines . . . Robt. S. Brain, Govt Printer, Melbourne.

206 × 115. Pp. 24. P. w. (title rptd).
Copies: AMAV, LNSW, ML, NL, SLV. 1925

Smith, Daniel
See Tichborne Case.

Smith, Sir Grafton Elliot
[From Vol. IX. (Series 2nd) of the "Proceedings of the Linnean Society of New South Wales" (October 31st, 1894).] A preliminary communication upon the cerebral commissures of the Mammalia, with special reference to the Monotremata and Marsupialia. ... [Text begins.]
204 × 135. Pp. 635–658 (l.b.). 1 pl. P. w.
'... a brilliant paper on the structure of the brain that laid the foundations, not only of his own later neurological researches, but of all future work upon the morphology of the mammalian brain.' (F. Wood Jones, 1938.)
Copies: ML, RACP, US. 1926

Thesis for presentation ... for the degree of M.D. at the University of Sydney, March, 1895. The comparative anatomy of the cerebrum of platypus. ... Redfern: Gornall, Printer, "Times" Office ... 1895.
209 × 135. Pp. 68. P. w. (cover title).
Author was first to graduate MD Syd.
US copy bears author's textual corrections.
Sir Grafton Elliot Smith (1871–1937) MD, DSc., FRCP, FRS, b. Grafton NSW, Prof. Anatomy at Cairo, Manchester, and Univ. Coll. Lond., was famed for his studies on the morphology of the brain and the concept of the diffusion of cultures. He published about 400 scientific papers and books. For biog., see Dawson, W. R. ed., *G.E.S. by his colleagues*, Lond., 1938; Wilson, J. T. (1936), *J. Anat.*, 71, pt 1 and *Obit. Notices Roy. Soc. Lond.*, no 6, vol. 2 : 323; Shellshear, J. L. (1937), *Med. J. Aust.*, 1 : 307. ML has bound coll. of obituaries, presented by his family.
Copies: FC, RACP, US. 1927

Smith, James
No. 14] [December, 1881. Australian Health Society, Melbourne. The nervous system: its use and abuse. ... A lecture delivered ... 3rd October, 1881. Reprinted from the "Victorian Review", November 1881. Melbourne: Mason, Firth & M'Cutcheon ... 1881.
212 × 139. Pp. 16. P. w. (title rptd).
Copies: AMAV, EF, ML, NL, SLS, SLV. 1928

See also Australian Health Society, Nos 103–4.

Smith, John
Chair of Experimental Philosophy and Chemistry, University College, Sydney. Testimonials in favour of John Smith, M.D., Fordyce Lecturer on Agriculture and Assistant in the Chemical Laboratory of Mareschal College, Aberdeen.
204 × 125. Pp. 18. ND. (1851.)
Copies: ML. 1929

Wayfaring notes. Sydney to Southampton by way of Egypt and Palestine. Printed for private distribution. Sydney: Sherriff & Downing ... 1865.
173 × 105. Pp. [iv] (ii blank), vi (l.b.), 340. Engr. frontis. Cloth.
Preface signed: J. S., University of Sydney. US and EF copies bear inscriptions of Prof. John Smith.
Copies: EF, FC, LNSW, ML, NL, SLV, US. 1930

Speech in opposition to the Medical Bill, delivered in the Legislative Council of N. S. Wales, May 13th, 1875. ... Sydney: Gibbs, Shallard, & Co. ...
212 × 138. Pp. 12.
Prof. Smith MLC, Dean of Medicine, opposes Bill for the control of unqualified practice and criticises qualified doctors. Pamphlet was published by his supporters after defeat of the Bill. An indignation meeting of doctors followed (No 1316).
ML copy bears ms. notes of Sir Alfred Stephen, who introduced the Bill. His further ms. note on Smith's speech appears in ML copy of his own speech on the Bill (No 2028); ends: 'I concur with the Profession in thinking that a gentleman with his opinions ... ought not to be Dean of the Faculty of Medicine.'
Copies: LNSW, ML. 1931

Wayfaring notes (Second Series). A holiday tour round the world. Reprinted, from the "Sydney Morning Herald". Aberdeen: A.

Brown and Co. 1876.

173 × 105. Pp. x (4 blanks), 406 (l.b.). Cloth. Preface signed: J. S., University of Sydney.

Another issue, 1876, with additions to title: 'Presented by the Author', and 'for private distribution.'

For John Smith (1821–85) MD, first Prof. Chem. and Dean of Med. Univ. Syd., see *Austsn med. Gaz.*, 1885, 5 : 54; Liversidge A. (1886), *J. & P. Roy. Soc. NSW*, 20 : 1; Le Fevre, R.J.W., *Roy. Aust. Chem. Inst Proc.*, Aug. 1959 : 348.

Copies: EF, LNSW, ML, SLT, SLV, US. 1932

Smith, John McGarvie

The biological laboratory of Mr. J. McGarvie Smith ... Woollahra, Sydney. From "The Sydney Mail", December 24th, 1892. Experimenting with live snakes. ... [Text begins.]

426 × 265. Pp. [4] (2, 3 blank).

Author collaborated with C. J. Martin in attempts to produce snake-bite antivenine and was said to have collected 500 snakes, from which venom was periodically extracted.

Copies: ML. 1933

Investigation of the composition of the air in the sewers of Sydney, with special reference to the presence of germs ... Sydney ... 1893. [Text begins.]

336 × 217. Pp. 12 (l.b.). Colophon—Syd.: Charles Potter, Govt Pr—1894. P. w.

Organisms cultured per litre of air from various points in the sewers. Discussed, *Austsn med. Gaz.*, 1894, 13 : 95.

J. McGarvie Smith (1844–1918), developed a vaccine for anthrax in sheep and cattle, which protected by single inoculation and kept indefinitely. This replaced the original Pasteur vaccine and found a large market in Australia and abroad. In 1918 the McGarvie Smith Institute was established for its manufacture in association with NSW Govt. Obit.: *J. & P. Roy. Soc. NSW*, 1919, 53 : 11.

Copies: ML. 1934

See also Nos 52–3.

Smith, Louis Lawrence

How to get thin, and how to get fat; or Banting superseded. ... Melbourne: Clarson, Shallard & Co. ... 1864.

208 × 135. Pp. 16 (2, 4 blank).

Weight reduction by restriction of fluids to 1 pint a day and food containing little water. Banting's system of reducing carbohydrate intake (No 159) is held to be more complex, and no more effective.

Copies: LNSW, SLV. 1935

Impotence and sterility. ... Melbourne: Published by L. L. Smith. 1864.

163 × 102. Pp. 132 (l.b.), [4] (advt).

Copies: CC, SLV. 1936

On obstacles to marriage. ... Melbourne: Published by the Author. 1864.

161 × 102. Pp. xii (l.b.), 13–138, [4] (advts). Cloth.

A popular work on sex, with anatomy and ailments.

'I shall be exposed to the slanders of my professional brethren, and ... they will do all in their power to throw odium upon me because I have dared to treat a subject of which the majority of them are totally ignorant ...'

Copies: ML. 1937

The means of prolonging life and avoiding diseases. ... Melbourne: Published by H. T. Dwight ... 1864.

163 × 102. Pp. vi (ii blank), 7–123, [2], [3] (advts). Cloth.

On the causes of disease, its nature, and prevention.

Copies: CC, EF, LNSW, ML, NL, RACS, SLT, SLV, UA. 1938

Dr. L. L. Smith's Medical Almanac for 1865. Guide to mothers and nurses and persons residing in the bush, and table of digestion of food. Printed by Clarson, Shallard, & Co.

204 × 145. Pp. 84. P. w.

Title of 1870 issue adds 'And vade-mecum for the profession.' Freely advertises author's practice.

Year of issue appears on title for 1874 (14th year), which places 1861 as date of first issue. Publication continued to 1925.

Copies: ML (1865–95, various), NL (1864, 1881), SLV (1863–1900, various). 1939

Concerning an insidious & deadly enemy. ... With a preface by Dr. L. L. Smith. Melbourne: ... H. Cordell. 1870.

201 × 132. Pp. 28.

Advt for a patent disinfectant (Chloro-Alkaline Deodorising Co.) containing articles contributed by Smith to *Australian Journal*, under pseudonym 'Colonial Lancet.'

Copies: ML. 1940

To the nervous. To those to whom married life is a burden. To those who have tried their family medical adviser, without ... relief. And to those who suffer from spermatorrhoea and other fearful results of indiscretion in youth. Dr. L. L. Smith ... begs to state he has devoted the whole of his life to the study and treatment of syphilitic diseases ... [Text continues.]

217 × 135. Single leaf, v.b. ND. NI. (Dated 1872 in pencil.)

Copies: E. M. Christie, Melb. 1941

Medical household sketches; popular treatises for parlour and bush-hut on the diseases prevalent in Australasia. ... Extracted from articles written by Dr. Smith in the "Australian Journal", under the name of "Colonial Lancet".

158 × 102. Pp. viii, 232 (l.b.). 4 figs. ND. (?1873.) Cloth.

Copies: NL, RACP, SLV. 1942

No. 2 Series of medical household sketches; or, popular treatises for parlour and bush-hut on the diseases prevalent in Australasia. ... Extracted from articles written by Dr. Smith in the "Australian Journal", under the name of "Colonial Lancet".

153 × 100. Pp. xvi, 120. 7 figs. London: Gregory and Co., Printers ... Hatton Garden. ND. [?1873.] Cloth.

Preface proposes publication of a third number of this series, on diseases to which mothers are subject. NS.

Copies: FC, ML, WLC. 1943

Discoveries in the nature and treatment of gout, with original notes and observations after twenty-six years' constant treatment of that disease. ... Melbourne: H. Cordell ... 1878.

178 × 122. Pp. 16. P. w. (title rptd).

Claims discovery of an un-named neutraliser and solvent of uric acid. He will divulge his method only after he has gained his reward. 'Those who like to avail themselves of my knowledge can do so, and reap the benefit,—those who do not, can bear their pain and keep their prejudices and their GOUT.'

Copies: CC, DOS, EF, KFR, LNSW, ML, NL, SLV, WLC. 1944

Our doctor; or, the colonial medical and surgical handybook. Containing reliable information and full instructions for families and those resident in the bush how to act in emergencies, accidents, and common sickness. ... Gibbs Shallard & Co. ... Sydney.

153 × 98. Pp. viii, 9–96. [1886.]

Copies: LNSW. 1945

The Brown-Sequard treatment of disease, by hypodermic injections of organic liquids. With obituary from "The Lancet". [Woodcut portrait of Brown-Sequard.] ... H. Cordell, Printer, Melbourne.

186 × 122. Pp. 48 (last—colophon). ND. [c. 1895.] P. w. (cover title).

Advocates treatment with orchitic and other glandular extracts, as introduced by Brown-Sequard.

L. L. Smith (1830–1910) LSA, MLA, prominent in the professional, commercial, political and sporting life of Melbourne, applied extensive advertising methods to practice, was proprietor of *Aust. Journal* and other papers, and his many interests included farms, vineyards, and racing stables. For biog., see Leavitt, T.W.H., *Aust. representative men*, Melb., 1887; Leavitt and Lilburn, *Jubilee history of Vic. and Melb.*, vol. 1, [1888].

NS: *Diseases of married life; The infirmities of age; Diseases incidental to various professions and trades* (all advertised as in press); *On the peculiarities of the Aust. climate in relation to health and disease* (1870 *Almanac* notes as shortly to be published); *Hints for emergencies—Bush almanac* ('for sale' in 1871 *Almanac*).

Copies: WLC. 1946

See also Royal Polytechnic Institute and

Museum.

Smith, Samuel

House of Commons, Session 1889. Speech of Mr. Samuel Smith, M. P. on moving his resolution relative to the opium trade with China ... Robert Barr, Printer ... Fitzroy, Melbourne. 1890.

214 × 138. Pp. 16. P. w. (title rptd).

Copies: ML. 1947

Smith, William

Testimonials, etc., of William Smith, M. B. (Lond. Univ.) M.R.C.S. Eng. ... [Qualifications] [Text follows.]

209 × 132. Pp. 4. ND. [c. 1870.] NI.

The following, with authorship noted in above, appear in *SGC*, ser. 1, under William J. Smith: *On the treatment of enlarged tonsils ... without operation of excision*, pp. vii, 55, Lond., 1865; *On ringworm; an inquiry into the pathology, causes, and treatment*, pp. iv, 75, Lond., 1865; another ed., Lond., 1867. (Both NS.)

For William Smith MB Lond. & Melb., MRCS, a founder of Children's Hosp. Melb., see *Aust. med. J.*, 1870, 15 : 286; Graham, H. B. (1953), 'Some memoirs of the Children's Hosp.', *Med. J. Aust.*, 2 : 517.

Copies: UM. 1948

———

On paralysis with apparent hypertrophy of the muscles. Melbourne: Stillwell & Knight.

8vo. Pp. 13. Repr. *Aust. med. J.*, 1871.

NS. Listed *SGC*, Ser. 1. Original paper (*Aust. med. J.*, 1871, 16 : 161) has 1 photo. laid down. 1948a

Smith, William Ramsay

... Breathing in singing. ... [Text begins.]

236 × 156. Pp. 6 (l.b.). Colophon—Witherly & Co. ... High Holborn, W. C. Repr., *J. Laryngology, Rhinology, & Otology*, June, 1894.

Copies: SLS. 1949

———

Angio-neurosis : being studies in diseases of the vaso-motor system. ... Bristol : John Wright & Co. ...

214 × 137. Pp. 78, [2] (book notices). 2 pl. ND. [1896.] Cloth.

Describes 'two very distinct and definite diseases' which he has differentiated, and names general angioneurotic oedema and erythema-urticaria. Etiology, pathology, treatment.

Copies: UA. 1950

———

The practical aspects of heredity and environment. ... Delivered before the Criminological Society of S. A., 1898 ... Adelaide: Whillas & Ormiston ... 1899.

180 × 124. Pp. 24 (last 2 blank). P. w. (title rptd).

Copies: CC, SLS, UA. 1951

———

South Australia. Central Board of Health. Report on bubonic plague by W. Ramsay Smith ... Chairman. Adelaide ... C. E. Bristow, Govt Printer ... 1900.

331 × 212. Pp. 22 (l.b.). 1 flg pl. P. w.

Reports submitted to Board from 15 Jan.–28 Feb. 1900, at the outset of the 1900–9 epidemic of plague in Australia.

Copies: NL, SPH, UA. 1952

———

Proof—Confidential Report on bubonic plague at Adelaide Hospital. (No. 2.) [Text begins.]

340 × 215. 4 leaves, printed on recto only. 1900.

Results of inquiries at Adelaide Hosp., following admission of three plague cases and discovery of plague rats. Signed as Chairman, Cent. Board of Health.

For William Ramsay Smith (1859–1937) MD, ChM Edin., DSc. Adel., Chairman Cent. Bd of Health, and Head of Health Dept of SA (1899–1929), see *Aust. Enc.*

Later works include: *A manual for Coroners*, 1904; *In Southern Seas*, 1924; and *Myths and legends of the Aust. aborigines*, 1930. NL (Cumpston coll.) has two vols of his pamphlets.

Copies: SPH. 1953

——— and Norwell, J. Stewart

Illustrations of zoology : invertebrates & vertebrates. ... Edinburgh and London : Young J. Pentland. 1889.

252 × 180. Pp. [12] (3 blanks), 70 litho. pl. (versos with notes of facing plate), [4] appendix, [2] book notes.

Copies: SLV, UA. 1954

Smyth, Mrs. B.

Love, courtship and marriage. A lecture delivered in the North Melbourne Town Hall

... October 17th, 1892, by ... the pioneer Australian lecturess and female instructor in matters pertaining to health and disease, and the improvement of the human race. Dr. W. Maloney, M.L.A. in the Chair. ... Melbourne: Austral Publishing Co. Ltd. ... 1892.

183 × 122. Pp. [14] (advts), 64 (last 12—advts). 48 text figs. P. w. (short title and portrait of author, advts other sides.)

Advice on the selection of marriage partners by physiognomical methods and 'the science of human nature.'

As with author's other publications, work includes advts for her practice of medical electricity, character delineation, and 'adaptation for marriage.'

Illustrated catalogue, including surg. and electric appliances, contraceptives and publications, inserted.

Copies: ML. 1955

———

Limitation of offspring ... Being the substance of a lecture ... in the North Melbourne Town Hall, and elsewhere, to large audiences of women only. Freely illustrated ... Melburne: Rae Bros. ... 1893.

183 × 122. Pp. xvi (advts), 44 (last 6—advts). 7 text figs. P. w. (variation of title, portrait of author, 8 ed.).

Discusses various contraceptive methods.

ML copy has blue card inserted, with price list of contraceptives and other items.

Copies: ML, SLV. 1956

———

The social evil: its cause and cure. ... Melbourne: Rae Bros. ... 1894.

181 × 115. Pp. xvi (advts), 38, ii (verso—colophon only). P. w. (variation of title, portrait; advts other sides).

Advice to parents on moral precept and guidance for children.

Copies: ML, US. 1957

———

What every woman should know. Diseases incidental to women. Their cause, prevention and cure. Being the substance of a lecture delivered at the Town Hall, North Melbourne ... Melbourne: H. J. Prender ... 1895.

183 × 120. Pp. viii (advts), 73, [74–82], [6] (advts). P. w. ('Women's diseases. Their cause, cure, and prevention ...', portrait of author). Illustns—text-book figs. Preface signed W. Maloney MRCSE.

Sections on anatomy and various diseases, in medical terminology.

Publications noted in various works: *Embryology; Stirpiculture, or the evolution of the sexes; The causes of sterility or barrenness.* NS.

Copies: EF. 1958

Smyth, James Carmichael

The effect of the nitrous vapour, in preventing and destroying contagion; ascertained, from a variety of trials, made chiefly by Surgeons of His Majesty's Navy, in prisons, hospitals, and on board of ships; with an introduction respecting the nature of the contagion, which gives rise to the jail or hospital fever; and the various methods formerly employed to prevent or destroy this. ... London: ... J. Johnson ... 1799.

229 × 140. Pp. xvi, 232 (l.b.). 1 flg plan, 1 flg table. Paper boards.

Contains three letters (pp. 166–177) from Samuel Hill, Surg. to hospital ship *Sincerity*, Langstone Harbour. They mention removal of patients with typhus and dysentery from convict transport *Hillsborough*, outward bound for Botany Bay on 21 Nov. 1798.

Hillsborough arrived in Sydney on 26 July 1799, after voyage on which 95 convicts of the 300 aboard, and 6 more on arrival, died of typhus.

Copies: ML, UA. 1959

Smyth, Robert Brough

The Aborigines of Victoria : with notes relating to the habits of the natives of other parts of Australia and Tasmania. Compiled ... for the Government of Victoria ... Vol. 1. ... John Ferres, Govt Printer. Published also by George Robertson ... Melbourne. London: Trübner and Co. ... and George Robertson ... 1878.

270 × 178. Vol. 1: pp. lxxii (ii, iv blank), 484 (last—colophon only), frontis., 246 figs, 1 map. Vol. 2 : pp. vi (ii, iv blank), 456, frontis., 52 figs, 1 map.

Sections on physical and mental characters, birth, food, diseases; notes on crania (G. B. Halford).

Copies: DL, EF, ML, NL, SLS, SLT, SLV, UM, US. 1960

Snyder, Harry

The chemistry of dairying An outline of the

chemical and allied changes which take place in milk, and in the manufacture of butter and cheese; and the rational feeding of dairy stock. ... Melbourne: E. W. Cole ... 1898.

183 × 125. Pp. viii, 110, [2] (advts), xviii (book notices). 2 pl., 21 figs. Cloth.

Reprint of US work. Includes testing, detection of adulteration, sanitary condition of milk, milk-borne diseases, sterilisation and preservation.

Copies: EF, ML, SLS, SLV, US. 1961

Society for Promoting Christian Knowledge

See Colonists' Handbooks.

Society for the Relief of Destitute Children, Sydney

Rules of the Society for the Relief of Destitute Children. Instituted in Sydney, A.D. 1852. Sydney: ... Joseph Cook ... 1852.

204 × 132. Pp. 12 (3 blanks).

First object of Society was to provide an Asylum for Destitute Children 'in consequence of the number of destitute and deserted children of all ages who crowd the streets and alleys of this city ...'

Copies: ML. 1962

———

First Annual Report of the Directors of the Society for the Relief of Destitute Children, for the year ended 30th June, 1853. Sydney ... Joseph Cook ... 1853.

201 × 130. Pp. 24. P. w. (title rptd).

1st meeting Feb. 1852; opened at Paddington June 1852; Randwick Asylum occupied 1858; Catherine Hayes Hosp. opened 1870. See Coulter, J. (1916), *Randwick Asylum: An hist. review*, Syd.; Oliver, T. J. (1871), 'Catherine Hayes Hosp.', *NSW med. Gaz.*, 1 : 142.

Copies: EF (1853–67, 1880), FC (1853–66), ML (1853–1915 incomplete), SLV (1853,–58,–62,–63). 1963

———

1875–6. New South Wales. Legislative Council. Randwick Asylum Board of Inquiry. Report ... and minutes of evidence. ... Sydney: Thomas Richards, Govt Printer. 1876.

323 × 204. Pp. 10 (l.b.).

Inquiry into management of Asylum.

Copies: LNSW, ML, NL, SLV. 1964

———

1879–80. Legislative Assembly. New South Wales. Report from the Select Committee on the Randwick Asylum for Destitute Children ... with the proceedings ... and minutes of evidence. ... Sydney: Thomas Richards, Govt Printer. 1880.

328 × 210. Pp. 8 (l.b.), 52. Chairman—Sir Henry Parkes.

Copies: LNSW, ML, NL, SLV. 1965

———

See also Brown, Alexander M.

Sohier, P.

The register of the size of the phrenological organs of the brain: shewing which to cultivate, and which to control; ... P. Sohier's Phrenological Museum, Great Bourke Street East, (at the Wax Works), where he may be consulted by parents, guardians, educators, teachers, and young people of both sexes. Melbourne: Shaw, Harnett & Co., ... 1861.

217 × 138. Pp. 16. P. w. (title rptd).

Copies: CC, EF, SLV. 1966

South Australia—Central Board of Health

[No. 38. South Australia. Report of Central Board of Health, 1874–5. Ordered by the House of Assembly to be printed, 20th May, 1875. [Text begins.]

305 × 204. Pp. 6 (l.b.).

Reports for 1874/5–1891/2 appear in *Proceedings of the Parlt of SA*, 1875–92.

Copies: LNSW, NL, SLS, SLV. 1967

———

South Australia. Central Board of Health Regulations. Ordered by the House of Assembly to be printed, August 18th, 1885. [Text begins.]

330 × 204. Single leaf, v.b. Double cols. NI. Signed H. T. Whittell, Pres.

Copies: LNSW, SLS. 1968

———

South Australia. Central Board of Health. Typhoid fever. [Text begins.]

340 × 215. Single leaf, v.b. ND. (1885.)

On typhoid infection from excreta of patients, with notes on preventive nursing.

Copies: EF. 1969

———

South Australia. Central Board of Health.

How to prevent the spread of scarlet fever. [Text begins.]

345 × 217. Single leaf, v.b. ND. (1886.)

Copies: EF. 1970

Earth closets. [Text begins.]

340 × 215. Single leaf, v.b. ND. (1886.)

Includes regulations on nuisances arising from improper night-soil disposal.

Copies: EF. 1971

See also Nos 1952–3.

South Australia—Parliament

The following items are selected from the *Proceedings of the Parliament of South Australia*, 1857/8–1900. See library catalogues for holdings. Detailed listing for NSW, NL, OL, US, appears in Cope, R. L., *Australian Parliamentary Serials*, Reference Monograph 9, Library of Parliament, Syd., 1973.

[No. 115. South Australia. Appointment of Colonial Surgeon. Ordered by the House of Assembly to be printed, November 3rd, 1858.

324 × 203. Single leaf, v.b. Blue paper. NI.

R. W. Moore MD appointed Col Surg.; outline of duties.

1972

[No. 165. South Australia. Report of the Select Committee of the Legislative Council, upon "The Aborigines"; together with minutes of evidence and appendix. Ordered by the Legislative Council to be printed, 16th October, 1860. Adelaide: . . . W. C. Cox, Govt Printer . . . 1860.

324 × 203. Pp. 8, 100, viii (l.b.). Blue paper.

Committee appointed to report on the present position of Aborigines and suggest measures by which these may be ameliorated. Includes medical evidence.

1973

No. 156. South Australia. Legally qualified medical practitioners. . . . Legislative Council, 11th October, 1864 . . . Amended return . . . for a list of the legally qualified medical men practising in the Colony . . .

340 × 210. Single leaf. Pp. 2. Blue paper. NI.

Signed: R. W. Moore, Pres. Med. Bd of SA.

1974

(No. 190. South Australia. Circular despatch on compulsory vaccination. Ordered . . . to be printed, 21st December, 1870. Despatch from the Secretary of State on the subject of the laws relating to vaccination. [Text begins.]

342 × 215. Pp. 2.

For history of vaccination in SA, see Cumpston, J.H.L. (1914), *The history of small-pox in Aust., 1788–1908*, Melb. : p. 145.

1975

[No. 154. South Australia. Prevention of nuisances in towns and villages. Ordered by the House of Assembly to be printed, 3rd November, 1871. [Text begins.]

330 × 204. Pp. 12 (l.b.).

Despatch from Sec. of State for Colonies on dry earth system of excreta disposal.

1976

(No. 59. South Australia. Children born and vaccinated—1854 to 1871. Ordered . . . to be printed, 9th April, 1872. [Text begins.]

342 × 215. Single leaf, v.b. From Central Vaccine Bd.

1977

(No. 153. South Australia. Vaccination return, 1854 to 1871. Ordered . . . to be printed, 23rd July, 1872. [Text begins.]

342 × 215. Single leaf, v.b.

1978

(No. 162. South Australia. Report from Central Vaccine Board. Ordered . . . to be printed, 7th August, 1872. [Text begins.]

342 × 215. Single leaf, v.b.

1979

(No. 183. South Australia. Non-supply of returns under Vaccination Act. Ordered to be printed . . . 20th September, 1872. [Text begins.]

340 × 213. Pp. 4 (l.b.).

Names of doctors who neglected to send returns, 1867–71.

1980

(No. 116. South Australia. Vaccination returns, 1873 to 1875. Ordered ... to be printed, 7th September, 1875. [Text begins.]

342 × 215. Single leaf, v.b.

1981

[No. 18. South Australia. Report of Commission appointed to inquire into the whole question of sanitation for the Province; together with minutes of evidence and appendix. Adelaide ... W. C. Cox, Govt Printer ... 1876.

331 × 204. Pp. xxviii (l.b.), 138 (l.b.), xxii. 2 flg pl.

Pollution from factories and noxious trades; city sanitation and drainage; water supply etc. of Yorke's Penin.; pollution of Torrens; health legislation.

For 'Public Health legislation: its evolution in SA', see Southwood, A. R. (1938), *Med. J. Aust.*, 1 : 726.

1982

South [Royal Arms] Australia. Report on Hospitals for the Insane for the year 1879. Adelaide: ... E. Spiller, Govt Printer ... 1880.

208 × 132. Pp. 32 (l.b.). P. w. (title rptd).

1983

[No. 75. South Australia. Report on ophthalmic cases at the Industrial School, Magill. Ordered by the House of Assembly to be printed, August 6th, 1884. [Text begins.]

330 × 204. Pp. 8 (l.b.). NI. Reports by Chas. Gosse MD; Alex. S. Paterson, Col Surg. and H. T. Whittell, Pres. Bd Health.

Examination of 127 inmates—free of eye disease 15, congestion of lids 20, granular disease of lids 82, admitted to Adel. Hosp. with purulent ophthalmia 10.

1984

No. 94. Report re small-pox at Bordertown. Ordered by the House of Assembly to be printed, August 14th, 1884. [Text begins.]

305 × 204. Pp. 4 (l.b.).

Includes report on suspected outbreak, to Cent. Bd of Health, by Dr. Alfred Austin Lendon.

1985

No. 115. South Australia. ... Ordered by the House of Assembly to be printed, September 4th, 1884. ... Report on the outbreak of diphtheritic sore throat at Elliston.

305 × 204. Pp. [2] (v.b.). Signed—G. Purcell Atkins.

G. P. Atkins was GMO Pt Lincoln.

1986

[No. 67. South Australia. Correspondence, etc., re alleged case of leprosy. Ordered by the House of Assembly to be printed, August 9th, 1898. [Text begins.]

338 × 204. Pp. 8 (l.b.).

Signs of suspected leprosy (appearance and sensory loss in area of leg) in a Chinese prove due to action of a Chinese plaster.

1987

South Australian Institute of Hygiene and Bacteriology

See No 481.

South Australian Instn for the Blind and Deaf and Dumb

See 'Vid', No 2429.

Southam, John Binns—

... The Australian guide to hydropathy, embracing the home hydropathic treatment of common complaints with chapter on diet. ... Brisbane: W. H. Wendt & Co. ... 1892.

181 × 117. Pp. vi (l.b.), 7–58. P. w. (title rptd).

Author was associated with Wickham House Hydropathic Establishment, Brisbane.

Copies: EF, OL. 1988

Spasshatt, Samuel Pierce

Sermon on the decease of Dr. Spasshatt, (20th October, 1874;) preached in St. Peter's Church, Armidale ... 25th October, 1874, by the Rev. S. Hungerford. ... Price—one shilling. The proceeds to go towards a memorial of the late Dr. Spasshatt. Armidale: Vincent Bros ...

220 × 140. Pp. 8. P. w. (title rptd).

S. P. Spasshatt MD practised at Armidale NSW for 12 years; died aged 43.

Copies: ML. 1989

Speculum, The

No. 1.] [July. 1884. The Speculum, A Journal of

the Melbourne Medical Students.

209 × 138. Pp. 20. Colophon—Rae Bros., Printers . . . Melbourne.

Journal of Melb. Medical Students' Soc. Published irregularly—(1 to 4 issues annually). Not published in 1893. Contains much information on the development of the Melb. Med. School and its personalities.

Copies: BG (1896–99), EF (1884–1900), ML (1891–98), NL (no 1, 1884), SLV (1884–1900), UM (1884–1900). 1990

Spence, Catherine Helen

Heredity and environment Delivered before . . . the Criminological Society of South Australia, October 23rd, 1897. . . . Adelaide: Webb & Son . . . 1897.

217 × 135. Pp. 16. P. w. (cover title).

Copies: EF, NL, SLS, SLV. 1991

Spencer, Edward

Public [Decoration] Hospitals. [Decoration] By Edward Spencer M. B., Ch.B. (Vict.) Late Resident Medical Officer, Perth Public Hospital. [Decoration] Perth: E. S. Wigg & Son, Printers . . . 1899.

8vo. Pp. 12.

Copies: SLW. 1992

Spencer, Sir Walter Baldwin and Gillen, Frances James

The native tribes of Central Australia . . . London Macmillan and Co. Limited New York: The Macmillan Company 1899.

222 × 140. Pp. xx, 672 (l.b.), [30] (book notices). Erratum slip., Profusely illustrated. Cloth.

Includes much information of medical interest on physical characters, native customs, childbirth and food; also chapter on medicine men, and physical measurements.

For later publications by authors, see *The health of Aust. Aborigines: an annotated bibliog.*, by P. M. Moodie and E. B. Pederson, Canberra, 1971.

Copies: DL, EF, ML, NL, SLS, SLT, SLV, UA, UM, UQ, US. 1993

Springthorpe, John William

No. 21.] [February, 1885. Australian Health Society . . . Unseen enemies and how to fight them . . . A lecture delivered . . . 27th October, 1884. Melbourne: Barton, Dunn & Wilkinson . . . 1885.

191 × 138. Pp. 16. P. w. (cover title).

Another ed., 1891.

On the bacterial origin of infectious diseases, the 'Sanitary Idea', and a plea for health education.

Copies: EF, ML, SLS, SLV. 1994

———

Two Australian foes . . . Melbourne: William Inglis & Co. . . . 1885

214 × 138. Pp. 8 (l.b.). P. w. (cover title).

On excessive meat eating and hydatid infestation—'two standing national dangers.' Aust. Health Soc. lecture.

Copies: ML. 1995

———

The typhoid germ: its recognition, propagation, and eradication. A lecture . . . Australian Health Society. . . . Melbourne: Stillwell & Co., 1889.

NS. Noted *Austsn med. Gaz.*, 1890, 9 : 109. 1996

———

Hygienic conditions in Victoria. . . . Reprinted from the "Intercolonial Medical Congress of Australasia Transactions". Melbourne: Stillwell and Co. . . . 1889.

244 × 153. Pp. 20 (l.b.). P. w. (cover title.)

A comprehensive survey, including personal hygiene: food, occupation, etc.; public hygiene: drainage, housing, sanitation, water supplies; legal hygiene: public health law, administration and statistics.

Copies: ML, UM. 1997

———

The nervous substratum of influenza. A series of cases illustrating localisation in nervous diseases. The hepatic element in disease. . . . Reprinted from the "Intercolonial Medical Congress of Australasia Transactions". Melbourne: Stillwell and Co. . . . 1889.

236 × 156. Pp. 20 (l.b.). P. w. (cover title).

Copies: ML, NL, UM. 1998

———

The Melbourne Hospital as a clinical school: being the inaugural lecture session 1890 Delivered at the Melbourne Hospital . . . Melbourne: Stillwell and Co. . . .

209 × 140. Pp. 16 (l.b.). Repr., *Aust. med. J.*, 1890.

Copies: SLV. 1999

Revised Edition.] [October, 1890. The Australian Health Society . . . Typhoid fever and diphtheria . . . [Text begins.]
212 × 138. Pp. 8. Colophon—Walker, May and Co. . . . Melb.
Another ed., 1889.
Copies: SLV, UA. 2000

A report on Koch's treatment of tubercular disease. . . . Reprinted from the "Australian Medical Journal", 1891. Melbourne: Stillwell and Co. . . . 1891.
214 × 135. Pp. 48. P. w. (title rptd).
Progress reports follow: 1st—pp. 12, 1891 (UM); 2nd—pp. 8, 1892 (UM).
Copies: CC, ML, SLV. 2001

Tuberculin as a diagnostic agent. . . . [Text begins.]
207 × 135. Pp. 14. 1 flg chart. Colophon—Stillwell and Co. . . . Melbourne. Repr., *Aust. med. J.*, March 1894.
Copies: UM. 2002

Republished by request. A perfect woman. A paper . . . read before the Melbourne Shakespeare Society . . . 1884.
168 × 102. Pp. ii (v.b.), 22 (l.b.). P. w. (cover title).
Another ed., 1907.
Copies: ML, SLV. 2002a

President's address Section of Public Health. The battle of life. . . . Delivered before the Intercolonial Medical Congress of Australasia . . . Stillwell and Co. . . . Melbourne.
217 × 140. Pp. 14 (l.b.). P. w. (cover title). Repr. *Intercol med. J. Austsia*, 1896, Mar. 20.
Copies: ML. 2002b

Further notes on typhoid. . . . Reprinted from the Australasian Medical Gazette, July 20, 1899. [Text begins.]
227 × 165. Pp. 4.
Copies: UM. 2002c

A new food for use in typhoid and other fevers. . . . Reprinted from the Australian Medical Journal, July 20, 1894. Stillwell and Co. . . . Melbourne.
217 × 138. Pp. 12. 1 flg sheet of charts. P. w. (cover title).
Results of trials of sterilised hopped malt extract as milk substitute.
Copies: EF, SLV, UM. 2003

Australasian Association for the Advancement of Science. Brisbane, 1895. The teaching of science in matters of health. . . . President of Section 1.
222 × 140. Pp. 12 (last 2 blank). P. w. (cover title).
Copies: ML. 2004

A plea for the re-use of tuberculin. . . . [Text begins.]
209 × 135. Pp. 6. Repr., *Glasgow med. J.*, Nov. 1896.
Copies: UM. 2005

The administration of chloroform in dentistry. . . . Melbourne: . . . J. T. Harty & Co. . . . 1898.
212 × 135. Pp. 8.
Copies: UM. 2006

The scope and operation of the proposed Anti-Tuberculosis Association. . . . Read before the medical profession of Victoria, July 27th, 1899 [Text begins.]
234 × 158. Pp. 4 (l.b.).
Copies: UM. 2007

Albuminuria from a life assurance point of view. . . .
183 × 117. Pp. 14. ND. Colophon—John Sands . . . Syd. Repr., *Austsn med. Gaz.*, Oct. 1899.
Copies: UM. 2008

Concerning influenza. . . . (. . . Australasian Association for the Advancement of Science, Melbourne, January 1900.) [Text begins.]
209 × 135. Pp. 10 Colophon—Stillwell and Co. . . . Melb.
Copies: UM. 2009

———

. . . The etiology of acute rheumatism. . . . [Text begins.]

209 × 135. Pp. 6. Colophon—Stillwell and Co. . . . Melb. Repr., *Intercol med. J. Austsia*, 1900, 5 : 517.

Copies: UM. 2010

———

List of addresses papers etc, 1883–1908.

222 × 178. Pp. [4] (1, 4 blank). NI. ND.

Lists 99 publications.

For J. W. Springthorpe (1855–1933) MD Melb., MRCP, prominent Melb. physician, see *Med. J. Aust.*, 1933, 2 : 26; Howard, G. T. (1933), *Melb. Hosp. Clin. Rep.*, 4 : 1.

Also published: *Verses in memory of Annie Constance Springthorpe*, illust. John Longstaff, Melb., 1897; *Therapeutics, dietetics and hygiene*, 2 vols, Melb., 1914.

Copies: UM. 2011

———

See also Australian Health Society, Nos 103–4; Brodribb, T. and Springthorpe, J. W.

——— **and Mullen, William Lowell**

On the plea of insanity in criminal trials . . . (Read before the Intercolonial Medical Congress, Sydney, September, 1892.) Sydney: Charles Potter, Govt Printer . . . 1892.

244 × 158. Pp. [ii] (v.b.), 20 (l.b.). P. w. (title rptd).

'. . . the present recognised legal test for insanity is false in theory and unsatisfactory in practice . . .'

Copies: CC, ML. 2012

———

The Same. Medical jurisprudence. On the plea of insanitary in criminal trials. Repr., *Amer. J. Insanity*, January, 1893. Pp. 28 (l.b.). Omits final paras. of Syd. ed.

Copies: ML. 2013

——— **and Mullins, George Lane**

Diet lists for Australian medical practitioners. Sydney: Angus & Robertson . . . Melbourne: James Little . . .

110 × 181. Oblong. Pp. [vi], [320] (perforated), [ii] (advts). ND. (c. 1896.) Cloth.

Tear-off diet lists for use in various stated ailments.

Copies: ML, US. 2014

Sprott, Gregory

Tuberculosis. Read at the Royal Society of Tasmania . . . August, 10th, 1896. . . .

210 × 136. Pp. 24. Colophon: 'The Mercury' Office, Hobart. P. w. (cover title).

Cause, mode of infection, prevention.

Copies: SLT. 2015

———

1896. . . . Parliament of Tasmania. Intercolonial Medical Congress, Dunedin, 1896; Report of Gregory Sprott, M.D., D.P.H., representative of Tasmania. Presented to both Houses of Parliament . . .

342 × 216. Pp. 8 (2, l.b.). Colophon—William Grahame, Govt Pr, Tas.

Copies: BG, LNSW, NL, SLT, SLV. 2016

———

The disposal of our dead by cremation. . . . Read July 12, 1897. [Text begins.]

204 × 127. Pp. 12 (l.b.). Repr., *Papers & Proc. Roy. Soc. Tas.*, 1897 : 13.

For Gregory Sprott (d. 1942) MD, DPH Glas., MOH Hobart, Hon. Surg. Hobart Hosp., see obit., *Med. J. Aust.*, 1942, 2 : 410.

Copies: EF (incomplete). 2017

———

Cause and prevention of typhoid fever. With special reference to the proposed metropolitan drainage scheme. . . . Read . . . Royal Society of Tasmania . . . August 8, 1898. Tasmania: Printed at the "Tasmanian News" Office . . . Hobart.

217 × 135. 15 leaves, numbered 1–15, printed on recto only. P. w. (cover title).

Principles of prevention; plans for sewerage of Hobart.

Copies: NL. 2018

———

1899. Parliament of Tasmania. Intercolonial Medical Congress, Brisbane, 1899: Report of . . . representative of Tasmania . . .

342 × 208. Pp. [ii] (l.b.), 4 (l.b.). Colophon—John Vail, Govt Pr, Tas.

Copies: LNSW, NL, SLT, SLV. 2019

Stanley, Edward

Euphorbia drummondii commonly known as "milk-weed", and reputed to be poisonous. Reports . . . on the Australian weed Euphorbia drummondii, with results of experiments therewith in the Urana District, and at Randwick. Sydney: Charles Potter, Govt Printer ... 1888.

212 × 132. Pp. 14.

Copies: ML. 2020

———

Department of Agriculture. Sydney ... Miscellaneous Publication, No. 109. Euphorbia drummondii, commonly known as "milk-weed", and erroneously reputed to be poisonous. Revised edition ... Sydney: Charles Potter, Govt Printer ... 1896.

247 × 158. Pp. [ii] (v.b.), 8. 1 pl. P. w. (title rptd).

John Reid MD described an extract of this plant, which he called 'drumine', as local anaesthetic. See No 1787.

Edward Stanley FRCVS was Chief Vet. Inspr, NSW.

Copies: EF, US. 2021

———

See N.S.W.—Anthrax Board.

Stawell, Sir Richard Rawdon

No. 6.] [Unabridged. Published by the Board of Public Health, Victoria, on behalf of the Australian Health Society. ... Infant feeding: The use and abuse of artificial foods. A lecture ... by a Member of the Staff of the Children's Hospital. ... Robt. S. Brain, Govt Printer, Melbourne.

214 × 140. Pp. 16. Flg graph. ND.

'Perhaps in no city in the world is the milk supply worse or more badly managed than in Melbourne.'

Authorship noted in Aust. Health Soc., *A 25 years record*, [1900].

Copies: EF, ML, NL, SLV. 2022

———

Some notes on the aetiology and pathological anatomy of summer diarrhoea in infants. (With chart). By R. R. Stawell, M.D. Melb., D.P.H. Lond., Honorary Medical Officer to Outpatient Department, Melbourne Hospital for Sick Children. Reprinted from the "Australian Medical Journal", February and March, 1895. Stillwell and Co. ... Melbourne.

204 × 127. Pp. 12 (l.b.). 1 flg chart.

For Sir Richard Stawell (1864–1935), distinguished physician and teacher, who was Hon. Phys. Melb. Hosp., 1st Pres. Assn of Phys. of Aust., see *Med. J. Aust.*, 1935, 1 : 63; *Melb. Hosp. Clin. Rep.*, 1935, 6 : 1.

Copies: CC, US. 2023

Stawell Hospital and Benevolent Asylum, Vic.

The First Annual Report of the ... Pleasant Creek Hospital, with the rules for the same for 1860 ... Ararat: Printed by Nuthall and Banfield ... 1860.

204 × 127. Pp. 24.

Established 1858; opened Feb. 1859; became Stawell Hosp. and Benevolent Asylum 1883; Benev. Asylum closed 1916/17; thereafter named Stawell Hosp. and later Stawell District Hosp.

Copies: ML (1877), SLV (1859–), Stawell Dist Hosp. (1859–), WLC (1864). 2024

Stayton, George H.

See Thompson, John Ashburton and Stayton, George H.

Steel, Freeman J.

Miscarriage of justice in Maryborough, and the Chinese octopus.

229 × 135. Pp. 22. Double cols. ND. Colophon —... Gearing and Son, Maryborough [Vic.]. P. w. (cover title). Author's name in preface.

Warns of dangers to health and morality from certain Chinese migrants.

Copies: FC. 2025

Steel, John

Testimonials in favour of Mr. John Steel, Bachelor of Medicine and Bachelor of Surgery, University of Melbourne ... [Qualifications]

198 × 165. Pp. [12]. ND. P. w. (cover title).

Testimonials dated 1878–81. John Steel LRCPE (1878), MB Melb. (1883), Dist Surg. Syd. Hosp., was reported as in China (1900).

Copies: ML. 2026

Stephen, Sir Alfred

Address on intemperance and the licensing system ... 11th December, 1869 ... His Excellency the Earl of Belmore in the Chair. John L. Sherriff ... Sydney. 1870.

178 × 122. Pp. 28.

Reviews social effects of drunkenness in NSW. Advocates establishment of hospital for inebriates, to which chronic alcoholics could be referred by courts.

Copies: DL, FC, LNSW, ML, NL, SLV. 2027

———

Sir Alfred Stephen's speech on the Medical Bill delivered in the Legislative Council of N. S. Wales, on ... May 6, 1875. Sydney: Gibbs, Shallard and Co. ...

212 × 138. Pp. 16 (last 2 blank).

Sir Alfred Stephen promotes Bill to regulate practice in NSW. The Bill was defeated, with Prof. J. Smith, Dean of Med. Univ. Syd., as main opponent. See Nos 1931 and 1316.

Author's copy, in ML, bears his ms. remarks.

Sir Alfred Stephen (1802–94) was Chief Justice of NSW.

Copies: FC, LNSW, ML. 2028

Stephen, Sir George

Suicide in Victoria. ... Melbourne: Samuel Mullen ... 1874. A. L. Henriques and Co., Printers ...

204 × 132. Pp. 24. P. w. (cover title).

Copies: CC, ML, NL, SLV. 2029

Stephen, George Milner

George Milner Stephen and his marvellous cures. By his son Harold W. H. Stephen, author of "The Golden Yankee", &c. ... Sydney: Turner and Henderson ...

186 × 115. Pp. 58, [2] (advts). ND. [?1881.] P. w. (title rptd).

Includes biog., healing by 'laying on of hands', cures.

Copies: DL, EF, FC, ML, NL, SLS, SLV. 2030

———

An essay on magnetic healing and some wonderful cures ... (Reprinted from the "Morning Herald", Dunedin, 12th and 26th April, 1884.) Published by Joseph Braithwaite ... Dunedin, N. Z.

171 × 112. Pp. 32. P. w. (cover title).

Includes testimonials of cures (including blindness and cancer), by a well-known Australian citizen.

For George Milner Stephen (1811–94), see Serle; Mennell. Fitts, C. H., 'Lines of communication', *Proc. Medico-Legal Soc. Vic.*, 1953–4, gives account of talented Stephen family, with special ref. to G.M.S. as healer.

Copies: LNSW, ML. 2031

———

A record of some wonderful cures (often instantaneous, by a word, or a touch,) by George Milner Stephen ... Barrister-at-Law, Mid. Temp.: Ex Acting Governor of South Australia: Ex Member Legislative Assembly, Victoria, &c., &c. "The Australian Healer". With a sketch of his eventful life; copious reports from the press ... Third edition, G. R. Smith ... Reading, 1889.

181 × 127. Pp. [ii], 46. Cloth.

Includes life of G.M.S. and testimonials to cures. For two years 'the Great Australian Healer has been healing ... the afflicted at 51 Baker Street, London W., by the marvellous magnetic power with which he is endowed.'

1000 copies were printed 'at the expense of a gentleman who has experienced ... (his) life restoring and healing powers ...'

Copies: ML. NL. 2032

Stephen, Harold W. H.

See Stephen, George Milner, No 2030.

Stephens, Alfred George

"Bulletin" Pamphlets. No. 11. The Suffield case. The evidence at the police court and at the trial ... and a commentary on the methods and manoeuvres of Botany Bay justice. ... Proceeds devoted to the fund for bringing the case to an open public enquiry. Sydney: The Bulletin Newspaper Co. ... 1897.

217 × 140. Pp. xxv, 26.

A plea for retrial, following sentence of ten years for attempted rape. Contains conflicting med. evidence; opinion of F. N. Manning MD that it would be possible for the woman, recovering consciousness after insensibility caused by attack of a bull, to be under the impression she had been sexually assaulted; and comments on med. evidence.

Copies: FC, ML, NL. 2033

Stephens, John

Sanitary reform: its general aspect and local importance ... a lecture delivered at ... Adelaide on ... 13th February, 1849. Together with practical observations on South Australia ... as affecting the sanitary condition of the Colony. ... Adelaide, South Australia: ... John Stephens ... 1849.

212 × 132. Pp. vi (l.b.), [ii] (v.b.), 64.

Facsimile ed., Adel.: Libraries Bd of SA, 1962.

Author was ed. and proprietor of *S. A. Register* and *Adel. Observer*, to readers of which this pamphlet was gratuitously presented.

Copies: ML, NL, SLS, SLV, UA. 2034

Stephenson, John

Medical zoology, and mineralogy; or illustrations and descriptions of the animals and minerals employed in medicine, and of the preparations derived from them: including an account of animal and mineral poisons. London: John Churchill . . . 1838.

247 × 155. Pp. vi, 350. 45 col. pl. Cloth.

Describes (with plate) the poison apparatus of platypus.

Copies: G. C. Ingleton, Sydney.

2035

Stevenson, Robert Louis

With Mr. R. L. Stevenson's compliments. Father Damien: an open letter to the Reverend Dr. Hyde of Honolulu from Robert Louis Stevenson. Sydney. 1890.

204 × 135. Pp. [ii] (v.b.), [3]–32. NI. [W. M. Maclardy, Sydney.]

The first printing of 'the Damien Letter', written during author's visit to Sydney—an angry defence of the late Father Damien, leper priest of the leper settlement at Molokai, from aspersions on his morals by a Honolulu clergyman, which were published in Sydney *Presbyterian.* See G. Mackaness: *The art of book-collecting in Aust.*, Syd., 1956.

Copies: DL, FC, ML. 2036

Stewart, William

Health in Australia: and how to preserve it, being a familiar treatise, grounded upon observations made in England, Ireland, East-Indies, Indian-Archipelago, Coast of Africa, and 25 years residence in Tasmania and Australia. By William Stewart, Surgeon, &c., &c. . . . Geelong: T. Higgins and Co. . . . 1861.

158 × 85. Pp. 118.

Chapters include: atmospheric influences, effects of diet, contingencies effecting health; predisposition to disease, prevalent diseases. Refers to septic infections at Geelong Hosp., ascribed to noxious vapours from a stagnant pool. Insanity is more prevalent in Aust. than in any other part of the world, 'nine-tenths being due to illicit liquor containing poisonous ingredients such as tobacco juice, sulphuric acid, helebore, mezereon, copperas, grains of paradise etc.'

Title shows authorship of prize treatise *How to govern the goldfields*. NS.

Copies: FC, ML, RACP, WLC. 2037

———

A practical treatise on pleuro-pneumonia, or catarrh in cattle, explanative of its causes, prevention, symptoms, and pathology. Founded upon post-mortem examinations. . . . Geelong: . . . Downie, & Thompson . . . 1864.

204 × 138. Pp. 16 (2,4 blank). P. w. (title rptd).

Copies: SLV. 2038

Stilwell, Charles

The rational treatment of insanity. . . . Newtown, Sydney: . . . Moss & Burford . . . 1878.

201 × 132. Pp. 12.

Advocates treatment of patients in small establishments under a physician and selected staff.

Charles Stilwell (1806–86) MRCS came to Aust. after practice in UK and US, was at Sandhurst Vic. in 1862, at Morpeth NSW in 1883.

Copies: ML. 2039

Stirling, Sir Edward Charles

Observations on certain eruptions of the skin which occur after recent operations and injuries: Thesis for the degree of M.D. in the University of Cambridge. . . . London, 1880.

205 × 132. Pp. 56 (l.b.). P. w. (cover title).

Copies: UA. 2040

———

With Dr. Stirling's compliments. The political franchise for women. Speech in the House of Assembly, South Australia . . . 22nd July, 1885. Reprinted from "Hansard". Adelaide: Burden & Bonython . . . Advertiser Office.

210 × 137. Pp. 24 (three blanks).

Author, who was MLA (SA), 1884–7, introduced the first Aust. bill for the franchise of women.

Copies: ML, SLS. 2041

———

'Hydatids', with J. C. Verco; chapter in Allbutt's *A system of medicine*, Vol. 2, Lond., Macmillan, 1897.

For Sir Edward Charles Stirling (1848–1919) MD Camb., FRCS, FRS, 1st Prof. Physiol. Univ. Adel., see obits, *Med. J. Aust.*, 1919, 1 : 298 and 309. 2042

———

Intercolonial Medical Congress of Australasia. . . . 1889. Address in surgery . . . Reprinted from the "Intercolonial Medical Congress of Australasia Transactions". Melbourne: Stillwell & Co. . . . 1889.

212 × 140. Pp. 24 (l.b.). P. w. (title rptd).

Presidential address to Section of Surgery.

Copies: SLS. 2043

———

See Horn Scientific Expedition.

Stirling, J.

Observations on the climate and geographical position of Western Australia, and on its adaptation to the purposes of a sanatorium for the Indian Army. In a letter addressed to J. R. Martin, Esq. London: Printed by J. C. Bridgewater . . . Oxford Street, W. 1859.

8vo. Pp. 8. Author's name on p. 7.

Copies: SLW. 2044

Stockdale, Harry

The legend of the petrified or marble man . . . with press extracts for and against. Sydney: F. Cunninghame & Co. . . . 1889

214 × 135. Pp. 40. Frontis. (marble figure).

Account of controversy, often humourous, as to whether a marble male figure, found in a quarry near Orange, was a sculpture or petrified human remains. Taylor, A. G. (1889), *The Marble Man*, Syd., also refers.

Copies: EF, FC, ML, NL, UM, US. 2045

Stockham, Alice B.

Tokology A book for every woman. . . . Illustrated. . . . Reprinted from the latest American edition. Melbourne: Pater & Co. . . . 1898.

186 × 125. Pp. 369 (misnumbered from 346—end). Cloth. Plates separate, in pocket. Title: *Plates illustrating Tokology* . . . Pp. 16 (l.b.), 18 figs.

Other Melb. eds, 1902, 1909.

Reprint of US work on reproduction and infant care.

Copies: EF. 2046

———

The Same. Pp. 368 (numbering corrected), 1898.

Copies: EF, KFR, SLV. 2047

Stokes, John Lort

The narrow escape Rear Admiral J. Lort Stokes, F.R.G.S. had of his life when Lieutenant in H.M.S. Beagle, discovering the Victoria River in North West Australia, 1839. Printed at "Potter's Newspaper" Office, H. West.

212 × 127. Pp. 12 (l.b.). ND. Haverfordwest, May 1870—in preface.

'The following Report of my Spear Wound in the lungs has . . . been found among the papers of the late Staff Surgeon Bynoe, and is now printed . . . with the Medical Opinions of Sir William Jenner . . . showing the very serious nature of that Wound, also the imminent danger to which it placed my life for some time . . .'

Copies: DL, ML, NL. 2048

Storie, John

The latest Presbytery scandal. A statement by the Rev. John Storie, A. M., Minister of St. Andrew's, and Colonial Chaplain. Reprinted from the "Launceston Examiner". Launceston . . . "Launceston Examiner" Office. 1878.

212 × 138. Pp. 14. P. w. (title, decorated, rptd).

Author justifies his opposition to the appointment of a US minister who had been indicted and acquitted (in US) of the murder of his wife. Trial evidence in the decision between murder and suicide is cited, with opinions of medicolegal experts.

Copies: FC, ML. 2048a

Stradbroke Island Lazaret, Qd

1898. Queensland. Report of the Medical Officer of the Lazaret, Stradbroke Island. Presented to both Houses . . . [Text begins.]

342 × 204. Pp. 4 (l.b.). Colophon— . . . Edmund Gregory, Govt Pr . . . Bris. Signed—P. Smith, MO.

Copies: LNSW, NL, OL, SLV. 2049

Stuart, Sir Thomas Peter Anderson

Testimonials in favour of T. P. Anderson Stuart . . . Candidate for the Chair of Anatomy and Physiology in Sydney University.

217 × 132. Pp. 46 (l.b.). Colophon—Edinburgh: Crawford and M'Cabe . . . ND. (1882.)

Addressed from Univ. Edin., where Stuart was Asst Prof. of Physiology.

Copies: EF, US. 2050

———

University of Sydney, June 5th, 1886. My Dear Chancellor [Text begins.]

331 × 209. Pp. 4, [2] (v.b.).

Letter, signed as Dean of Medicine, recommending commencement of teaching in diseases of children, psychological medicine and diseases of eye.

Copies: US. 2051

University of Sydney. Memorandum to the Senate from Professor Stuart, June 16th, 1888. [Text begins.]

339 × 214. Pp. 4 (2, 4, blank).

Urges division of combined Dept of Anat. and Physiol. and recommends appointment of J. T. Wilson as Lecturer in Anatomy.

Copies: US. 2052

Catalogue of the scientific serial literature in the following libraries in Sydney, N.S.W. viz.: The Australian Museum, Free Public Library, Linnean Society of N.S.W., Observatory, Parliamentary Library, Royal Geographical Society of N.S.W., Royal Society of N.S.W., Technological Museum and the University of Sydney. Compiled under the direction of T. P. Anderson Stuart, M.D. ... By W. T. Dayton. Sydney: Charles Potter, Govt Printer. 1889. ...

247 × 156. Pp. vi (l.b.), 146. P. w. (title rptd).

Copies: EF, LNSW, ML, SLV, UM, US. 2053

Intercolonial Medical Congress Melbourne, 1889. Address by ... President of the Section of Anatomy and Physiology. Melbourne: Stillwell and Co., Printers ... 1889.

212 × 135. Pp. 20. P. w. (title rptd).

Includes: 'The new medical curriculum of the Univ. of Sydney.'

Copies: EF, ML, NL. 2054

[From the Pharmaceutical Journal, December 13, 1890.] On the so-called "eucalyptus honey". ... [Text begins.]

239 × 156. Pp. 8. Double cols. Colophon—W. L. Richardson ... London.

Author investigated claims of Caraman, Ch. T. *(q.v.)* that the eucalyptus-containing honey of certain Tasmanian bees had unique medicinal properties. He finds that such honey does not occur naturally, but as sold in France, is made by addition of eucalyptol to native honey.

Copies: EF. 2055

'A simple mode of demonstrating how the form of the thorax is partly determined by gravitation". ... Received January 12, 1891. [Text begins.]

212 × 135. Pp. 2. Repr., *Proc. Roy. Soc. Lond.*, 1891, 49 : 143.

Copies: EF. 2056

"On the connexion between the suspensory ligament of the crystalline lens and the lens capsule". ... [Text begins.]

212 × 135. Pp. 2. Repr., *Proc. Roy. Soc. Lond.*, 1891.

Copies: EF. 2057

1891. New South Wales. Report to the Governments of New South Wales, South Australia, and New Zealand, on the Koch method of treating tuberculosis ... Sydney: George Stephen Chapman, Acting Govt Printer. 1891. ...

245 × 152. Pp. vi, 110. 3 coloured pl. Morocco or p. w.

Report of official mission to Germany to enquire into Koch's tuberculin treatment. 'We cannot at present regard the lymph as a successful curative agent, yet ... it is the first example of a new method of treatment which opens up a wide field ... and by which eventually, not only tuberculosis, but also such diseases as diphtheria, tetanus and others, may possibly be prevented, cured, or even annihilated.'

Copies: DOS, EF, ML, RACP, SLS, UA, US. 2058

The Same. 325 × 210. Pp. iv, 76. 3 coloured pl. Morocco or p. w. (title rptd).

Copies: AMAN, EF, HDN, ML, UM. 2059

A review of university life in Australasia with its conditions and surroundings in 1891 ... A paper read before the Royal Colonial Institute January 12, 1892 ... Reprinted by permission from the 'Proceedings of the Institute'

212 × 138. Pp. 44. Colophon— ... Spottiswoode & Co. ... London. P. w. (title rptd) or cloth.

Copies: DL, EF, ML, NL, RACP, SLS, SLV, UM, US. 2060

———

The Same. Title at head of p. 1, prefixed: 'To be read at a Meeting of the Royal Colonial Institute ...' 35 numbered leaves, v.b. Lacks last 7 pp. of above. Author's copy, with his ink erasures and marginal notes (as delivered).

Copies: EF. 2061

———

The "mika" or "kulpi" operation of the Australian aboriginals. ... (Read before the Royal Society of N. S. Wales, June 3, 1896.) [Text begins.]

217 × 147. Pp. 10 (l.b.). 1 pl. P. w. (title rptd). Repr., *J. & P. Roy. Soc. NSW*, 1896.

Describes ritualistic subincision of penis, with views on its effect on fecundity. Reprinted in Mathews, R. H. (1905), *Ethnological notes on the aboriginal tribes of NSW and Vic.*, Syd.

Copies: EF, UQ. 2062

———

An artificial larynx ... Reprinted from the Lancet, April 17, 1897.

217 × 138. Pp. 12. 11 figs.

Copies: EF, ML, US. 2063

———

Royal Society of New South Wales. Sydney. Anniversary address by the President ... May 2nd, 1894. Sydney: F. W. White ... 1894.

217 × 138. Pp. 38, [ii] (colophon, v.b.). Repr., *J. Roy. Soc. NSW*, 1894.

Reviews recent local work on artesian waters; poisons of platypus, Aust. spiders, ticks and snakes; hydatids; anthrax.

Copies: EF, NL. 2064

———

"Medicine as a career". ... The Annual Lecture, delivered before the Medical Students' Society of the Melbourne University ... Melbourne: The Austral Publishing Co. ... 1898.

220 × 143. Pp. 16. P. w. (title rptd).

Copies: EF, FC, ML, SLS. 2065

———

The bubonic plague A popular lecture ... (Sydney, May, 1900.) ... Sydney: William Applegate Gullick, Govt Printer. 1900.

178 × 122. Pp. [iv] (ii, iv blank), 36. Frontis. P. w. (title rptd).

Delivered at outset of Aust. plague epidemic of 1900–1909.

For Sir Thomas Anderson Stuart (1856–1920) Prof. of Physiol., Dean of Medicine, and founder of Med. School, Univ. Syd., see Epps, W., *Anderson Stuart M.D.*, Syd., 1922; obits, *Med. J. Aust.*, 1920, 1 : 244 and *Syd. Univ. Med. J.*, Mar. 1920 : 181; also Blackburn, Sir Charles (1948), 'The life and work of Sir T.A.S.', *BPCMUS*, 1948, 4 : 107. Author's copies of complete publications, 2 vols, with bookplate, are in EF coll.

Copies: DL, EF, ML, NL, SLS, SLV, SLW, US. 2066

——— **and MacCormick, Sir Alexander**

The position of the epiglottis in swallowing. ... [Text begins.]

220 × 143. Pp. 8. P. w. Repr., *J. Anat. & Physiol.*, 1892.

For Sir Alexander MacCormick (1856–1947), of Sydney, surgical leader of his day, see obit., *Med. J. Aust.*, 1948, 1 : 118 (with bibliog.); Skirving, R. S. (1949), 'Sir A. M.', *BPCMUS*, 5 : 1; Miller, D. (1969), 'Sir A. M., man and Surgeon', *Aust. NZ J. Surg.*, 38 : 189.

Copies: EF, ML, US. 2067

Sturt, Thomas James

Female physiology; a treatise of the diseases of women, their causes, symptoms, and means of cure: with hints on the management of health during pregnancy and in the lying-in room, &c., forming a complete ladies' guide. Illustrated with fifty engravings on steel. ... London: James Gilbert ... 1854.

NS. Written long before its time, this work was violently criticised by *Lancet*, 1854, 2 : 103 as a pernicious book intended to 'unblushingly give to the ladies of England, drawings of the vagina, uterus, various stages of labour, spermatozoa &c. ... and obscene descriptions of things they should never hear of ... such disgusting rubbish has never before been put into type and we blush to think ... that the author is a brother-practitioner and a Doctor of Medicine of the University of London.'

T. J. Sturt MD Lond. & Melb., Accoucheur to W. Lond. Lying-in Hosp., arrived in Melb. in 1868 and was at once appointed Lect. Mat. Med. Melb. Univ., relinquishing the post after two years. In 1883 he was in practice at Bulli NSW, and after 1892 retired to Kogarh NSW.

2068

Surgeons-Superintendent of Convict Ships

Instructions for the guidance of Surgeons Superintendent and Masters of convict ships, arriving in the River Derwent with prisoners, and which are to be strictly observed. [Text begins.]

245 × 155. Single leaf, v.b. ND. [c. 1826.] NI.

12 numbered instructions on procedures at arrival and disembarkation. Tas. State Archives copy (GO 33/1/p657) is in file dated 1826.

Copies: Tas. State Archives. 2069

Convict vessels. Copies of instructions to the Surgeons-Superintendents and the Masters of convict vessels, during their voyage to foreign settlements. ... Ordered, by the House of Commons, to be printed, 4 March 1834.

338 × 213. Pp. [ii], 16.

Includes: Admiralty letter (23 June 1832): instructions; instructions for Surgeons-Supt and Masters of ships arriving in River Derwent.

Establishment of the post of surgeon-supt reformed the infamous state of early convict transport and abated its heavy toll of death and disease. This arose from adoption of a notable report by William Redfern (1778–1833), ex-convict Asst Col Surg. at Sydney, to Governor Macquarie in 1814. The master-stroke of this was the appointment of experienced naval surgeons to all ships, with supreme powers in all matters relating to the convicts. In addition they were responsible for hygiene, medical care, welfare, and discipline. The system was later applied to Govt emigrant ships.

For Redfern's report, see *HRA*, ser. 1, 8 : 274; also Ford, E. (1953), 'The life and work of Wm Redfern', *BPCMUS*, 9 : 1; Bateson, C. (1959), *The convict ships*, Glasgow.

Copies: ML. 2070

Instructions for Surgeons-Superintendent on board convict ships proceeding to New South Wales, or Van Diemen's Land; and for the Masters of those ships. London: Printed by William Clowes and Sons ... for Her Majesty's Stationery Office. 1838.

223 × 149. Pp. [36] (5 blanks), 46 (appendix, 19/20 flg chart). Cloth.

Admiralty letter (1 March 1838) precedes instructions for Surg.-Supts (47 clauses), and is repeated before Master's instructions (16 clauses). Appendix includes scales of stores, medicines, clothing, victualling etc.; forms and accounts.

ML copy inscribed 'J. Denham Pinnock, Sydney.'

Copies: CC (lacks title p.), ML. 2071

The Same, 1840. Pp. [40], 50 (appendix). Cloth. NL copy has ms. amendments and additions; inserted memo. (1842) precedes appendix.

Copies: LNSW, NL. 2072

The Same, 1846. Pp. 114 (69/70, flg chart). Cloth. DL copy has additional instructions in ink on half title.

Copies: DL. 2073

Instructions for the guidance of Surgeons Superintendent and Masters of convict ships, arriving in the River Derwent with prisoners. [Text begins.]

325 × 196. Single leaf, v.b. ND. NI. [Hobart, c. 1845.] At foot: Colonial Secretary's Office, 184

14 numbered instructions. Tas. State Archives copy, bound with correspondence dated 1845, has ms. deletions and amendments.

Copies: Tas. State Archives (CSO 16/22/585). 2074

Surgeons-Superintendent of Emigrant Ships

Instructions for Surgeons Superintendent on board emigrant ships proceeding to New South Wales or Van Diemen's Land. [London, 8 Jan. 1838.]

300 × 209. Pp. 16–24. NI. Pale blue paper.

Included in: Emigration. Letter from ... Agent Gen. for Emigration ... [London], 22nd March 1838. Pp. 24. From *NSW*, *Leg. Council*, *V&P*, [1838].

Copies: LNSW, ML, NL. 2075

Instructions for the Surgeons Superintendent of Government emigrant ships going to New South Wales. London: Printed by W. Clowes and Sons ... for Her Majesty's Stationery Office. 1839.

231 × 150. Pp. 58 (l.b.), [ii] (colophon, v.b.). Cloth. Issued by Agent Gen. for Emigration.

Details duties during embarkation, on voyage, and upon arrival. Appendices include: regulations, medicines, medical comforts, hospital

equipment, stores and utensils, victualling scale, hints on dietary.
Copies: DL, FC, ML. 2076

South Australian Commission. Instructions for the Surgeons-Superintendent of emigrant ships proceeding to South Australia. London: Printed by W. Clowes and Sons ... for Her Majesty's Stationery Office. 1839.
231 × 150. Pp. 28. Cloth. Signed in ms. : S. Walcott, Sec.
Copies: ML. 2077

Remuneration of private surgeons, serving as Superintendents of emigrant ships. [Text begins.] The following are the terms of remuneration to a Surgeon, not belonging to the Royal Navy, employed in the superintendence of a Government emigrant ship to New South Wales. ...
331 × 209. Single leaf, v.b. Lond., 20 March 1839. NI. Signed: T. Frederick Elliott, Agent Gen. for Emigration.
Copies: FC. 2077a

Instructions to Surgeons of emigrant ships sailing under Government superintendence. [Royal Arms] London: Printed by W. Clowes and Sons ... for Her Majesty's Stationery Office. 1847.
209 × 135. Pp. 32. Issued by Col Land and Emigration Office.
Copies: ML. 2078

Great Britain, Colonial Land and Emigration Commissioners. Instructions to Surgeons of emigrant ships sailing under the superintendence of Her Majesty's Colonial Land and Emigration Commissioners. London: ... Her Majesty's Stationery Office. 1854.
8 vo. Pp. 73.
Copies: SLW. 2079

Instructions to Surgeons Superintendents of Government emigrant ships. [Royal Arms] London: Printed by George E. Eyre and William Spottiswoode ... for Her Majesty's Stationery Office. 1858.
227 × 147. Pp. 78 (l.b.), [ii] (r.b., colophon). Signed: Sec., Col Land and Emigration Office. Cloth.
Copies: ML. 2080

The Same. Pp. 114, [ii] (colophon, r.b.). 2 plans. London: Eyre and Spottiswoode. 1866. Cloth. ML copy inscribed: Wm Donaldson, Surgeon Supt.
Copies: ML. 2081

Instructions to Surgeon-Superintendents of Queensland ships sailing under the direction of H. M. Queensland Government. [Royal Arms] London: ... Rees & Company, Printers to H. M. Government of Queensland. ... 1869.
236 × 152. Pp. [ii], viii (ii blank), 108 (l.b.). Stiff p. w. (title rptd), linen backstrip.
OL copy has amendments in ink, substitutions by over-pasted cuttings, and date on title altered to 1872.
For voyages and mention of surgeons and epidemics, see Davies, A. G. (1935), 'Immigration and immigrant ships (Moreton Bay)', *J. Hist. Soc. Qd*, 2 : 305.
Copies: OL. 2082

Instructions to Surgeons-Superintendent of South Australian Government emigrant ships London Spottiswoode & Co., Printers ... 1873
229 × 150. Pp. [iv], (ii, iv blank), 80 (l.b. 1 flg chart, 3 figs. Limp leather.
Copies: ML. 2083

Instructions to Surgeon-Superintendents of Queensland ships sailing under the direction of H. M. Government of Queensland. [Royal Arms] London: A. A. Russell & Co. ... 1883.
239 × 147. Pp. [ii], viii, 110 (l.b.). P. w. (title rptd). Issued by Govt Emigration Office, London.
Copies: ML. 2084

Surgical Appliance Aid Society, Sydney

The Surgical Appliance Aid Society. For the supply of mechanical supports to the afflicted poor. First Annual Report, 1888–99. Offices: 293 Crown St., Surry Hills. Sydney: Samuel E. Lees ... 1899.
220 × 138. Pp. 16 (l.b.). P. w. (title rptd).
Assistance includes provisions of artificial

limbs, trusses, splints, crutches, spectacles, bandages and articles for use in sick-room.

An reps issued to 25th, 1923.

Copies: ML. 2085

Suter, R. George

Queensland Philosophical Society. (From the *Queensland Guardian*, July 2, 1866.) The construction and arrangement of hospitals ... [Text begins.]

217 × 138. Pp. 8 (l.b.). Double cols. Colophon —G. Wight, 'Guardian Office', Brisbane.

Copies: FC. 2086

Sutherland, Alexander

No. 15.] [January, 1882. Australian Health Society, Melbourne. Little stomachs. Written for the Australian Health Society ... [Woodcut figure of parents and sick child] Melbourne: Walker, May & Co. ... 1881.

212 × 136. Pp. 8.

A moral tale on the diet of children.

Copies: EF, ML, SLS, SLV. 2087

———

Victoria and its Metropolis past and present [Vignette] Vol. 1. ... With two hundred and fifty-eight illustrations Melbourne: McCarron, Bird & Co., Publishers ... 1888.

275 × 214. 2 vols. Vol. 1 : pp. xii, 594, frontis., figs. Vol. 2 : pp. xii, 824 (l.b.), frontis., flg map, figs.

Chap. 24 (vol. 2, pp. 779–85), 'The medical profession in Vic.', by J. E. Neild MD, contains history of profession from first settlement, including med. societies and journals.

Copies: ML, SLS, SLV, SLW, US. 2088

———

See Australian Health Society, No 104.

Sutherland, Miss

See Charity Organization Society of Melbourne.

Swan Hill District Hospital, Vic.

Report for the year 1864, of the Committee of Management of the Lower Murray District Hospital, Swan Hill, with the rules of the institution ... Sandhurst: Printed by Maurice Moran, Advertiser Office ... 1865.

204 × 127. Pp. 14. P. w. (sketch of hosp. on front).

Founded 1860; name changed to Swan Hill District Hosp., 1872.

Copies: SLV (1864–71). 2089

———

Swan Hill District Hospital Board Room, Swan Hill, 29th March, 1872. In accordance with a proclamation declaring the "Lower Murray District Hospital" to have been incorporated under the name ... of the "Swan Hill District Hospital" ... [Notice continues.]

201 × 135. Single leaf, v.b.

Copies: SLV. 2090

———

Bye-laws. Swan Hill District Höspital. 1872. Incorporated ... 11th March 1872. Melbourne: Stillwell & Knight, Printers ... 1872.

204 × 127. Pp. 14 (l.b.).

Copies: SLV. 2091

Swift, Harry

Diphtheritic paralysis: with special reference to the prognosis. ... Read at Cambridge, June, 1887, as subject of thesis for M.D. degree. Adelaide: J. H. Sherring & Co. ... 1889.

204 × 135. Pp. vi (l.b.), 7–34.

A study, made prior to author's arrival in Aust., to which is added review of a few local cases.

Harry Swift (1858–1937) MD Camb. & Adel., who came to Adel. from London in 1887, was Hon. Phys. Adel. Children's and Adel. Hosp. and Dean of Med. Univ. Adel. In 1914 he described a new disease entity he named erythroedema, later termed pink disease or Swift's disease (*Trans. Austsn Med. Cong.*, 1914 : 547). Obit.: *Med. J. Aust.*, 1937, 2 : 976.

Copies: LNSW, UA. 2092

Syder, Charles Broady Mingay

A series of lectures on the most approved principles and practice of modern surgery; principally derived from the lectures delivered by Astley Cooper, Esq. F.R.S. ... Interspersed with numerous cases. By Charles William Jones. Second edition. By Charles Mingay Syder, Surgeon. London: Printed for Samuel Highley ... and Otridge and Rackham ... 1821.

8vo. Pp. viii, 9–438. Portrait (John Hunter).

1 ed. of this work (Lond., 1819) shows author as Charles William Jones. 2 ed. (above) has introductory letter to Astley Cooper, signed by Syder, with apologies for 1 ed. having appeared in the name of his student, C. W. Jones, without acknowledgement 'that the original ideas of this

series were derived from your lectures ...'

BMC lists other early publications: *The chemical decompositions of the London Pharmacopoeia*, Lond., 1821; *A series of questions and answers, for ... examination at Apothecaries Hall*, Lond., 1821. NS.

Copies: Roy. Coll. Surg., London. 2093

The voice of truth in defence of nature; and opinions antagonistic to those of Dr. Kilgour, upon the effect of the climate of Australia upon the European constitution in health and disease. By Mingay Syder, M.D., ... of above thirty years practice "at home"; and of five years "colonial" experience. Geelong: Heath and Cordell, Market Square. 1855.

212 × 138. Pp. [iv] (ii, iv blank), 56. P. w. (title rptd, book notice—v. of back wrapper).

A refutation of Kilgour's pamphlet (No 1086) on adverse Aust. climatic effects. Author ascribes 'the fearful amount of disease and mortality' to imported disease and weakness. 'This Colony was not a nursery for the idle, dissipated, scofulous, phthysical ... worn out constitutions; or for the "prostitutes", and the other fungi of Europe.'

Advt on back wrapper invites subscriptions for: *A treatise on the causes and prevention of diseases, under the influence of the climate of Victoria*, 8vo, 300 pp. NS.

C.B.M. Syder (d. 1871) MD, LSA (1820) practised and taught in London; settled in Geelong about 1850. He died—the oldest doctor in the colony—in Melb. Hosp. Obit.: *Aust. med. J.*, 1871, 16 : 312.

Copies: ML, RACP, SLV. 2094

The Same. New ed., 1861.

Copies: EF, LNSW, ML, NL, SLV, US. 2095

Sydney Biological Station

Rules of the Biological Station, Sydney. Trustees appointed by the Government: ... 1. The use of the Sydney Biological Station shall be granted to bona fide biologists only ... [Text continues.]

209 × 171. Pp. 4 (2, 4 blank). NI. ND. (?1882).

Copies: ML. 2096

Sydney Biological Station. The number of biological stations throughout the world is increasing yearly. [Text continues.]

344 × 214. Pp. 4 (l.b.). 3 figs (plans). NI. ND. (P. 4, addressed for mailing, is postmarked 'Ap 19, 82'.)

Plans, description and brief history of station on Port Jackson between Watson's Bay and Camp Cove. This centre for biological study was established by the efforts of Miklucho-Maclay (later biologist in charge), supported by Linnean and other societies, with Govt and public aid. See Miklucho-Maclay, N. N. No 1381; also Aust. Biol. Station.

Copies: ML. 2097

Sydney City Council

Minutes of evidence taken before the Special Committee of the City Council ... to consider the best means of affording a permanent supply of water to the City of Sydney. ... 12th March, 1850. [Text begins.]

305 × 204. Pp. 64. Blue tinted paper. Colophon—Syd.: Printed by E. Alcock.

Copies: ML. 2098

Sydney Dispensary

See Sydney Hospital.

Sydney Foundling Hospital and Home for Destitute Infants

Second Annual Report of the Sydney Foundling Hospital and Home for Destitute Infants, for the year ending 1st June, 1876. Sydney: Robert Bone ... 1876.

204 × 130. Pp. 16 (l.b.).

Report claims that 'since the opening of the charity, infanticide has almost if not entirely ceased.' Name changed to Infants' Home, Gorton, Ashfield, in 5th an. rep. (1879).

Copies: ML (2, 3, 5; 1876,–77, –79). 2099

Sydney General Hospital

Hospital of the penal settlement ('the Convict Hospital'), established on Syd. Cove in 1788, was precursor of Sydney Hosp. *See* Nos 306–7. 2099a

Sydney Homoeopathic Dispensary

The First Annual Report of the Sydney Homoeopathic Dispensary. Established July, 1858. With a list of subscribers and rules of the institute. Sydney, N.S.W.: ... Reading and Wellbank ... 1859.

204 × 135. Pp. 14.

For Syd. Homoeopathic Hosp., established

1902 in Cleveland St, Redfern, see circular and subscription leaflets (1902) and an. reps, 1906–26. (ML.)

Copies: ML (1, 1859; 3, 1861), SLT (3, 1861). 2100

Sydney Hospital

The First Report of the Committee of the Sydney Dispensary, established in the month of August, 1826; with a list of subscriptions and donations received. Sydney: Printed by A. Hill ...

183 × 110. Pp. 12 (l.b.). ND. (1828).

Dispensary was established 1826, by public subscription, for care of the indigent sick. On reduction of the convict population, the south wing of the General Hospital was made available to the Dispensary in 1843, and an associated hospital, named Sydney Dispensary and Infirmary, opened in 1845. Assumption of the main central block in 1848 completed replacement of the convict institution by the public charity, the name of which was changed to Sydney Hospital in 1881. Present buildings opened 1894. For history, see Watson, J. F. (1911), *The history of the Syd. Hosp.*, Syd.; Peyser, D. (1939), 'History of welfare work in Syd.', *JRAHS*, 25 : 89.

An. reps issued 1828—present. Dispensary: separate series; Syd. Hosp. continues numbers of Infirm. and Dispensary.

Copies: EF (1844), LNSW (1828–44), ML (1828–44), SLV (1834–5, 1842). 2101

Report of the Sub-Committee appointed by the General Committee of the Sydney Dispensary, by minute of 17th April, 1844, to draw up regulations for the management of the Hospital when brought into operation. Submitted to the General Committee 4th June, and revised July 1844.

220 × 138. Pp. 16. [Sydney, 1844.] NI.

Copies: ML. 2102

Rules and regulations of the Sydney Infirmary and Dispensary: Instituted in the year 1844. Sydney: Printed by D. L. Welch ... 1844.

222 × 138. Pp. 16, [ii] (inserted leaf with amended rules). P. w. (title rptd, engraved fig.).

Editions: 1844, ND [1845], 1853, 1858, 1862, 1863, 1867, 1875.

Copies: EF (1853), LNSW (1853,–62,–67), ML (1844,–45,–62,–67,–75), SLV (1853,–58, –63). 2103

The First Report of the Board of Directors of the Sydney Infirmary and Dispensary, established in the month of July, 1845. With a list of subscriptions and donations, received during the year 1845. Sydney: Printed by D. Wall ... 1846.

214 × 140. Pp. 16. P. w. (title rptd).

Numbering of series was continued when rebuilt instn was renamed Syd. Hosp. (from 38th an. rep., 1883).

Copies: EF (1850–63), ML (1845–), NL (1858), SLV (1848,–57,–62), UM (1846–55). 2104

1866. Legislative Assembly. New South Wales. Sydney Infirmary. (Appointment of a Commission to inquire into.) ... "Copies of all correspondence and minutes ..." ... [Text begins.]

330 × 210. Pp. 10. Colophon—Syd.: Thomas Richards, Govt Pr—1866.

In response to Board of Directors' demand for Govt inquiry into accounts, stores, inefficient nursing, bad order and discipline, etc., Commission was appointed 'to inquire into the state of the Infirmary.' Directors, now also subject to inquiry, complain of Govt interference, and refuse cooperation. Governor's minute: 'Whenever money is granted by Parlt, the right of inspection follows as a matter of course.'

Copies: LNSW, ML, NL, SLV. 2105

1870. Legislative Assembly. New South Wales. Sydney Infirmary. (Report from Sub-Committee relative to charges against the management of.) ...

325 × 210. Pp. 26. Colophon—Syd.: Thomas Richards, Govt Pr—1870.

Copies: LNSW, ML, NL, SLV. 2106

Sydney Infirmary. Reports of Sub-committees on the capabilities of the nursing staff, &c., and on expenses of the institution generally. ...

209 × 135. Pp. [ii]–44 (l.b.). Colophon: Mason, Firth, and M'Cutcheon ... Melb. ND. [1870.]

Included in: Melb. Hosp. Report of the Sub-Committee of Enquiry on Trained Nurses. July, 1871. No 1348.

For introduction of trained nurses and estab-

lishment of School of Nursing, see Nightingale, Florence.
Copies: NL. 2107

By-laws of the Sydney Infirmary and Dispensary passed ... 28th May, 1875. Sydney: F. Cunninghame & Co., Printers ... 1875.
209 × 135. Pp. 32 (l.b.). P. w. (title rptd).
Copies: ML. 2108

Correspondence with reference to the grant of the land on which the Sydney Infirmary is built, and to the erection of a permanent modern hospital. Printed by order of the Board of Directors ... 1878. Sydney ... F. Cunninghame and Co. ...
214 × 132. Pp. [iv], 28 (l.b.). P. w. (cover title).
Copies: ML. 2109

1882. The Thirty-eighth Annual Report of the Sydney Hospital. Established in the month of July, 1845. Sydney: F. Cunninghame and Co., Printers ... 1883.
217 × 140. Pp. 48. P. w. (title rptd).
An. reps of renamed, rebuilt hosp. continue series of Syd. Infirmary (No 2104).
2110

1883. Legislative Assembly. New South Wales. Management of the Sydney Hospital. (Report of Committee of Inquiry into certain complaints.) ... [Text begins.]
328 × 206. Pp. 28 (l.b.).
Copies: LNSW, ML, NL, SLV. 2111

Rules and regulations of the Sydney Hospital. 1888. Sydney: Turner & Henderson ... 1888.
209 × 110. Pp. 40 (l.b.). P. w. (cover title).
Copies: ML. 2112

The Same. 1895. Pp. 48 (last—colophon).
Copies: ML. 2112a

Sydney Hospital. Report to Directors.
217 × 138. Pp. 8. 1891. Colophon—Turner and Henderson, Syd.
'I feel compelled to plainly place before the Board ... the disgraceful conditions under which its officers have to conduct the treatment of its patients.' Signed: Walter Hall, (Med. Supt). This report, and its 'scandalous and cruel facts', are discussed in *Austsn med. Gaz.*, 1891, 11 : 59.
Copies: ML. 2113

Sydney Hospital. Honorary medical staff's report on present condition of Hospital.
217 × 138. Pp. 8. (1891.) Colophon—Turner and Henderson, Sydney.
'The Honorary Medical and Surgical Staff ... desire again to protest against the disgraceful nature of the accommodation provided ...'
Copies: ML. 2114

Formal opening of the Sydney Hospital ... 10th August, 1894.
220 × 138. Pp. 16 (l.b.). Colophon—Sydney: F. Cunninghame ... P. w. (title rptd).
Copies: ML. 2115

By-laws of the Sydney Hospital, 1894. With copy of the Sydney Hospital Act of 1881. Sydney: Turner and Henderson ... 1894.
217 × 140. Pp. 28. P. w. (title rptd).
Copies: ML. 2116

See No 604.

——— **— Pharmacopeia**

According to J. F. Watson, an edition compiled in 1870 was printed but not at once adopted. An amended version was used in late 1870s. NS.
7 ed., 1911; 8 ed., 1921; 9 ed., 1937.
2117

Sydney Hospital for Sick Children

Sydney Hospital for Sick Children. Rules. Sydney: Turner & Henderson, ... 1878.
212 × 130. Pp. 12. P. w. (cover title).
Another ed., 1880.
For history, see Hipsley, P. L. (1952), *The early history of the Royal Alexandra Hosp. for Children*, Syd. Hosp. opened at Glebe Point 1880; transferred to Camperdown as Royal Alexandra Hosp. for Children, opened 1906.
Copies: EF (1880), LNSW (1878). 2118

———

Fourth Annual Report of the Hospital for Sick Children, Glebe Point, Sydney, for year ending 31st December, 1883. Sydney: Gibbs, Shallard, & Co. . . . 1884.

209 × 135. Pp. 16. P. w. (cover title).

Copies: ML (1883, 1891, 1895–), Roy. Alexandra Hosp. (1880–). 2119

———

Sydney, September, 1887. To the benefactors and subscribers of the Sydney Hospital for Sick Children, Glebe. [Text begins.]

260 × 209. Pp. [4] (l.b.).

Circular, signed 'Subscriber', supports Miss F. G. Holden in controversy which led to her dismissal as Lady Supt. See: Holden, Miss, F. G.

Copies: EF. 2120

———

The New Sydney Hospital for Sick Children. Leading article appearing in the Sydney Morning Herald of 15th August, 1900.

138 × 105. Pp. [4]. Brown paper. Colophon—William Brooks & Co. . . . Sydney.

Appeal for new hospital building.

Copies: ML. 2121

———

The New Sydney Hospital for Sick Children. . . . William Brooks & Co., Printers . . . Sydney.

147 × 247. Oblong. Pp. 16, [8] (last—colophon). 6 illustns of old hospital. (1900.) P. w. (short title, fig. of nurse and child).

Appeal for funds for building new hospital.

Copies: ML. 2122

Sydney Infirmary and Dispensary
See Sydney Hospital.

Sydney Institute of Medicine and Electricity
See Watson, Walter Carter.

Sydney Ladies' Sanitary Association

The Sydney Ladies' Sanitary Association. Annual Reports.

12 an. rep., 1900–1901 only seen. Earlier reports published. Formed in 1888 'to bring before women the laws of health and hygiene.' In 1908 Assn became the Health Soc. of NSW, reviving the name of earlier extinct body.

2123

Sydney Magazine of Science and Art, The

The Sydney Magazine of Science and Art. Containing . . . the Proceedings of the Australian Horticultural and Agricultural Society and the Philosophical Society of New South Wales. Volume 1. Edited by Mr. Joseph Dyer. Sydney: James W. Waugh, Publisher . . . 1858.

331 × 236. Vol. 1: pp. [vi] (ii, iv blank), 274 (l.b.). Vol. 2, 1859: pp. vi, 250. Vols 1 and 2 only published.

Vol. 1 contains Phil. Soc. papers: C. Rolleston 'Sanitary condition of Sydney'; Dr. Bland, 'Sanitary reform of towns and cities'; Isaac Aaron, 'Sanitary reform.'

Vol. 2: C. Rolleston, 'On the mortality of Sydney', and 'Means of deodorising and utilising the sewage of towns.'

Copies: DL, FC, ML, NL, SLV. 2124

Sydney Medical Association Defence Fund
See New South Wales Medical Union.

Sydney Ophthalmic Institution
See Berncastle, Julius (note).

Sydney Sanitarium
See 1822a (note).

Sydney Strangers' Friend Society

Report of the Sydney Strangers' Friend Society, instituted January, 1835, for the purpose of visiting and relieving sick and distressed strangers, and other poor, at their respective habitations, in Sydney and its vicinity, with an account of some of the cases visited . . . for the year ending 31st December, 1841. . . . Sydney: . . . James Reading, General Printing Office . . . 1842.

8vo. Pp. 16 (l.b.).

Copies: ML. 2125

Sydney United Friendly Societies' Dispensary

Rules & regulations for the government of the Sydney United Friendly Societies' Dispensary. Inaugurated August 13th, 1886. . . . Sydney: Boore & Long, Printers . . . 1886.

153 × 102. Pp. 16. Cloth.

Copies: ML. 2126

Sydney University
See University of Sydney.

Sydney University Medical Society. Journal of the

Hermes Medical Supplement. The Journal of the Sydney University Medical Society. Vol. 1, No. 1. August 20th, 1895. Contents. ... [Text begins.]

244 × 173. Pp. 16. P. w.

Published once each academic term. Later twice a year or annually. 1895-date.

Appeared as *Hermes Medical Supplement* (1895–1907), thence as *J. Syd. Univ. Med. Soc.*, *Univ. of Syd. Med. J.*, and latterly as *Syd. Univ. Med. J.*

Copies: See *SSAL*. 2127

Sydney Water Supply

Minutes of evidence taken before the Special Committee of the City Council ... to consider the best means of affording a permanent supply of water to the City of Sydney. ... 12th March, 1850. [Text begins.]

326 × 204. Pp. 64. Blue tinted paper. Colophon—Syd.: Printed by E. Alcock.

Copies: ML. 2128

———

1869. New South Wales. Sydney Water Supply. Report of the Commission appointed to inquire into the supply of water to Sydney and suburbs. Presented to both Houses of Parliament ... Sydney: Thomas Richards, Govt Printer. 1869.

336 × 206. Pp. 64 (l.b.), 190. 52 maps and plans. Stiff p. w. (title rptd). Pres.—Prof. John Smith MD.

Reports supply as 'inadequate and uncertain' and recommends a new 'Upper Nepean scheme.'

Copies: HDN, LNSW, ML, NL, SLV, US. 2129

———

The water supply of the City of Sydney. Sydney ... J. Degotardi, "Sydney Printing House" ...

212 × 140. Pp. 16 (l.b.). ND.

Three letters from *Syd. Morning Herald* complaining of state of Syd. water supply—two signed 'Senex', a third G. Allen Mansfield.

Copies: DL, ML, SLV. 2130

Syme, David

On the modification of organisms ... Melbourne: George Robertson and Co. London: Kegan Paul, Trench and Co.

191 × 127. Pp. viii (3 blanks), 164, [2] (book notices). ND. [1890.] Cloth.

A critical examination of Darwinian theory.

For David Syme (1827–1908), newspaper proprietor and 'father of protection in Australia', see Mennell (with note on above work).

Copies: CC, EF, FC, LNSW, ML, NL, SLV, UA, UM. 2131

Syme, Sir George Adlington

The nature and treatment of typhlitis, so-called. By G. A. Syme ... Surgeon to Out-patients, Melbourne Hospital ...

212 × 135. Pp. 14. Colophon—Melbourne: Stillwell and Co. ... Repr., *Aust. med. J.*, 1891, ns 13 : 230.

Advocates operative treatment for appendicitis. For author's influence, and report of second Aust. appendicectomy, see Lee, A. E. (1944), *Med. J. Aust.*, 2 : 653.

For Sir George Syme (1859–1929) a leading Aust. surgeon, see obit., *Med. J. Aust.*, 1929, 1 : 712; Kenny, A. L. (1932), 'G.A.S.: the man and the surgeon', *Med. J. Aust.*, 1 : 215.

Copies: UM. 2132

T

Tait, George
See Hulme, Edward and Tait, George.

Tarban Creek Lunatic Asylum, NSW
See Gladesville Hospital for the Insane.

Tarrant, Harman John
Functional derangements of the nervous system and diseases of the generative organs ... 151 Elizabeth Street ... Sydney. Second edition.] [Illustrated by 31 wood engravings.

173 × 120. Pp. vi, [ii] (v.b.), 264. Frontis. (portrait), 4 pl., 10 page figs (v.b.), text figs. ND. (testimonials dated 1898). Colophon—McCarron, Stewart & Co., Printers, Syd. Cloth.

Mainly on spermatorrhoea, impotence, venereal diseases.

H. J. Tarrant (1844–1900) FRCSE, MLC, Hon. Surg. Syd. Hosp., who was financially ruined in the depression of the '90s, went abroad. He later returned; above work is of latter days of stress and ill health. For obit. see *Age*, 2 Oct. 1900 (reprinted on red slip in Freeman and Wallace, *Clin. experiences on nervous and private diseases*, 1900); also Deane, R. E., *Cosmos*, 1898 : 687.

Copies: AMAV, EF. 2133

Tart, Quong
A plea for the abolition of the importation of opium. By Quong Tart. Sold in aid of the Bulli Relief Fund. Sydney. John Sands, Printer ... 1887.

209 × 135. Pp. 8. P. w. (title rptd).

Indicates evils of opium smoking upon individuals and community.

For author, Chinese merchant and philanthropist, see *The life of Quong Tart* by his wife, Margaret Quong Tart, Syd., 1911; *Aust. Enc.*

Copies: NL. 2134

———

The Same. Pp. 8. Syd., H. T. Dunn, 1890.
Copies: ML. 2135

———

Official report of anti-opium demonstration held at Congregational Church, Pitt Street, Sydney, on ... April 5th, 1894. Dr. T. Storie Dixson in the Chair. ... Sydney: T. J. Houghton & Co., Printers ... 1894.

217 × 138. Pp. 22 (l.b.). Cover title.

Meeting convened by Mr. Quong Tart, with the object 'of urging upon the Government the immediate necessity for restricting the sale of opium ... to purposes strictly medicinal.'

Copies: ML, NL. 2136

Tasmania—Central Board of Health
(No. 92.) [Royal Arms] 1886. Parliament of Tasmania. Central Board of Health. Interim Report ...

331 × 217. Pp. 8 (l.b.). Colophon—William Thomas Strutt, Govt Pr ...

Board established in 1886 under Public Health Act 1885. Annual reports, issued till Board succeeded by Dept of Health in Jan. 1904, appear in Parliamentary Papers of Tasmania.

Copies: LNSW, SLT, SLV. 2137

———

Tasmania. Report of the Central Board of Health for the year 1886. With appendices and diagram. Tasmania: William Thomas Strutt, Govt Printer, Tasmania, 1887.

323 × 214. Pp. 14. 1 flg graph. P. w. Signed: H. A. Perkins MD, President.

1st Annual Report.

Copies: LNSW, SLT, SLV. 2138

———

Central Board of Health. Instructions, regulations, and model by-laws for the guidance of Local Boards of Health and others, under "The Public Health Act, 1885" ... [Royal Arms] Tasmania: William Thomas Strutt, Govt Printer. 1886.

216 × 135. Pp. 68. P. w. (title rptd).

Copies: SLT. 2139

———

The Same. ... Regulations, &c. for the guidance

and instruction of Local Boards . . . 1886. Pp. 30.
Copies: NL. 2140

See also items under Mault, Alfred.

Tasmania—Convict Department

Convict Department, Tasmania. Rules and regulations for the Penal Settlement on Tasman's Peninsula. Tasmania: Pratt and Son . . . Hobart. 1858.

178 × 107. Pp. 62 (l.b.). Paper boards.

Another ed., 1868. W. Fletcher . . . Hobart Town.

Includes duties of medical officers and ration scales.

Copies: ML, SLV. 2141

Tasmania—Metropolitan Drainage Board

Metropolitan Drainage Board, Hobart. Correspondence respecting water supply and river pollution. [Royal Arms] Tasmania: William Grahame, Jun., Govt Printer, Hobart. 1896.

344 × 204. Pp. 8.

Copies: NL. 2142

Tasmania—Parliament

The following items are selections from the Parliamentary Papers of Tasmania, 1856/7–1900. See library catalogues for holdings. Detailed listing for LNSW, NL, OL, US appears in Cope, R. L., *Australian Parliamentary Serials*, Reference Monograph 9, Library of Parliament, Syd., 1973.

No. 1. [Royal Arms] 1858. Tasmania. Military sanitarium. Report of the Board of Commissioners. . . . ordered by the House to be printed, 7 September, 1858.

330 × 205. Pp. [ii] (v.b.), 44. 2 coloured graphs (v.b.) included in pagination. Colophon—James Barnard, Govt Pr, Tas.

Climate, access from India, expense and available accommodation, in connection with proposed establishment of a centre for treatment and convalescence of British Army patients. Appendix by E.S.P. Bedford FRCS on climate includes admissions and deaths in military hospitals in Tas. (1843–58), seasonal influence in troops, and lower morbidity and mortality compared with other British stations.

2143

The Same. Report of the Board of Commissioners appointed by His Excellency Sir Henry Young, on the 1st July, 1858, to consider the probable benefits which would result from the establishment in Tasmania of a military medical sanitarium, and post for convalescents. Published by the Hobart Town Mercury, 12th August, 1858.

4to. Pp. 44, 5 meteorological tables.

NS. Reviewed by E. Swarbreck Hall, *Aust. med. J.*, 1858, 3 : 285–312, who states 100 copies printed. He severely criticises Board: 'Not one has ever publicly evinced, either a special knowledge of vital statistics and sanitary science, or shown any zeal in the cause of sanitary improvement', and writes of their 'grievous errors and pernicious recommendations.'

2144

(No. 90.) [Royal Arms] 1863. [Second Session.] Tasmania. Vaccination. Report from the Select Committee. . . . ordered by the House to be printed, 3 September, 1863.

332 × 206. Pp. 16. Colophon—James Barnard, Govt Pr, Tas.

Reports law as unsatisfactory and large proportion of children unprotected.

2145

(No. 16.) [Royal Arms] 1864. Tasmania. Vaccinations. Report of Superintendent for 1863. . . .

344 × 214. Pp. 8 (l.b.). Colophon—James Barnard, Govt Pr, Tas. Signed: E. Swarbreck Hall.

Annual reps (1863–1887), from commencement of 'public gratuitous vaccination.'

2146

Royal Commission on Charitable Institutions. Report of the Commissioners, together with the evidence taken, and various returns. Presented to both Houses . . . Tasmania: James Barnard, Govt Printer, Hobart Town. 1871.

344 × 217. Pp. [ii] (title, v.b.), xlii (l.b.), 108.

2147

(No. 93.) 1875. Tasmania. House of Assembly. Public Health. Correspondence between the

Government and the Health Officers. Hobart Town and Launceston ...

342 × 214. Pp. 6 (l.b.). Colophon—James Barnard, Govt Pr.

Reports on the sanitary condition of the two cities, ordered on account of the increased death rate and typhoid incidence. Geo. Turnley (Hobart) recommends establishment of a Public Health Dept; J. L. Miller (Lcstn) improved sanitation and inspection. The latter notes an alarming increase of typhoid, diphtheria, erysipelas and puerperal fever in the past 20 years. Measles was 'followed by more deaths than any other similar epidemic in my colonial experience.'

2148

(No. 23.) [Royal Arms] 1877. ... Tasmania. House of Assembly. Officer of Health. Report on the Towns of New Town, Sandy Bay, and Wellington Hamlets. ...

344 × 204. Pp. 6 (l.b.). Colophon—James Barnard, Govt Pr, Tas.

An. reps 1876–86; printed 1877–87.

2149

Royal Commission on the State of the Lunatic Asylums in Tasmania. Report of the Commissioners with the evidence ... and other documents. Tasmania: William Thomas Strutt, Govt Printer, Hobart. 1883.

346 × 217. Pp. xxii (l.b.), 68 (l.b.).

2150

(No. 90.) [Royal Arms] 1888. Parliament of Tasmania. Quarantine: memorandum by the Secretary of the Central Board of Health. Presented to both Houses ...

331 × 204. Pp. 6 (l.b.). Colophon—William Thomas Strutt, Govt Pr, Tas.

Supports med. inspection of incoming vessels, and urges abandonment of quarantine (detention) of ships.

2151

(No. 7.) [Royal Arms] 1888. Federal Council of Australasia. Quarantine: papers relating to. ...

331 × 204. Pp. 16. Colophon—William Thomas Strutt, Govt Pr, Tas.

Refers to correspondence between Tas. and Austsn Boards of Health, and attempts to secure uniformity in quarantine procedure. 'Federal Council' apparently refers to continuation of meetings following the Austsn Sanitary Conference of Sydney, 1884, which initiated federal action.

2152

(No. 24.) [Royal Arms] 1890. Parliament of Tasmania. Government Medical Officer: Report for 1889. Presented to both Houses ...

344 × 214. Pp. 6. Colophon—William Thomas Strutt, Govt Pr, Tas.

1st an. rep. Duties: med. care of New Town Charitable Instn; visiting sick poor; boarding vessels from infected ports; supervision of Hosps for Insane; Med. Adviser to Cent. Bd of Health. Reports 1889–1900.

2153

(No. 20.) [Royal Arms] Melbourne Plague Conference. 11th to 15th April, 1900 ... [Text begins.]

326 × 204. Pp. 6 (l.b.). Colophon—John Vail, Govt Pr, Tas.

Report by Tas. delegates.

2154

Tasmanian Phrenological Society

See Sheridan, John J.

Taylor, Alfred Joseph

Overpressure in education as inevitable consequence of payment by results: a protest and a warning to parents. ... Mr. Girling, at ... the National Union of Elementary Teachers, referred to the case of a child who had then just died of brain-fever, whose continual cry in his last delirium was, "I can't get it right! I can't get it right!" Hobart ... "The Mercury" Office ... 1885.

212 × 132. Pp. 8. Double cols. P. w. (title rptd).

A warning against overstudy induced by an English system of grading financial support of schools by the pass rates of pupils, with opinions on possible resultant ailments.

Copies: ML, NL, SLV. 2155

Some facts and figures relating to vaccination. Illustrating errors of the anti-vaccinationists. ... Hobart: Calder, Bowden & Co. ... 1891.

214 × 138. Pp. 20 P. w. (title rptd).
Copies: FC, ML, NL, SLT, UA, WLC. 2156

———

The germ theory of disease, with special reference to the dangers to be guarded against in cases of consumption. ... A lecture ... [Reprinted from the Tasmanian News, August 9th, 1893.]
212 × 135. Pp. 8. Double cols. P. w. (title rptd).
A. J. Taylor was Librarian of Public Library of Tas.
Copies: FC, ML, NL, SLT. 2157

Taylor, William Frederick
1885. Queensland. Report on water supply and sewage disposal . . . Presented to both Houses . . . Brisbane: . . . James C. Beal, Govt Printer . . . 1885.
320 × 204. Pp. 42.
On water storage and purification, sewage disposal, house sanitation and refuse control.
Copies: LNSW, ML, NL, OL, SLV. 2158

———

Public abattoirs and the prevention of tuberculosis ... Read before the Royal Society of Queensland, December 16, 1899. I propose to show ... what effect public abattoirs should have in checking disease caused by the tubercle bacillus. [Text continues.]
204 × 132. Pp. 16 (l.b.). Colophon: H. Pole & Co. . . . Brisbane.
For W. F. Taylor (1840–1927) MD, DPH, MLC, MOH Brisbane, Hon. Surg. Brisbane Hosp., see obit., *Med. J. Aust.*, 1927, 2 : 171.
Copies: US. 2159

Techow, Gustav
Manual of gymnastic exercises, for the use of schools and at home. . . . Melbourne: Blundell & Ford . . . 1866.
200 × 125. Pp. xiv, [ii] (v.b.), 144 (last—colophon). 2 flg pl. Cloth.
Includes chapters on medical gymnastics.
Also published: *Memorandum on the teaching of gymnastics in state schools*, Melb., Govt Pr, ND.
Copies: ML, NL, SLV. 2160

Tegg, Thomas
Tegg's handbook for emigrants; containing useful information & practical directions on domestic, mechanical, surgical, medical, and other subjects, calculated to increase the comforts, and add to the conveniences of the colonist. London: Printed for Thomas Tegg . . . ; R. Griffin and Co., Glasgow; Tegg and Co., Dublin; and J. and S. A. Tegg, Sydney and Hobart Town. 1839.
173 × 107. Pp. viii, 212. 3 figs. Cloth.
Medical section (6 chapters) occupies more than half the book. Comprehensive med., surg., and obstet. advice.
Copies: FC, ML, SLV. 2161

———

The Same, 1843.
Copies: FC. 2162

———

The Same, 1844.
Copies: ML. 2163

Temperance Book Depot
The human body and its structure; with hints on health. A practical treatise on the design, nature, and functions of the various parts ... Melbourne: Temperance Book Depot.
183 × 120. Pp. viii, 176 (l.b.), [8] (book advts). 86 figs. Colophon: J. Ogden . . . London.
Copies: RACP. 2164

Temperance Society of New South Wales
Half an hour's reading from the Temperance Society of New South Wales. Sydney: . . . Stephens and Stokes . . . 1834.
196 × 127. Pp. 8.
An early temperance tract. 'Drunkenness expels reason, drowns memory, distempers the body, defaces beauty, diminishes strength, corrupts the blood, inflames the liver, and weakens the brain; turns men into walking hospitals; causes internal, external, and incurable wounds; is a witch to the senses, a devil to the soul, a thief to the purse, the beggar's companion, a wife's woe, and children's sorrow; makes man become a beast and self-murderer, who drinks to other's good health, and robs himself of his own . . .'
Copies: LNSW. 2165

Temple, R. C.
The Australasian colonies, considered with regard to sick and general leave. By Lieutenant R. C. Temple, 21st Royal North British Fusiliers. Madras: Higginbotham and Co. 1874.
163 × 102. Pp. [iv] (l.b.), 58 (l.b.). Frontis.

(flg map). Paper boards.

Guide book for invalid and other visitors. Author visited Australia on sick leave in 1872.

Copies: ML. 2166

Tench, Watkin

See No 2495 (note).

Terry, W. H.

W. H. Terry's general catalogue comprising the literature of spiritualism, mesmerism, psychology, phrenology, dietetics, physiology, chromopathy, social science, secularism and free religious thought ... Imported and on sale wholesale and retail, at "The Harbinger Light" Publishing Office ... Melbourne.

171 × 102. Pp. 88 (l.b.). ND. ML copy dated by hand 1886. Colophon—J. C. Stephens ... Melbourne.

Copies: ML. 2167

Thirlmere Home for Consumptives, NSW

Second Annual Report of the Thirlmere Home for Consumptives for the year ending the 31st August, 1895. W. E. Smith ... Sydney, also at Newcastle and London. 1895.

212 × 138. Pp. 16 (cover title).

1st an. rep. issued with 2 an. rep. of Queen Vic. Homes for Consumptives Fund *(q.v.)*.

Founded by Mr. Goodlet in 1878, Home was transferred to a public committee in 1893, and still operates in association with Sydney Hosp.

Copies: FC, ML (2–5, 1895–8). 2168

Thomas, David John

Medical Society of Victoria. April 23rd, 1862 [Text begins.]

204 × 132. Pp. 20 (l.b.).

Includes papers on 'Lithotomy' and 'Loose cartilages in joints' (*Aust. med. J.*, 1862), and 'Excision of the foot by a new method' (*ibid.*, 1864). SLV copy inscribed to Sir Redmond Barry by author.

Copies: SLV. 2169

———

On the reproduction of bone, with an interesting specimen ... [Text begins.]

204 × 135. Pp. 8 (l.b.). Repr., *Aust. med. J.*, 1864.

Copies: SLV. 2170

———

Medical Society of Victoria. Wednesday August 3, 1864. Ordinary monthly meeting. [Text begins.]

204 × 127. Pp. 10.

Paper on 'The general and local deposit of fat', by D. J. Thomas. Includes report of operation considered by O'Sullivan (*Med. J. Aust.*, 1956, 1 : 1065) to be the first performance of laparotomy in Australia.

Copies: SLV. 2171

———

On a case of intestinal obstruction treated by chloroform. ... [Text begins.]

212 × 135. Pp. 8. ND. Colophon—Wilson and Mackinnon ... Melb. Repr., *Aust. med. J.*, 1865.

Reports relief of intestinal obstruction following chloroform anaesthesia, which 'has not been hitherto recommended or tried.' Contains also: 'On dislocations of the hip ... and the value of chloroform in such cases.'

Copies: ML. 2172

———

Medical Society of Victoria. On the excision of joints. By the President of the Society ... [Text begins.]

217 × 135. Pp. 8 (l.b.). ND. (1865.) Colophon—Wilson & Mackinnon ...

Three cases of successful joint excision—'substantial instances of the triumph of conservative surgery.' From *Aust. med. J.*, 1865, 10 : 16. SLV copy inscribed by author to Sir Redmond Barry.

Copies: ML, SLV. 2173

———

Medical Society of Victoria. Annual Meeting. Wednesday, January 11, 1865. The valedictory address of the President ... [Text begins.]

209 × 132. Pp. 24 (l.b.). Colophon—Wilson and Mackinnon ...

On recent advances in medicine. From *Aust. Med. J.*, 1865, 10 : 40 and 70. SLV copy inscribed by author to Sir Redmond Barry.

Copies: ML, SLV. 2174

———

A paper read before the Medical Society of Victoria, Tuesday, August 7th 1866 ... On a case which recently formed the subject of inquiry in the Supreme Court, and in which the cause of death was variously accounted for by the medical witnesses. ... [Text begins.]

204 × 132. Pp. 22. (1866.) Colophon—Wilson

and Mackinnon . . .

Review of path. evidence in trials of J. G. Beaney for the murder of Mary Lewis. Criticises Crown med. evidence and holds that reasonable cause of death was not given. See Reeves, C. E., No 1776.

Copies: AMAV. 2175

———

Address of the President, Dr. D. J. Thomas, at the Eisteddfod, held at the Theatre in Ballarat, on the 25th of December, 1867. [Text begins.]

202 × 133. Pp. 8. Colophon—Stillwell and Knight . . . Melb.

Copies: AMAV, SLV. 2176

———

Medical Society of Victoria. The following paper was read . . . on the 10th of June. On the deposit of fat. By D. J. Thomas, M.D., F.R.C.S. . . . [Text begins.]

209 × 132. Pp. 8 (l.b.). Colophon—Stillwell and Knight . . . Melbourne. Repr., *Aust. med. J.*, 1868, 13 : 202.

For D. J. Thomas (1813–71) MD St And. & Melb., FRCS, Surg. Melb. Hosp., an outstanding figure in the medical history of Victoria and an Aust. pioneer of surgery and anaesthesia, see obit., *Aust. med. J.*, 1871, 16 : 187; Russell, K. F. (1948), 'The Royal Melb. Hosp. and its early surgeons', *Roy. Melb. Hosp. Clin. Rep.*, Centenary Vol.; O'Sullivan, D. M. (1956), 'D.J.T., a founder of Vic. medicine', *Med. J. Aust.* 1 : 1065 (with bibliog.).

Copies: AMAV, ML. 2177

———

Memoir of Dr. David John Thomas. (From "The Australian Medical Journal" of June, 1871.)

217 × 143. Pp. 8. Cover title within black rules. Colophon—Stillwell and Knight . . . Melbourne. Author: J. E. Neild.

Copies: KFR, UM. 2178

Thomas, John

(No. 5.) Odology: An antidote to spiritualism, being an analysis of the claims of spirit rapping. By John Thomas, M.D. [Text begins.]

204 × 132. Pp. 16 (l.b.). (1869.) Colophon— . . . A. R. Ford, at St Kilda Advertiser Office . . .

Copies: ML. SLV. 2179

Thomas, John Davies

A consideration of the respective merits of chloroform and vinic ether as general anaesthetics. . . . Resident Surgeon of the Clunes District Hospital . . . (Read before the Medical Society of Victoria, May 1875).

217 × 140. Pp. 24 (l.b.). Cover title. Colophon—Stillwell and Knight, Printers . . . Repr., *Aust. med. J.*, 1875, 20 : 375.

Considers ether safer and more convenient than chloroform.

For further paper: 'Questioning the preference shown by British surgeons for chloroform', *Aust. med. J.*, 1876, 21 : 13.

Copies: AMAV, DOS, EF, ML, UA. 2180

———

From the Australian Medical Journal, November, 1875. Ether and chloroform as anaesthetics. . . . [Text begins.]

200 × 128. Pp. 20. Colophon—Stillwell and Knight, Printers . . .

Copies: DOS. 2181

———

Hydatid disease of the lungs. . . . Adelaide: Frearson's Printing House . . . 1884.

217 × 138. Pp. 90 (last—colophon). 3 pl. Errata slip. P. w. (title rptd). Repr., *Proc. SA Branch BMA*, Sep. 1884.

Describes radical operation and reports 30 cases, of which 25 recovered—'a larger number than any other previous author.' Review, *Aust. med. J.*, 1884, ns 6 : 561.

Copies: LNSW, ML, SLS, UA, US. 2182

———

Hydatid Disease, with special reference to its prevalence in Australia . . . Adelaide: E. Spiller, Govt Printer . . . 1884.

214 × 138. Pp. [iv], vi, 220 (l.b.). 5 litho. pl. (titles on recto of interleaves), 1 graph, 88 figs. Errata slip. Cloth, or bound with No 2186, with covering title.

First work in English devoted wholly to hydatid disease. Deals with preventive aspects. Appendix describes experiments on development of worms in dogs, following ingestion of human material. Review, *Aust. med. J.*, 1884, ns 6 : 126.

Copies: AMAV, CC, DOS, EF, ML, MLWA, NL, RACP, RACS, SLS, SLV, UA, UM US. 2183

———

Echinococcus of the brain: hydatids of the brain. ... (Reprinted from Transactions of the Intercolonial Medical Congress, held in Adelaide, 1887.)

224 × 140. Pp. 36 (l.b.). P. w. (cover title). Reviews 97 published cases.

Copies: UA, US. 2184

———

The operative treatment of hydatid cysts of the liver and lungs. ... Melbourne: Stillwell & Co. Printers ... 1889.

206 × 135. Pp. [vi] (3 blanks), 112. P. w. (title rptd).

Advances 'evidence which has induced me to view with disfavour tapping, as a routine treatment for ... cysts of the internal organs, and to adopt ... direct incision of the sac ...'

Copies: AMAV, UA, US. 2185

———

Hydatid Disease, Vol. 11. By the late John Davies Thomas, M.D. (Lond.) ... A collection of papers on hydatid disease. Edited and arranged by Alfred Austin Lendon, M.D. (Lond.) ... Sydney: L. Bruck ... London: Bailliere, Tindall, & Cox ... 1894.

212 × 135. Pp. xii (ii, iv blank), 166, [ii] (colophon only, on verso). Cloth; or bound with No 2183, with covering title.

On clinical aspects and operative treatment. Review, *Aust. med. J.*, 1894, ns 16 : 145.

Copies: AMAV, BG, CC, EF, KFR, ML, NL, RACP, RACS, SLS, UA, UM, US. 2186

———

Hydatid disease with special reference to its prevalence in Australia, by the late John Davies Thomas ... to which is added a collection of papers on hydatid disease, by the same author. Edited and arranged by Alfred Austin Lendon ... Sydney: L. Bruck ... London: Bailliere, Tindall, & Cox ... 1894.

212 × 135. Title (v.b.) of vol. containing Nos 2183 and 2186. Cloth.

For John Davies Thomas (1844–1893) MD Lond., FRCS, Hon. Phys. Adel. Hosp., original worker on hydatid disease and author of first Aust. contribution on biliary tract surgery (1888), see obits, *Aust. med. J.*, 1893, ns 15 : 90, *Austn med. Gaz.*, 1893, 12 : 66; also Graham, H. B. (1953), *Med. J. Aust.*, 1 : 869 for hydatid studies; Gandevia, B. (1952), *Roy. Melb. Hosp. Clin. Reps*, 22 : 19 for biliary surg. UA has 12 vols of author's ms. notes on hydatid disease.

Copies: AMAV, BG, EF, KFR, ML, RACP, SLS, SLV, UA, UM, UQ, US. 2187

———

In memoriam. [Cross] John Davies Thomas, M.D. (Lond.), F.R.C.S. (Eng.) Adelaide: W. K. Thomas & Co., Printers ... 1894.

180 × 120. Pp. 14. P. w. (title rptd).

Copies: SLS, UA. 2188

'Thomas, Julian'

See James, Stanley.

Thomas-Caraman, Ch.

See Caraman, Ch. Thomas—

Thomas Walker Convalescent Hospital, Concord, NSW

Opened Sep. 1893. 2 an. rep. noted in *Austsn med. Gaz.*, 1896, 15 : 187; an. rep. reviewed: *ibid*, 1897, 16 : 154. NS.

2189

Thomassen, E. S.

A biographical sketch of Nicholas de Miklouho Maclay, the explorer. Communicated to the Royal Geographical Society by E. S. Thomassen, F.R.G.S. Brisbane, 1882.

214 × 135. Pp. 46, viii. Colophon—G. & J. Black, Printers ... Brisbane. Flg map (New Guinea). P. w. (title rptd).

US copy has note on title p. by Margaret Miklouho Maclay.

Copies: ML, NL, SLV, US. 2190

Thompson, Sir Henry

Sir Henry Thompson, F.R.C.S. Eng. on cremation. From "The Argus" of March, 1874. [Text begins.]

214 × 140. Pp. 6. Colophon—Stillwell and Knight ... Melbourne.

Copies: ML. 2191

Thompson, John Ashburton

Free phosphorus in medicine: with special reference to its use in neuralgia: a contribution to materia medica and therapeutics. ... London: H. K. Lewis ... 1874.

220 × 138. Pp. xiv (l.b.), 276 (l.b.). Cloth.

Pharmacology and clinical application.

Copies: HDN. 2192

Concealed accidental haemorrhage. A paper presented to the Harveian Society of London. London: M'Gowan & Co. 1876.

183 × 120. Pp. 30.

Author had 'considerable reputation' as an obstetrician in London prior to departure for Australia, and was Councillor of the Obstet. Soc. of London.

Copies: EF. 2193

1885–6. New South Wales. Dengue fever. (Report of the Chief Medical Inspector to the Board of Health.) Presented to Parliament by Command. [Text begins.]

326 × 204. Pp. 6 (l.b.). Colophon—Sydney: Thomas Richards, Govt Pr—1885.

Dengue on ship from Fiji, with account of the disease.

Copies: HDN, LNSW, ML, NL, SLV. 2194

1885–6. Legislative Assembly. New South Wales. Report to the President of the Board of Health upon an outbreak of typhoid fever in the municipal district of Leichhardt, due to polluted milk. With an account of the state of certain dairies . . . and remarks upon the legislation necessary to protect the purity of public milk-supplies. . . . Sydney: Thomas Richards, Govt Printer. 1886.

324 × 212. Pp. 24. 1 flg pl., 1 graph, 1 flg map. P. w. (title rptd).

Reports milk-borne typhoid epidemic of 38 cases, with 5 deaths. Preface by H. N. MacLaurin, Pres. Board of Health, states this to be the first investigation of the kind in this country.

HDN copy inscribed: 'This outbreak led to passing of Dairy Supervision Act in 1886 . . .'

Copies: EF, HDN, LNSW, ML, NL, SPH, SLV. 2195

A report to the President of the Board of Health: containing photographs of a person suffering from variola discreta, and an account of the case; to which is added a clinical report and diagnosis of the five cases with which the outbreak of small-pox of 1884–5 began. . . . Sydney: Thomas Richards, Govt Printer. 1886.

377 × 270. Pp. [2] (v.b.), 6 (l.b.). 1 graph, 11 leaves each with 2 mounted photographs (v.b.), numbered I-XI. Paper boards or leather.

For instruction of doctors, since 'it was impossible to give these gentlemen an opportunity of examining the cases for themselves, since the patients were isolated in the Quarantine hospital-ship.' Photographs show stages of eruption from 3–25 days.

Copies: AMAV, AMAN, BG, EF, HDN, ML, NL, SLV, UA, UM, US. 2196

Sanitary Section of the Royal Society of New South Wales, October 19th, 1886. The late case of the M.M.S.S. 'Oceanien". [Text begins.]

326 × 204. Pp. 2. Single leaf. NI.

Another issue, 1887. Pp. 6 (l.b.). Syd: Charles Potter, Govt Pr.

Criticism of quarantine procedures for vessel in which smallpox occurred during voyage to Sydney.

Copies: ML, NL. 2197

Quarantine and small-pox. . . . [Read before the Sanitary Section of the Royal Society of N.S.W., 18 Oct., 1887.] [Text begins.]

209 × 135. Pp. 6. NI. P. w. (title rptd).

Copies: NL. 2198

1889. New South Wales. Report on an outbreak of fever at Balranald, caused by polluted water . . . Sydney: Charles Potter, Govt Printer. 1889.

331 × 214. Pp. 26 (l.b.). 2 flg maps.

Epidemic, probably due to pollution of river water, was responsible for 120 cases of typhoid, with 15 deaths, in a population of 670.

Copies: LNSW, ML, NL, SLV, SPH. 2199

A district hospital: its construction and cost. This pamphlet is published . . . with the view of assisting . . . in designing hospital buildings. It is not intended . . . to limit or stereotype the form which these buildings should take, or to prescribe the exact material or the degree of architectural embellishment, but to set out some general principles . . . F. Norton Manning, Medical Adviser to the Government. Sydney: Charles Potter, Govt Printer. 1890.

246 × 150. Pp. 12. 5 pl. (incl. 2 flg plans). P. w. (cover title). Author's name at head of p. 1; also 'Amended and reprinted . . . from a paper read before . . . the Royal Society, N.S.W., 12 July, 1887.'

Includes plans for hospital of 11 or 21 beds, constructed of iron, and costing £2000; photo. and details of Kiama Hosp.

Copies: HDN, LNSW, ML, SLV, UM. 2200

1890. Legislative Assembly. New South Wales. Epidemic of influenza. (Report on, in New South Wales during 1890.) ... [Text begins.]

331 × 212. Pp. 16 (l.b.). 1 flg map.

Based on replies to a questionnaire sent to all doctors in NSW.

Copies: EF, HDN, LNSW, ML, NL, SLV, SPH. 2201

A record of the sanitary state of New South Wales, on 31 December, 1887: ... Reprinted from the Transactions of the Intercolonial Medical Congress of Australasia, January, 1889. Sydney: Charles Potter, Govt Printer. 1890.

244 × 150. Pp. [iv] (ii, iv blank), 24 (l.b.).

Reprinted 'with important amendments and additions.' Includes: public health laws and administration, quarantine station, Coast Hosp., vaccination, water supply, sewerage, quarantine, infectious diseases, hosp. accommodation, med. practice, statistics.

Copies: ML, NL, UM. 2202

1890. Legislative Assembly. New South Wales. Typhoid fever. (Report by Board of Health on outbreak of, at Waverley and Randwick.) Ordered by the Legislative Assembly to be printed, 20 August, 1890. [Text begins.]

336 × 212. Pp. 14 (l.b.). 2 maps. Colophon—Charles Potter, Govt Pr—1890. Signed: J. Ashburton Thompson.

Milk-borne epidemic (112 cases, 9 deaths). It is stated that 'had the Municipal Council of Randwick properly carried out the provisions of the Dairies Act, and paid ordinary heed to the advice and admonition of the Board, the catastrophe which resulted in so much suffering and loss of life would not have occurred.'

Copies: EF, HDN, LNSW, ML, NL, SLV, SPH. 2203

Australasian maritime quarantine: theory and practice. By J. Ashburton Thompson ... Official Delegate of the Government of New South Wales to the International Congress of Hygiene and Demography, London, 1891. ... reprinted with ... additional notes ...

217 × 135. Pp. 12. Colophon—Syd.: Charles Potter, Govt Pr—1892. Stiff p. w. (Royal Arms and short title).

Copies: ML. 2204

Paper relating to the collection and disposal of night-soil in un-sewered municipal districts. [Text begins.]

320 × 206. Pp. 8. Colophon—Syd.: Charles Potter, Govt Pr—1892.

Copies: HDN, ML. 2205

1892. New South Wales. Epidemic of influenza. (Report on, in New South Wales during 1891.) [Text begins.]

331 × 212. Pp. 56. Colophon—Syd.: Charles Potter, Govt Pr—1892.

Final report on influenza epidemic of 1890–91. Appendices include: Bd of Health circular on influenza; Remarks on shearing shed fever (sometimes called fog-fever).

Copies: EF, HDN, LNSW, ML, NL, SLV, SPH. 2206

Australian Association for the Advancement of Science, Brisbane, 1895. Is leprosy a telluric disease? ... [Text begins.]

222 × 140. Pp. 12 (l.b.).

On epidemiology of leprosy.

Copies: NL. 2207

A contribution to the history of leprosy in Australia. ... London: Published by Macmillan & Co. ... Printed by Adlard & Son. 1897.

214 × 132. Pp. 238. 1 flg map. Cloth.

The Same. In *Prize essays on leprosy. Thompson. Cantlie.* Lond.: New Sydenham Soc., 1897.

Cook, C. E. (1927), *The epidemiology of leprosy in Aust.*, Canberra, states that Thompson's 'acute powers of observation and moderation in inference earned him a world-wide reputation as a leprologist.'

Copies: AMAQ, BG, DOS, EF, FC, HDN, ML, MLWA, NL, RACS, SLV, SLW, SPH, UM, US. 2208

———

. . . Department of Public Health, New South Wales. 1. Prevention of tuberculosis in cattle. 2. Application of the tuberculin test to the ox.

247 × 150. Pp. 24. Colophon—Syd.: William Applegate Gullick, Govt Pr—1898.

Copies: BG, ML. 2209

———

Leprosy in Hawaii: a critical inquiry . . . [Map of Molokai] Sydney: William Applegate Gullick, Govt Printer. 1898.

244 × 156. Pp. vi, [ii], 40. Frontis. P. w. (title rptd).

Copies: ML, US. 2210

———

On the history and prevalence of lepra in Australia. . . . Reprinted from the "Intercolonial Medical Journal of Australasia", February 1898. Melbourne: Stillwell and Co., Printers . . .

250 × 158. Pp. 12.

Copies: NL. 2211

———

Prevention of consumption (tuberculosis). The following suggestions for prevention . . . are published for general information and guidance. . . . [Text begins.]

355 × 250. Single leaf, v.b. Colophon—Syd.: William Applegate Gullick, Govt Pr—1899.

Copies: EF, ML. 2212

———

On the guidance of public effort towards the further prevention of consumption. An address . . . Medical Congress of Australasia . . . Brisbane, September 1899. . . . Reprinted from the 'Intercolonial Medical Journal of Australasia', October 20th, 1899. Melbourne: Stillwell and Co. . . . 1899.

244 × 153. Pp. 20. Stiff p. w. (cover title).

Copies: ML. 2213

———

1900. Legislative Assembly. New South Wales. Outbreak of plague at Sydney, 1900. (Report of the Chief Medical Officer on.) Ordered . . . to be printed, 4 December, 1900. [Text begins.]

336 × 214. Pp. 82 (l.b.). 5 pl., 1 flg chart, 1 flg map. Colophon—William Applegate Gullick, Govt Pr—1901. Signed: J. Ashburton Thompson.

First of a series of classical reports issued during the plague epidemic of 1900–9. Reports on 303 cases, with 103 deaths, occurring 19 Jan.–8 Aug. 1900. Includes bact. report by F. Tidswell.

For discussion of Thompson's (and Tidswell's) work on transmission and control during this epidemic, which gained world acknowledgement, see Hirst, L. B., *The conquest of plague*, Lond., 1953; also *Trans Roy. Soc. Trop. Med. & Hyg.*, 1925, 19 : 224.

For J. Ashburton Thompson (1846–1915) MD Brux., LRCP, MRCS, DPH Camb., administrator and epidemiologist, Pres. NSW Bd Health and head of Pub. Health Dept, see *Med. J. Aust.*, 1915, 2 : 307; Armstrong, W. G. (1925), *Health*, 3 : 97; Sutton, H. (1950), *J. Roy. San. Inst*, 70 : 73.

Copies: EF, HDN, ML, SLV. 2214

———

See also NSW—Board of Health.

——— **and Stayton, George H.**

1889. New South Wales. Legislative Council. Report . . . upon an outbreak of typhoid fever in the municipalities of Newtown and Macdonaldtown; with a description of the cause and modes of spread of this disease, and suggestions for its prevention . . . Sydney: Charles Potter, Govt Printer. 1889.

331 × 212. Pp. [ii] (v.b.), 28. 2 flg maps. P. w. (title rptd).

Information to support legislative action for metropolitan sewerage.

G. H. Stayton was Engineer, NSW Dept of Public Works.

Copies: BG, EF, HDN, ML, NL, SLV, SPH. 2215

Thompson, Rezin

The medical adviser: a full and plain treatise on the theory and practice of medicine. Especially adapted to family use. By Rezin Thompson, M.D. . . . Twentieth edition . . . Standard Publishing Company, Melbourne. 1884.

229 × 145. Pp. xxvi, [25]–1035. Title p. tipped in. Frontis., 14 pl.

Aust. issue of US work. 1 ed., Cincinatti, 1870.

Copies: AMAN. 2216

Thomson, J. Bruce

The psychology of criminals : a study.

204 × 140. Pp. 30. ND. (1871.) Colophon—... Gibbs, Shallard, and Co. ... Sydney. P. w. (title rptd). Repr., *J. Mental Sci.* 1870. Preface by F. Norton Manning.

Copies: DL, ML, NL, RACP. 2217

Thomson, Rev. John—Editor

See Franks, Lizzie.

Thomson, William

Not man, but man-like. A reply to "Not like man" of Professor of Anatomy in the University of Melbourne. ... (Reprinted with additions from "The Argus".)

210 × 130. Pp. 32 (l.b.). Frontis. ND. [?1863.]

Criticises anti-evolutionary pamphlet of Prof. G. B. Halford.

Copies: LNSW, SLV. 2218

———

Some points of interest in a medico-legal enquiry. Being a paper read before the Medical Society of Victoria. June 1863. ... Reprinted from the "Australian Medical Journal".

204 × 135. Pp. 24. Colophon—Wilson and Mackinnon ... Melb. P. w. (cover title).

Copies: NL. 2219

———

The development of the question. [Text begins.]

209 × 130. Op. 4. Double cols. ND.

Letter to *The Argus*, signed 'Opifer', opposes Halford's evidence against Huxley's views on evolution.

Copies: SLV. 2220

———

The transversalis pedis in the foot of the gorilla. ... (Read before the Medical Society of Victoria).

210 × 130. Pp. 18 (l.b.). P. w. (title rptd).

Supports Huxley in evolution controversy. Repr., *Aust. med. J.*, 1864.

Copies: LNSW, NL, SLV. 2221

———

The gorilla on its last legs. [Text begins.]

209 × 130. Pp. 4. Double cols. ND.

Letter signed 'Opifer', supporting theory of evolution.

Copies: SLV. 2222

———

Testimonials in favour of Mr. W. Thomson, South Yarra.

204 × 135. Pp. 12. ND. Colophon—Melb: Stillwell and Knight ...

SLV copy bears ms. note: 'Candidate for lectureship in Materia Medica.'

Copies: SLV. 2223

———

Consumption in Australia: a review. ... Reprinted from the "Medical and Surgical Review".

217 × 135. Pp. 32. Colophon—Fergusson and Moore ... Melb. ND. (1864.) P. w. (title rptd).

Unfavourable review of S. Dougan Bird's *On Australasian climates* (1863).

Copies: ML. 2224

———

On phthisis and the supposed influence of climate being an analysis of statistics of consumption in this part of Australia with remarks on the causes of the increase of that disease in Melbourne. ... Melbourne: Stillwell & Knight ... 1870.

221 × 138. Pp. 160. 1 flg map (coloured). Cloth.

Opposes theory that Aust. climate has especially favourable influence in preventing and arresting tuberculosis.

Copies: BG, EF, ML, NL, SLV, UA, UM. 2225

———

A consumptive voyage to the Medical Society. Melbourne: Fergusson & Moore, Printers ... 1870.

206 × 132. Pp. 16 (l.b.). P. w. (cover title). Repr., *The Age*.

Attacks Med. Soc. Vic. for its views on consumption, with reasons for his expulsion; evils of sending advanced phthisis patients to Aust.

Copies: SLV. 2226

———

Digest of the return ordered by the Legislative Council of all the deaths (2143) from phthisis in Melbourne and suburbs, during the years 1865–1869, and first half of 1870, forming a sequel to the essay on phthisis, etc. etc. ... Melbourne: Stillwell & Knight ... 1871.

222 × 140. Pp. [iv], 42. P. w. (title rptd).

Some copies lack leaf (iii, iv).

Further statistics in support of his disputed thesis that phthisis was highly prevalent in Victoria.

Copies: BG, DOS, EF, LNSW, ML, SLV, UA, UM. 2227

The appointment of a Lecturer on Materia Medica at the Melbourne University. To the Editor of the "Australian Medical Gazette". [Text begins.]

247 × 183. Pp. 4. Double cols. ND. (1871.) NI.

Not published in *Aust. med. Gaz.*, probably for legal reasons; apparently distributed with number of July 1871. AMAV and US copies are bound with journal for 1871. Former bears 'South Yarra, July 1871' in W. T.'s hand; latter pencilled initials.

On author's rejection for lectureship, attacking University authorities.

Copies: AMAV, US. 2228

Remarks on the introduction of diphtheria into Victoria. ... Melbourne: Stillwell and Knight ... 1872.

206 × 135. Pp. 28. Repr., *Aust. med. J.*, July 1872.

Recommends isolation, as in smallpox, the only contagious fever to which this had been applied.

Copies: AMAV, LNSW, ML, SLV. 2229

Ship yachts and full-power steamers.

165 × 102. Pp. 22. (1872.) Melb.: Fergusson and Moore ... P. w. (cover title).

Urges use of fast sailing vessels, rather than steamers, for passenger traffic on long voyages.

Copies: FC. 2230

On typhoid fever ... Melbourne George Robertson 1874.

260 × 168. Pp. [vi] (ii, vi blank), 7–214, [ii] (book notice, v.b.). Errata slip. Cloth.

Author's report to Board of Health (Vic.) on typhoid appeared in its 15th rep. (1874), with Board's conclusion that his case for contagiousness was suggestive but unproved—a decision here criticised.

Copies: BG, CC, DOS, EF, FF, ML, NL, RACS, SPH, UA, UM, US. 2231

The Same. 2 ed., 1874. Pp. [vi], 7–218 (l.b.), [ii] (v.b.). Errata slip. Cloth. Added text has circular dated 20 Jan. 1875.

Copies: EF, SLV. 2232

The Same. 3 ed., revised, 1878. Title: Typhoid fever its cause and extent in Melbourne based on the report ... Pp. [xxxvi], 348 (l.b.). Frontis. (graph), 1 flg table, 2 figs. Cloth.

Copies: BG, DOS, EF, ML, MLWA, NL, SLV, UA, UM, US. 2233

On the analogy of epizootic pleuro-pneumonia to epidemic measles. ... Melbourne: Stillwell and Knight ... 1874.

224 × 150. Pp. 40.

Suggests diseases identical.

Copies: BG, NL. 2234

Review. From "The Argus" of January 30, 1875. On typhoid fever. [Text begins.]

239 × 153. Pp. 4. Colophon—Stillwell and Knight ... [Melb.].

Ends: 'Mr. Thomson might ... abate these evils if he only combined a moderate amount of tact and temper, sobriety of language, self-restraint and conciliation, with his perfervid zeal and professional ability.'

Copies: EF. 2235

The histochemistry and pathology of tubercle ... Melbourne Stillwell & Knight ... 1876

210 × 134. Pp. 54 (2, 4 blank), [2] (book advt, v.b.).

Published before Koch's demonstration of tubercle bacillus (1882) and subsequent clarification of the pathology. The author states: 'The idea of micrococci being ... associated with ... tuberculosis is a recent one; and the explanation of their mode of operation is, at least, as far as I am aware, now for the first time in the history of pathology attempted ...'

For Thomson's views on relationship of organisms to tuberculosis see Gandevia, B. (1953), *Med. J. Aust.*, 1 : 398.

Copies: BG, CC, DOS, LNSW, ML, NL, SLV. 2236

A third analysis of the statistics of phthisis in Victoria completing the series to which are prefixed remarks on one of the modern modes of medical treatment ... Melbourne Stillwell & Knight ... 1876

212 × 139. Pp. [ix] (4 blanks), x–xii, 96 (last—book notice). P. w. (title rptd).

Copies: BG, EF, ML, NL, SLV. 2237

A third analysis of the statistics of phthisis in Victoria ... Melbourne Stillwell & Knight ... 1877

209 × 139. Pp. [iv] (ii, iv blank), 58 (l.b.).

As item above, omitting section on treatment.

Copies: BG, LNSW, NL. 2238

On phthisis and the supposed influence of climate being a fourth fasciculus of statistics of consumption in this part of Australia shewing the steady increase of that disease in Melbourne. ... Melbourne: Stillwell & Knight ... 1877.

210 × 139. Pp. 18 (2 blank).

Copies: BG, DOS. 2239

On phthisis and the supposed influence of climate being an analysis of statistics of consumption in this part of Australia with remarks on the cause of the increase of that disease in Melbourne ... [Quotation] Melbourne Stillwell and Co. 1879

224 × 145. Pp. xii (ii, iv blank), 124 (l.b.). P. w. (title rptd, quotation on v. of back wrapper), or cloth. Some copies have pp. ix, x cancelled and revised leaf inserted.

Though often regarded as 2 ed. of No 2225 above, from similarity of titles ('cause' for 'causes' and author's qualifications the main variations), this is an entirely different work.

Author's copy, bound with his other works on phthisis, is in Gandevia coll.

Copies: BG, EF, NL, SLV. 2240

"The Lancet" review of Mr. Thomson's report on typhoid fever, Melbourne. First notice. (June 14th, 1879.)

213 × 133. Pp. 30 (last—colophon), [2] ('Times' letter of 12 May 1879, book notice on verso).

Copies: AMAV, BG, CC, NL. 2241

Remarks on a review of the report on the cause & extent of typhoid fever in Melbourne ... George Robertson Melbourne, Sydney and Adelaide 1879

218 × 143. Pp. 80. P. w. (title rptd, quotations on back); or bound with *Typhoid fever*, 3 ed. (1878). Cloth.

Following variations occur: pp. 80; pp. 80, [ii] (v.b.); pp. 80, [ii] (v.b.), viii.

Copies: AMAV, BG, DOS, EF, ML, NL, SLS, SLV, UA, UM, US. 2242

Typhoid fever in Melbourne in 1878. [Text begins.]

208 × 136. Pp. viii. Colophon—Stillwell and Co. ... ND. (1879.)

Issued separately, or as addendum to *Remarks on a review of the Report* (1879).

Copies: AMAV, DOS, EF, LNSW, NL, SLV, UA. 2243

Sir, In the hope and belief that you feel interested in discussing the feasibility of quite destroying every germ of typhoid fever in Melbourne, where ... the rate of sickness and mortality is greater than any city, town or district of Great Britain, a few remarks ... [Text continues.] William Thomson. South Yarra, September 1879.

188 × 115. Single leaf, v.b. NI.

Copies: AMAV. 2244

Excerpts from The abolition of zymotic diseases and of other similar enemies of mankind. By Sir Thomas Watson, Bart., M.D., F.R.S. London: C. Kegan Paul & Co. ... 1879.

218 × 145. Pp. 12 (last—colophon). Colophon—Printed for private circulation, by Stillwell and Co., Melb.

Cites Thomson on typhoid.

Copies: BG, SLV. 2245

Contagion alone the cause of typhoid fever in Melbourne ... [Quotation] Melbourne Stillwell and Co. 1880.

228 × 148. Pp. 22 (2 blank), [2] (book notice, v.b.). P. w. (title rptd).

Copies: BG, FC, LNSW, ML, SLV, UM. 2246

A ten years' retrospect of phthisis in Victoria. [Text begins.]

224 × 147. Pp. 24 (l.b.). No title p. ND. (1880.) Colophon—Stillwell and Co. . . .

Emphasises role of bacteria in the disease. This is 'no mere scientific curiosity, but a practical rule guiding the means of preventing phthisis . . .'

Copies: ML, SLS. 2247

Bacon and Shakespeare on vivisection In reply to Dean Plumptre Controversies in religion hinder the progress of science Melbourne: Sands & McDougall 1881

223 × 137. Pp. [ii], 1–3, [ii], 4–40 (l.b.). P. w. (title rptd).

Thomson was an ardent supporter of the theory that Bacon wrote the Shakespearian works, and developed this in the following: *The political purpose of the Renascence drama*, (by Cerimon), Melb., 1878; *On Renascence drama*, Melb., 1880; *William Shakespeare in romance and reality*, Melb., 1881; *Bacon, not Shakespeare*, Melb., 1881 (2 issues); *The political allegories in the Renascence drama of Francis Bacon*, Melb., 1882; *A minute among the amenities*, Melb., 1883.

Copies: FC, ML, NL, RACS, SLS, SLV, UA. 2248

The "Lancet" & The "Argus" on typhoid fever in Melbourne . . . Melbourne: Sands & McDougall 1882

225 × 150. Pp. 32. Flg graph. P. w. (title rptd, press extracts inside back wrapper).

The Same, with new title: "*Lancet and Argus*" . . . Pp. 32.

The Same, 1882. Pp. 50. Also pp. 52 (added postscript).

Further ed., 1882, with the title: *Typhoid fever in Melbourne*. (Item below.)

Reply to *Argus* accusation of 'spreading false reports about the extent of typhoid fever in Melbourne.'

Copies: BG, ML, NL, SLV, UM. 2249

Typhoid fever in Melbourne . . . [Quotation] Melbourne: Sands & McDougall 1882

228 × 140. Pp. 32. P. w. (title rptd, press notices inside back wrapper).

Re-titled ed. of *The "Lancet" & The "Argus"* (above). Though varied, text literally follows enlarged ed. of latter in great part.

Copies: BG, ML. 2250

Typhoid fever at Whittlesea stopped and the poisoning of the Yan Yean reservoir with all its consequences prevented . . . Melbourne: Sands & McDougall 1882

209 × 136. Pp. 20 (2 blank).

Copies: SLV. 2251

The germ origin of tubercle illustrated from the history of phthisis in Victoria . . . Melbourne: Stillwell and Co. 1882

221 × 142. Pp. [iv] (ii, iv blank), 132. P. w. (title rptd).

Following Koch's announcement of discovery of the tubercle bacillus in 1882, author claims priority for his *Histochemistry and pathogeny of tubercle* (1876) as the pioneer work on the germ theory of tuberculosis.

Copies: AMAV, LNSW, ML, NL, SLV. 2252

The germ theory of phthisis verified and illustrated by the increase of phthisis in Victoria. . . . Melbourne: Sands & McDougall 1882

226 × 139. Pp. 96. P. w. (title rptd).

Similar in content to *The germ origin of tubercle* (above) and could be regarded as another ed.

Copies: AMAV, ML. 2253

For private circulation. [The Journal of Science: London, December, 1882.] The germ theory and its latest conquest. [Text begins.]

210 × 133. Pp. 16.

Reprints review of *The germ theory of phthisis verified* . . . (1882), which gives priority to Thomson for his thesis on the bacterial origin of tuberculosis, published 1876.

Copies: ML. 2254

The germ theory of disease applied to eradicate phthisis from Victoria . . . Melbourne: Sands & McDougall 1882

240 × 218. Pp. 78 (l.b.). P. w. (title rptd).

Urges 'adoption of the germ theory of phthisis, in its application to the immediate control and eventual eradication . . .'

Copies: ML, SLV. 2255

A very "startling novelty" in current medical literature. To the Editor of the Age [Text begins.]

289 × 201. Single leaf, v.b. Double cols. ND.

Letter signed 'Asclepiades', criticising local ignorance of contagiousness of tuberculosis.

Copies: SLV. 2256

(From the Melbourne Herald). It is only when fell disease knocks at our doors, and that the weekly bills of mortality swell inordinately . . . [Text continues.]

230 × 150. Pp. 4. ND. NI.

Reprints article on typhoid outbreak at Hamilton.

Copies: SLV. 2257

"Figuring in the newspapers". [Text begins.]

207 × 133. Pp. 8. (1883.) NI.

Strong rejoinder to criticisms of certain works of author, which were among the most vituperative of the time.

Copies: ML. 2258

The Freeman's Journal. Dublin: Wednesday, Nov. 23. [Text begins.]

232 × 147. Pp. 4. ND. NI.

Includes article on two pamphlets by Thomson. H. Boyd Graham regards this as Thomson's last publication. Concludes: 'So now my work does cease, I'll break my staff, drown my book, retire to my cell, and requite all readers with a welcome.'

William Thomson (1819–83) FRCSE, FLS, a fervent advocate of contagionist doctrine and germ theory of disease, engaged in vivid controversy on these and other subjects. His ultimate influence was great, but the enmity roused caused him to receive scant acknowledgment in his day. See obit., *Aust. med. J.*, 1883, ns 5 : 315; also Gandevia, B. (1953), 'W. T. and the history of the contagionist doctrine in Melb.', *Med. J. Aust.*, 1 : 398; Ford, E. (1954), *Bibliog of W. T.*, Syd.

Copies: H. Boyd Graham, Melb. 2259

Tichborne Case

1878. Legislative Assembly. New South Wales. William Creswell. (Correspondence, minutes, &c.) . . . [Text begins.]

326 × 209. Pp. 28 (l.b.). Colophon—Syd.: Thomas Richards, Govt Pr—1878.

Arthur Orton, who under the name of Castro had settled in Wagga NSW in the 1860s, claimed to be Sir Roger Tichborne, lost heir to the Tichborne estate, brought suit in England (1871–2), and was proved an imposter. Partisans later claimed that Wm Creswell, patient in Parramatta Lunatic Asylum, was Orton and pressed for his transfer to England 'to obtain justice for the imprisoned Sir Roger.' Local enquiries confirm Creswell's identity.

Copies: LNSW, ML, NL, SLV. 2260

Tichborne trial. Startling affidavit of Lady Tichborne, mother of Sir Roger Tichborne, now a prisoner in Portsea Gaol, whom she unmistakeably recognized as her long lost son. All persons desirous of seeing justice done . . . should read this pamphlet. Price threepence. The proceeds to be devoted towards repaying the expenses of taking Arthur Orton, now a lunatic in the Parramatta Asylum, to England, so that Sir Roger Tichborne's identity may be clearly established. Published by Daniel Smith, of London, now of . . . Castlereagh-street, Redfern, and printed by James Miller & Co. . . . Sydney.

8vo. Pp. 10, [2] (advt). Cover title. ND. [1883.]

Copies: FC. 2261

Twenty-three letters . . . (published by the "National Independent" from June to November, 1886). Proving on medical evidence that the Parramatta lunatic is Arthur Orton. . . . To be had of G.B., Elm Dean, Surbiton. . . .

183 × 122. Pp. 32. [?1886.] Colophon—H. Blacklock & Co. . . . London, E. C. P. w. (cover title, preface on verso).

Supporter of Tichborne claimant (Georgiana Baring) attempts to prove, from certificates of Australian doctors, that Wm Creswell is Orton.

Copies: DL. 2262

1899. (Third Session.) Legislative Assembly. New South Wales. Progress Report from the Select Committee of case of William Creswell . . . and minutes of evidence. . . . Sydney: William

Applegate Gullick, Govt Printer. 1900.
330 × 210. Pp. 30 (l.b.).
Includes medical evidence of identity.
Copies: LNSW, ML, NL, SLV. 2263

Tidswell, Frank

1895. Legislative Assembly. New South Wales. Antitoxic serum for the cure of diphtheria. (Report by Board of Health.) . . . [Text begins.]
336 × 212. Pp. 20 (l.b.).
Results of first diphtheria anti-toxin used in NSW.
Copies: EF, HDN, LNSW, ML, NL, SLV, SPH. 2264

1896. Legislative Assembly. New South Wales. Insanitary state of the town of Parkes. (Return respecting.) Printed . . . 18 June, 1896. [Text begins.]
331 × 212. Pp. 8.
On the prevalence of typhoid and unhealthy state of town.
Copies: HDN, LNSW, ML, NL, SLV. 2265

1896. Legislative Assembly. New South Wales. Insanitary state of the town of Forbes. (Report on.) Printed . . . 6 August, 1896. [Text begins.]
331 × 212. Pp. 4 (l.b.). Colophon—Syd.: Charles Potter, Govt Pr—1896. Signed: Frank Tidswell.
Copies: HDN, ML, NL, SLV. 2266

A brief sketch of the history of small-pox and vaccination in New South Wales . . . Read before the Australasian Association for the Advancement of Science . . . 1898.
212 × 140. Pp. 8. Colophon—Syd. . . . Govt Pr—1899. P. w. (cover title).
Reprinted in Cumpston, J.H.L. (1914), *The history of small-pox in Aust., 1788–1908*, Melb.
Copies: NL. 2267

1899. Legislative Assembly. New South Wales. Department of Public Health. Report on protective inoculation against tick fever. An account of an experimental inquiry into its effect on cattle, and on meat and milk; together with some notes on protective measures other than inoculation. . . . Sydney: William Applegate Gullick, Govt Printer. 1899. . . .
339 × 214. Pp. [ii] (v.b.), [ii], 16. P. w. (title rptd).
Copies: EF, HDN, ML, NL, SLV, SPH. 2268

Department of Agriculture, Sydney . . . Miscellaneous Publication, No. 321. Some further observations on protective inoculation against tick-fever. Sydney: William Applegate Gullick, Govt Printer. 1899.
273 × 255. Pp. [ii] (v.b.), 16. P. w. (title rptd).
Includes report by J. Sydney Hunt.
Copies: ML. 2269

New South Wales. Department of Public Health. Second report on protective inoculation against tick fever. An account of an experimental inquiry concerning the protective value of inoculation; together with some observations upon cattle ticks and upon the practice of inoculation. . . . Sydney: William Applegate Gullick, Govt Printer. 1900.
336 × 212. Pp. 18 (l.b.). P. w. (title rptd).
Copies BG, EF, HDN, ML, NL, SPH. 2270

On plague and its dissemination . . . An address . . . Reprinted from "The Australasian Medical Gazette", May 21, 1900. Sydney: John Sands . . . 1900.
236 × 183. Pp. 12 (l.b.). Double cols. P. w. (cover title).
Includes role of rat and flea.
For Frank Tidswell (d. 1941) MB, ChM Syd., DPH Camb., founder and Director of Govt Bureau of Microbiology, Syd., see obit., *Med. J. Aust.*, 1941, 1 : 594; also Hirst, L. F. (1953), *The conquest of plague*, Oxford, for his first confirmation of the disputed role of fleas in plague transmission, which 'opened a new and important chapter.'
Copies: EF, ML. 2271

The Same. 214 × 140. Pp. [ii] (v.b.), 40. 3 pl. Syd., Govt Pr, 1900. Stiff p. w. (title rptd).
Copies: EF, ML, NL. 2272

See also Thompson, John A., No 2214; NSW—Bd of Health, No 1505.

——— **and Dick, James Adam**

Bubonic plague in 1141 B.C. ... Reprinted from "The Australasian Medical Gazette", October 20, 1899. Sydney: John Sands ... 1899.

244 × 158. Pp. 8 (l.b.). P. w. (title rptd).

Identifies Biblical epidemic among the Philistines (*Samuel* 1) as bubonic plague.

J. A. Dick (d. 1943) MD Edin., FRCSE, practised at Randwick NSW. Obit.: *Med. J. Aust.*, 1943, 1 : 289.

Copies: ML, NL, US. 2273

———

The Same, with variation in title. Pp. 8 (l.b.). Title at head p.1. ND. NI. Repr., *Trans Intercol Med. Cong. Austsia*, 1899.

Copies: CC, EF, NL. 2274

Tiffin, C.

The Queensland Philosophical Society. (From the *Queensland Guardian*, August 29, 1866.) [Text begins.]

217 × 138. Pp. 4. Double cols. Colophon— . . . 'Guardian Office', Bris.

'On the use of earth closets as a means of preventing the vitiation of the air.' Advocates for Brisbane, where heavy rains fill cesspits.

Copies: FC. 2275

———

Ventilation. A paper on the ventilation of buildings, read ... before the Queensland Philosophical Society ... at ... the Brisbane Hospital. [Text begins.]

217 × 138. Pp. 6. Double cols. (1869.) Colophon—W. C. Belbridge ... Bris.

Expounds miasmatic theory of disease, with reference to Brisbane.

Copies: FC. 2276

Tomlins, P. Stanley

The Coroner's Guide. A summary of the duties, powers & liabilities of coroners from the most approved authorities by P. S. Tomlins. Chief Clerk of Police. V. D. Land. 1837.

Manuscript. 161 × 100. Pp. 104.

Printed copy not seen. Publication announced in *Hobart Town Courier*, Dec. 1837, as ready for delivery the following Monday at the *Courier* Office—Price 10s. (Ferguson, 2 : 2250a, where author's name appears as Tomkins.) Above title is from a finely written ms. in ML, probably copy of the printed work. Text begins at p. 5 with : 'General outline of the duties, powers and liabilities of Coroners as applicable to Van Diemen's Land, &c.'

Copies: ML (ms.). 2277

Tomlins, William Henry

The Droitwich brine baths as therapeutic agents in various diseases. London: H. K. Lewis, 1895.

NS. Listed in *SGC* (Ser. 2). 8vo. Pp. 22.

W. H. Tomlins MRCS (1884), late Ballina Dist. Hosp., was in practice at Alstonville NSW in 1911. 2277a

Toowoomba Asylum for the Insane, Qd

See Goodna, Ipswich and Toowoomba Asylums.

Toowoomba Hospital, Qd

Toowoomba Hospital rules [Text begins.]

204 × 127. Pp. 8. Colophon—Printed at the "Darling Downs Gazette" Office. 1871.

Copies: FC. 2278

Topinard, Paul

Étude sur les races indigènes de l'Australie par le Docteur Paul Topinard ... Paris Typographie A. Hennuyer ... 1872

220 × 140. Pp. 120. P. w. (title rptd).

Includes physical characters, fertility, causes of depopulation.

Copies: FC, ML, NL, OL, SLT, SLV, SLW, US. 2279

Towle, William Bentley

The sexual system in health and disease 11th edition [Cut of premises] Illustrated with 19 wood engravings Reviewed by Dr. W. B. Towle ... Sydney.

178 × 120. Pp. xvi, 164. 19 figs. ND. (c. 1897.) Limp cloth.

Sexual diseases, electricity in their therapy. Advertises author's practice.

W. B. Towle MD, ChM Montreal, practised at Gympie Qd in 1896, and later in Sydney, where he died, aged 43, in 1898.

Copies: ML. 2280

Tracy, Richard Thomas

University of Melbourne. Inaugural lecture of the course on obstetrics and diseases of women and children. ... (Delivered ... March 9, 1865.) [Text begins.]

204 × 127. Pp. 12. From *Aust. med. J.*, 1865, 10 : 113.

Copies: UM. 2281

[Emblem] . . . Nov. 27, 1874 . . . Catalogue of the library of medical and general literature and surgical instruments, the property of the late Dr. Tracy . . . Gemmell, Tuckett & Co. . . . Mason, Firth and M'Cutcheon . . . Melbourne.

204 × 125. Pp. 10, [2] (colophon, v.b.).

For R. T. Tracy (1826–74) MD Glas., LRCPI, first Aust. obstet. specialist, a founder of Melb. Lying-in Hosp., 'the brightest name in the history of ovariotomy in these Colonies', see obits, *Aust. med. J.*, 1874, 19 : 364 and *NSW med. Gaz.*, 1875, 5 : 97; also Forster, F.M.C. (1964), 'R.T.T. and his part in the history of ovariotomy', *Aust. NZ J. Obst. Gynaec.*, 4 : 128; Forster, F.M.C. (1967), *Progress in obstetrics and gynaecology in Aust.*, Syd.

Copies: SLV. 2282

Trotter, Thomas

Medical and chemical essays. Containing [Contents follow in double cols] additional observations on scurvy . . . Communications from New South Wales, on scurvy, and other interesting subjects. . . . Thoughts on the decomposition of water, and a method of preserving it pure and sweet in long voyages . . . By Thomas Trotter, M.D., Physician to His Majesty's Fleet under the command of Admiral Richard Lord Howe. The second edition. . . . London: Printed for J. S. Jordan . . . 1796.

214 × 130. Pp. [iv] (3 blanks), 5–156 (l.b.).

Includes letter of Edward Laing, Surgeon, Sydney, Dec. 1792 (pp. 64–105), describing voyage of transport *Pitt*, Eng. to VDL, 17 July 1791–14 Feb. 1792, with 600 aboard, and occurrence of smallpox, remittent fever and scurvy. (*HRNSW*, 2 : 459 shows 49 deaths.) Health and climate in NSW are described, and local antiscorbutics etc. mentioned.

Edward Laing, Surgeon's Mate to NSW Corps, acted as Asst Col Surg. in NSW for a time; returned to England Dec. 1794.

Copies: ML. 2283

True Copy of the Depositions (Case of Susan Nixon)

See Bruck, Ludwig.

'Truth'

See [Wilmot, Dr.].

Tryon, Henry

Plants poisonous to stock. A review: . . . Brisbane: . . . Warwick & Sapsford . . . 1887.

244 × 153. Pp. 8. Double cols.

Review of Bailey, F. M. and Gordon, P. R. (1887), *Plants reputed poisonous and injurious to stock* (No 121).

Copies: ML. 2283a

Tucker, George Alfred

Testimonials presented to George A. Tucker, late partner and superintendent of the Cremorne Private Lunatic Asylum, Melbourne. [Text begins.]

255 × 198. Pp. 4 (l.b.). ND. (1865.) Colophon —Clarson, Shallard, & Co. . . . Melb.

Testimonials (dated 1865), also extracts from visitors' book of Cremorne Asylum.

Copies: SLV. 2284

A treatise on psychology, insanity, and medicine . . . by G. A. Tucker, M.D. Sydney: Gibbs, Shallard, and Co. . . . 1872.

217 × 135. Pp. 36 (l.b.). P. w. (shortened title).

According to *Austsn med. Gaz.*, 1883, 2 : 184, author was PhD. MD was not used in subsequent publications.

Copies: LNSW, ML, SLV. 2285

The Gheel Lunatic Colony. . . . Birmingham: Cornish Brothers . . . 1884.

217 × 138. Pp. vi (l.b.), 20 (last—emblem). P. w. (title rptd).

Belgian method of mental care, by distributing patients among local residents, is severely criticised. For review, see Weale, J. Cyril M.

Copies: NL. 2286

Lunacy in many lands. Being an introduction to the reports on the lunatic asylums of various countries, visited in 1882–5, by G. A. Tucker, and presented by him to the Government of New South Wales . . .

214 × 138. Pp. [ii] (v.b.), 136. 1 engr. pl., 1 coloured litho. flg pl. NI. ND. (Birmingham, 1855.) Paper boards or cloth.

Copies: EF, ML, NL, SLV. 2287

1885–6. Legislative Assembly. New South Wales. Hospitals for the Insane. (Report of Dr. Tucker on the hospitals for the insane visited by him, under the circular letter of the Colonial Secretary ...) Ordered ... to be printed, 16 February, 1886. [Text follows.]

331 × 204. Pp. 40. Colophon—Syd.: Thomas Richards, Govt Pr—1886.

Dr. J.H.L. Cumpston notes that, according to accounts of the time, author complained of the heavy abridgement of his report herein. Unaware of its bulk and over-ruling his advisers, Premier ordered full printing of the massive work below.

Copies: LNSW, ML, NL, SLV. 2288

———

Lunacy in many lands ... Sydney: Charles Potter, Govt Printer. 1887.

236 × 153. Pp. xvi, 1564. 17 pl., 2 figs. Cloth, leather spine.

Detailed information on mental instns, from world survey. Claimed by author to be the most comprehensive report of its kind ever issued.

Author was associated with J. T. Harcourt *(q.v.)* at his Harbury House private mental home at Pascoe Vale Vic. and Cremorne Asylum at Richmond Vic. In 1865 he established Bay View Lunatic Asylum at Cook's River NSW. See also Bay View Hosp.

Copies: EF, HDN, ML, NL, SLV, UQ, US. 2289

Tuckett, Frederick

Do not emigrate, until you can possess that portion of the land which should be your's. Being a few remarks on the sufferings of emigrants in ships and colonies; addressed to the people. ... London: Charles Gilpin ... Edinburgh: A. and C. Black. Dublin: J. B. Gilpin. 1850. ...

214 × 132. Pp. 16, 4. P. w. (cover title).

Attacks conditions, inadequate for health, comfort and decency, existing in emigrant ships. Conditions in the colonies, and 'the suffering and murder of natives in countries colonised by the British' are also discussed.

Author travelled in NSW, Port Phillip and SA in 1845.

Copies: CC, ML. 2290

Tuckey, James Hingston

An account of a voyage to establish a colony at Port Philip in Bass's Strait, on the south coast of New South Wales, in His Majesty's Ship Calcutta, in the years 1802–3–4. By J. H. Tuckey, Esq. first lieutenant of the Calcutta. ... London: Printed for Longman, Hurst, Rees, and Orme ... and J. C. Motley, Portsmouth. 1805.

222 × 135. Pp. xvi (last—errata), 240 (last—book advts). Paper boards.

Includes observations on convict transport and means of preserving health on voyage (pp. 231–39).

Copies: DL, FC, ML, NL, SLV, UA, US, WLC. 2291

Tumut Cottage Hospital, NSW

Rules of the Tumut Cottage Hospital. Adopted in February 14, 1900. Tumut: S. Groves, Printer, "Times" Office ...

193 × 122. Pp. 8. P. w. (cover title).

Hospital opened 1900. Minute book (1898–1905) in ML.

Copies: ML. 2292

Turkish Bathing

Health is happiness. Turkish bathing; by various authors. Edited by R.N.H. An appeal to the sensible. Melbourne: Turkish Bathing Establishment, Royal Arcade. ... 1870.

186 × 117. Pp. 38.

Includes section on medical value, with testimonials from Melb. doctors.

Copies: SLV. 2293

Turnbull, Adam

Letter, Adam Turnbull, M.D., Clerk of the Council, Van Diemen's Land, to the Secretary of State for the Colonies, London. And appendix.

204 × 122. Pp. 34. ND. (c. 1853). Colophon—Dumfries: Printed at the Courier Office ... P. w. (cover title).

Author defends his resignation from Leg. Council in protest against continuance of transportation, for which he was dismissed from official posts.

Adam Turnbull (b. 1803) MD Edin., settled in Hobart in 1825, farmed and practised there, and subsequently became Sec. to Governors Franklin and Wilmot. He later entered the Presbyterian ministry. See Mackay, E. A. (1934), 'Med. men as pastoral pioneers', *Med. J. Aust.*, 2 : 476.

Copies: ML. 2294

Turnbull, William Mackie

Testimonials in favour of Dr. William Mackie Turnbull, Licentiate of the Royal College of Surgeons, Edinburgh ...

193 × 125. Pp. 12 (l.b.). ND. NI.

Letters from Edin. teachers, dated 1841.
Copies: ML. 2295

To the subscribers of the Melbourne Lying-In Hospital.
209 × 130. Pp. 16 (l.b.). ND. (?1861.)
Disagrees with memorial complaining of non-admission of a single girl of disorderly life.
For W. M. Turnbull MD Edin. & Melb., Hon. Phys. to Lying-in Hosp., Melb., see obit., *Aust. med. J.*, 1867, 12 : 312.
Copies: SLV. 2296

To the Ladies' and Gentlemen's Committees of the Melbourne Lying-in Hospital. [Text begins.]
339 × 212. Pp. [2]. Blue paper. 14 March 1863. NI. Signed at foot.
Protest against establishment of an outdoor wet nursing service, in which women delivered at Hospital, would be maintained as visiting nurses.
Copies: Royal Women's Hosp., Melb. 2297

Turner, Alfred Jefferis and Ashworth, Louis Naish
The value of antitoxin in the treatment of diphtheria. By A. Jefferis Turner ... and L. N. Ashworth ... [Text begins.]
247 × 153. Pp. 36. Repr., *Intercol med. J. Austsia*, 1896.
For A. J. Turner (1861–1947) MD Lond., DPH Camb., paediatrician and entomologist of Brisbane, see obit., *Med. J. Aust.*, 1948, 1 : 517; Mackerras, I. M. (1949), *Proc. Roy. Soc. Qd*, 60 : 69 (with bibliog.)
Copies: ML. 2298

Turner, Duncan
A manual of diet for the invalid and dyspeptic, with a few hints on nursing. Second edition. London: J. Churchill & Sons. 1870.
NS. Listed *SGC*, ser. 1. 8vo. Pp. 96. 2299

Notes on the treatment of typhoid fever ... Melbourne: Stillwell and Co. Printers. 1883.
220 × 143. Pp. 62 (l.b.). P. w. (title rptd).
Copies: AMAV, NL, UM. 2300

The Same. Another ed., 1884. Pp. 50 (l.b.). Melb.: Samuel Mullen. Cloth.
Copies: ML, SLV. 2301

The Same. 2 ed. 1895. Pp. [ii], [4], 5–100. Melb.: Melville, Mullen and Slade. Cloth.
Copies: SLV, UM. 2302

Air and diet in chronic chest diseases ... Melbourne: Melville, Mullen & Slade ... 1893.
183 × 122. Pp. viii, 80 (l.b.). P. w. (title rptd), or cloth.
UM copy has author's inscription and a few ms. corrections; EF copy, pencilled amendments.
Copies: AMAV, EF, ML, NL, SLV, UM. 2303

The Same. 2 ed., 1896. Melb., George Robertson & Co. Pp. xii, 146, [ii] (colophon, v.b.). Stiff p. w. or cloth.
Copies: CC, EF, ML, NL, SLV, UM. 2304

Is consumption contagious? ... Melbourne: Melville, Mullen & Slade ... 1894. ...
183 × 122. Pp. 54 (4 blank), [2] (book notice, v.b.). P. w. (title rptd).
Tuberculosis is not contagious and there is no danger from close contact with sufferers. He hopes to break down the 'unnecessary barrier between the healthy and afflicted.'
Also published: *A new treatment of consumption and other chronic chest diseases*, Melb., 1904.
For Duncan Turner (1839–1918) MRCP, Hon. Phys to Melb. Benev. Asylum, see obit., *Med J. Aust.*, 1918, 1 : 525.
Copies: ML. 2305

The Same. 2 ed., 1900, with title: *Consumption not contagious*. Melb.: George Robertson & Co. Pp. x (iv, l.b.), ii (v.b.), 5–104 (last—colophon only), [2] (advts, v.b.).
Copies: ML, SLS. 2306

Turner, Frederick
The supposed poisonous plants of Western Australia. By Fred. Turner, F.L.S., F.R.H.S., &c. (Read before the Australasian Association for the Advancement of Science ... January 10, 1898.) [Text begins.]
212 × 135. Pp. 10. Colophon—Syd.: William Applegate Gullick, Govt Pr—1899.
Copies: NL. 2307

U

Unbeliever in the 'Argus'
See Bowie, Robert, No 377.

Underwood, Charles
Antidote for the bite of snakes and other venomous reptiles. Price, ten shillings per bottle. ... The undersigned, being in possession of a certain antidote against the bites of snakes, and other venomous reptiles and insects, tested in various experiments during a period of twenty years, is desirous ... [Text continues.]

280 × 153. Single leaf, v.b. ND. (c. 1860.) Colophon—J. C. Hall & Co., Printers ... Hobart Town.

Wrapper for phial of Underwood's secret cure, with directions and testimonials dated 1850–59. For Underwood and his antidote: Crowther, W.E.L.H. (1956), *Med. J. Aust.*, 1 : 83. Underwood died after snake-bite, his agent stating that his antidote had been improperly applied, 'he being under the influence of liquor at the time' (*The Mercury*, 29 Jan. 1881). But Dr. L. Gray Thompson (*ibid*, 19 Feb. 1881) states that the snake was harmless, and death due to heat apoplexy.

Copies: Roy. Soc. Tas. 2308

University of Adelaide
Adelaide Medical School, third Australian foundation, was established in 1885. For history: Lendon, A. A., *Jubilee of the Medical School*, Adel., 1935; Poulton, B., "The Adelaide Medical School", *Austsn med. Gaz.*, 1913, 34 : 21; also Hughes, J. Estcourt, *A History of the Royal Adelaide Hospital*, Adel., 1967. *See* the *Calendar* of the University, published annually, from 1885. 2308a

University of Melbourne
Scheme for the institution of a Faculty of Medicine. 1. That the Faculty of Medicine be established in the University, before the seventeenth day of April next; and that, during the ensuing year, arrangements be made for opening a school of medicine on the first day of May, 1858 ... [Text continues.]

247 × 196. Single leaf, v.b. Blue paper. ND.

Includes recommendations on staffing, dissection, accommodation.

Copies: UM. 2309

Letter from James Paget, F.R.S. ... to the Hon. Hugh Culling Eardley Childers, on medical education and medical examinations in the Colony of Victoria. Read at a meeting of the Council of the University of Melbourne ... June 28th, ... [Text follows.]

255 × 204. Pp. 4 (l.b.). Blue paper. 1858.

Outlines medical course. H.C.E. Childers (1827–96) was one of the founders and first Vice-Chancellor of University.

Copies: UM. 2310

The University of Melbourne. Special regulations for conferring degrees in Medicine. [Text begins.]

255 × 204. Pp. 4 (l.b.). Blue paper. ND. (1861.)

Admits to examination persons who held qualifications and had practised for 5 years.

Copies: UM. 2311

The University of Melbourne. Regulations for degrees in Medicine and Surgery, framed by the Professorial Board and proposed for the adoption of the Council. [Text follows.]

255 × 204. Pp. 4 (l.b.). Blue paper. ND. (1861.)

Copies: UM. 2312

University of Melbourne. Report of the Medical School Committee. [Text begins.]

255 × 204. Pp. [4] (last 3 blank). 24 June 1861.

Recommends establishment of Medical School; erection 'of a plain structure to be used temporarily ... at a cost not exceeding four thousand pounds.' Signed: A. C. Brownless MD, Chairman.

School established 1862; teaching began 1863. See also the annually published *Calendar* of the University, from 1863.
Copies: UM. 2313

The University of Melbourne. Rules for the conduct of examinations for the degrees of M.B. and M.D., under special regulations. [Text begins.]
331 × 209. Single leaf, v.b. Blue paper. ND. (c. 1863.)
Copies: UM. 2314

Melbourne University, 29th September, 1881. The Chancellor, Vice-Chancellor, and Members of the Council of the University of Melbourne. [Report from Faculty continues.]
212 × 138. Pp. 12. Colophon—Fergusson and Moore . . . Melb.
Report (signed: George B. Halford MD, Dean) drawing 'attention . . . to the rapid growth of the Medical School, and to the necessity for modifying and extending the curriculum . . .'
Copies: EF. 2315

Report of the Committee of the Faculty of Medicine concerning medical education. The report of the Committee is embodied in the following letter to the Council . . . 25th November, 1884. Melbourne: Fergusson & Moore, Printers . . .
158 × 138. Pp. 16.
Details courses and recommends improvements.
Copies: SLV. 2316

Report of the Faculty of Medicine concerning medical education. 20th December, 1884. Melbourne : Fergusson & Moore, Printers . . .
217 × 140. Pp. 16.
Suggestions for extension of teaching and revised curriculum.
Copies: EF, SLV. 2317

University of Melbourne. 9th December, 1897. Dear Sir, The vacancy in the Council of the University caused by the lamented death of the late Sir Anthony Colling Brownless is of especial importance to . . . the welfare of the Medical School. . . . [Text continues.]
339 × 214. Single leaf, v.b. NI.
An appeal for support of Prof. H. B. Allen in Council election; signed by senior teachers.
Copies: UM. 2318

University of Melbourne. Report of the Faculty of Medicine concerning the medical curriculum. (Provisionally adopted November 8, 1898). [Report to Council continues.]
357 × 217. 5 numbered leaves, each v.b. Double cols. NI.
Proposes new curriculum and other measures for improvement.
Copies: EF. 2319

See also Brownless, Sir Anthony Colling; Wilson, Edward J.

University of Sydney

University of Sydney, July 19, 1879. [Text begins.]
229 × 181. Pp. 12. Colophon—Gibbs, Shallard, & Co. . . . Syd.
Address by Chancellor, mentioning projected establishment of medical school and Prince Alfred Hospital.
Copies: ML. 2320

University of Sydney. Medical School. . . . [Staff list follows.]
214 × 135. Pp. 16 (last—colophon only). Colophon: Gibbs, Shallard and Co. . . . Syd. Feb. 1884.
Includes by-laws, fees, time tables. Signed: T. P. Anderson Stuart, Dean.
School established May, 1883. See also the annually published *Calendar* of the University, from 1883.
Copies: EF. 2321

1883–4. Legislative Assembly. New South Wales. School of Anatomy. (Reports, minutes, &c.) Ordered . . . to be printed, 18 June, 1884. [Text begins.]
339 × 217. Pp. 16. Colophon—Syd.: Thomas Richards, Govt Pr—1884.
Papers on anatomy studies at new school. Differences between Prof. Stuart and Inspr of Anatomy (T. B. Belgrave MD), had led to a proposed inquiry into conduct of the school.

Minister considers that the post of Inspr is no longer required.

Copies: EF, ML, NL, SLV, US. 2322

University of Sydney. Challis Chair of Anatomy. [Text begins.]

209 × 130. Single leaf, v.b. July, 1889.

Leaflet notifying terms of appointment.

Copies: US. 2323

Reprints of papers from the science laboratories of the University of Sydney, 1894–5. Part 1. From the Departments of Anatomy, Biology, Geology and Physiology. For private circulation only. Sydney, 1896.

201 × 135. Pp. [iv] (2 blanks), 18 papers with own pagination. Stiff p. w. (title rptd).

Includes papers by C. J. Martin, F. Tidswell, G. Elliot Smith, J. T. Wilson, W. J. Stewart McKay.

Further ed. (1897–1903) published 1903.

Copies: ML, US. 2324

University of Sydney. July, 1896. School of Dentistry. Proposed by-laws. [Text begins.]

300 × 173. Pp. [2]. Single leaf. Signed: A. Stuart.

School opened March 1901. See University *Calendar*, from 1901.

Copies: US. 2325

See Nicholson, Sir Charles, and Woolley, John.

University of Sydney Medical Journal

See *Sydney University Med. Society. Journal of*

Upper Goulburn District Hospital, Woods Point, Vic.

Fifth Annual Report of the Upper Goulburn District Hospital, Woodspoint with the financial statement ... Melbourne: Evans Brothers Printers ... and at Ballarat.

198 × 127. Pp. 16 (l.b.).

Copies: SLV (5–7; 1870–2). 2326

Urquhart, David and Barter Dr.

The Turkish Bath established June, 1860, by the Oriental Bathing Company. Extract from lectures by David Urquhart, Esq. & Dr. Barter. Melbourne: Charlwood & Son ...

204 × 127. Pp. 8. ND. [1860.] P. w. (cover title; advts inside both wrappers, view of the Baths on back).

Copies: ML. 2327

Usher, John Edward

The perils of a baby ... Melbourne: Samuel Mullen ... 1888.

156 × 102. Pp. 32. P. w. (title rptd).

Advice to mothers on infant care.

J. E. Usher MD New York, LRCP, MO to Qd Immigration Service and later of Toorak Vic., returned to Britain about 1892.

Copies: ML, SLV. 2328

Usher, Joseph Francis

... The School of Mines and Industries Ballaarat. A lecture on human physiology: delivered ... 30th August, 1882. ... Ballaarat: Printed by F. W. Niven & Co. ... 1882.

191 × 125. Pp. 28 (l.b.). P. w. (cover title).

For J. F. Usher (1832–1909) LAH Dub., MD New York (1872), of Ballaarat, see obit., *Austsn med. Gaz.*, 1909, 28 : 454.

Copies: NL, SLV. 2329

The Same. Human physiology: Body and bones. In *Ballaarat Science Lectures*, 1st ser., 1882. Ballaarat: James McHutchison, 1883.

Copies: ML. 2330

V

Vaccination Question, The
The vaccination question. Lymph or liberty? An attempt to educate a Minister of Education. [Quotation] Caldr, Bowden, & Co., Printers . . . Hobart.
212 × 140. Pp. 60. ND. P. w. (title rptd).
Copies: CC, WLC. 2331

Vaccination, Instructions for Public
Instructions for public vaccinators. We have been requested to publish the following . . . duties and responsibilities of Government vaccinators.—Eds N.S.W.M.G. [Text continues.]
217 × 140. Single leaf. Pp. [2]. (1871.)
Arm to arm vaccination, and preservation of human lymph when lack of a succession of cases requires this. Lymph obtainable from Vaccine Instn, Sydney.
Copies: EF. 2332

'The Vagabond'
See [James, Stanley].

Valentine, Ferdinand C.
600 medical don'ts by Ferd. C. Valentine, M.D. Published and sold . . . at Cole's Book Arcade, Melbourne . . .
174 × 127. Pp. 90, [4]. ND. P. w. ('Fifty dozen medical don'ts', on front). Colophon—Troedel & Co., Melbourne.
Reprint of US publication—with 'New York, 1887' at end of text.
Copies: EF, ML. 2333

Van Diemen's Land—Comptroller General of Convicts
Regulations for the penal settlement at Port Arthur. [Royal Arms] Hobart Town : Printed by William Pratt . . .
178 × 115. Pp. 22 (l.b.). ND. Limp vellum.
Includes duties of medical officer.
Change of name of Van Diemen's Land to Tasmania, authorised 21 July 1855, became effective from 1 June 1856.
Copies: ML. 2334

———
General regulations for houses of correction under the orders and control of the Comptroller-General of Convicts. [Royal Arms] Hobart Town: Printed by William Pratt . . .
196 × 122. Pp. 32, [2]. (1845.) Limp vellum.
Includes duties of medical officer.
Copies: ML. 2335

———
Regulations of the Probationary Establishment for Female Convicts in Van Diemen's Land. [Royal Arms] Hobart Town: Printed by William Pratt . . .
188 × 120. Pp. 24. (1845.) Vellum wrappers (title rptd).
Includes duties of medical officer.
Copies: ML. 2336

Van Diemen's Land—Inspector Gen. of Hospitals
Instructions for the management of the convict hospitals. Hobart Town, V. D. Land : Printed at the Advertiser Office . . . 1845.
234 × 158. Pp. 48, [24] (l.b.), 1 flg leaf.
Rules for convict hospitals and medical officers of probation stations and road parties. Includes diet tables, medicines, table of diseases for returns. Signed: J. Robertson MD, Dep. Inspr Gen. of Hospitals.
Copies: ML, SLV. 2337

Van Diemen's Land—Lieutenant Governor
Act of Parliament (12 & 13 Vict. Cap. 33) for regulating the carriage of Passengers in Merchant Vessels. Also Her Majesty's Order in Council; and the Proclamation of His Excellency the Lieutenant Governor. [Royal Arms] Van Diemen's Land : James Barnard, Government Printer, Hobart Town. 1850.
8vo. Pp. 62. P. w. (title rptd).
Includes English statute of 1849 which makes detailed provision for health and safety of passengers on voyages from UK; rules and regulations, arising from the above, for maintenance of health on voyages to British

colonies; and proclamation of Lieutenant Governor of VDL, Sir Wm Denison (pp. 56–62), implementing the statute in detail with quantities of water, food, medicines, stores, and other requirements for medical care on voyages to the colony.

Copies: CC, ML. 2337a

Van Diemen's Land Asylum

Van Diemen's Asylum. Instituted 1848. Hobart Town: H. and C. Best, Printers, "Courier" Office. 1848.

168 × 100. Pp. 12.

Objects and rules of newly founded 'Asylum for the Protection of Destitute and Unfortunate Females.'

Copies: FC, ML, NL. 2338

———

First Annual Report of the Van Diemen's Land Asylum. Instituted 1848. Hobart Town: H. and C. Best, Printers, "Courier" Office. 1849.

175 × 117. Pp. 16.

Copies: CC, ML, NL, SLT. 2339

Van Hemert, Francis Thomas

(From the Australian Medical Journal, July, 1869.) On a recent case of small-pox. ... [Text begins.]

209 × 130. Pp. 4 (l.b.).

Copies: SLV. 2340

———

On "What a surgeon may suffer in Victoria" from trial by jury; being a report of the suit-at-law, Turner v Van Hemert, in the Supreme Court of the Colony of Victoria, with articles, correspondence, &c. &c. and remarks. By Chirurgeon. ... Melbourne: Stillwell and Knight ... 1872.

212 × 135. Pp. 72 (l.b.). P. w. (title rptd).

Damages for malpraxis in treatment of fractured femur; a verdict considered unjust by Melb. doctors.

F. T. Van Hemert MRCS, of St Kilda Vic., moved to Dunedin NZ soon after. Here in 1876, he and his wife died within a week of each other, leaving nine children unprovided for.

Copies: DL, ML, NL, SLV. 2341

Varley, Henry

Second edition. Mr. Varley's full address on the "Social Evil" ... Town Hall, Melbourne. Revised and enlarged. With a preface by the publisher ... C. T. Scown, Publisher. Melbourne: W. H. Williams, Printer ... 1878.

217 × 127. Pp. 22 (l.b.).

1 ed., 1878. NS.

On sexual incontinence, with references to prostitution in Melbourne.

Copies: ML, LNSW, NL, SLT. 2342

———

... Private address to boys and youths on an important subject. Containing invaluable information for boys, youths, and parents. ... "Be not deceived: neither fornicators, nor adulterers, nor effeminate (those guilty of self-abuse), nor abusers of themselves with mankind; shall inherit the kingdom of God" ... Varley Bros. ... Melbourne. 1893. ...

183 × 122. Pp. 16. P. w. (title rptd).

On 'the terrible evils which attach to the sin of self-pollution.' Advertises Melb. ed. of *The curse of manhood*, 1893. NS.

Copies: ML, SLV. 2343

———

... Lecture to men on a vitally important subject, containing invaluable information for young men, and those who are married. ... This lecture has been delivered to 300,000 men in various parts of the world. ... Varley Bros. ... Melbourne. 1894.

186 × 125. Pp. 40. P. w. (title rptd; book notices on back wrapper).

On physical and moral evils of incontinence.

For Henry Varley (1835–1912), evangelist and social reformer, see *Henry Varley's life story*, by H. Varley, Lond., ND.

Copies: EF, FC, ML. 2344

Vegetarian, The

The Vegetarian The Organ and Property of the New South Wales Vegetarian Society. Vol. 1. No. 1. March 10, 1896. Price gratis.

222 × 143. Pp. 4.

Society was established in 1891.

Copies: ML. 2345

Vegetarian Society of Australia

Constitution and manifesto of the Vegetarian Society of Australia. Melbourne. Walker, May & Co., Printers ... 1886.

212 × 138. Pp. 12.

Soc. established 1886. Advertised in *Health and Home (q.v.)*. See also Jones, Robert.

Copies: SLV. 2346

Verco, Sir Joseph Cooke

The South Australian statistics of consumption. [From the Transactions of the Philosophical Society of Adelaide, 1879.] . . . [Text begins.]

209 × 127. Pp. 22. NI. P. w. (title rptd).

Copies: ML, NL. 2347

———

Should a medical man practice midwifery, while in charge of puerperal fever? . . . [Text begins.]

242 × 153. Pp. 8. Repr. *Trans Intercol Med. Cong. Austsia*, 1889 : 684.

Also published: 'Hydatids', with E. C. Stirling; chapter in Allbutt's *A system of medicine*, vol. 2, Lond., 1897.

Later publications: *Cat. of marine Mollusca of SA*, Adel., 1908; *Combing the Southern Seas*, Adel., 1935.

For Sir Joseph Verco (1851–1933) MD, FRCS, Hon. Phys. Adel. Hosp., Dean of Med. and later Dent. Univ. Adel., see obit., *Med. J. Aust.*, 1933, 2 : 390; *SA Naturalist*, 1933, 14 : 121 (for conchological bibliog.); Ludbrook, A. M. *Notable hymns and their authors*, Melb., 1935.

Copies: US. 2348

Viavi Hygiene

See Law, Hartland and Law, Herbert E.

Victoria—Board of Public Health

1891. Victoria. Board of Public Health. Report of the Board, 1890–91. Presented to both Houses of Parliament . . . By Authority: Robt. S. Brain, Govt Printer, Melbourne.

320 × 206. Pp. 90.

Board was established by Public Health Act 1889, which abolished former Central Board of Health. Reports 1890/91 to 1908/9/10—all issued.

Copies: AMAV, HDV, LNSW, ML, NL, SLV. 2349

———

Vaccination. Memorandum. Vaccination from the tubes should be prepared in the following . . . [Text continues.]

349 × 214. Single leaf, v.b. 2 figs. ND.

Directions for vaccination with calf lymph.

Copies: NL. 2350

———

Resolution of the Board of Public Health of Victoria, on 11th September, 1895, on the subject of compulsory infantile vaccination. [Text begins.]

344 × 220. Pp. 4. Colophon— . . . Robt S. Brain, Govt Printer, Melb.

Compulsory vaccination of infants should be continued. Statistical evidence of efficacy and safety presented.

Copies: EF, NL. 2351

———

Vaccination. Board of Public Health, Victoria. Facts about small-pox and vaccination.

165 × 107. Pp. 14. ND [1898.] Colophon— . . . Robt S. Brain, Govt Pr.

Issued by BMA, 19 Jan. 1898; reissued by Board.

Copies: NL. 2352

———

Board of Public Health, Victoria. Bubonic plague. Translation of medical circular, issued by the German Imperial Board of Health. June, 1900. . . . Robt. S. Brain, Govt Printer, Melbourne.

165 × 102. Pp. 14 (l.b.).

Clinical features, bacteriology, treatment and epidemiology of plague.

Copies: NL, SLV. 2353

———

See also items under Gresswell, Dan Astley.

Victoria—Central Board of Health

1855–6 Victoria. Central Board of Health . . . First annual report. Laid upon the Council table by the Chief Secretary . . . and ordered by the Council to be printed, 26th February, 1856. . . . John Ferres, Govt Printer, Melbourne.

329 × 201. Pp. 12. Blue paper. Signed: W. McCrea, Pres.

Central Board of Health was established in 1855, abolished by Public Health Act 1889, and succeeded by Bd of Public Health. Reports (irregular) 1855–6 to 1889. After 1877–8, no reports till 1885, when publication resumed to 1889.

Copies: AMAV, BG, EF, HDV, ML, NL, SLV. 2354

———

Central Board of Health, Melbourne, 6th January 1871. Circular. The attention of the Central Board of Health having been called to the desirability of placing in the hands of persons in charge of factories, mines, and other places where machinery is used, some instructions for the preliminary treatment, pending the arrival of surgical aid, of persons accidentally injured . . . [Text continues.]

339 × 212. Single leaf, v.b. NI.

Circular distributed with copies of following item. Ms. note on ML copy states that copies were sent to Local Boards of Health, Vic. Railways, and Hobson's Bay Railway Co.

Copies: ML. 2355

Rules for the course to be followed by the bystanders in case of injury by machinery, when surgical assistance cannot be at once obtained. Prepared by John H. Packard, M.D. . . . [Text begins.]

510 × 377. Single leaf, v.b. 5 woodcut figs, decorated frame. ND. (1871.) Colophon— . . . John Ferres, Govt Pr, Melb. At foot: Reprinted for and circulated by the Central Bd of Health of Victoria for general information.

Poster for display in work places.

Copies: ML. 2356

1880. Victoria. Diphtheria at Oakleigh. Return to an order of the Legislative Assembly . . . 22nd September 1880. . . . [Text begins.]

344 × 217. Pp. 4 (l.b.). Colophon— . . . John Ferres, Govt Pr, Melb.

Central Bd of Health opposes a claim that a fatal case of diphtheria was milk-borne. Richard Youl MD, Pres., states he had never traced an outbreak to milk, the usual causes being 'contagion, bad drainage, filth (especially cesspits), impure water, and bad ventilation.'

Copies: AMAV, BG, EF, HDV, LNSW, NL, SLV. 2357

1880–81. Victoria. Vaccination. Memorandum by the Central Board of Health on the advantages of vaccination, the alleged danger of transmitting disease, etc. Presented to both Houses of Parliament. . . . [Text begins.]

346 × 220. Pp. 2. Colophon—Robt S. Brain, Acting Govt Pr, Melb.

For history of vaccination in Aust., see Cumpston, J.H.L. (1914), *The history of small-pox in Aust.*, Melb., 1914 : p. 130.

Copies: AMAV, HDV, LNSW, ML, NL, SLV. 2358

Instructions, etc., for the use of Local Boards of Health and others, under "The Public Health Amendment Statute 1883", No. 782. . . . John Ferres, Govt. Printer, Melbourne.

181 × 120. Pp. 42. (Central Bd of Health, 1884.)

Copies: DL. 2359

1887. Victoria. Typhoid fever. Report by the Central Board of Health. . . . Robt. S. Brain, Govt Printer, Melbourne.

331 × 212. Pp. 24. 1 flg chart, 1 map.

States that contagiousness of typhoid is now generally accepted. Necessary factors in prevention: compulsory notification, isolation, proper excreta disposal, destruction of typhoid excreta, general hygiene, protection of water supplies. Legislation for these is recommended.

Copies: AMAV, HDV, LNSW, ML, NL, SLV. 2360

1887. Victoria. Small-pox on board the S. S. "Preussen". Report of the President of the Central Board of Health . . . Presented to both Houses . . . John Ferres, Govt Printer, Melbourne.

339 × 214. Pp. 8 (l.b.).

1 death on voyage, 29 cases with 3 deaths in quarantine.

Copies: AMAV, BG, EF, LNSW, ML, NL, SLV. 2361

Victoria—Department of Mines and Water Supply

The mineral springs of Victoria. Extract from the Annual Report of the Secretary for Mines on the Mineral Statistics for 1887. . . . Robt. S. Brain, Govt Printer, Melbourne. 1889.

163 × 102. Pp. 28. P. w. (title rptd).

Copies: ML. 2362

Victoria—Hospitals for Insane

Regulations for attendants and nurses.

180 × 122. Pp. 6. Colophon— . . . Robt S. Brain, Govt Pr, Melb. ND. [1898.]

Copies: SLV. 2363

Victoria—Legislative Council

1852 Victoria. Health Officer. . . . Report of the Health Officer. Williamstown, May 4th, 1852. [Text begins.]

316 × 200. Pp. 4. Blue paper. *V&P*, 1852–3.

Health rep. on 81 overseas vessels entering Port of Melb. in 1851. All vessels healthy except *Eagle*, with small-pox and dysentery aboard—quarantined.

Copies: LNSW, ML, NL, SLV. 2364

1852. Victoria. Colonial Surgeon and Assistant Colonial Surgeon. Return to address, No. 47 on the motion of Dr. Thomson, 28th October, 1852. ... Melbourne: ... John Ferres, at the Govt Printing Office, 1853.

311 × 198. Pp. 8. Blue paper. *V&P*, 1852–3.

Medical reports on Melb. Gaol, House of Correction, Lunatic Asylum, lunatics in Melb. Gaol, with duties of Col Surg.

Copies: AMAV, BG, ML, NL, SLV. 2365

1852–1853. Victoria. Sewerage & Water Supply. Report from the Select Committee on the Sewerage of and Supply of Water for Melbourne, together with the ... evidence. Ordered by the Council to be printed, 11th January, 1853. Melbourne: ... John Ferres ... Govt Printing Office. 1853.

305 × 212. Pp. xii (l.b.), 46, 6, 47, 80 (l.b.), [ii] (fig. on recto). 1 flg map. J. F. Palmer, Chairman.

Copies: AMAV, LNSW, ML, NL, SLV. 2366

1853. Victoria. Inquests. ... ordered by the Council to be printed, 6th September, 1853. ... John Ferres, Govt Printer, Melbourne.

340 × 208. Pp. 32 (l.b.). Blue tinted paper. *V&P*, 1853–4.

Abstract of inquests (Vic.), 1 Jan.–30 June 1852.

The Same, 1854. 1 July–31 Dec. 1853. *V&P*, 1854–55.

Copies: LNSW, ML, NL, SLV. 2367

1853–4. Victoria. Health Officer. Return of diseases most prevalent on board ships performing quarantine during the half-year ending ... 31st December, 1852. Report of the Health Officer ... to 30th June, 1853. ... John Ferres, Govt Printer, Melb.

331 × 217. Pp. 10. Blue paper.

Reports half-yearly 1852–1859, then annually to 1880.

Copies: AMAV, ML, NL, SLV. 2368

1853–4. Victoria. Report from the Select Committee of the Legislative Council on Intemperance, together with the proceedings ... minutes of evidence, and appendices. Ordered ... to be printed 31st March, 1854. ... John Ferres, Govt Printer, Melbourne.

340 × 208. Pp. 38. Blue tinted paper.

On the 'alarming increase and destructive effects of Intemperance in this Colony and the best means of restraining such ...'

Copies: LNSW, ML, NL, SLV. 2369

1854. Victoria. Health report of immigrants, prisoners, and the public force of the Colony, by the Chief Medical Officer, for the half year ending 30th June, 1854. ... John Ferres, Govt Printer, Melb.

344 × 217. Pp. 10. Blue paper. *V&P*, 1854–5.

Includes statistics of morbidity, mortality, and prevalent diseases in immigrants (from landing till leaving Depot), police, military, and prisoners. Signed W. McCrea MB.

Copies: HDV, LNSW, ML, NL, SLV. 2370

1855–6. Victoria. Lunatic confined within goals or other prisons in Victoria. ... Laid upon the Council table, by the Chief Secretary ... 6th March, 1856.

340 × 210. Single leaf, v.b. Colophon—John Ferres, Govt Pr. Blue tinted paper.

Report 68 patients so confined (1856). Further report, 1856–7 (for 1857).

Copies: LNSW, ML, NL, SLV. 2371

Victoria—Parliament

The following items are selections from the *Votes and Proceedings of the Legislative Assembly of Victoria*, 1856/7–1900. See library catalogues for holdings. Detailed listing for LNSW, NL, OL, US, appears in Cope, R. L. *Australian Parliamentary Serials*, Reference Monograph 9, Library of Parliament, Syd., 1973. Separately issued papers of the series occur in various collections, notably in AMAV.

1857–8. Victoria. Chief Medical Officer. Return of diseases in the various establishments under the charge of the Chief Medical Officer, for the year 1857. Presented to both Houses . . . John Ferres, Govt Printer, Melbourne.

298 × 193. Pp. 8. Blue paper.

Statistics and notes on sickness and deaths from Immigration Hosp., penal establishments, and Immigrants' Depot, Geelong. Signed: W. McCrea, CMO. Annual, 1857–78.

2372

Chief Medical Officer. Report on the Sanitary Station, for the year 1857. Presented to both Houses . . . John Ferres, Govt Printer, Melbourne.

339 × 212. Pp. 4. Blue paper.

Termed 'Sanatory' Station in later reports. Annual, 1857–83.

2373

1858–9. Victoria. Report of the Select Committee of the Legislative Council on the Aborigines, . . . with proceedings . . . evidence, and appendices. . . . John Ferres, Govt Printer, Melbourne.

331 × 209. Pp. viii, 106 (l.b.), 1 litho. pl. Blue tinted paper.

On 'the present condition of the Aborigines . . . and the best means of alleviating their absolute wants.'

2374

1858–9. Victoria. Report from the Select Committee upon water from the Yan Yean Reservoir . . . with . . . proceedings . . . minutes of evidence and appendices. . . . John Ferres, Govt Printer, Melbourne.

310 × 195. Pp. xiv, 108 (l.b.). Blue paper.

2375

1859–60. Victoria. Yan Yean water. Report and supplementary report of analysis of two samples of water . . . by Alfred Swaine Taylor, M.D., F.R.S., Professor of Chemistry, Guy's Hospital, London; and William Thomas Brande, F.R.S., Royal Mint, London. . . . John Ferres, Govt Printer, Melbourne.

310 × 195. Pp. 8. Blue paper.

2376

1861. Victoria. First Report of the Central Board appointed to watch over the interests of the Aborigines in the colony of Victoria. Presented to both Houses . . . John Ferres, Govt Printer, Melbourne.

346 × 214. Pp. 36.

Medical notes and reports throughout.

Central Board was succeeded by Board for Protection of Aborigines in 1870. Annual reports, 1861–1900.

2377

1862–3. Victoria. Report of the Commissioners appointed to enquire into the municipalities and the charitable institutions in Victoria. Presented to both Houses . . . John Ferres, Govt Printer, Melbourne.

342 × 220. Pp. [viii] (versos blank), 74, xc (xiii-xxi, xxvi-xxx—flg leaves, numbered consecutively, rectos blank). Blue tinted paper.

2378

1864. Victoria. Health Officer. Report for the year ending 31st December, 1863. Presented to both Houses . . . John Ferres, Govt Printer, Melbourne.

331 × 220. Pp. 14. Blue paper.

Return of quarantine officer, Queenscliff: vessels boarded, deaths and causes on voyage, vessels in quarantine.

Annual reports, 1852–80.

2379

1864. Victoria. Hospitals and Lunatic Asylums. Copy despatch from . . . Secretary of State, with enclosures relative to public hospitals and lunatic asylums. Presented to both Houses . . . John Ferres, Govt Printer, Melbourne.

367 × 217. Pp. 36.

Based on enquiry from all British colonies, requested on account of 'flagrant abuses and cruelties' in certain institutions in Jamaica, to provide information on general condition of hospitals and lunatic asylums. Scanty information on Tas., Vic. and WA institutions appears at pp. 12, 30, with general suggestions.

2380

1864–5. Victoria. Quarantine Regulations. Return to an Order of the Legislative Assembly . . . Instructions for the guidance of the Resident

Surgeon, Sanatory Station. [Text begins.]
344 × 217. Pp. 4 (l.b.). Colophon— . . . John Ferres, Govt Pr, Melb.
2381

1864–5. Victoria. Report from the Select Committee on Castlemaine and Sandhurst water supply . . . John Ferres, Govt Printer, Melbourne.
336 × 217. Pp. xii, [ii], 134, 46.
2382

1864–5. Victoria. Quarantine—"Golden Empire". . . . Legislative Assembly . . . Report of the Commission appointed to enquire into the quarantine of the "Golden Empire", and . . . the management of the Sanatory Station.
352 × 214. Pp. 4. Colophon— . . . John Ferres, Govt Pr, Melb.
Criticises procedure and accommodation at Sanatory Stn (Pt Nepean) and recommends removal to site nearer Melbourne.
2383

1864–5. Victoria. Quarantine. . . . appendices to the Report of the Board . . . to enquire into the Quarantine Regulations, and . . . the *Golden Empire* . . .
371 × 214. Pp. 24 (l.b.). Colophon— . . . John Ferres, Govt Pr, Melb.
2384

1864–5. Victoria. Quarantine—"Golden Empire". Remarks by the Chief Medical Officer on the report of the Board appointed to enquire into the Quarantine Regulations and in regard to the "Golden Empire". . . . [Text begins.]
344 × 217. Pp. 6 (l.b.). Colophon— . . . John Ferres, Govt Pr, Melb.
Opposes removal of Sanitary Stn from Point Nepean to Sandridge (Pt Melb.). Discusses typhus, the limited chances of its spread in Vic., and the frequent occasions of its importation in ships in the past 13 years (including the case of the *Ticonderoga*, in which, of 795 aboard, 98 died on voyage and 75 after arrival). In 12 years only 4 persons had contracted typhus while caring for the sick, the disease never extending beyond these or establishing itself. Signed: W. McCrea, CMO.
2385

1866. Victoria. Quarantine. Report of the Chief Medical Officer on . . . quarantine. Presented to both Houses . . . John Ferres, Govt Pr, Melbourne.
344 × 217. Pp. 8. Signed: W. McCrea.
CMO states that there is 'much alarm . . . created by . . . typhus fever in Melbourne among passengers of the *Golden Empire*'—hence this report.
2386

1866. Victoria. Chief Medical Officer. Return of vessels placed in quarantine during the year 1864 and report on the Sanitory Station for . . . 1865. . . . John Ferres, Govt Printer, Melbourne.
342 × 217. Pp. 8 (l.b.).
2387

1866. [Second Session.] Victoria. Report from the Select Committee on Night Soil, Melbourne. Together with the proceedings . . . evidence, and appendices. . . . John Ferres, Govt Printer, Melbourne.
344 × 209. Pp. 6, 36, 42.
Recommends use of earth closets and abolition of all cesspits in Melbourne and Geelong.
2388

1869. Victoria. Small pox. Copy of correspondence relating to the recent introduction of small pox into the Colony and the steps taken to arrest its progress. Ordered by the Legislative Assembly to be printed, 9 March, 1869.
357 × 244. Pp. 20 (l.b.). Colophon— . . . John Ferres, Govt Pr, Melb. Signed: W. McCrea CMO.
Additional report of CMO. 6 April 1869. Pp. 4 (l.b.).
A further report of CMO. 20 July 1869. Pp. 2.
2389

1869. Victoria. Report of the Inspector of Asylums on the Hospitals for the Insane for the year 1868. Presented to both Houses . . . John Ferres, Govt Printer, Melbourne.
344 × 222. Pp. 26.
Annual reports, 1868–1900, include notes on establishments, statistics. Later termed: Rep. of Inspector for Lunatic Asylums.
2390

1869. Victoria. Report from the Select Committee upon Victorian Water Supply; together with the proceedings ... evidence and appendices. ... John Ferres, Govt Printer, Melbourne.

314 × 196. Pp. 194 (last—colophon only).

2391

1870. ... Victoria. Progress Report of the Royal Commission on Noxious Trades, etc.; with minutes of evidence. Presented to both Houses ... John Ferres, Govt Printer, Melbourne.

309 × 201. Pp. xii (iv blank), 94.

Final rep., 1871. Pp. xviii, 30.

Chairman—Wm McCrea CMO. On health hazards and nuisance due to 'pollution of the atmosphere or waters in and around Melbourne', their causes and prevention. Recommendations include : improved siting and processing in certain industries; scheduling, licensing and inspection of noxious trades; control of river pollution; replacement of earth closet system of excreta disposal by sewerage.

2392

1871. Victoria. Charitable institutions. Report of the Royal Commission appointed ... to ... report upon the condition and management of the charitable institutions of the colony ... together with minutes of evidence and appendices. ... John Ferres, Govt Printer, Melbourne.

342 × 214. Pp. xxii, [ii] (v.b.), 146 (129–136—consecutively numbered flg leaves, v.b.).

2393

1871. Victoria. Victorian water supply. Report of the Board appointed to ... report upon and advise the Government in respect of the ... recommendations made by Lieut.-Colonel Sankey, R. E., in his several reports ... John Ferres, Govt Printer, Melbourne.

344 × 217. Pp. 14, 1 map.

2394

1872. Victoria. Diphtheria. Report of the Royal Commission appointed ... to enquire into the origin of ... diphtheria, the best mode of treatment ... etc. ... with minutes of evidence, etc. Presented to both Houses ... John Ferres, Govt Printer, Melbourne.

339 × 212. Pp. xx, 164.

Commissioners—Wm McCrea CMO (Pres.), J. W. Gunst MD, F. Lloyd LRCS, D. B. Reid MRCS.

For the violent objection of Med. Soc. Vic. to the provocative appointment of all members excepting Pres.—'a burlesque on commissions, a ridiculous abortion of a court of medical enquiry ... a board bursting with confident ignorance, an alliance of ridiculous incapacity etc. ...'; libel action against its organ *Aust. med. J.*; and refutation of Report's selection of sulphurous acid as a specific remedy; see numerous refs, *Aust. med. J.*, 1872, vol. 17.

2395

1872. Victoria. Industrial Schools and Sanatory Station. First Report of Royal Commission on Industrial and Reformatory Schools and the Sanatory Station. Presented to both Houses ... John Ferres, Govt Printer, Melbourne.

344 × 212. Pp. 66 (l.b.).

1874, 2nd and final rep., pp. 16.

Recommends transfer of Pt Nepean Quarantine Stn to a more suitable site; opposed by CMO (W. McCrea).

2396

1873. Victoria. Ararat Water Supply. Report. presented to both Houses ...

342 × 214. Pp. [2] (v.b.). Colophon— ... John Ferres, Govt Pr, Melb.

2397

1873. Victoria. Report on the Geelong Water Supply. Presented to both Houses. ... John Ferres, Govt Printer, Melbourne.

346 × 217. Pp. 6 (l.b.). Signed: G. Gordon, Chief Engineer.

2398

1873. Victoria. Beechworth Water Supply. Memorandum. Presented to both Houses ... To the ... Minister for Mines.

346 × 217. Pp. 2. Colophon— ... John Ferres, Govt Pr, Melb. Signed: G. Gordon, Chief Engineer.

2399

1877. Victoria. Royal Commission on the Aborigines. Report of the Commissioners appointed to inquire into the present condition of the Aborigines of this Colony, and ... the best means of caring for, and dealing with them, in the future ... with ... evidence and appendices. ... John Ferres, Govt Printer, Melbourne.

344 × 209. Pp. xviii (l.b.), [ii] (v.b.), 130 (l.b.).

2400

1879. Victoria. Aborigines. Report ... relative to the mortality amongst the residents of the aboriginal stations of Victoria, etc. Presented to both Houses ... John Ferres, Govt Printer, Melbourne.

305 × 217. Pp. 6.

Aborigines Bd reports rapid decrease in aboriginal population due to lung disease, with spitting of blood, peculiar to Aborigines and inevitably fatal. Those born on aboriginal stations or entering them in childhood mostly die at ages 12–25. CMO (W. McCrea) holds that unhealthy living conditions 'in wretched hovels' were conducive to lung diseases and recommends improved hygiene, diet and accommodation.

2401

1880–81. Victoria. Report from the Select Committee upon Vaccination Law; together with the proceedings of the Committee ... Ordered by the Legislative Assembly to be printed, 24th March 1881. ... Robt. S. Brain, Acting Govt Printer, Melbourne.

344 × 244. Pp. vi, [ii], 32 (l.b.).

Recommends that animal vaccination be tried, and 'depots established for supplying animal lymph from young heifers.'

2402

1880–81. Victoria. Yan Yean water supply. Report of the Board ... to enquire into the present condition of the Yan Yean water, and to suggest any immediate remedy. Ordered by the Legislative Assembly ...

344 × 217. Pp. 4 (l.b.). Colophon—... Robt S. Brain, Acting Govt Pr, Melb.

2403

1881. Victoria. Public Charities. Report of Inspector for the half-year ended 30th June, 1881, and rough draft of proposed Amending Bill; together with additional reports. Presented to both Houses ... John Ferres, Govt Printer, Melbourne.

214 × 143. Pp. 88.

Reports contain comprehensive information on all Vic. public hospitals and charitable institutions. Annual to 1900.

2404

1882. Victoria. Southern Board. Report of the Board ... upon the ... claims of compensation arising from the action of the Sanatory Authorities in connection with ... small-pox case in Swanston Street, Melbourne, and the alleged neglect to afford the patient proper attendance and treatment. Presented to both Houses ... John Ferres, Govt Printer, Melbourne.

344 × 217. Pp. vi (l.b.), 82.

2405

1885. Victoria. Tuberculosis in cattle. Report of the Board appointed to inquire relative to the existence and extent in Victoria of the disease in cattle known as tuberculosis, whether its existence is likely to be detrimental to the Public Health, and what preventive means should be adopted; together with ... evidence. ... John Ferres, Govt Printer, Melbourne.

346 × 217. Pp. xliv, 80 (l.b.).

Gives current views on contagiousness of tuberculosis and discusses local prevalence, identity of human and bovine infections, and danger from infected meat and milk. Recommendations include: declaration of bovine tuberculosis as infectious disease (no country had yet so legislated); advice on prevention; safe meat supply; safety of milk, including inspection of herds and destruction of infected cattle.

Progress Rep., 1884, pp. viii, includes symptoms, course, and pathology.

2406

1885. Victoria. Report of the Noxious Fumes Board. Presented to both Houses ... John Ferres, Govt Printer, Melbourne. No. 105.

349 × 220. Pp. x, 124.

On alleged injurious effects to miners from nitro-glycerine compounds—to which no permanent injury is attributed, and compressed air—reported as harmless. Ventilation is stressed. Includes much med. evidence.

2407

1886. Victoria. Hospitals subsidized by Government. Return to an Order of the Legislative Assembly. . . . 22nd June, 1886.

357 × 217. Pp. [2] (v.b.). Colophon— . . . John Ferres, Govt Pr, Melb.

Names of hospitals, average yearly patients 1884–5.

2408

1886. Victoria. Royal Commission on Asylums for the Insane and Inebriate. Report. Presented to both Houses . . . John Ferres, Govt Printer, Melbourne.

342 × 216. Pp. clxx (report), 602 (evidence). Chairman—E. L. Zox.

Review, *Aust. med. J.*, 1886, ns 8 : 221. For current criticism of asylums, see 'Victorian lunatic asylums', *Austsn med. Gaz.*, 1883, 3 : 44.

2409

1887. Victoria. First Report of the Chief Inspector of Factories, Workrooms, and Shops, for the period from 1st March to 31st December, 1886. Presented to both Houses . . . Robt. S. Brain, Govt Printer, Melbourne.

346 × 217. Pp. 16 (15–16 flg chart, v.b.).

Issued under Factories and Shops Act 1885, which requires registration, regulates working hours for women and children, and provides for proper sanitation, ventilation, and safety precautions. Annual reps onwards from 1886.

2410

1888. Victoria. Report of the Ventilation of Mines Board. Presented to both Houses . . . Robt. S. Brain, Govt Printer, Melbourne.

344 × 217. Pp. xii (l.b.), 94, 7 plans (1 flg).

Inquiry was established on urgent appeal of miners on account of widespread lack of ventilation, even in many deep quartz mines with shafts to 2000 ft. Recommends ventilation methods and dust-laying sprays.

2411

1889. Victoria. Typhoid fever cases. Return to an order of the House. . . . 20 June, 1889 . . . A return showing all the cases of typhoid fever reported . . . during the last six months . . . [Text begins.]

344 × 217. Single leaf, v.b. Colophon—Robt S. Brain, Govt Pr, Melb.

Cent. Bd Health notifies 5159 cases reported in previous 6 months.

2412

1890. Victoria. Royal Commission on Vegetable Products. No. 2. Perfume plants and essential oils. Facts from the evidence . . . Robt. S. Brain, Govt Printer, Melbourne

214 × 135. Pp. 64.

Includes evidence on cultivation of medicinal plants in Vic., and table of those grown at Ballarat by J. F. Usher MD.

2413

1891. Victoria. Charitable institutions. Report of the Royal Commission on Charitable Institutions. Presented to both Houses . . . Robt. S. Brain, Govt Printer, Melbourne.

349 × 220. Pp. xxiv.

1890, 1st progress rep., pp. 16 (l.b.). 1892, synopsis, evidence, appendix, pp. xlvi (l.b.), [ii] (v.b.), 1488, 9 charts (1 flg). 1895, supplementary rep., pp. 8 (l.b.).

Chairman: E. L. Zox. Reports detailed investigation of all Vic. instns, and recommends wide reorganisation. Proposals include appointment of RMOs and Hon. MOs to all hospitals; employment of female nurses wherever possible; provision of nursing training and better accommodation, status and relief from menial tasks for nurses.

2414

1896. Victoria. Royal Commission on Water Supply. Minutes of evidence. Presented to both Houses . . . Robt. S. Brain, Govt Printer, Melbourne.

323 × 212. Pp. vi, [ii] (v.b.), 534 (l.b.).

2415

1899. Victoria. Report of the Board appointed to inquire into the question of the treatment of habitual drunkards, with appendices and synopsis of evidence. ... Robt. S. Brain, Govt Printer, Melbourne.

326 × 204. Pp. 36 (2, 4 blank).

SLV copy bound with minutes of evidence; pp. [2] printed title, 274 (l.b.) type-written with ms. corrections.

Chairman: E. L. Zox MP. Recommends commitment for institutional treatment—work, deprivation of liquor, payment on release—and suggests French Island as centre. Drug addicts should be similarly treated.

2416

Victoria Medical Association

Rules and regulations of the Victoria Medical Association. Instituted at Melbourne, June 1852. Melbourne: Printed by Benjamin Lucas, Collins Street. 1852.

209 × 127. Pp. 8.

Established 7 May 1852, following dissolution of Port Phillip Medical Assn; combined with the Medico-Chirurgical Soc. of Vic. 18 July 1855 to form Medical Soc. of Vic.

Copies: SLV. 2417

———

Victoria Medical Association. Rules for the circulation of books and periodicals. ... Library, T. M. Buzzard ... Melbourne. Slater, Williams, & Hodgson, Printers ...

186 × 117. Single leaf, v.b. ND. Signed: J. Black, Hon. Sec.

Used as label in books of Library.

Copies: AMAV, BG, EF. 2418

Victorian Asylum and School for the Blind

The Victorian Asylum & School for the Blind. Temporary premises: Commercial Road, Prahran. Committee & Officers ... Melbourne: Wilson and Mackinnon ... 1866.

171 × 105. Pp. 12.

Includes constitution and rules, report of provisional committee.

Copies: SLV. 2419

———

The First Annual Report of the Committee of the Victorian Asylum and School for the Blind. Presented ... August 23, 1867. ... Temporary premises : Commercial Road, Prahran. ... Melbourne: Fergusson and Moore ... 1867.

204 × 127. Pp. 14, [2].

Copies: SLV. 2420

———

Minutes of evidence taken at the Blind Asylum respecting the case of Mary Ann Grace, and the management of the institution. Melbourne: M'Carron, Bird & Co., Printers ... 1877.

210 × 133. Pp. 98.

Copies: SLV. 2421

Victorian Benevolent Society

See Melbourne Benevolent Asylum

Victorian Cremation Association

See Rusden, Henry Keylock.

Victorian Deaf and Dumb Institution, Melbourne

The Sixth Annual Report of the Committee of the Victorian Deaf and Dumb Institution, presented ... September 3, 1868. ... Melbourne: Fergusson and Moore, Printers ...

204 × 127. Pp. 16.

Copies: SLV (1864–93 various). 2422

Victorian Eye and Ear Hospital

Twelfth Annual Report of the Committee of Management of the Victorian Eye and Ear Hospital, Melbourne (Incorporated 1876), for the year ending 31st December, 1878. Melbourne: A. H. Massina & Co., General Printers ... 1879.

209 × 135. Pp. 16.

Formed by amalgamation of Melb. Instn for Diseases of the Eye and Ear (A. S. Gray), and Ophthalmic and Orthopaedic Instn (T. A. Bowen), under the name of the Eye and Ear Hospital. This was prefixed 'Victorian' in 1873, and later 'Royal.' For history, see Gardiner, L., '*The Eye and Ear*'. *The Royal Vic. Eye and Ear Hospital*, Melb., 1968.

Copies: FC (1878), SLV (1867–74). 2423

Victorian Institute for the Advancement of Science

Transactions and Proceedings of the Victorian Institute for the Advancement of Science. For the sessions 1854–1855. Melbourne: Published for the Society by George Robertson ... 1855.

212 × 135 (trimmed). Pp. viii, 168, xxiv.

Founded 1854; amalgated with Philosophical Soc. 1855 to form Philosophical Inst of Vic., which assumed title of Royal Soc. of Vic. in 1860. Transactions of parent body appear in this single volume.

Contains papers on 'Statistical sanitary

processes' (W. A. Archer); 'On the water supply of Melbourne' (M. E. Jackson); 'On the mineral waters of Vic.' (J. Maund MD), 'The water of the Plenty River' (J. Maund).
Copies: EF, ML, NL, SLV. 2424

Victorian Medical Association
See Medical Association of Victoria.

Victorian Medical Benevolent Association
Fourth Report of the Committee of Management of the Victorian Medical Benevolent Association, for the year ending June 30th, 1869. Melbourne: Stillwell & Knight . . . 1869.
204 × 127. Pp. 8 (last—colophon).
Founded 1865; still active. See Graham, H. B. (1952), *Med. J. Aust.*, 2 : 213; *ibid*, 1956, 1 : 564.
Copies: CC (20th), SLV (1–14, 36). 2425

———

Rules of the Victorian Medical Benevolent Association. (July 1879.) [Text begins.]
209 × 132. Pp. 4 (l.b.). Colophon—Stillwell and Co. . . .
Copies: SLV. 2426

Victorian Sanatorium for Consumptives
Twelfth Annual Report of the Victorian Sanatorium for Consumptives (with notes on the treatment and prevention of consumption), Echuca & Macedon, for the year ending 30th June, 1901. Melbourne: Varley Brothers . . . 1901.
209 × 165. Pp. 40. P. w. (title rptd, decorated and rearranged).
See Serjeant, Mrs. G., for Echuca establishment.
Copies: SLV. 2427

Victorian Tract Distribution Society
Australasian text-book of temperance, with six diagrams of the stomach, marking the stages and progress of alcoholic disease. Published by the Victorian Tract Distribution Society. . . . Melbourne: Mason, Firth, & M'Cutcheon . . . 1873.
183 × 117. Pp. 60. Coloured litho. frontis. P. w. (cover title).
Copies: EF, ML. 2428

'Vid'
A visit to the South Australian Institution for the Blind and Deaf and Dumb on . . . Nov. 4, 1880 by "Vid" . . . Adelaide: R. Kyffin Thomas, Printer . . .
157 × 100. Pp. 16. P. w. (title rptd, decorated).
Copies: SLS. 2429

———

See also Adel. Children's Hosp.; Belair Inebriates' Retreat.

Vines, Edward Prince
(No. 56.) [Royal Arms] 1879. Tasmania. House of Assembly. Bass's Straits : report of Dr. Vines upon the fever in the islands. Laid upon the table by the Colonial Secretary . . .
342 × 214. Pp. 6. Colophon—James Barnard, Govt Pr, Tas.
On a 'low malignant fever', regarded as typhus, in workers gathered for the mutton bird season in conditions of crowded squalor.
Copies: NL, SLT, SLV. 2430

Vitadatio
An interesting address, as delivered by Mr. S. A. Palmer . . . at Launceston, Tasmania, March 2, 1897. [Text begins.]
204 × 138. Pp. 16. Colophon—Echo Publishing Co. . . . Melb. Advt for Vitadatio patent medicine.
Copies: DL. 2431

———

A wonderful discovery is the great Tasmanian herbal remedy Vitadatio for all diseases of the blood. It will cure (without operation) even when eminent doctors of London and Melbourne . . . have failed, be it Bright's disease, cancer, hydatids, consumption . . . [Text continues.]
342 × 212. Single leaf. Pp. [2]. Woodcut fig. ND. Colophon—Echo Publishing Company . . . Melb.
Copies: DL. 2432

———

Vitadatio sick room cookery book and general recipes Melbourne Echo Publishing Company . . .
183 × 122. Pp. 76. Portrait (S. A. Palmer), figs. (1899.) P. w. (illustrated title).
Includes life of S. A. Palmer, 'Agent-General for Vitadatio'.
Copies: EF, ML. 2433

———

The crucifixion of Phillip Strong by Charles M. Sheldon . . . with trustworthy information regarding the renowned Vitadatio the healer of diseases 1899 Vitadatio Series issued by S. A. Palmer, Melbourne. Printed by T. Shaw Fitchett . . .

178 × 117. Pp. [ii], viii, 118. P. w. (shortened title, decorated).

Advertises positive cure for cancer, consumption, Bright's disease—and most other ailments. Rep. *Roy. Com. on Secret Drugs, Cures and Foods*, Melb., 1907, states that this medicine was mainly gin.

Copies: ML. 2434

Vogan, Arthur James

A day spent in learning this may save you fifty years' regret. Household ambulance rules. By Arthur James Vogan, F.R.G.S., . . . [Text begins.]

566 × 296. Single leaf, cloth backed. 4 cols. [1898.] NI.

Wall sheet of first aid rules.

Copies: ML. 2435

Vox E. Deserto

See Campbell, Francis, No 483.

W

Waite, Edgar Ravenswood

A popular account of Australian snakes with a complete list of the species and an introduction to their habits and organisation. . . . Illustrated with sixteen colored plates and numerous figures . . . by the author. Sydney: Thomas Shine . . . 1898.

178 × 120. Pp. 72. 16 coloured pl., figs. Cloth.

Includes: treatment of snake-bite, recognition of venomous species.

Copies: FC, ML, NL, SLS, SLV, UM, US. 2436

Walker, M. Docetti

Domestic guide to the use of Dr. Schüssler's new remedies. The more common diseases and their treatment. By M. Docetti Walker, M.D., Edited by W. Corrie Johnston. . . . Truth and Health Supplies Company, Christchurch. N. Z. . . . Melbourne: Head Office at A. J. Smith and Co.'s . . . 1893.

181 × 122. Pp. 52, [xl] (testimonials etc.). Cloth.

Another issue, 1893, pp. 52. Bound with W. E. Forest's *Health, the new method* (No 684) under covering title.

Schüssler's 'biochemic treatment': 'the body consists of twelve inorganic salts . . . disease arises from deficiency or lack of distribution of these . . . the very element required is given as a medicine.'

Copies: ML, SLV. 2437

Walker, Thomas

The reign of Bacchus . . . First series. Sydney: Websdale, Shoosmith and Co., Printers . . . 1892.

178 × 120. Pp. 140, [4] (advts). P. w. (title rptd).

Alcohol drinking; includes history, adulteration, effects.

Copies: EF, FC, NL, SLT, SLW. 2438

[Walker, William], 'Tom Cringle'

The Hand. By Tom Cringle. "As is the mind so is the form." Melbourne: Stillwell & Knight. 1867.

204 × 140. Pp. 16. 16 pl. Double cols. P. w. (cover title).

Copies: FC, ML, NL, SLV. 2439

The Same. 2 ed., 1868. *The hand, and physiognomy of the human form, in relation to the mind*, Melb.: Clarson, Massina and Co., Syd.: Gibbs, Shallard, and Co. Pp. 40, 18 pl.

Copies: ML, NL, SLV. 2440

On the philosophy of stinks which do not affect public health, whilst the neglect of house ventilation fills our grave-yards. Read before the Royal Society of Victoria, April 11, 1870 . . . Melbourne: Clarson, Massina, and Co. . . . 1870.

217 × 135. Pp. 32. P. w. (title rptd).

'. . . energies of our present Health Officers are directed against wandering goats, city stinks, smoky chimneys, and unswept channels—all of them bad enough in their way—but wholly innocuous when compared with the monster of non-ventilation.'

Copies: ML, NL, SLS, SLV. 2441

Walker, William, of Windsor, NSW

History of the Hawkesbury Benevolent Society. Sydney: Turner and Henderson, 1887.

204 × 135. Pp. 12 (last—colophon only).

Also in Walker's *Miscellanies*, 2 ed., Syd., 1887.

Copies: ML, NL. 2442

Wallace, Francis Lascelles

A catalogue of elegant household furniture, engravings, paintings . . . valuable collection of books, medical works, to be sold by auction, by Mr. T. S. Mort, at the residence of Dr. Wallace . . . who is about leaving the Colony for a short period, on account of ill health . . . Sydney: . . . Statham & Forster, "Australian" Office . . . 1845.

201 × 127. Pp. 8.

F. L. Wallace MD was member of 1st NSW

Med. Board (appointed 1838), Phys. Benev. Soc. NSW. He was in Syd. in 1827, and still practised in 1848.

Copies: ML. 2443

Wallace, Richard

Homoeopathy: the substance of a lecture delivered before "The Assistant Chemists' Association of New South Wales" ... 1895. ... Darlinghurst Road, Sydney. To be had at Fisher's Homoeopathic Pharmacy ...

220 × 137. Pp. 24. P. w. (title rptd).

Recommends establishment of homoeopathic hospital in Sydney—'the only city with over 300,000 inhabitants which has not' one.

For Richard Wallace, see Freeman, Howard and Wallace, Richard.

Copies: EF. 2444

Walsh, George

Manhood perfectly restored. The Civiale urethral treatment a prompt, painless and certain cure for impotence, lost manhood, spermatorrhoea, losses, weakness and nervous debility. Also for prostatitis and varicocoele. No stomach drugging. The Civiale Remedial Agency Dr. George Walsh, L.R.C.P. & S. et L. M., Supt. 131 Collins Street, Melbourne.

165 × 102. Pp. [2] (portrait of author, v.b.), 3–52. ND. Colophon—J. T. Harty & Co., Printers, Melb. P. w. (title on v. of front wrapper; 'The Bright Side' (decorated) on r.).

Advertises treatment of practically all ailments of the male genital tract by medicated 'urethral tapers' attributed to Civiale of Paris, and electrical stimulation.

Copies: CC. 2445

Wardley, Edward

The confessions of Wavering Worthy, or the great secret of success in life: an ethical and autobiographical essay, edited by his most intimate friend, E. Wardley, M.R.C.S.L. and inscribed to the rising generation of Australia by the author. Sydney: Sherriff & Downing ... 1864.

186 × 122. Pp. xii (l.b.), 262 (last—colophon only), [2] (publisher's notices). Paper boards or cloth.

Thoughts and reminiscences of a fictional doctor, probably with autobiographical basis, including life on Vic. goldfields and Riverina, and arrival in Sydney. Includes verses, and letters on various subjects including homoeopathy and insanity.

Copies: AMAV, EF, ML, NL, OL, SLT, SLV, UM, UQ, US. 2446

———

Confessions of Wavering Worthy; a true story of Australian life. Life on the gold diggings—Strange story of his life—threatens to kill his wife—Landlord murdered. House on fire—Six women burned—He jumps overboard— Stuck up by bushrangers. Scott's trial. Is he insane?—Prisoner at the Bar—Judge's summing up—Sentence of death—Farewell to confessor. Price, 2s 6d.

Varies from above ed. only by replacement of title p., which is poorly printed, tipped in, and has v.b. ND.

Copies: NL, OL. 2447

———

The abolition of capital punishment considered. By "Fiat Justitia". Sydney: Gibbs, Shallard, & Co. ... 1869.

204 × 132. Pp. 20. P. w. (cover title).

Library of NSW identifies author.

Copies: LNSW, ML, NL. 2448

———

Lectiones Tarbanae; or, tall talk at Tarban. ... Sydney: Gibbs, Shallard, and Co. ... 1870.

214 × 135. Pp. vi, 7–176 (l.b.).

Verse and essays, read at meetings of selected patients at Tarban Creek Asylum. Author states: 'It was my first experience of the capacity of the lunatic mind to join in intellectual occupation and be diverted.' US copy has textual corrections and inscription by author.

Copies: ML, US. 2449

———

Some phases of insanity and its treatment, popularly considered. ... Read at ... Philosophical and Literary Society of Parramatta. Together with a brief notice of some of the most eminent statesmen of the present century. ... Parramatta: John Ferguson, "Cumberland Times" Office ... Sydney. 1871.

212 × 135. Pp. [ii] (v.b.), 38, [ii] (v.b.), 14 (l.b.). P. w. (title rptd).

Refers to conditions in NSW. Review, *NSW med. Gaz.*, 1871, 1 : 223.

For Edward Wardley (1817–72) MRCS, Supt Parramatta Lun. Asylum, see obit., *NSW*

med. Gaz., 1872, 2 : 287; also Dawson, W. S. (1965), *Annals of psychiatry in NSW 1850–1900*, Syd., typescript (ML, RACP).
Copies: LNSW, ML. 2450

Warner , H. H. and Co.
This book is the most valuable work ever issued for free circulation. H. H. Warner & Co., Limited, Australasian Branch: ... Melbourne, Vic. ...
129 × 92. Pp. 62, [ii]. ND. (1900.) P. w. ('Warner's Blue Book' on front).
Advertises Warner's Safe Cure.
Copies: ML. 2451

Warnings of The Present Season of Sickness and Mortality, The
The warnings of the present season of sickness and mortality. [Quotation] Hobart Town: Printed by William Pratt & Son ... 1852. While this tract has been passing through the press, the epidemic to which it refers has, by God's mercy, abated. But the warning remains; and any notice of it under His blessing, must still be timely.
8vo. Pp. 12.
Wholly devotional.
Copies: SLT, SLV. 2452

Warren, Stewart
The wife's guide and friend being plain and practical advice to women on the management of themselves during pregnancy and confinement, and other matters of importance that should be known by every wife and mother. ... Seventh edition Will Andrade ... Melbourne ... McCutchan & Co., Printers ... Richmond.
143 × 120. Pp. 112. 43 figs. ND. [1898.] P. w. (title rptd; 'The Prosecuted Work!' added).
Reproductive system, pregnancy and infant care. Includes advice on contraception, for which publisher was prosecuted in Melb. in 1898. Dismissal of the charge removed such literature from the class of 'obscene books' in Vic. Includes catalogue of contraceptive and other appliances.
Copies: SLV. 2453

Warwick Hospital, Qd
Rules and by-laws of the Warwick Hospital, as adopted by the subscribers at a special general meeting, held at Warwick, on Monday, April 12, 1875. Warwick. Printed by Cowton & Irwin, at the "Examiner and Times" Office. 1875.
12mo. Pp. 12 (l.b.).
Copies: T. P. Walker coll. 2454

Watson, Archibald
Mrs. L.'s Case. Statement by Professor Watson. This statement is so perfectly simple that anyone can understand it. Adelaide: W. K. Thomas & Co., Printers ... 1896.
214 × 132. Pp. 26 (l.b.). 3 pl. (coloured anatomical diagrams).
Earlier ed.—noted on verso of title. NS.
Preface: letter to Chairman Adel. Hosp. Board. A defence of his criticism of operative procedure, for which author was dismissed from posts of Hon. Cons. Surg. and Pathologist in Oct. 1896. For Hosp. inquiry, see Adel. Hosp., No 16.
For Archibald Watson (1849–1940) MD Paris & Göttingen, FRCS, Elder Prof. of Anatomy Univ. Adel., see obit., *Med. J. Aust.*, 1940, 2 : 361; also Cleland, J. B. (1950), 'The naturalist in medicine', *Med. J. Aust.*, 1 : 549; Smith, J. O. (1967), *S. G. Watson and his sons especially Archibald*, *Watson Mem. Lect.*, RACS, Melb.
Copies: ML, SLS, UA. 2455

See also Horn Scientific Expedition; NSW—Parlt Nos 1561–2.

Watson, Sir Thomas
See Thomson, Wm, No 2245.

Watson, Walter Carter
Maladies of mankind Compiled by Dr. Walter Carter Watson ... Chief Physician and Surgeon to the St. Aubyn's Private Hospital Hunter Street, Sydney.
177 × 115. Pp. [iv], 288. Frontis. (portrait of author), 3 pl., 16 figs. ND. Colophon—McCarron, Stewart & Co. ... Sydney. Cloth.
A popular work, with descriptions of diseases and prescriptions.
Walter Carter Watson MD Bellevue Med. Coll. USA (1888) practised at Newtown NSW in 1892, and later at Richmond and Cangai NSW.
Copies: ML, US. 2456

The Same. ND. Pp. 224. Colophon—Arthur Norwood, Syd. A copy has appointments on title covered by label: 'Late Chief Physician

and Surgeon to St. Aubyn's Private Hospital.'
Copies: AMAV, CC, EF. 2457

The Same. ND. Pp. [iv], 300, vi. Colophon—John Andrew, Syd. Adds: 'and Sydney Institute of Medicine and Electricity' to title. A further ed. contains testimonials dated 1904.
Copies: DOS, EF. 2458

Way, Edward Willis
A concise history of the Royal Infirmary, Edinburgh. Edinburgh, 1872.
NS. Noted by E. A. Petherick. Repr., *Edin. med. J.*
2459

Healthy households. . . . A lecture . . . Adelaide: Printed at the Advertiser, Chronicle and Express Offices . . . 1878.
214 × 140. Pp. 12.
Domestic hygiene, with appeal for Adel. Children's Hosp., then under construction.
For E. W. Way (1846–1901) MB, MRCS, Hon. Surg. Adel. Hosp. and Adel. Children's Hosp., see *Austsn med. Gaz.*, 1901, 20 : 452.
Copies: ML, SLS. 2460

Weale, J. Cyril M.
A colony of lunatics. A review of Dr. Tucker's pamphlet on "The Gheel Lunatic Asylum". Reprinted by permission of the proprietors of the "Express". Sydney: . . . "Express" Office . . . 1884.
217 × 178. Pp. 10.
See Tucker, George A.
Copies: ML. 2461

Weatherby, Lionel A.
Ambulance lectures; what to do in cases of accident or sudden illness. . . . Melbourne: E. W. Cole, Book Arcade . . .
156 × 117. Pp. [2] (advts), [viii], 9–88, [ii]. 23 figs. ND. Preface dated 1882. Cloth.
Reprint of Eng. publication, first issued 1880.
Copies: ML. 2462

Webb, G. F.
The art of dentistry A useful and comprehensive treatise on the teeth—natural & artificial By G. F. Webb, registered surgical and mechanical dentist . . . Prahran, and . . . Armadale, . . . Melbourne: Griffith and Spaven . . . Fitzroy. 1885.
163 × 105. Pp. 36. P. w. (title rptd).
Preface notes as 7 ed. (1 Aust. ed.); previously issued in England.
Copies: ML. 2463

Webb, John Holden
The treatment of spinal curvature and abscess by inflation. . . . Melbourne: Stillwell and Co. . . . 1880.
217 × 135. Pp. 32. 1 litho. pl. P. w. (cover title). Reprinted with amendments from series of papers *Aust. med. J.*, 1879–80.
Treatment of early Pott's disease by head suspension, late stages by plaster jacket, sinuses and abscesses by inflation with carbolised air.
J. H. Webb (d. 1908) MRCS, LRCP, Hon. Surg. Melb. Hosp., suggested appendicectomy for appendicitis very early in the history of the operation and described McBurney's point five years before McBurney (Russell, *infra*). See obit., *Austsn med. Gaz.*, 1909, 28 : 50; also Russell, K. F. (1939–40), 'J. H. Webb and the early history of appendicectomy', *Aust. NZ J. Surg.*, 9 : 333.
Copies: LNSW, ML, SLV, UM. 2464

Treatment of hip disease . . . From the "Australian Medical Journal", February 15, 1889. Melbourne: Stillwell and Co. . . . 1889.
217 × 127. Pp. 12. P. w. (title rptd).
Copies: SLV. 2465

Welch, Robert Porter
A familiar treatise on the diseases of the eye. By Robert Porter Welch, M.R.C.S. &c. late one of the Surgeons of the Taunton and Somerset Hospital. Author of "The Married Woman's Adviser and Young Mother's Guide". Sydney: Printed by T. Trood, King Street, East. 1840.
177 × 108. Pp. 24. P. w. (title rptd, price 1s 6d added; book notice on verso of back wrapper).
The first medical work separately printed and published in Australia. Discusses structure of the eye, its ailments, and their domestic treatment.
The married women's adviser and young mother's guide (in title), NS. Advt on back wrapper: Price 6d. 'This little book is what it professes to be—no lady's medicine chest is complete without it', &c.—Paris and London Advertiser.
Copies: ML. 2466

———

The Australian medical & surgical adviser. For the use of families, settlers, schools, &c.

NS. Announced in *The Atlas*, 8 Feb. 1845, p. 132, as to be published 'by subscription, price 10s 6d.' Address: Dr. Welch's Dispensary and Drug Establishment, George-st, Sydney. 2467

———

Observations on convict and free labour for New South Wales. ... (Reprinted from the Colonial Magazine for July, 1847.) London: Simmonds and Ward, Colonial Publishers ... 1847.

205 × 133. Pp. 30 (l.b.), [2] (book notices).

Also published: *Songs, ballads, and rhymes.* By R.P.W., Syd.: T. Trood, 1841. The Same, 1841, author's name (Robert Porter Welch) replaces initials in title.

For R. P. Welch MRCS, see Ford, E. (1973), 'R.P.W. and his first Aust. med. publication', *Med. J. Aust.*, 1 : 503.

Copies: FC, LNSW, ML, NL. 2468

Wellington, J. H.

—"Man Know Thyself."—Self-explanatory phrenological—and—physiological chart & register as given, by J. H. Wellington, phrenologist & physiognomist ... Published by Messrs Wellington & Thomas, phrenologists & physiognomists. Rae Bros., Printers ... Melbourne.

242 × 153. Pp. [ii] (chart, v.b.), errata slip, 104. Figs. ND. [c. 1886.] P. w. (cover title).

Copies: NL. 2469

Wells, Arthur Lucadou—

A treatise on the preservation of children's teeth ... Tasmania: ... "The Launceston Examiner" Office. 1882.

185 × 120. Pp. 12 (l.b.). P. w. (title rptd).

Copies: ML, SLT, SLV. 2470

Wentworth, William Charles

A statistical account of the British settlements in Australasia; including the Colonies of New South Wales and Van Diemen's Land: with an enumeration of the advantages which they offer to emigrants, ... The third edition. ... In two volumes. Vol. 1. By W. C. Wentworth, Esq. A native of New South Wales. London: Printed for Geo. B. Whittaker ... 1824.

2 vols. 216 × 135. Vol. 1 : pp. viii (3 blanks), 485, [3] (book notices), frontis., 1 flg map; vol. 2 : pp. [ii] 416. 1 flg map. Paper boards.

The first work published by an Australian born author. Two earlier single vol. eds, 1819 and 1820, and later 4 ed., 1840, bear title: *A statistical, historical, and political description of the Colony of New South Wales* ... These include notes on diseases. Enlarged 3 ed. (above) has lengthened section (vol. 1, pp. 309–12), probably by Wm Redfern.

Dysentery was the most prevalent disease, catarrhal and pulmonary affections rare, and only two or three cases of phthisis had occurred in native born youths. Epidemic catarrhal fever (influenza) appeared in 1820. Typhus, repeatedly introduced, was rarely transmitted to colonists. Infantile diseases were almost unknown, and measles, whooping cough and small-pox entirely so.

Copies: ML, NL, SLT, SLV, UM, UQ, US. 2471

West Australian Settler's Guide and Farmer's Handbook

Part 1. The West Australian settler's guide and farmer's handbook. ... Issued by ... the Bureau of Agriculture. Edited by L. Lindley-Cowen ... 1897 E. S. Wigg & Son. ... Perth.

204 × 135. Pp. 818, 24 (l.b.). 6 parts, each with title; running pagination. Illustrated. Pts 1–4, 1897; 5–6, 1898.

Pt 2 includes: 'Medical and surgical hints' (Dr. O'Connor, Perth); Pt 3 : 'The poison plants of W. A.' (Dr. Alex. Morrison).

Copies: EF, ML, SLW. 2472

Western Australia—Medical Department

1899. Western Australia. Rules and regulations for the Medical Department, Western Australia. [Arms] Perth: ... Richard Pether, Govt Pr. 1899.

209 × 138. Pp. 42. P. w. (title rptd).

Copies: EF, LNSW, NL, SLV, SLW. 2473

Western Australia—Parliament

The following items are selections from the *Votes and Proceedings of the Parliament of Western Australia*, 1870/1–1900. See library catalogues for holdings. Detailed listing for LNSW, NL, OL, US, appears in Cope, R. L., *Australian Parliamentary Serials*, Reference Monograph 9, Library of Parliament, Syd., 1973.

1873. Western Australia. Report upon the quarantine laws and regulations in force in this Colony. ... Perth: ... Richard Pether, Govt Printer. 1873.

325 × 204. Pp. 8 (l.b.).

2474

1877. Western Australia Suggestions by the Central Vaccine Board relative to the enforcement of the vaccination ordinances. ... Perth: Richard Pether, Govt Printer. 1877.

339 × 214. Pp. 6 (l.b.).

For history of vaccination in WA, see Cumpston, J.H.L. (1914), *The history of small-pox in Aust., 1788–1908*, Melb. : p. 142.

2475

1877. Western Australia. Report by the Colonial Surgeon on the Public Health of the Colony, for the year 1876. ... Perth: ... Richard Pether, Govt Printer. 1877.

323 × 204. Pp. 4. Signed: Alfred R. Waylen MD.

Annual, 1876–89.

2476

1879. Western Australia. Correspondence and reports upon the sanitary condition of the Colony. ... Perth: ... Richard Pether, Govt Printer. 1879.

317 × 204. Pp. 18 (l.b.).

On sanitation, water pollution, typhoid.

2477

1883. Western Australia. Report by the Colonial Surgeon on the condition of the sick native prisoners at Rottnest Prison. ... Second Session. Perth: ... Richard Pether, Govt Printer. 1883.

323 × 204. Pp. 4 (l.b.). Signed Alfred R. Waylen, M.D.

2478

1884. Western Australia. Report of a Commission appointed ... to inquire into the treatment of aboriginal native prisoners of the Crown in this Colony: and also into certain other matters relative to aboriginal natives. With appendices and a map. ... Perth: ... Richard Pether, Govt Printer. 1884.

326 × 204. Pp. 18. 1 map.

Includes: present state of the race; medical and poor relief; missions; Rottnest Island Prison.

2479

1884. Western Australia. Report of the Select Committee appointed to consider the question of sanitation. ... Perth: ... Richard Pether, Govt Printer. 1884.

325 × 204. Pp. 2 (l.b.).

Recommends appointment of Commission on subject.

2480

1885. Western Australia. Report of the Commission ... upon the sanitary condition of the City of Perth and the town of Fremantle, especially with regard to ... water supply and the disposal of sewage. Presented to the Legislative Council ... Perth: ... Richard Pether, Govt Printer. 1885.

346 × 220. Pp. 16. 3 flg plans. A. R. Waylen MD, Chairman.

Recommends establishment of Board of Health, pan system for nightsoil, reticulated water supply.

2481

1886. Western Australia. Despatches on the subject of the establishment of a sanitarium in Western Australia for the British troops serving in India. ... Perth: ... Richard Pether, Govt Printer. 1886.

317 × 204. Pp. 4.

2482

1888. Western Australia. Report of the health of residents at Rottnest Island for the year 1887, by the Medical Officer ... Perth: ... Richard Pether, Govt Printer. 1888.

331 × 204. Pp. 4 (l.b.). Signed: James W. Hope, FRCP.

2483

1891. Western Australia. Report of the Select Committee of the Legislative Assembly appointed to inquire into the nature, extent and results of the adulteration of liquors, wines, beer, and other beverages ... Perth: ... Richard Pether, Govt Printer. 1891.

317 × 204. Pp. 4.

'... tobacco, snuff, the plant locally known as "droke" and other substances are used by unscrupulous publicans', and are often used for drugging men with much money in their pockets. All cheap brands are adulterated. Recommends public analyst, analyses, legislation.

2484

———

1898. Western Australia. Legislative Assembly. Petition of medical practitioners of Perth, with regard to the immediate establishment of a system of deep drainage in the City ...

323 × 204. Single leaf, v.b. Colophon—... A. Curtis, Acting Govt Pr, Perth.

20 doctors submit that typhoid, diphtheria and scarlatina, then prevalent, would worsen in the absence of adequate sanitation, and recommend sewerage.

2485

———

1898. Western Australia. Report of the Select Committee of the Legislative Assembly appointed to inquire into the Perth Water Supply and administration of the Metropolitan Water Works Board. ... Perth: ... A Curtis, Acting Govt Printer. 1898.

323 × 204. Pp. 58. Chairman—Sir John Forrest.

2485a

———

1900. Western Australia. Venice International Sanitary Convention, 1897. General sanitary regulations to prevent the introduction and spread of bubonic plague. Translated by Ernest Black President-Central Board of Health. ... Perth: ... Richard Pether, Govt Printer. 1900.

305 × 204. Pp. 10.

2486

———

1900. Western Australia. Report of the Acting Principal Medical Officer on the Medical Department ... 1st July, 1899, to 30th June, 1900. ... Perth: ... Richard Pether, Govt Printer. 1900.

305 × 204. Pp. 8.

Reports 1899, 1900.

2487

Western Suburbs Cottage Hospital, Sydney

Third annual report of the Western Suburbs Cottage Hospital Committee, 1894. Ashfield: G. Watson ... 1895.

217 × 138. Pp. 8. P. w. (title rptd).

Established 1891; opened 1894. Name changed to Western Suburbs Hosp. 1923. Above is first printed report.

Copies: ML (1894); Western Suburbs Hosp. (1894–). 2488

Westgarth, William

A report on the condition, capabilities, and prospects of the Australian aborigines. Melbourne: ... William Clarke, at the Herald Office. 1846.

216 × 132. Pp. [vi] (l.b.), 40. 1 flg table. Errata slip. P. w. (title rptd).

Includes notes on causes of decrease of aboriginal population (diseases, infant mortality, diet); infanticide; racial admixture; aptitude for instruction and mental capacity.

Copies: DL, ML, NL, SLS, SLV, US. 2489

Weston, Frank

For gratuitous distribution. Frank Weston's sixth edition Australian companion [Litho. portrait] A selection of valuable recipes ... with much information ... Published by Frank Weston ... Charles Troedel, Lith, Melb. & Sydney.

140 × 110. Pp. 32. Figs. ND. [?1876.] P. w. (cover title).

Advertises patent remedies of Frank Weston, 'Wizard Oil Prince', American travelling lecturer and medicine seller.

Copies: SLV. 2490

Westrum, Wilhelm Adolph

Austsn med. Gaz., 1894, 13 : 216 notes that Dr. Westrum (MD Munich, 1886), after practising at Nyngan NSW for 7 years, had returned to Germany to publish 'an exhaustive work in German on diseases peculiar to Australia.' No reference to this has been found. *SGC*, ser. 2, lists—Wilhelm Westrum: *Klinische Beitrage zur Kenntnis der Syringomyelie*, pp. 50, Erlangen, 1901.

2491

Wheeler, Henry

On some common affections incidental to city life, together with remarks on children's ailments and some infectious diseases, with their appropriate homoeopathic treatment. . . . Melbourne: Martin & Pleasance, homoeopathic chemists . . .

147 × 84. Pp. 94, [6] (advts). ND. Limp cloth.

2 ed. of Eng. work, adapted 'to the needs of colonial life.'

'The hurry and bustle of business, the keen competition of trade, compelling men nowadays to work in such a manner as our forefathers never dreamed of, have their . . . effects upon the organism, health, and comfort.'

Henry Wheeler MRCS, LRCP, of Hawthorn Vic., formerly Phys. to Lond. Homoeopathic Hosp., was Hon. Phys to Homoeopathic Hosp., Melb. in 1892.

Copies: BG, EF, FC, ML. 2492

Whitby Falls Lunatic Asylum, WA

See No 704.

White, J. C.

Queensland the progressive! An account of the Colony, its soil, climate, productions & capabilities, with a description of every phase of life and occupation, advice to immigrants, &c. By J. C. White, forty years in Australia. . . . London: . . . S. W. Silver and Co. . . .

204 × 125. Pp. vi, [7]–80, [2] (advts, r.b.). 1 map. ND. [1870.] P. w. (title rptd).

Includes lay advice to migrants on the availability of doctors, and colonial diseases and ailments (pp. 46–49).

Copies: FC, ML, NL, SLS. 2493

[White, J. H.], 'The Shroff'

The box seat or Medicus and the Shroff by the Shroff Melbourne Melville and Mullen . . .

183 × 122. Pp. viii, 9–120 (l.b.). ND. [1900.] Paper boards.

Account of holiday at Beechworth Vic., interspersed with discussions by 'Medicus' (Patrick Moloney MB), including: bathing, massage, tobacco, sleep, simples and other remedies. See also: Moloney, Patrick.

Copies: AMAV, DOS, EF, ML, NL, SLS, SLT, SLV, US. 2494

White, John

Journal of a voyage to new South Wales with sixty-five plates of non descript animals, birds, lizards, serpents, curious cones of trees and other natural productions by John White Esqre. Surgeon General to the Settlement. [Vignette—view of Port Jackson] London—Printed for J. Debrett, Piccadilly 1790

305 × 239. Pp. [xviii] (l.b.), 300 (l.b.), [36] (l.b.), [iv] (advts). 65 engraved pl., mainly of flora and fauna, hand coloured in some copies. Boards. For variations of plates and cancelled leaf (p. 240), see Ferguson, 1 : 97; for general appreciation, Davidson, R., *A book collector's notes*, Melb., 1970.

Another ed., 1962. Ed. by Alec. H. Chisholm, biog. by R. Rienits. Syd.: Angus & Robertson; Roy. Aust. Hist. Soc. Includes index, bibliog. and notes.

The first Australian work by a medical author, Surg. General of the First Fleet and the new settlement on Sydney Cove. An account of the voyage and the colony to 11 Oct. 1788, with appendix on flora and fauna. Ed., T. Wilson.

This work is third of the six earliest contemporary accounts of the new settlement. These, the incunabula of Australiana, published in London, comprise: Arthur Phillip, *The voyage of Governor Phillip to Botany Bay; with an account of the establishment of the Colonies of Port Jackson and Norfolk Island*, 1789; Watkin Tench, *A narrative of the expedition to Botany Bay; with an account of New South Wales*, 1789; John White, *Journal . . .*, 1790; John Hunter, *An historical journal of the transactions at Port Jackson and Norfolk Island*, 1793; Watkin Tench, *A complete account of the settlement at Port Jackson*, 1793; and David Collins, *An account of the English colony in New South Wales*, 1798. All are of prime importance to medical historians, giving the background to earliest practice, as well as incidental references of medical interest.

For John White (1757–1832) Surg. RN, see Anderson, D. (1933), 'John White, Surgeon-General to the First Fleet', *Med. J. Aust.*, 1 : 183; Cleland, J. B. (1950), 'The naturalist in medicine', *Med. J. Aust.*, 1 : 549; Ford, E. (1955), 'Med. practice in early Syd.' *Med. J. Aust.*, 2 : 41; Rienits, R., Intdn to 1962 Syd. ed.

Copies: BG, DL, DOS, EF, ML, NL, RACP, RACS, SLT, UA, UM, US, WLC. 2495

Reisen in der Sudsee von John White, erstem wundarzte der Kolonie in Neu-Holland, und von William Bligh, Befehlshaber das Schiffes Bounty . . . Aus dem Englischen übersetzt. Mit Anmerkungen von Johann Reinhold Forster . . . Mit Kuppern und einer Karte. Berlin, 1791. In der Vossichen Buchhandlung.

8vo. Pp. viii, 232.

Copies: ML. 2496

---

1. Tagebuch eine Reise nach Neu-Südwallis von John White Esq., erstem Wundarzte der in Port Jackson angelegten neuen Kolonie. 11. William Bligh's Bericht von dem Aufruhre an Bord des Schiffes Bounty . . . [Wien, gedruckt und verlegt bey F. A. Schrämbl. 1792.]

158 × 100. Pp. xxvi, 378. 4 engr. pl.; 1 flg map. No title p. Titles precede sections; imprint from series title. Cloth.

From *Magazin von merkwürdigen neuen Reisebeschreibungen*, Bd 9. Ed. and transl. by J. R. Forster. White's *Journal*, pp. 1–222, and 4 plates.

Copies: NL, RACP. 2497

John Whites Resa till Nya Holland, Åren 1797 och 1788. I Sammandrag af Samuel Ödmann. [Emblem] Upsala, Tryckt hos dir. J. Edmans enka, 1793.

172 × 98. Pp. xii, 148. 4 pl. Stiff p. w., marbled.

Includes Swedish abridgment of White's *Journal*.

Copies: ML, NL. 2498

Voyage a la Nouvelle Galles du Sud, a Botany-Bay, au Port Jackson, en 1787, 1788, 1789; . . . Ouvrage ou l'on trouve de nouveau détails sur le caractere et les usages des habitans du ćap de Bonne-Espérance, . . . et de la Nouvelle Hollande, ainsi qu'une description exacte de plusiers animaux inconnus jusq'à present. Traduit de l'Anglais, avec des notes critiques et philosophiques sur l'histoire naturelle et les moeurs; par Charles Pougens. A Paris, Chez Pougin, Imprimeur-Libraire, . . . An 3 de la Republique, 1795 (vieux style.)

200 × 122. Pp. xii (iv blank), 206, [ii], 256, [iv]. Some copies with 2 engr. pl. by Monnet and Clement, as in Guillaume ed. (below).

Copies: DL, DOS, EF, FC, ML, NL, OL, UQ, WLC. 2499

The Same. Paris, Chez Guillaume, libraire, 1798. Pp. xii, 206, [ii], 256, [iv]. 2 engr. pl. Title as item above, with addition—'et enrichi de deux vignettes, dessinées par Monnet et gravées par Clement.'

Copies: ML, SLT. 2500

Whittell, Horatio Thomas

Practical observations on diphtheria; comprising an epitome of the most recent European experience and opinions on its causes, pathology, and treatment. . . . Adelaide: Shawyer, Printer and Publisher . . . 1859.

178 × 106. Pp. 36 (two blanks). P. w. (title rptd).

Advice 'to those called upon for the first time to combat one of the most insidious and dangerous diseases of modern times, which has of late invaded our Colony.'

For H. T. Whittell (1826–99) MD Aberd., MRCS, Surg. Adel. Hosp. and Pres. Bd Health, see 'A South Australian sanitarian', *Health*, 1925, 3 : 161.

Copies: SLS. 2501

Why do doctors vaccinate?

. . . Why do doctors vaccinate? Common-place comments on a surgeon's assertions. [Quotation] Tasmania: Printed by Calder, Bowden, & Co., Hobart.

175 × 107. Pp. 8. ND. (c. 1889.) P. w. (title rptd).

Opposes pamphlet (NS) by Dr. C. E. Barnard, Supt of Vaccination, Tas.

Copies: ML. 2502

Wicken, Mrs. H. F.

The Australian home, a handbook of domestic economy . . . Edwards, Dunlop & Co., Limited, Sydney, Brisbane and London. 1891

178 × 122. Pp. [6] (advts, l.b.), x, 260, [4] (advts, v.b.). Cloth.

Includes chapters on physiology, diet, hygiene and sanitation, sick nursing, common ailments and simple remedies, care of children and old people.

Copies: ML, NL, OL, US. 2503

Wigg, Henry Higham

Milk and milk supplies. A lecture delivered in connection with the Institute of Hygiene and Bacteriology, at the University . . . August 2nd, 1899. . . . Adelaide: W. K. Thomas & Co., Printers . . . 1899.

180 × 106. Pp. 24 (l.b.).

H. H. Wigg, MD Brux., FRCSE, was MOH Unley at time of publication.

Copies: SLS. 2504

Wilkie, David Elliott

The failure of the Yan Yean reservoir. Being a paper read before the Philosophical Society of Victoria. . . . Melbourne: James J. Blundell & Co. . . . 1855. . . .

186 × 110. Pp. 52. Frontis.—map. P. w. (title rptd).

Wilkie's enlightened interest in Melb. water supply and his objections to the early Yan Yean scheme are noted by H. B. Graham (infra).

FC copy has author's inscription to Dr. Bland.

Copies: FC, ML, NL, SLV. 2505

———

On the expected water supply of the City of Melbourne from Yan Yean. Being a paper read before the Philosophical Society of Victoria. . . . Melbourne: James J. Blundell & Co. . . . 1855.

186 × 110. Pp. 30. P. w. (title rptd).

See *Aust. facts and prospects*, by R. H. Horne, Lond., 1859, for controversy on purity and other information.

For D. E. Wilkie (1815–85) MD Edin. & Melb., MLC, a leading doctor of early Melb., see obits, *Aust. med. J.*, 1885, ns 7 : 170 and *Austsn med. Gaz.*, 1885, 4 : 178; also Graham, H. B. (1956), *Med. J. Aust.*, 1 : 557 (with bibliog.).

Copies: FC, ML, NL, SLV. 2506

———

On a double-jointed uterine pessary. . . . (Read before the Medical Society of Victoria, 1st July, 1863.) [Text begins.]

212 × 130. Pp. 8 (l.b.). 1 pl. Colophon—Wilson & Mackinnon . . .

Copies: SLV. 2507

———

On delivery on the right side. . . . (Read before the Medical Society, 7th October, 1863.) From the Australian Medical Journal, October, 1863. [Text begins.]

210 × 130. Pp. 12. Colophon—Wilson and Mackinnon . . .

'The object . . . is to show that . . . delivery is more speedily, and more safely accomplished with the patient lying on her right side than on her left.'

Copies: ML, SLV. 2508

——— **and Mueller, Sir Ferdinand von**

White men's graves in the Interior. [Read before the Royal Society, 10th October, 1864.]

210 × 135. Pp. 10. Title at hand p. 1. Colophon—Wilson and Mackinnon, Printers . . . Melbourne. Signed at foot.

Inquiry into evidence on certain graves which could not be identified with any travellers known to have perished in or near the locality. Includes consideration of fate of Leichhardt.

Copies: OL, SLV. 2509

Wilkins, John

On the treatment of diphtheria by local remedies only . . . Melbourne: . . . Stillwell & Knight . . . 1870.

212 × 135. Pp. 24. P. w. (title rptd).

Local treatment with potassium iodide, iodine, or tannic acid prevents simple cases from becoming complicated and dangerous.

Copies: CC, EF, ML, NL, SLV. 2510

———

On some cases of squint, with comments, and on the successful operation of cleft palate in a little child. Together with a few remarks on the case of a child operated upon two years since. . . . [Text begins.]

217 × 135. Pp. 12 (l.b.). Colophon—Stillwell and Knight . . . Collins Street East. ND.

At publication, John Wilkins FRCS Edin., MRCS Eng., of Melb., was Hon. Surg. Alfred Hosp. and Self-supporting Infirm. for Diseases of Throat, Chest, Eye and Ear. He was later Hon. Oculist and Aurist, Christchurch Hosp. NZ.

Copies: ML. 2511

Wilkinson, George Blakiston

South Australia: its advantages and its resources. Being a description of that colony, and a manual of information for emigrants. London: John Murray . . . 1848.

201 × 117. Pp. xii (l.b.), 392 (l.b.), [4] (advts). Flg map.

Notes on prevailing diseases, pp. 186, 196–198. 'The climate is famous for the cure of pulmonary and asthmatic disease.'

Copies: DL, ML, NL, OL, SLS, SLV, SLW, UM, US. 2512

Wilkinson, William Camac

Intercolonial Medical Congress Melbourne, 1899. Address by W. Camac Wilkinson . . . Lecturer on Pathology in the University of Sydney. President of the Section of Pathology. Melbourne: Stillwell and Co. . . . 1889.

209 × 135. Pp. 26 (3 blanks). P. w. (title rptd). Includes review of work of Koch and Pasteur.

For W. C. Wilkinson (1857–1946) MD Lond., FRCP, a leading protagonist of tuberculin in treatment and diagnosis, who left Sydney to practise in London in 1909, see obit., *Med. J. Aust.*, 1946, 1 : 488. Publications include: *The treatment of consumption*, Lond., 1908; *Tuberculin in the diagnosis and treatment of tuberculosis*, Lond., 1912; *The tuberculin dispensary for the poor*, Lond., 1923; The *principles of immunity in tuberculosis*, Lond., 1926.

Copies: US. 2513

Wilkinson, William Percy

A short bibliography of Chinese medical, botanical and alchemical literature ... Melbourne, 1896.

178 × 122. Pp. 8. Colophon—McCarron, Bird and Co. ... Melbourne. P. w. Extract from *Chemist and Druggist of Austsia*, 1 Sep. 1896.

Copies: KFR, SLV. 2514

———

An examination of the beer retailed in Melbourne and suburbs. ... Reprinted from the "Intercolonial Medical Journal of Australasia," June 20, 1900.

212 × 138. Pp. 8 (l.b.).

Report to Board of Health, Vic., recommending legislation to prevent adulteration.

Copies: ML. 2514a

Wilks, Stephen Geary

Observations on the diseases, medical and surgical, of New South Wales, more particularly in their relation to the systems of European and of tropical nosology, including remarks on the various effects of snake-bitten wounds, and some account of the cutaneous affections and other maladies prevalent among the Aborigines. To which is appended, a manual of instructions, to persons who reside at a remote distance from the medical stations, ... for ... cases of acute disease, sudden illness, and serious accident, which most frequently occur in the interior of the colony. By S. G. Wilks, M.D. ... author of the Life-preserving Manual, &c. &c; and during five years, a resident surgeon at Bathurst, in the colony of New South Wales.

NS. Advertised, Syd. *Gazette*, 5 Dec. 1828, p. 1, as 'speedily will be published.'

2515

Will the Coming Man Drink Wine?

See [Parton, James].

Williams, Dr.

The therapeutic & phenomenal application of mesmerism, or extracts from the note-book of a practical mesmerist, being a series of lectures by Dr. Williams, M.A., for ten years honorary lecturer on mesmerism, and Professor of Psychological Science, to the Brighton Psychological Society, England. Melbourne: W. H. Terry ... 1882

186 × 120. Pp. viii, 96.

Part 1 of a future 'guide and practical work of reference to the psychological student.' Includes history, curative and anaesthetic uses, phenomena and principles, somnambulism and clairvoyance, and 'valuable hints to those who study psychology and mesmerism for the cure of disease.'

Copies: EF. 2516

———

The Same. 2 ed., 1884. *The text book of mesmerism, or extracts from the note-book* ..., pp. viii, 64.

Copies: ML. 2517

Williams, John

Abdominal pulsation, simulating aneurism of the abdominal aorta. ... Reprinted from the Australian Medical Journal of October 15th, 1880.

204 × 127. Pp. 14, [ii] (colophon, v.b.). Colophon—Melb. : Stillwell and Co. ...

Copies: CC, EF, ML, NL. 2518

———

A guide to medical case-taking in the wards of the Hospital ... Melbourne: Samuel Mullen ... 1885.

163 × 102. Pp. 24 (l.b.). P. w. or leather (title rptd).

Another ed., 1901. (NL.)

Copies: BG, CC, EF. 2519

———

Intercolonial Medical Congress held at Adelaide ... 1887. Address in medicine. Some characteristics of modern medicine ... Stillwell & Co. ... Melbourne.

217 × 138. Pp. 16 (last 2 blank). P. w. (title rptd).

Copies: CC, EF, NL, SLV. 2520

President's address delivered at the Annual Meeting of the Medical Society of Victoria, January 11, 1888. ... Melbourne: Stillwell and Co. ... 1888.

209 × 132. Pp. 14, [ii] (colophon, v.b.). P. w. (title rptd).

For John Williams (d. 1914) MD Edin. & Melb., Hon. Phys. Melb. Hosp., see obit., *Austsn med. Gaz.*, 1914, 35 : 403; also Stawell, Sir R. R. (1932), *Melb. Hosp. Clin. Rep.*, 3 : 1.

Copies: NL. 2521

Williamson, William Cotter

Lectures on the care and treatment of the insane for the instruction of attendants and nurses. ... Sydney: Thomas Richards, Govt Printer. 1885.

217 × 140. Pp. 74. Limp morocco.

W. C. Williamson (1856–1945) MD QUI, Surg. RN, joined staff of Parramatta Asylum in 1884 and became Med. Supt of other NSW mental instns. See Dawson, W. S. (1965), *Annals of psychiatry in NSW*, Syd., typescript. (ML, RACP.)

Copies: EF, HDN, ML. 2522

Willis, T.R.H.

See Australian Health Society, No 103.

Willows, Anthony

See No 1552.

Willson, Rt Rev. Robert William

A few observations relating to the Yarra Bend Lunatic Asylum, by the Right Rev. R. W. Willson, D. D., Catholic Bishop of Hobart Town; together with remarks on an hospital for the insane. Reprinted from the Australian Medical Journal. Melbourne: ... Wm. Goodhugh & Co. ... 1859.

217 × 138. Pp. 14.

For life of author, see Kelsh, T. His experience in care of the insane appears in evidence before Joint Com. on New Norfolk Hosp. for Insane (1859).

Copies: ML, SLV. 2523

See also: Browning, Colin Arrott and Willson, Robt Wm.

[Wilmot, Dr.], 'Truth'

Education: thoughts on the mental condition to which it is applicable. [Quotation] Melbourne: Wilson, Mackinnon and Fairfax, General Printers ... 1856.

8vo. Pp. 36.

Author states his only name was 'Truth'. Craig copy, formerly in library of Dr. J. E. Neild, Melb., has 'Dr. Wilmot' written on title p., apparently noting authorship.

Copies: CC. 2524

Wilmot, Sir John Eardley Eardley—

Government House, Sept. [3d] 1846. Sir The Secretary of State having instructed me to institute an immediate enquiry into the state of the Convict Population in this Island, I request you ... to convey to me your opinion, founded ... on your own observation, and ... knowledge ... on the following points, and if you will do so ... I shall be able to obtain a ... satisfactory report on this momentous subject. [Letter continues.]

247 × 204. Single leaf, v.b. Main body of text and subscription in cursive script; requirements listed in usual type; signed by hand.

Letter requires information on convicts of both sexes under headings: Health of convict population; their industry; moral and intellectual culture; religious knowledge and habits; personal habits—temperance and decency; occupation; daily average labour; leisure; reading and amusements; estimate of improvement or increase of bad habits and evil practices.

In 1847 convicts in VDL numbered 29,000 of a total population of 66,000.

Copies: CC. 2524a

Wilson, Edward John

Statements addressed to the Council of the Melbourne University, relative to the general and special regulations for conferring degrees in medicine. ... Melbourne: Wm. Goodhugh & Co. ... 1862.

206 × 132. Pp. 8.

Objections by meeting of practitioners to new regulations on medical degrees.

E. J. Wilson (1820–87) MRCS practised at Richmond Vic.

Copies: ML, SLV. 2525

Wilson, James Thomas

Notes on the innervation of the musculus sternalis, with remarks on its morphology, and notes on the stephanion and on various descriptions of the temporal lines of the skull. ...

Reprinted from the Proceedings of the Intercolonial Medical Congress of Australasia—Fourth Session. Dunedin: ... Otago Daily News Office ... 1897.

228 × 140. Pp. 8. P. w. (cover title).

Copies: EF, US 2526

(From the Proceedings of the Linnean Society of New South Wales, 1899, Part 1, March 29th.) Presidential Address. ...

222 × 143. Pp. 30 (l.b.). P. w. (cover title).

On 'vitalism' versus 'mechanism.'

J. T. Wilson (1861–1945) MB, ChM Edin., FRS, Prof. Anat. Univ. Syd., in 1920 became Prof. Anat. Univ. Camb. See obit., *Med. J. Aust.*, 1945, 2 : 512; also *J. Anat.*, 1941/2. vol. 76 (dedicated to him); Smith, S. A. (1950), 'The life and work of J.T.W.', *BPCMUS*, 6 : 1.

Copies: EF, ML, US. 2527

Wilson, John Bracebridge

Comparative methods of digestion, circulation & respiration in fishes, amphibia & mammals. Geelong: ... Geo. Mercer, Malop Street. 1891.

212 × 138. Pp. 16. Cloth.

Author was Headmaster, Geelong Grammar School.

Copies: EF, CC, FC, ML, SLV. 2528

Wilson, Thomas Braidwood

Narrative of a voyage round the world; comprehending an account of the wreck of the ship "Governor Ready", in Torres Straits; a description of the British settlements on the coasts of New Holland, more particularly Raffles Bay, Melville Island, Swan River, and King George's Sound; also, the manners and customs of the aboriginal tribes; with an appendix, containing remarks on transportation, the treatment of convicts during the voyage, and advice to persons intending to emigrate to the Australian colonies. By T. B. Wilson, M.D. Surgeon R. N. ... London: Printed for Sherwood, Gilbert, & Piper, 1835.

224 × 140. Pp. xvi (l.b.), 350, [ii] (errata, v.b.), 8 (book advts). 2 litho. pl., 1 flg chart. Cloth.

Facsimile ed., 1968. Lond., Dawsons.

Author, who had made 8 voyages to Aust. as surg.-supt of convict ships, describes return voyage of *Governor Ready*, its wreck, and visits to N. Aust. settlements at Raffles Bay and Melville Is. Appendix includes routine of surg.-supt and observations on convict health.

Copies: DL, FC, ML, NL, SLS, SLV, SLW, SPH, UA, UM, WLC. 2529

Wilson, William S.

The ocean as a health resort A handbook of practical information as to sea-voyages for the use of tourists and invalids ... With a chart showing the ocean-routes and illustrating the physical geography of the sea. London J & A Churchill ... 1880

183 × 122. Pp. xii, 260, [12] (advts). Cloth.

Includes: curative effect of ocean climate; health voyages; management of health at sea; Aust. climate, cities and health resorts.

Copies: AMAV, US. 2530

The Same. 2 ed., 1881.

Copies: SLS. 2531

Windeyer, Sir William Charles

Ex parte Collins. A judgment by W. C. Windeyer, LL.D., Senior Puisne Judge of the Supreme Court of New South Wales. Sydney: W. M. Maclardy ... 1889.

212 × 135. Pp. 24 (l.b.). P. w. (title rptd).

A notable judgement (12 Dec. 1888) that a pamphlet describing contraceptive methods (Annie Besant's *The law of population*) was not an obscene publication.

Annie Besant, an autobiography, Lond., 1893, regards this as 'one of the most luminous and cogent statements on the Neo-Malthusian position.' See also Robinson V. (1919), *Pioneers of birth control*, N.Y.: 82 (notes ed., published by Bradlaugh and Besant); Coleman, P. (1962), *Obscenity, blasphemy, sedition*, Bris.: 71.

Copies: EF, FC, ML, NL, SLS, SLV, UA. 2532

Is limitation of the family immoral? A judgement of Annie Besant's 'Law of Population', delivered in the Supreme Court of New South Wales. London, Freethought Publishing Company, 1889.

NS. Noted in *British birth control ephemera, 1870–1947*, Leicester, 1969.

2533

Witt, J. B.

Lecture on ventilation, delivered by Mr. J. B. Witt (Managing Director of the Victorian

Atmospheric Refrigerating Company Limited ...), under the auspices of the Australian Health Society. Melbourne: Tyzack & Picken, Printers and Stationers ... 1888.

215 × 140. Pp. 16 (l.b.). P. w. (cover title).

Copies: SLT. 2534

Women's Hospital, Melbourne

The Melbourne Lying-In Hospital, and Infirmary for Diseases of Women & Children. 41, Albert Street. [Text follows.]

252 × 198. Pp. [4] (l.b.). ND. (1856.) Colophon—Campbell, Printer ...

Includes report of opening (19 Aug. 1856).

Copies: AMAV. 2535

———

First Annual Report of the ... Melbourne Lying-in Hospital and Infirmary for Diseases of Women and Children, for the year ending 30th June, 1857; with the rules of the institution ... Melbourne: Printed by Goodhugh & Hough ... 1857.

198 × 130. Pp. 16.

Name changed to 'The Hospital for Women', 1884; rapidly translated to 'The Women's Hospital'; and to 'Royal Women's Hospital', 1954.

See Cunningham, E. S. (1940), *The history of the Women's Hosp.*, Melb.; Sayers, C. E. (1956), *The Women's ... a social history*, Melb.; Macdonald, C. (1957), *Med. J. Aust.*, 1 : 25; Forster, F.M.C. (1967), *Progress in obst. and gynaec, in Aust.*, Syd.; also nos 2296–7.

Copies: LNSW (1856/7–60), ML (1856/7, 1860), SLV (1856/7–73, 1877–87), Roy. Women's Hosp. (1856/7–). 2536

———

Thirtieth Annual Report of the Committee of Management of the Women's Hospital, and Infirmary for Diseases of Women, for the year ending 30th June, 1887 ... Melbourne: Andrew Kerr & Co., Printers ... 1887.

206 × 135. Pp. 32 (last—colophon only).

Copies: See above. 2537

Women's Hospital, Sydney

Objects and rules of the Women's Hospital and Dispensary. Adopted at meeting of subscribers ... 13th August, 1895. Sydney: H. Hely & Co. ... 1895.

127 × 90. Pp. 8. P. w. (title rptd).

Objects—to provide a maternity hospital for poor and necessitous women, domiciliary obstetric service, indoor and outdoor gynaecological treatment, and midwifery nursing school.

Copies: FC, ML. 2538

———

The Women's Hospital. Report and statement of receipts and expenditure account for the year ended 30th June, 1896. Notice is hereby given that the Annual General Meeting ... will be held on ... 31st day of August, 1896 ... David Fell, Hon. Secretary. ... Sydney, 4th August, 1896. H. Hely & Co., Printers ... Sydney.

331 × 209. Pp. 4. P. w. (with title transversely on back wrapper, for folding).

1st annual report.

Hospital was situated in Hay St., Sydney. 2 an. rep. notes acquisition of building in Crown St, Surry Hills, whence moved in 1897.

Copies: ML (1895/6–). 2539

———

The Women's Hospital, 207 Hay Street, Sydney. Inaugurated 1st October, 1893. Board of Directors: [List of Officers.]

209 × 127. Pp. [4]. 1896. P. w. (cover title). Colophon—H. Hely & Co. ... Sydney.

Copies: ML. 2540

Wood, Arthur C. J.

Practical embalming, (scientific and sanitary,) by Arthur C. J. Wood, of (Wood and Company,) first certified embalmer of New South Wales ... A. O'Toole & Co., Printers ... Balmain.

153 × 102. Pp. 12. (1896.) P. w. (decorated cover title).

Copies: ML. 2541

Wood, W.

Eye-sight, good, bad & indifferent Defects and remedies. ... Sydney and Melbourne: ... Alf. Hughes (Victorian Printing Works) ...

183 × 122. Pp. [2], 30, [4] (advts). 7 figs. (1895.) P. w. (title rptd).

Advertises firm of opticians.

Copies: ML, SLV. 2542

Wood, William Atkinson

Practical household hygiene ... With fourteen illustrations. Melville, Mullen & Slade ... Melbourne. Rae Bros., Polygraphic Printers ... Melbourne.

133 × 107. Pp. 140 (last—colophon). 14 figs. (1893.) Cloth.

An elementary text-book on hygiene for popular education.

W. A. Wood (d. 1945) MD, MS Melb., DPH Lond., practised in South Yarra Vic., was Hon. Surg. to Children's and Austin Hosps.

Copies: EF. 2543

Australian Health Society. Animals as a cause of scarlet fever and diphtheria. Melbourne. 1893.

8vo. Pp. 4.

NS. Noted in *25 years record* ..., Melb., Aust. Health Soc., [1900]. 2544

Woodward, George Paul Minchin

New South Wales Railways ambulance handbook. Copiously illustrated. Accidents and their treatment, aids in cases of injuries, sudden illness, &c., &c. Enlarged edition, issued by the Commissioner for Railways. ... Sydney Charles Potter, Govt Printer. 1887. ...

156 × 105. Pp. xvi (l.b.), 184. Flg pl., 72 figs. Morocco.

2 ed., 1892; 3 ed., 1898; 5 ed., 1904; 6 ed., 1911.

G. P. M. Woodward (d. 1908) MD Brux., FRCSI, a former Army surgeon (DDGMS) with service in Indian Mutiny, Crimea and Abyssinian Wars, was MO to NSW Railways. Obit.: *Austsn med. Gaz.*, 1908, 27 : 555.

Copies: EF, ML, NL, RACP, SLV, UA, US. 2545

Woogaroo Lunatic Asylum, Qd

1868–9. Queensland. Legislative Assembly. Lunatic Asylum, Woogaroo. Report from ... the Commissioners appointed to inquire into the Lunatic Asylum, Woogaroo. ... Brisbane: ... James C. Beal, Govt Printer ... 1869.

325 × 203. Pp. [ii] (v.b.), 4, 74. Blue paper.

Woogaroo Lunatic Asylum, at Goodna, was about 1881 renamed Goodna Asylum for the Insane. For period thereafter, see Nos 750 and 751.

Copies: LNSW, ML, NL, OL, SLV. 2546

1869. Queensland. Legislative Assembly. Report from the Joint Select Committee on the Woogaroo Lunatic Asylum ... Brisbane: ... James C. Beal, Govt Printer ... 1869.

326 × 204. Pp. 74 (l.b.). 9 pl. (maps and plans). Blue paper. Recommends wide reforms, improved facilities.

Copies: LNSW, ML, NL, OL, SLV. 2547

1870. Queensland. Woogaroo Asylum. (Report of the Acting Surgeon-Superintendent of) ... [Text begins.]

320 × 203. Pp. 10 (l.b.). Colophon—James C. Beal, Govt Pr, Bris.

Annual reports of Surg.-Supt, 1870–79. For continuation, see Goodna and Ipswich Asylums, No 750.

Copies: LNSW, NL, OL, SLV. 2548

1877. Queensland. Woogaroo Commission. Report ... the Royal Commission ... into the management of the Woogaroo Lunatic Asylum and the Lunatic Reception Houses of the Colony ... Brisbane: James C. Beal, Govt Printer ...

320 × 205. Pp. 20, xvi, 126.

Copies: LNSW, NL, OL, SLV. 2549

1880. Queensland. Board of Inquiry, Woogaroo Asylum. Report of the Board appointed to inquire into certain charges made against Dr. Patrick Smith, Surgeon-Superintendent of Woogaroo Lunatic Asylum ... and the general management of the institution ... Brisbane: ... James C. Beal, Govt Printer ... 1880.

318 × 200. Pp. 88. 1 plan.

Copies: LNSW, NL, OL, SLV. 2550

Woolls, William

A contribution to the flora of Australia ... Sydney: F. White ... Parramatta: J. Ferguson ... Melbourne: G. Robertson ... 1867.

206 × 132. Pp. x, 256 (l.b.). Cloth.

Contains 'Medicinal plants of the Parramatta District' (94–101).

Copies: FC, ML, NL, OL, SLS, SLT, SLV, UA, UM, UQ, US. 2551

Woore, Thomas

Supply of water from the Warragamba River, sewerage of Sydney, irrigation of Cumberland, relief of Hawkesbury, suburban railway, and defence of the north shores of Botany Bay, combined in one scheme by Thomas Woore, a member of the Water Commission of 1872. Sydney: ... F. White ... 1876.

217 × 140. Pp. 28 (l.b.). P. w. (title rptd).
Copies: ML, NL. 2552

Workman, Francis

The ocean as a health resort. Letter ... to the Reading Pathological Society. Reading: ... J. J. Beecroft ...

204 × 135. Pp. 12 (l.b.). ND. (1884.) P. w. (cover title).

Describes voyage from Plymouth to Melb. as surgeon of clipper ship *Sabraon*, then a 'hospital ship', providing health voyages for invalids. Warns of possible hardships and risks of such voyages for seriously ill and tubercular.

Francis Workman MRCS arrived in Vic. from Eng. in 1884, practised in W. Melb., died at Hamilton Vic. in 1897, aged 63. See Thomas, B. and Gandevia, B. (1959), *Med. J. Aust.*, 2 : 1.
Copies: Reading Path. Soc. 2553

World's Dispensary Medical Association

See Parker, William R.

Wormald, F. G.

... Analyses, testimonials of medical profession and dentists ... regarding the "pure carbolic and toilet soap" known as "sapo acidi carbolici". Detergent, antiseptic, disinfectant ... F. G. Wormald, Chemist and Druggist ... Carlton.

181 × 107. Pp. 24. ND.
Copies: SLV. 2554

Worsnop, Thomas

The prehistoric arts, manufactures, works, weapons, etc., of the aborigines of Australia. Compiled ... by Thomas Worsnop, Town Clerk, Adelaide. South Australia: C. E. Bristow, Govt Printer ... 1897.

209 × 132. Pp. xvi (4 blanks), 172. Frontis., 85 pl. Cloth.

Includes section on native medicine and surgery, with sketch of fixation of fractured humerus.

Copies: ML, NL, SLS, SLV, SLW, UM, US. 2555

Worthy, Wavering

See Wardley, Edward.

Wylde, R. T.

A lecture on cremation by R. T. Wylde, Surgeon, J. P. ... Adelaide: W. K. Thomas & Co., Printers ... 1890.

210 × 140. Pp. 16, inserted enrolment form.

Introduction to foundation of Cremation Soc. of SA.
Copies: SLS. 2556

Wynne, Edward Thomas

See Hunt, James Sidney, Collins, W., and Wynne, E. T.

Y

Yarra Bend Lunatic Asylum, Vic.

Regulations for the guidance of the officers, attendants, and servants, of the Lunatic Asylum, Port Phillip. Published by authority. Melbourne: ... E. Wilson, Govt Printer ... 1849.

188 × 120. 20 un-numbered leaves (11 blank). P. w. (short title).

First Victorian mental hospital; established 1848.

Copies: Parlt Library of Vic. 2557

1852. Victoria. Report from the Select Committee of the Legislative Council on the Yarra Bend Lunatic Asylum ... Melbourne: ... John Ferres, at the Govt Printing Office.

328 × 197. Pp. x, 86. Blue tinted paper.

On condition and management. States that patients are 'subjected to all the coercion and punishments usually had recourse to in Madhouses, at the will and caprice of uncontrolled Attendants ... and were much more likely to have their malady hopelessly confirmed, than to have a fair chance ... of being cured ...'

For history of administration, see Benn, K. M. (1957), 'The moral versus the medical controversy: an early struggle in Vic. psychiatry', *Med. J. Aust.*, 1 : 125.

Copies: AMAV, LNSW, NL, SLV. 2558

1855. Victoria. Lunatic Asylum at Yarra Bend. Return to address—Mr. Mollison ... ordered by the Council to be printed, 18th December, 1855. [Report begins.]

340 × 210. Pp. 2. Colophon— ... John Ferres, Govt Printer, Melb. Blue tinted paper.

Two reports on instn, signed W. McCrea, Chairman, Bd of Visitors.

Copies: LNSW, ML, NL, SLV. 2559

1855–6. Victoria. Yarra Bend Lunatic Asylum. Return to address. Mr. Mollison—22nd January, 1856. ...

340 × 210. Pp. [2]. Blue tinted paper. Colophon— ... John Ferres, Govt Pr, Melb.

Inspection report with recommendations. Signed: J. F. Palmer, Redmond Barry, W. McCrea.

Copies: LNSW, NL, SLV. 2560

1856–7. Victoria. Report on the Yarra Bend Lunatic Asylum for the year 1856. Presented to both Houses ... John Ferres, Govt Printer, Melbourne.

342 × 210. Pp. 12. Blue tinted paper. Signed—W. McCrea CMO.

Copies: BG, LNSW, ML, NL, SLV. 2561

1857–8. Victoria. Report from the Select Committee upon the Lunatic Asylum ... Ordered by the Legislative Assembly to be printed, 20th April, 1858. ... John Ferres, Govt Printer, Melbourne.

343 × 214. Pp. xiv (l.b.), 82 (l.b.). Blue tinted paper.

Copies: AMAV, BG, LNSW, ML, NL, SLV. 2562

Yarra Bend mismanagement. Petition to the Honourable the Chief Secretary and the Members of Parliament ... [Text begins.]

8vo. Pp. 8. ND. Colophon—R. Bell, Printer ... Melb.

Copies: SLV. 2563

The late inquiry at the Yarra Bend Asylum; describing in the words of the witnesses, the Western Gaol, the Yarra Bend, and the proceedings of the Board of Visitors: from notes by a shorthand reporter. [Quotation] Richmond: ... Richmond General Printing Office, ... 1859.

204 × 127. Pp. 32.

Report of coroner's inquiry following death of a patient.

Copies: EF. 2564

1858–9. Victoria. Report from the Select Committee upon the Yarra Bend Lunatic Asylum ... with the proceedings of the Committee. Ordered by the Legislative Assembly to be printed, 16th February, 1859. ... John Ferres, Govt Printer, Melbourne.

343 × 215. Pp. vi (iv blank). Blue tinted paper.

Further reports : 1859–60, progress rep., pp. [iv] (l.b.). 1859–60, 2nd progress rep., pp. [iv] (l.b.). 1860–1, progress rep., pp. [vi] (l.b.), [5]–64, 74, x. 1861–2, progress rep., pp. [iv] (l.b.). 1861–2, 2nd progress rep., pp. [iv] (l.b.). 1861–2, 3rd progress rep., pp. [vi], 77 (l.b.). 1862–3, progress rep., pp. [vi] (l.b.).

On condition, management, and criminal lunatics.

Copies: AMAV, LNSW, ML, NL, SLV. 2565

1861–2. Victoria. Report from the Select Committee on the Lunatic Asylum ... Ordered by the Legislative Assembly to be printed, 20th May, 1862. ... John Ferres, Govt Printer, Melbourne.

344 × 216. Pp. xiv, [ii], 16 (l.b.), viii. Blue paper.

On management of patients in Asylum, and gaols in which patients committed through courts were confined till transfer arranged. Recommendations include temporary accommodation in hospitals; erection of asylums at Beechworth, Sandhurst and Ballarat; separation of criminal lunatics.

Copies: AMAV, LNSW, ML, NL, SLV. 2566

See also Bowie, Robert; Willson, Robt. W.; No 1006.

Young, Mrs. I. S. Hunter

One of the many marvels of the nineteenth century. Vocal speech & lip reading for the deaf mute: giving the experience and opinions of some of the greatest living authorities. ... Melbourne: M'Carron, Bird & Co. ... 1883.

212 × 135. Pp. 30. P. w. (title rptd).

Copies: ML, SLV. 2567

Z

Zimmermann, F.
See Nos 52–3.

APPENDIX

CHRONOLOGICAL LIST OF PUBLICATIONS TO 1850

THE NECESSITY for an alphabetical presentation of items listed herein is regretted, since this precludes ready appreciation of the development of Australian medical publication during its formative years. To resolve this in part, titles of the early period to 1850, chronologically arranged, are shown below. Certain omissions occur, including papers of the New South Wales Legislative Assembly and recurring items such as annual reports.

Settlement to 1800

Medicine in the period of the first settlement on Sydney Cove to 1800 is represented by John White's *Journal of a Voyage to new South Wales*, Lond., 1790, one of the six great contemporary accounts describing these years of struggle with disease, starvation and isolation. For a full appreciation of the medical background of this time, reference to the companion volumes of Arthur Phillip, Watkin Tench, John Hunter and David Collins is also necessary. Items of Australian interest occur also in Kite, Charles, *Essays and observations, physiological and medical*, Lond., 1795; Trotter, Thomas, *Medical and chemical essays*, Lond., 1796; and Smyth, James Carmichael, *The effect of nitrous oxide in preventing contagion*, Lond., 1799.

The First Ten Years

The first decade of the new century marked the firm establishment of Australian publication when, in 1802, George Howe issued the *New South Wales Standing Orders*, the first book printed in Australia, and the next year the first issue of *The Sydney Gazette and New South Wales Advertiser*, the earliest newspaper. Medical journalism began in the *Gazette* of 14 Oct. 1804 with a short article, 'General observations on the small-pox', by Principal Surgeon Thomas Jamison. In 1805, Tuckey, James H., *An account of a voyage to establish a colony at Port Philip*, Lond., including health in convict ships, and in 1807 Péron, Francois A., *Voyage de découvertes aux Terres Australes*, Paris, with experiment on strength of Aborigines, appeared.

Published 1810–19

Benevolent Society of New South Wales, earliest Australian charity, 1st an. rep., Syd., 1819; Haslam, John, *Convict-ships*, Lond., 1819, first of a series of works by surgeons-superintendent of convict vessels following reform of the transport service; Wentworth, William Charles, *A statistical, historical, and political description of New South Wales*, Lond., 1819, earliest work by an Australian author, with notes on current diseases.

Published 1820–29

Bigge, John Thomas, *Report of the Commissioner of Inquiry into the state of the Colony of New South Wales*, Lond., 1822; Reid, Thomas, *Two voyages to New South Wales and Van Diemen's Land*, Lond., 1822; Bigge, John Thomas, *Report of the Commissioner of Inquiry, on the state of agriculture and trade in the Colony* ..., Lond., 1823; *Instructions for the guidance of surgeons superintendent and masters of convict ships arriving in the River Derwent*, [1826], earliest of a series of official instructions (1826–45);

Cunningham, Peter Miller, *Two years in New South Wales*, Lond., 1827; *Female Friendly Society, Rules of*, Syd., 1827; Sydney Dispensary (established 1826), 1st an. rep., Syd., 1828; two pamphlets relating to Henry Grattan Douglass MD, Syd., 1828; Cameron, Charles, *Copy of a letter from Mr. Charles Cameron, a surgeon in His Majesty's Navy*, Lond., 1829; Lesson, R. P., *Voyage médical autour du mond*, Paris, 1829.

Published 1830–34

Jeanneret, Henry : *Hints for the preservation of the teeth*, Syd., 1830, the first Australian dental publication; Bland, William, *Journal of discovery to Port Phillip . . . by Messrs. W. H. Hovell, and Hamilton Hume*, Syd., 1831, the first book on Victoria; Goodridge, Charles Medyett, *Narrative of a voyage to the South Seas*, Lond., 1832, includes notes on health: Goodridge, Charles Medyett, *Statistical view of Van Diemen's Land*, Lond., 1832, separately published section of above; *Australian chivalry; or fire-side knight errantry*, Syd., [1832], an anonymous poem involving Sir John Jamison MD; Osborne, Alick, *Notes on the present state and prospects of society in New South Wales*, Lond., 1833; Bennett, George, *Wanderings in New South Wales*, Lond., 1834; Lang, John Dunmore, *An historical and statistical account of New South Wales*, Lond., 1834; Temperance Society of New South Wales, *Half an hour's reading*, Syd., 1834.

Published 1835–39

Bennett, George and Others : *Reports on the epidemic catarrh or influenza . . .*, Syd., 1835; Wilson. Thomas B., *Narrative of a voyage round the world*, Lond., 1835; Launceston Benevolent Society, 2nd an. rep., Launceston, 1836; Browning, Colin Arrott, *An address to the prisoners debarked from the "Surry" . . .*, Hobart Town, 1836: Tomlins, P. Stanley, *The coroner's guide*, Hobart Town, 1837; Mitchell, James, *Statement of the case of Jas. Mitchell, Esq.*, Syd., 1838; *Instructions for surgeons superintendent on board emigrant ships proceeding to New South Wales or Van Diemen's Land*, Lond., 1838, first of a series of official instructions (1838–83); Adelaide Hospital, appeal for funds prior to foundation, Adel., 1839; Goodwin, John, *Testimonials . . .*, Syd., 1839; Melbourne Union Benefit Society, *Articles and rules . . .*, Melb., 1839, the first pamphlet published in Victoria; Butler, Samuel, *The hand-book for Australian emigrants*, Glasgow, 1839; Tegg, Thomas, *Tegg's handbook for emigrants*, Lond., 1839.

Published 1840

Australia as it is . . . Climate and diseases, Bristol; Hawkesbury Benevolent Society and Hospital, an. rep., Syd.; St Mary's Hospital, prospectus, Hobart; Welch, Robert Porter, *A familiar treatise on diseases of the eye*, Syd., the first medical work separately published in Australia.

Published 1841

Adelaide Hospital, *Some account of the . . .*, [Adel.]; Bland, William, *Paper on the present epidemic scarlatina*, Syd., earliest Aust. contribution to clinical medicine; Bright, John, *Hand-book for emigrants*, Lond.; Browning, Colin Arrott, *An address to the women who debarked at Sydney . . .*, Syd.; Clark, Sir James, *The sanative influence of climate*, Lond.; Fitzpatrick, Adolphus, *A guide to the preservation of health in South Australia*, Adel.; St Mary's Hospital, rep., Hobart.

Published 1842

Baker, W., *The New South Wales Medical Act; together with a list of the legally qualified medical practitioners of the Colony*, Syd., the earliest Aust. med. directory; Browning, Colin Arrott, *England's exiles*, Lond.; Lee, William, *Brandy and salt . . . remedy for most of the diseases that afflict humanity*, Syd.;

Little, Robert, *Practical observations on the treatment of the epidemic scarlet-fever, recently so prevalent in New South Wales*, Syd.; *Sydney Strangers' Friend Society*, rep. for 1841, Syd.

Published 1843

Bartlett, Thomas, *New Holland*, Lond., with notes on diseases and climate; Bland, William, *Suppression of spontaneous combustion in wool ships*, Syd.; Browning, Colin Arrott, *A brief word of advice to the men . . . from the ship "Earl Grey"*, Hobart Town.

Published 1844

Browning, Colin Arrott, *The convict ship*, Lond.; Sherwin, William, *On the primum mobile of the blood in the lungs at birth*, Syd., the first medical publication by a native-born Australian; Simpson, Stephen, *Journal of an excursion to the Bunya Country*, Lond.

Published 1845

Bathurst Dist. Hospital, an. rep. 1844, Syd.; Dredge, James, *Brief notices of the Aborigines of New South Wales*, Geelong; Henderson, Andrew, *Scraps and facts of convict ships*, Devonport; McCrae, Farquhar, *Election of medical officers to the Sydney Infirmary*, Syd.; Melbourne Hospital, report of meeting for foundation, Melb.; Pugh, William Russ, *A letter to the medical profession of Van Diemen's Land : accompanied by the particulars of an operation for strangulated congenital hernia*, Launceston, earliest publication on a surgical subject; Van Diemen's Land—Comptroller Gen. of Convicts, 3 items containing duties of med. officer, Hobart Town; Van Diemen's Land—Inspector Gen. of Hospitals, *Rules for convict hospitals*, Hobart Town; Wallace, Francis L., sale catalogue, Syd.

Published 1846

Australian Medical Journal (1846–7), earliest Aust. medical periodical; Bland, William, *Correspondence between Dr. Farquhar M'Crae and Mr. Surgeon Bland*, Syd., reply to McCrae's pamphlet (below); Campbell, Francis, *An abstract of the letters of Iatros, on lunatic asylums and the treatment of lunatics*, Syd.; Claridge, R. T., *Hydropathy*, Launceston; McCrae, Farquhar, *Correspondence between Dr. Farquhar M'Crae and Mr. Surgeon Bland*, Syd.; St John's Hospital, letter to subscribers, Launceston; *Sydney Infirmary and Dispensary*, 1st an. rep., Syd.; Tarban Creek Lunatic Asylum [Gladesville], Syd., first of numerous reports; Westgarth, William, *A report on the condition, capabilities and prospects of the Australian Aborigines*, Melb.; Wilmot, Sir J. Eardley, letter seeking information on health etc. of convicts, [Hobart].

Published 1847

Best, John, *A review of the letter addressed to the householders of Hobart Town by the Reverend H. P. Fry*, Hobart Town: Browning, Colin Arrott, *The convict ship, and England's exiles*, Lond.; *Hobart Town General Dispensary and Humane Society*, Hobart Town; Pocock, Zachary P., *Transportation and prison discipline*, Lond.

Published 1848

Lunatic Asylum, New South Wales [Gladesville], regulations, Syd.; *Van Diemen's Land Asylum. Instituted 1848*, Hobart Town; Wilkinson, George Blakiston, *South Australia : its advantages and resources*, Lond.

Published 1849

Goulburn District Hospital, an. rep. (7th) for 1848, Goulburn; Melbourne Hospital, an. rep.

(1st) for 1848, Melb.; Parramatta Benevolent Society, rep. for 1848, Parramatta; Ray, James, *A voice from the inquest room*, Hobart Town; Stephens, John, *Sanitary reform*, Adel.; *Van Diemen's Land Asylum*, objects and rules, Hobart Town; *The same*, 1st an. rep.; [Yarra Bend Asylum], *Regulations . . . of the Lunatic Asylum, Port Phillip*, Melb.

Published 1850

Australian Medical Subscription Library, rules and regulations, Syd.; Bright Richard, *An address to the inhabitants of Van Diemen's Land*, Hobart Town; Campbell, Francis, *A commentary on the use and abuses of tobacco*, Syd.; Clutterbuck, James Bennett, *Port Phillip in 1849*, Lond.; Duncan, Handasyde, *The Colony of South Australia*, Lond.; Gorringe, Thomas F., *Short dissertations on diarrhoea, dysentery, cholera morbus, scarlatina and erysipelas*, Hobart Town; H, J. B., *A catechism of mesmerism*, Melb.; Medini, Michael, *Statements and correspondence relative to the case of . . .*, Syd.; Port Phillip Medical Association, *Rules and regulations*, Melb.,—first Aust. medical society.

INDEX

All references are to entry numbers and not to pages

ADDENDA

Items listed below are not included in the Index

Abramowski, Otto Louis Moritz

The proposed Mildura and Darling River railway. Criticism of the Parliamentary Railway Committee's report. ... Issued by ... the Mildura and Darling River Railway Extension League ... 1896: The Mildura Irrigationist ...

212 × 143. Pp. 8. P.w. (cover title). Signed: O.L.M. Abramowski, Chairman.

O.L.M. Abramowski MD, ChD Berlin (1875) practised at Terowie SA and later as Med. Supt Mildura Dist Hosp. (1894–1908). He advocated a purely vegetable diet, on which he wrote and lectured, and after 1908 conducted the Sun Sanitorium at Sandringham Vic. He died in 1910. For obit.—*Austsn med. Gaz.*, 1911, 30:47.

He published: *The no-food treatment and fruit diet at Mildura District Hospital*, Mildura, 1908; *Vitalism, the art of eating for health*, Melb., 1908; 2 ed., 1910; 3 ed. (with title *Eating for health*), 1913; *Fruitarian diet and physical rejuvenation*, Lond., 20th thousand, [1916].

Copies: ML. 1a

Blair, John

On injuries of the skull and its contents. ... [Text begins.]

205 × 130. Pp. 4. Colophon—Stillwell and Knight ... Melb. P.w. (cover title). Repr. *Aust. med. J.*, 1873.

Copies: SLV. 325a

———

On a case of gunshot wound of the hand, and one of ankle joint disease. ...

205 × 130. Pp. 4 (l.b.). 2 figs. Colophon—Stillwell and Knight ... Melb. P.w. (cover title). Repr. *Aust. med. J.*, 1873.

Copies: SLV. 325b

———

On a tumour removed from the femoral region. ... [Text begins.]

205 × 130. Pp. 4 (l.b.). 1 litho. pl. Repr. *Aust. med. J.*, 1873.

Copies: SLV. 325c

Bohemian University Student, A

The happy delivery of a legal lady in Jolop Street East. A dramatic episode. Price sixpence. By a Bohemian University Student. Printed and published by the Author, at the University Steam Works ... 1866.

218 × 140. Pp. 10.

A medico-legal farce.

Copies: LNSW, ML, SLV. 349a

Bonwick, James

Notes of a gold digger and gold diggers' guide ... Melbourne: R. Connebee ... and sold by all booksellers. 1852.

12mo. Pp. 42. Frontis., map. P.w. (title rptd).

Another ed., 1942. Melb.: Hawthorn Press. (250 copies.)

Includes short chapter, 'Health at the diggings', with general advice on living conditions, hygiene, diet, water, and care in illness, particularly diarrhoea and dysentery. Notes for this were supplied by author's 'friend and mate at the diggings', R. T. Tracy (see No 2282), who had accompanied him from Adel. to the Loddon and Bendigo fields, where he combined practice with digging.

Copies: DL, FC, ML, NL, SLV, SLW. 358a

Buchanan, David

Donkey worship v. hero worship; or, cricket & boat-pulling amongst Australians. By David Buchanan, M.P. (of the Middle Temple), Barrister-at-Law. Sydney: Batson & Atwater ... 1882.

204 × 132. Pp. 20.

On Australian obsession with sport, dedicated to 'the larrikans and donkeys of NSW and their instructors, the Press'. Refers to 'the insane folly of the people running in droves after cricketers and boat-pullers ... which threatens to submerge the land in deluges of humbug, triviality, frivolity, and all manner of delirious absurdity'.

For David Buchanan (1832–90) MLC, barrister and orator, see Mennell.

Copies: FC, ML, NL. 461a

Candler, Samuel Curtis

[*Additional note*] According to Bowden, K. M., *Doctors and diggers of the Mount Alexander Goldfields*, Collaroy, 1974, Candler was registered in Vic. and was at Fryer's Creek in 1853. He was Coroner, Wedderburn, in this year; District Surg. Maryborough 1854; and Coroner, Melb., 1863. 494

Davy, Edward

An experimental guide to chemistry. Printed for the Author: London, 1836.

8vo. Pp. iv, 98. NS.

Edward Davy (1806–85) LSA, MRCS, a pioneer in the development of the electric telegraph, came from London to SA in 1839 and was ed. Adel. *Examiner* and later Manager of Yatala copper smelters. In 1853 he moved to Vic., and practised at Malmsbury to his death. Obits, *Aust. med. J.*, 1885, ns 7 : 77 and *Roy. Soc. Vic.*, *Trans. & Proc.*, 1884, 21 : 150; also *Aust. Enc.*, 3 : 211.

Copies: British Museum. 606a

Duchatelet, Parent, and a Doctor of Medicine

Prostitutes and prostitution in Paris from the celebrated work of M. Parent Duchatelet and a Doctor of Medicine. Comprising the whole system of police surveillance, the actual lives of these unfortunates, &c. Sydney ... H. J. Franklin ...

214 × 135. Pp. 32. ND. P.w. (extended title).

From preface: 'Common and numerous as prostitutes have ever been in the Aust. colonies, little has been done to mitigate this scourge ... except to improve their morality by committing them pretty often to prison. ... In Brisbane, the evil has been brought under some sort of control, partly to follow the system adopted in Paris ...'

Copies: ML. 635a

Fairfax, William

Handbook to Australasia; being a brief historical and descriptive account of Victoria, Tasmania, South Australia, New South Wales, Western Australia, and New Zealand: edited by William Fairfax. ... Melbourne: ... William Fairfax and Co. ... 1859.

173 × 112. Pp. [2] (advts), cxl (misnumbered clx), 244, [34] (advts). Flg map. Cloth.

Vic. section contains chapter on Med. Dept, including information on Cent. Bd of Health, Benev. Asylum, Yarra Bend Lunatic Asylum, and Point Nepean Sanitary Stn; also accounts of Melb. medical instns.

List of published works on Australia (pp. 229–44), prepared by Public Library of Vic., has been described as 'the first steps towards an Australian bibliography'.

Copies: DL, EF, FC, LNSW, ML, NL, OL, SLS, SLT, SLV, SLW, UM, US. 660a

Greene, John S.

"In vino veritas". A tilt at teetotalism; or a refutation of the "Refuter refuted" ... Geelong: Wise & Downie, Printers ... 1868.

171 × 107. Pp. 24. P.w. (title rptd).

Attacks teetotal views of Benjamin Wilkins (2509a, Addenda).

Copies: ML. 766a

Haig, William

On a case of tumour in the neck. ...

206 × 130. Pp. 4. 1 litho. pl. ND. Colophon—Stillwell and Knight. Repr. *Aust. med. J.*, 1874.

Copies: SLV. 804a

Hutchinson, John

The spirometer, the stethoscope, & scale-balance; their use in discriminating diseases of the chest, and their value in life offices; with remarks on the selection of lives for life assurance companies. London, John Churchill ... 1852.

8vo. Pp. 79. 1 pl. NS.

John Hutchinson MRCS, MD Giessen (1811–61), Asst Phys. Brompton Chest Hosp., Lond., inventor of the spirometer for estimation of the vital capacity of the lungs, arrived in Melb., suffering from tuberculosis, in 1851. He practised in Bendigo and was Hon. MO to Bendigo Hosp. to 1861, when he left for Fiji, where he died the same year. For his life in Vic., see Bowden, K. M., *Doctors and diggers on the Mount Alexander Goldfields*, Collaroy, 1974.

Copies: British Museum 973a

Krefft, Gerard

Letters & testimonials from distinguished men of science, addressed to Mr. Gerard Krefft, Curator and Secretary of the Australian

Museum. [Text begins.]

339 × 204. Single leaf. Blue paper. Pp. [2]. (Sydney.) ND.

Letters (dated 1858–74) include Richard Owen FRS to Dr. George Bennett (1874); Charles Darwin to Krefft (1873.)

For Krefft as a local champion of Darwin, see Mozley, Ann (1967) 'Evolution and the climate of opinion in Aust., 1840–76', *Victorian Studies*: 429.

Copies: SLV. 1111a

Maconochie, Alexander

Thoughts on convict management and other subjects connected with the Australian Penal Colonies by Captain Maconochie, R. N., K. H. [Quotation] Hobart Town: Printed by J. C. Macdougall . . . 1838.

212 × 132. Pp. [vi] (versos blank), viii (l.b.), [ii], 222. Errata slip. Cloth.

Includes: 'On the prevalence of drunkenness in VDL' (pp. 149–54).

Copies: ML, NL, SLT, WLC. 1247a

Macgillivray, Paul Howard

From "The Australian Medical Journal", May 1869. On a case of abscess of the spleen. . . . [Text begins.]

224 × 138. Pp. 2.

Copies: ML. 1219a

Meymott, Charles

New truths and their reception: A lecture . . . School of Arts, Sydney . . . 1858, by Charles Meymott, Esq., M.R.C.S., L.A.C. . . . Sydney . . . J. R. Clarke . . . 1858. Printed at the "Spectator" Office.

178 × 107. Pp. 30 (l.b.). Errata slip. P.w. (title rptd).

Copies: FC, ML, NL, SLV. 1375a

Moore, William [Surgeon]

[*Additional note*] See also Rank, Sir Benjamin K., *Jerry Moore and some of his contemporaries*, Melb., 1975, for biog. and appreciation as surgeon. Moore's book, *Plastic Surgery*, 'one of the first on the subject in the English language', though well in advance of its time, was virtually unknown. It is described by author, present-day Australian leader in plastic surgery, as 'a lost classic'. 1407

New South Wales—Board of Health

1890. Legislative Assembly. New South Wales. Borough of Redfern. (Report of the Board of Health on the deposit of garbage in . . . Ordered . . . to be printed, 15 October, 1890. [Text begins.]

327 × 210. Pp. 4. 1 flg map, 6 pl. Colophon—Sydney: Charles Potter, Govt Pr.—1896.

Copies: EF, HDN, ML, SPH. 1500a

New South Wales—Government Asylums for Infirm and Destitute

By-Laws of the Board for Managing the Government Asylums for the Infirm and Destitute. Sydney: Thomas Richards, Govt Printer . . . 1862.

204 × 130. Pp. 8 (l.b.). Signed—Chris. Rolleston, Chairman, Hyde Park Asylum, Sydney.

Copies: LNSW. 1511a

———

Regulations for the internal management of the Government Asylums for the Infirm and Destitute. 1862. Sydney: Thomas Richards, Govt Printer . . . 1862.

204 × 130. Pp. 8. Signed—Chris. Rolleston, Chairman, Hyde Park Asylum, Sydney.

Copies: LNSW, ML. 1511b

New South Wales—Parliament

1879–80. Legislative Assembly. New South Wales. Deodorization of sewage matter. (Correspondence.) Ordered . . . to be printed, 22 June, 1880. [Text begins.]

344 × 217. Pp. 4. Colophon—Sydney: Thomas Richards, Govt Pr—1880.

Prof. John Smith's copy, with ms. letters and notes, is in EF coll.

1547a

———

1881. Legislative Assembly. New South Wales. Vaccination in Darlinghurst Gaol. (Correspondence.) . . .

339 × 217. Pp. 8 (l.b.). Colophon—Thomas Richards, Govt Pr . . .

It was directed, contrary to advice, that vaccination should not be compulsory in gaols.

1881. . . . (Further correspondence) . . .

1549a

———

New South Wales Parliament. Notes on the Medical Bill, 1892.

244 × 204. Pp. 12 (l.b.). Colophon—Sydney:

Charles Potter, Govt Pr—1892. P.w. (cover title). 1571a

New South Wales Contingents for South Africa

The New South Wales Contingents for South Africa being a pictorical record of the organisation of the Colonies' forces for active service, and the scenes ... marking their departure for the front. ... New South Wales Bookstall Co. ... Sydney. 1900. Printed by John Sands ...

280 × 220. Pp. 24. P.w. (decorated title: 'The Transvaal War ...', with cut; advts all other sides).

Includes portraits of 11 medical officers, personnel of medical units, and nurses.

Copies: ML, SLV, US. 1583a

Pell, Morris Birkbeck

Rates of mortality and increase of the population of New South Wales. ... Reprinted from the "Sydney Morning Herald". William Maddock ... Sydney. Wilson & Harris ... Newcastle.

209 × 135. Pp. 36 (l.b.). ND. P.w. (cover title).

Based on figures for 1868–74. Author was the first Prof. of Mathematics at Univ. Syd. See *Aust. Enc.*

Copies: ML. 1657a

Rochlitz, Koloman

See 2219a (Addenda); also 1814.

Royal Society of New South Wales, Medical Section

Report of the sub-committee of the Medical Section of the Royal Society of New South Wales on the properties of the "Carica papaya". Sydney. 1887.

NS. Summary in *Austsn med. Gaz.*, 1887, 6 : 124. Discusses trials on action as galactogogue, digestive and escharotic.

See also Hirschfeld, E. (Brisbane), 'The therapeutic value of Carica papaya in cancer', *Austsn med. Gaz.*, 1893, 12 : 336—application to exposed cancers had no effect on the growth, but showed antiseptic and analgesic properties. Current use of paw-paw juice for digestion of false membrane in diphtheria and for gastric juice deficiency is noted. See also items under Lucas, T. P., an advocate of its curative value in various ailments, including cancer, who issued a range of paw-paw remedies from his Vera Papaw Hosp., Brisbane. 1828a

Rusden, Henry Keylock

Royal Society of Victoria. Cremation and burial in relation to death certification. ... Ford & Son ... Carlton, Melbourne.

214 × 138. Pp. 4. P.w. (cover title). Repr. *Proc. Roy. Soc. Vic.*, 1894.

Copies: ML. 1851a

Schomburgk, Richard Moritz

Paper read by Dr. Schomburgk on ... July 20, 1869. Subject:- "The use and properties of plants". [Text continues.]

204 × 127. Pp. [4] (l.b.). Title—head of p. 1. Colophon: Andrews, Thomas, & Clark ... Adelaide. Read ... Adel. Phil. Soc.

The Same. No 11. Read (Adel. Phil. Soc.) November 16, 1869. Pp. [2]. Title—head of p. 1. Colophon: Andrews, Thomas, & Clark ... Adel.

Also in 'Papers read before the Phil. Soc. and the Chamber of Manufactures', 1873.

Describes many plants of medical interest.

Copies: EF, FC, LNSW, ML, NL, SLS, SLV, SLW, UQ. 1879a

Smelfisic Smelfee

See Thomson, William, 2219a (Addenda).

Smith, Charles

Treatise on the medical treatment of children and females in New South Wales, by Charles Smith M.D.

NS. Title from advt in *The Colonist*, vol. 3, 1847, p. 19 (noted by E. A. Petherick). Price—'not to exceed 5s per copy payable on receipt'; publication to proceed 'as soon as 1000 copies ordered'.

'The great mortality amongst the children ... of NSW, has induced the author, during nearly eight years practice, to enquire the causes, and ... to apply such remedies, as the diversified forms of the diseases required ... Female diseases—ages 10–50 varied from European by climate, habits, and endemic diseases'.

1925a

Smith, Louis Lawrence

Our criminal classes. Concluding article. Reprinted from the Australian Journal. Dedicated to my fellow-members of both Houses of the Legislature, and to the ratepayers of Victoria, who bear the cost of our present expensive and ineffective penal system. ... Melbourne: Clarson, Massina, & Co. ... 1872.

209 × 138. Pp. 17–56 (l.b.). P.w. (cover title).

Copies: ML, SLS, SLV. 1941a

[*Additional note*] See also, for biog. details, Churches, Kelvin, 'The Tracy-Maund Memorial Lecture', *The Age*, Melb., 24 April 1976, pp. 13, 14. 1946

Smith, Robert Greig

[From the Proceedings of the Linnean Society of New South Wales, 1900, Part 1, April 25th.] The mechanism of agglutination. ... The flocculation of bacteria.

220 × 135. Pp. 20 (l.b.). P.w. (cover title).

R. G. Smith (1866–1927) MSc Dur., DSc Edin. was Macleay Bacteriologist of Linnean Soc. NSW (1898–1927). On his arrival from Scotland in 1898, a laboratory, 'with every modern appliance for bact. investigation', was fitted for him at Linn. Soc. Hall, Elizabeth Bay. He published on a wide range of bact. techniques and problems. For biog., see *J. & P. Roy. Soc. NSW*, 1928, 62: 5; *Proc. Linn. Soc. NSW*, 1928, 53: v; also *Austsn med. Gaz.*, 1889, 18: 455.

Copies: NL. 1946a

South Australia—Parliament

(No. 81. South Australia. Return of cases of vaccination. Ordered ... to be printed, June 15th, 1859. [Text begins.]

342 × 215. Pp. 2. Blue paper.

Signed R. W. Moore, Col Surg. and Chairman of Vaccine Board. 1972a

---

(No. 146 South Australia. Correspondence with vaccination officer. Ordered ... to be printed 14th September, 1877. [Text begins.]

342 × 215. Single leaf, v.b.

On selection of Quarantine Station. 1977a

(No. 130. South Australia. Petition against compulsory vaccination. Ordered ... to be printed, November 6th, 1900. [Text begins.]

342 × 215. Single leaf, v.b.

Preamble to petition of 1,149 names. 1987a

State Vaccination

State vaccination. Reprinted from the "Intercolonial Medical Journal of Australasia", August 20, 1896. Stillwell and Co. ... Melbourne.

239 × 150. Pp. 8. P.w. (cover title).

On 'the value of vaccination, and the obligation of the State in regard to it'.

Copies: NL. 2021a

Stirling, Sir Edward Charles

South Australian Museum. Directions for collecting and preserving specimens of natural history. Prepared by E. C. Stirling, M.D., ... J. W. Haache, Ph.D., ... and Geo. Beazley. ... Adelaide: E. Spiller, Govt. Printer ... 1882.

8vo. Pp. 8 (l.b.).

Copies: SLS. 2040a

Stuart, Sir Thomas Peter Anderson

Nickle and cobalt: their physiological action on the animal organism. Part 1. Toxicology ... [Text begins.]

210 × 132. Pp. 34 (l.b.). P.w. From *J. Anat. Physiol.*, 1882, 17: 89–123.

From author's MD thesis, Univ. Edin. His further paper on subject appeared in *Archiv. Exp. Path. Pharmacol.*, 1884, 18: 151–73.

Copies: US. 2050a

Thomson, John

Intercolonial Medical Congress of Australasia. Fifth Session ... Brisbane ... 1899. Presidential Address ... Our craft in the Queen's reign. ... Brisbane: ... E. Gregory, Govt Printer ... 1901.

236 × 147. Pp. 16. Repr. *Trans Intercol Med. Cong. Austsia*, 5 Sess.

Outlines medical developments (1837–99), including anaesthesia, antiseptic surgery, bacteriology, hygiene, specialism, nursing, med. education, hospitals, and the position of the medical man.

John Thomson (1847–1909) MB, ChM Edin., of Brisbane, doyen of Queensland doctors at the turn of the century, was Hon. Surg. Bris. Hosp., Member Med. Bd and Bd of Health Qd and Pres. BMA Qd. For obit., see *Austsn med. Gaz.*, 1909, 28: 273.

Copies: EF. 2217a

Thomson, William

Appendix. Reprinted from the Herald of ... July 20, 1861. The Australian Medical Journal. To the Editor of the Herald. [Text begins.]

210 × 132. Pp. 4. Signed at foot: Wil. Thomson, Late Editor *Australian Medical Journal*. 19th July, 1861. Colophon—Wilson and

Mackinnon, Printers . . .

Author announces his resignation as editor, *Aust. med. J.*, following altercation with his editorial committee, who disagree with his 'rather free expression [written and spoken] on the proceedings of the University Council' in regard to certain arrangements for establishment of the Melb. Med. School.

RACS copy inserted between pp. 218/9 of *Aust. med. J.*, vol. 6 [Thomson's personal copy].

Copies: RACS. 2218a

———

A "Rechauffage", spicy, piquant, saucy, of Pudding Homoeopathic, never before cooked. By Smelfisic Smelfee, M. B. et M. D., Melb. [Quotation].

212 × 125. Pp. 42. ND (c. 1864). Colophon—Tomlinson and Co., Printers . . . St Kilda. Copy inscribed 'from the author, William Thomson'.

Title covers three contributions to the vivid homoeopathy controversy of the time. Thomson attacks 'the great medical heresy' in two anonymous articles—*One fire burns out another's burning* (pp. 3–20); *The therapeutic phantasy* (pp. 21–32). These are opposed in *Similia similibus curantur* (pp. 33–42), a letter of 15 Aug. 1864 to Ed., *Med. and Surg. Review* signed Koloman von Rochlitz, MD, ChD, Vienna, with appended pungent editorial comment—which is obvious reason for its inclusion.

Copies: Private coll. 2219a

———

Mr. Thomson's work. From "The Argus" of February 6, 1875. [Text begins.]

242 × 156. Single leaf, v.b. Signed: Henry Plow Kane. Corrects statement of reviewer of *Typhoid fever*.

Copies: EF, ML. 2235a

Victoria—Parliament

1879. Victoria. Safety mining cages. Report of the Board of Inquiry on Safety Mining Cages 1878–9; . . . with proceedings . . . and appendices. Presented to both Houses . . . John Ferres, Govt Printer, Melbourne.

339 × 209. Pp. 40 (l.b.), 4 pl.

2401a

———

1889. Victoria. Deaths from typhoid fever. . . . All deaths . . . registered during last six months . . .

342 × 204. Pp. [2] (v.b.). Colophon— . . . Robt S. Brain, Govt Printer, Melb.

Deaths: typhoid—457; diseases of typhoid nature, including enteric fever, colonial fever, asthenic fever, febris gastrica, gastric fever, low fever,—332. Population not shown.

2412a

Webb, John Holden

Two cases of psoas abscess. . . . From the "Australian Medical Journal", March 15, 1889. Melbourne: Stillwell and Co. . . . 1889.

217 × 127. Pp. 12. P.w. (title rptd).

Copies: CC, EF, NL. 2465a

Welsh, David Arthur

On the parathyroid glands of the cat: a preliminary study in experimental pathology. By D. A. Welsh, M. A., M. D., Assistant to the Professor of Pathology in the University of Edinburgh; Pathologist to the Royal Hospital for Sick Children, Edinburgh. [Text begins.]

245 × 158. Pp. 20 (l.b.). 2 pl. P.w. (short title). Repr. *J. Path. Bact.*, 1898, 5.

D. A. Welsh (d. 1948), first Prof. of Path. Univ. Syd., Dean of Med. (1927–9), published a large body of scientific work—that on the cytology of the parathyroids and the precipitin reaction being especially notable. See obit., *Med. J. Aust.*, 1948, 2 : 24 (with bibliog.).

Copies: EF. 2470a

Wilkins, Benjamin

The "Refuter" refuted: or, T. A. Sidders "Weighed in the balance and found wanting". . . . Geelong: Henry Thacker . . . 1868.

171 × 107. Pp. 24 (l.b.). P.w. (title rptd).

Denies advantages of alcohol as stated in No 1907, and discusses its evils, including claim that present-day physical degeneracy results from heavy ancestral drinking. Attacked by Greene, J. S. (766a, Addenda).

Copies: ML. 2509a